MEDICAL DICTIONARY
FOR THE
NONPROFESSIONAL

Charles F. Chapman

Coordinator, Editorial Office
Louisiana State University
School of Medicine
New Orleans, Louisiana

McDowel - To
 # Wild Rose, To
A water Lilly

ESTRALITA

BARRON'S

BARRON'S EDUCATIONAL SERIES, INC.
Woodbury, New York / London / Toronto / Sydney

From *Mosby's Medical and Nursing Dictionary.* © 1983 The
C. V. Mosby Company. Reprinted by permission. Pages 36,
77, 122, 136, 152, 219, 232, 308, 360, 377 (right), 391,
413, 414

From *The Human Body* by The Diagram Group, © 1980
Diagram Visual Information Ltd. Reprinted by permission of
Facts on File Publications. Pages 110 (top), 146 (bottom),
158, 220, 275, 306, 386, 397 (top).

All inquiries should be addressed to:
Barron's Educational Series, Inc.
113 Crossways Park Drive
Woodbury, New York 11797

International Standard Book No. 0-8120-2247-5

PRINTED IN THE UNITED STATES OF AMERICA

567   550   987654

Table of Contents

PREFACE

Language is organic; it grows with specific communication needs. Today English is increasingly the lingua franca, the universal language, especially in the sciences. English-speaking persons should not become too complacent, however, for languages have had great acceptance in the past, only to be supplanted during changes in both commerce and science. Much of today's international acceptance of English stems from technical achievements by which English-speaking scientists have extended the horizons of research and applicability.

But language is also archaic, with roots in the tongues of the ancients, Greeks, Romans, and others. Indeed, we are not remote from the lessons of Hippocrates, a Greek physician who lived in the fourth century B.C., as his writings admonish us about matters that today's media present as *current* needs and *recent* findings, including cautions about abuse of the environment, occupational hazards, misuse of foods and drugs, and the like.

In medicine and the health sciences, terminology derives largely from Greek and Latin. Interestingly, just as English has borrowed, so the Latin of the ancient Romans was enriched by the Greek language to fulfill needs of a changing society. The need to identify structures, functions, processes, symptoms, and states has not changed in the millenia since Athens ruled the world. A bone by any other name remains a bone, whatever the era; pains, blotches, coughs, and fractures were problems long ago as they are now, and each age has found words to describe such phenomena.

Some terms survive; others do not. Who today knows that *hucklebone* referred to either the hipbone or the anklebone? And probably most of those called lepers in Biblical times suffered from diseases other than leprosy.

Naming diseases has not been easy. A condition once called *Parkinson's disease* was renamed *paralysis agitans,* until, after many years, the medical community protested that no paralysis was involved. Furthermore, many argued, Parkinson had not had the disease, so the older term was misleading, if not altogether a misnomer. (Parkinson had reported on the condition; hence the credit to him.) The common wisdom then held that *no* disease should bear anyone's name. To complete the cycle, it was later decided that eponyms (names based on or derived from those of persons should be preferred, because most eponyms provide single terms for otherwise multiple-word designations. A consequence of the process is that Parkinson retains his identity in what is now called *parkinsonism.*

An interesting old argument is whether a single term can properly have both Latin and Greek roots. Formerly, *phlebogram,* meaning a picture-record of a vein (Greek, *phleps,* vein + *graphein,* to write), competed with *venogram* (Latin *vena,* vein + Greek *graphein,* to write); today, the latter is preferred. When medical personnel knew Latin and Greek, they could delight in such "correct root" questions. In our time, however, the argument has no practical importance. Having absorbed some Greek and Latin into English, users of English find some Latin-Greek or Greek-Latin combinations more comfortable to say or to hear. Hence both *vena* and *phleps* survive in our medical glossary.

Health specialists have compounded some terms that have opposite or tangential meanings. *Bacteriotoxin,* for example, means that the bacterium both is poisoned and does the poisoning. Even in common usage we refer to the mosquito *bite*, when what the pesky creature does is more akin to *sting*.

Notable today is the breakdown (*lysis*, if you will) of the autonomy of divisions of science (called "disciplines"). Now the physicist and the physician communicate about such matters as the fluid dynamics of the body's vascular system, and the philosopher and the cleric try with the health-care professional to resolve difficult questions on the quality of life, the ethics of human experimentation, and the definitions of personhood, parenthood, and death. Terminology thus comes to medicine from many sources in addition to the basic and clinical sciences.

Scientists and other professionals have jargons, specific "within-group" vocabulary. In medical terminology one finds definitions on three levels of use: colloquial (sometimes including vulgarities), professional-modern, and professional-classic. Thus the "heelbone" is the "calcaneus" and the "os tarsi fibulare." Knowing the subject matter is largely a question of learning terms and definitions. Often, knowing the terminology of a specialty group yields great understanding of the complexities involved.

This book is not definitive. Intended as a reference for the nonprofessional, it includes selected entries and materials for those whose need is other than for a comprehensive work. The definitions are deliberately simple; here, too, the contents have been selected to answer the needs of persons not trained specifically in the medical sciences. In many cases, additional helpful information—for example, symptoms of a disease, usual treatment procedures for a disorder, or side effects of a treatment—are provided.

As John Locke wrote, "A taste of every sort of knowledge is necessary to form the mind, and is the only way to give the understanding its due improvement to the full extent of its capacity." Here, then, is a tool to help form the mind, to bring greater knowledge and, through that knowledge, fulfillment.

Charles F. Chapman

ACKNOWLEDGMENTS

Many persons gave me encouragement and suggestions for writing this book. Several helped specifically in providing organizational ideas and recommendations for entries. I am deeply indebted to Virginia I. Howard, Assistant Coordinator, Editorial Office, Louisiana State University School of Medicine, New Orleans, for her preparation of many of the preliminary entries and for her scholarly interest, good counsel, and sustaining friendship as the book evolved. Marcia J. Thompson, formerly Editorial Director, Alton Ochsner Medical Foundation, New Orleans, contributed several suggestions and samples that helped to set the style for the entries. Lynny Steiner, formerly Editorial Assistant, LSU Editorial Office, enthusiastically assisted with the preliminary selection of terms to be defined and with the typing of those selections.

My gratitude extends to members of the faculty of Louisiana State University School of Medicine, New Orleans, whose individual interests and recommendations added greatly to the contents. Included are Barbara Y. Legardeur, M.S.; Alfredo Lopez, S., M.D., Ph.D.; Chandan Prasad, Ph.D.; Henry Rothschild, M.D., Ph.D.; Charles V. Sanders, M.D.; and Elijah T. Sproles III, M.D.

Sadie Smalls, Director of Nursing Education and Assistant Director of Nursing, Woodhall Medical and Mental Health Center, New York, served as a Consultant for the Barron's editorial staff and helped improve the contents of the book. The Barron's editor Ruth Flohn contributed greatly to the preliminary editing and styling of the book, and editor Barbara Tchabovsky worked tirelessly and effectively toward the preparation of all copy, proofs, illustrations, tables, and front matter in accordance with professional standards.

My daughters Anne, Sara, and Elizabeth aided me with copy preparation, library research, proofreading, and correspondence. But the greatest measure of acknowledged gratitude goes to Kathy Chapman, financial records manager in LSU Medical School's Department of Medicine. Often working late into evenings, on weekends, and through holidays, she typed, questioned, rewrote, corrected, and gave a wife's devotion to sharing her husband's interests and to succeeding with this "togetherness" project.

Charles F. Chapman

Key to Effective Use of This Dictionary

Overall View: To obtain an overall view of this book that will enable you to use it effectively, follow these steps:

1. Refer to the Table of Contents and turn to each section, familiarizing yourself with the general content and purpose of each.

2. Read the Preface.

3. Study the Table of Abbreviations to avoid misinterpretations.

4. Read several main entries in the alphabetical listings. Note that all main entries are given in **BOLDFACE CAPITALS** and are singular, except as indicated. Each entry lists the part of speech; provides a clear and concise definition of the term, often with an example; and where appropriate provides related parts of speech and plural forms, also given in **boldface.**

Alphabetization: The reader should note that all entries have been alphabetized letter by letter rather than word by word.

Cross References: *Italic type* is used within the text of an entry to call attention to terms that are defined as separate entries and that should be understood to assure comprehension of the term whose definition is sought. Terms given in italics may appear as entries having different forms or as different parts of speech. For example, although the term *antigens* may appear in the text of a definition, the dictionary entry is **ANTIGEN.**

The appearance of a word in regular type does not preclude the possibility of its having been included as a separate entry. Many terms that represent basic and commonly understood concepts or substances—for example, bone and muscle—are often printed in regular type, though they are listed as separate entries.

Sub-Entries: In several instances a main dictionary entry includes several sub-entries. These sub-entries are terms logically understood in the context of the broader term or most likely to be looked up under the main entry. For example, **habitual abortion** is a sub-entry under **ABORTION** and **compound fracture** is a sub-entry under **FRACTURE.**

Table of Abbreviations

adj.	adjective
adv.	adverb
comb. (form)	combining form
e.g.	(*exempli gratia*) for example
esp.	especially
i.e.	(*id est*) that is
n.	noun
pert.	pertaining
pl.	plural
sing.	singular
v.	verb

a

A: BLOOD TYPE n. one of four blood groups (the others being AB, B, and O) in the *ABO blood group system* for classifying human blood based on the presence or absence of *antigen* A and/or B on the surface of *red blood cells.* A person with type A blood produces antibodies against B antigens that cause the blood cells to agglutinate, or clump together. A person with type A blood must receive *blood transfusions* only from others with type A blood or from those with type O blood (see also *blood typing*).

A: VITAMIN n. fat-soluble chemicals (retinol and carotene) essential for the development and proper function of the eyes and *epithelium;* found in liver, cream, butter, egg yolk, some green and yellow vegetables; deficiency can result in *night blindness* and *xerophthalmia* (see *vitamin*; Table of Vitamins).

A-, AN- prefix meaning "without" or "not" (e.g., *aspecific*, not specific, not associated with a specific cause or organism).

AB: BLOOD TYPE n. one of four blood groups (the others being A, B, and O) in the *ABO blood group system* for classifying human blood based on the presence or absence of two *antigens*—A and B—on the surface of *red blood cells;* it is the least common of the four groups in the U.S. population. A person with type AB blood has both antigens and does not produce antibodies against either. A person with type AB blood can receive *blood transfusions* from any other type (A, B, or O) and is sometimes called the "universal recipient" (see also *blood typing*).

AB- prefix meaning "from," "away from" (e.g., *abduct*); "departing from" (e.g., *abnormal*).

ABARTICULATION n. dislocation of a joint (e.g., a "pulledout shoulder").

ABASIA n. inability to walk. adj. **abasic, abatic**

ABDOMEN n. the part of the body between the chest and the *pelvis;* the belly, including the stomach, liver, intestines, and other organs called the *viscera.* adj. **abdominal**

ABDOMINAL BREATHING n. breathing in which *diaphragm* muscle action is reinforced by the abdominal muscles. Such breathing occurs more in men than in women and is commonly practiced by singers.

ABDOMINAL DELIVERY n. delivery of a child through an incision in the abdomen (see *Cesarean section*).

ABDOMINAL PREGNANCY n. pregnancy in which the *conceptus* develops in the abdominal cavity, not in the *uterus;* occurs in about 2% of *ectopic* (extrauterine) *pregnancies* and usually results in fetal death (see *ectopic pregnancy*).

ABDOMINO- comb. form indicating an association with the abdomen (e.g., **abdominothoracic,** pert. to the abdomen and chest).

ABDOMINOCENTESIS n. surgical puncture into the belly, generally to remove fluid or other material for diagnosis (see *paracentesis*).

ABDOMINOVESICAL adj. pert. to the abdomen and *urinary bladder.*

ABDUCENS n. 1. the VIth *cranial nerve;* a motor nerve, it originates in the *brain stem* and supplies the lateral rectus muscles of the eye; 2. the lateral rectus muscle of the eyeball, responsible for turning the eye outward.

ABDUCT v. to move a body part (e.g., an arm) away from the center line of the body, as in testing range of motion or general function.

ABDUCTION n. the act of abducting, drawing away from, as a limb being drawn away from the center of the body.

ABDUCTOR n. a muscle that causes a body part to *abduct*.

ABERRANT adj. deviating from the typical or normal state (e.g., having an abnormal chromosome number); wandering (e.g., in relation to a person's speech).

ABERRATION n. an imperfection, a deviation from normal; a mental disorder.

ABETALIPOPROTEINEMIA n. a rare, inherited disorder of fat metabolism characterized by severe deficiency or total absence of beta-lipoproteins, abnormally low *cholesterol* levels, and the presence of abnormal red blood cells; symptoms include malnutrition, growth retardation, degeneration of the retina, and progressive neurological dysfunction (compare *hypobetalipoproteinemia*).

ABIENT adj. avoiding a stimulus (e.g., a research animal avoiding a flash of light).

ABIOTROPHY n. loss of vitality, degeneration of cells and tissues, esp. those involved in hereditary degenerative disorders.

ABLACTATION n. *weaning;* the cessation of milk secretion.

ABLATE v. to remove, esp. by suction or cutting, or a combination of the two (as is sometimes done in removing part of an organ, e.g., damaged tissue in the brain).

ABLATION n. removal of a part by suction and/or cutting.

ABLEPHARIA n. a condition in which the eyelids are small or absent; also: **ablephary.** adj. **ablepharous**

ABNORMAL adj. unusual in placement, development, structure, or condition.

ABO BLOOD GROUP SYSTEM n. the most important of several systems for classifying human blood, used in *blood transfusion* therapy. Based on the presence or absence of two *antigens*—A and B—on the surface of *red blood cells,* the system classifies blood into four groups: type A, which contains antigen A and antibodies against antigen B; type B, which contains antigen B and antibodies against antigen A; type AB, which contains both antigens; and type O, which contains neither antigen but has antibodies against both (see also *blood typing*).

ABOCCLUSION n. a condition in which, in biting, the upper jaw teeth do not touch the lower jaw teeth.

ABORTIFACIENT n. an agent that acts to produce *abortion*.

ABO BLOOD GROUPS

Name of group	Agglutinogens in red blood cells		Agglutinins in serum	
	A	**B**	**anti-A**	**anti-B**
Group O	none	none	present	present
Group A	present	none	none	present
Group B	none	present	present	none
Group AB	present	present	none	none

ABORTION n. termination of *pregnancy;* expulsion or removal of the *embryo* or *fetus* before it has reached full development and can normally be expected to be capable of independent life. It may be spontaneous or induced. adj. **abortive**

habitual abortion n. the reported spontaneous expulsion of the products of *conception* in three or more pregnancies, often for no known cause.

imminent abortion n. the appearance of symptoms, including bleeding from the *vagina* and colicky pains, that signal impending loss of the products of conception.

incomplete abortion n. termination of pregnancy in which some of the products of conception are not expelled but rather are retained in the uterus. It usually leads to heavy bleeding, is occasionally complicated by infection, and almost always requires surgical intervention; also: **partial abortion.**

induced abortion n. deliberate termination of pregnancy. The conception product may be removed by suction, *curretage* (scraping of the uterus), the induction of uterine contractions, or hysterotomy (cutting into the uterus).

spontaneous abortion n. noninduced, natural loss of the product of conception. Common causes include faulty development of the embryo; abnormality of the *placenta;* or disease, injury, or trauma in the expectant mother. Symptoms include bleeding from the *vagina* and abdominal pain; also: **miscarriage.**

therapeutic abortion n. a legal, induced abortion done for medical reasons, as when the pregnancy threatens the pregnant woman's life.

threatened abortion n. the appearance of symptoms, including bleeding from the *vagina* and sometimes abdominal cramps, that signal that the products of conception may be lost. Rest and careful medical observation are usually advised.

ABORTUS n. a *fetus* whose weight is below $\frac{1}{2}$ kilogram (a little more than 1 pound) at the time it is removed or expelled from the mother's body.

ABRACHIA n. a condition of having no arms (see also *phocomelia*).

ABRADE v. to rub off, as a skin or covering layer, deliberately or accidentally.

ABRASION n. 1. rubbing or wearing away by some frictional, mechanical process; 2. the area of body surface that has lost its outer layer of skin or mucous membrane because it has been rubbed off or worn away, as in scraping the knee in a fall.   adj. **abrasive**

ABREACTION n. esp. in psychoanalysis, working out a repressed disagreeable experience or emotion through reliving it in speech and action (see *catharsis*). If feelings are worked out through muscular (motor) use, the process is motor abreaction.

ABRUPTIO PLACENTAE n. a disorder of *pregnancy* in which the *placenta* prematurely separates from attachment to the wall of the *uterus;* marked by *hemorrhage* (concealed or evident), pain, and *fetal distress*.

ABSCESS n. an accumulation of *pus* that results from a breakdown of tissues (a common problem being tissue breakdown around a tooth, producing an "abscessed tooth").

ABSOLUTE THRESHOLD n. the lowest level of stimulus that can be sensed (e.g., the lowest intensity of a sound that a person can hear).

ABSORPTION n. the incorporation of matter by other matter, as in the dissolving of a gas in a liquid or the taking up of a liquid by a porous solid; the passage of substances into tissues, as in the passage of digested food into the intestinal cells (compare *adsorption*).

ACANTHOCYTE n. an abnormal *red blood cell* with irregular projections of *protoplasm*, giving it a spiny or thorny appearance.

ACANTHOCYTOSIS n. the abnormal presence of acanthocytes in the blood, as in *abetalipoproteinemia*.

ACANTHOLYSIS n. breakdown of the thorny-cell layer of the *epidermis* (e.g., in the skin disorder *pemphigus vulgaris*).

ACANTHOMA n. a tumor of outer-skin cells.

ACANTHOSIS n. overdevelopment and thickening of the prickle-cell layer of the outer skin, as in *psoriasis*. adj. **acanthotic acanthosis nigricans** n. a skin disease characterized by *hyperpigmentation* and warty lesions of the body folds; can be *benign* or *malignant*.

ACAPNIA n. a condition in which the carbon dioxide level in the blood is less than normal, sometimes caused by very deep or very rapid breathing; also: **hypocapnia.** adj. **acapnic, acapnial**

ACARDIA n. *congenital* absence of the heart, as in some *monsters*.

ACARIASIS n. infestation with mites (e.g., the itch mite, which causes *scabies*); also: **acaridiasis, acariosis.**

ACARYOTE see *prokaryote*.

ACATALEPSIA n. 1. lowered capacity or inability to understand; 2. an uncertain diagnosis; also: **acatalepsy.** adj. **acataleptic,** not able to understand easily; mentally deficient.

ACATAPHASIA n. a condition in which a central nervous system *lesion* leaves one unable to express thoughts in an organized manner.

ACATHEXIA n. inability to retain bodily secretions. adj. **acathectic**

ACATHEXIS n. an abnormal psychological condition in which objects, thoughts, and memories that ordinarily have great significance to an individual arouse no emotion.

ACCESSORY adj. aiding or serving to supplement; for example, the eyebrow is an accessory of the eye, helping to protect it.

ACCESSORY NERVE n. XIth *cranial nerve;* a motor nerve supplying muscles involved in speech, swallowing, and certain movements of the head and shoulders.

ACCIDENT n. an unexpected happening, esp. one that results in injury (see also *cerebrovascular accident*).

ACCIDENT-PRONE adj. having a greater-than-average incidence of accidents.

ACCLIMATION n. state of adaptation to new conditions or environment; also: **acclimatization.**

ACCOMMODATION n. adjustment, esp. adaptation of the eye to change in the distance of an object from the viewer.

ACCOMMODATION REFLEX n. reflex changes that enable an object to be focused on the *retina*. In adjusting for near vision, the *pupils* constrict, the lenses become more convex, and the eyes converge; in adjusting for far vision, the reverse changes occur. The ability of the eye to accommodate decreases with age.

ACCOUCHEMENT n. an old term for *childbirth,* obstetrical delivery.

ACCRETIO n. an abnormal joining of parts that are normally separate (e.g., two fused organs).

ACCRETION n. addition of new material, resulting in growth; an accumulation.

ACELLULAR adj. not containing cells; not having a cell structure.

ACEPHALIA n. absence of the head, as in the development of some *monster* fetuses; also: **acephalism, acephaly.**

ACETABULUM n. the cup-shaped hollow in the hipbone into which the head of the thighbone (*femur*) fits and rotates in a ball-and-socket joint.   adj. **acetabular**

ACETAMINOPHEN n. a widely used nonprescription drug, sold under many trade names (e.g., Tylenol), that relieves mild-to-moderate pain (*analgesic*) and reduces fever (*antipyretic*); it contains no *aspirin* and is frequently used in place of aspirin (e.g., to avoid the side effects of gastrointestinal upset sometimes associated with aspirin use).

ACETANILID n. a pain-relieving, fever-reducing drug; its use has been largely discontinued because of its toxicity.

ACETONE n. a colorless liquid with a characteristic sweet, fruity odor present in small amounts in normal urine but in increased amounts in the urine of those with faulty glucose and fat metabolism (e.g., in *diabetes mellitus* and certain other metabolic disorders). Commercially available specially treated paper and sticks that turn a certain color when wet with urine containing acetone are used by some with diabetes mellitus to test for acetone production as an indication of the course of their disorder.

ACETONE BODIES   see *ketone bodies*.

ACETONURIA   see *ketonuria*.

ACETYLCHOLINE n. a chemical that is an important *neurotransmitter* in the body, functioning in the transmission of impulses between nerve cells and between nerve cells and muscle.

ACETYLSALICYLIC   ACID see *aspirin*.

ACHALASIA n. failure of a muscle, particularly a sphincter (muscular ring or valve), to relax, esp. in the gastrointestinal tract (e.g., cardiac sphincter of the stomach; also: **cardiospasm**).

ACHE n. a dull, usually moderately intense, persistent pain, as in *headache*.

ACHILLES TENDON n. the large tendon that connects the calf muscles to the heelbone.

ACHLORHYDRIA n. an abnormal condition characterized by the absence of *hydrochloric acid* in the *gastric juice*, often associated with *pernicious anemia*, other severe anemias, and cancer of the stomach.   adj. **achlorhydric**

ACHOLIA n. 1. a condition in which little or no *bile* is secreted; 2. a condition in which the normal flow of bile into the digestive tract is obstructed.

ACHONDROPLASIA n. an inherited disorder in which a defect in cartilage and bone formation results in a form of *dwarfism* characterized by short limbs on a normal trunk; also: **chondrodystrophy.**   adj. **achondroplastic**

ACHROMASIA n. a condition in which there is less pigment in the skin than is normal; pallor (see also *albinism, vitiligo*).

ACHROMATISM n. the state of seeing gray tones instead of colors; colorlessness.

ACHROMIA n. absence of normal color, as in *albinism*.   adj. **achromic**

ACHROMYCIN n. tradename for the antibiotic *tetracycline*.

ACHYLIA n. absence or severe deficiency of *hydrochloric acid, pepsinogen,* or other digestive secretions. adj. **achylous**

ACID n. 1. a chemical that has at least one hydrogen atom, tastes sour, turns *litmus paper* pink or red, and forms a salt when combined with a *base* (*hydrocholoric acid* is normally a part of the digestive juice produced in the stomach); 2. a colloquialism for *LSD*, a drug that causes *hallucinations* (a person using LSD is called an "acid head"). adj. **acidic**

ACIDITY n. a condition of having an acid content, or of being an acid, or of tasting sour.

ACID-BASE BALANCE n. the normal equilibrium between *acids* and alkalis (*bases*) in the body maintained by buffer systems in the blood and the regulatory activities of the lungs and kidneys in excreting wastes to prevent the buildup of excessive acids (*acidosis*) or alkalis (*alkalosis*) in the blood and other tissues. With a normal acid-base balance in the body, the blood is slightly alkaline, registering 7.35–7.45 on the *pH scale* (where 7 is neutral and above 7 alkaline).

ACIDEMIA n. a condition in which there is an increased concentration of hydrogen ions in the blood and hence the blood is more acid than normal (below 7 on the *pH scale*.)

ACID-FAST adj. term describing microorganisms whose stained color resists decolorization after treatment with an acid solution, esp. the tubercle bacillus *Mycobacterium tuberculosis*.

ACIDOPHIL n. 1. a cell that readily stains with acids; 2. a microorganism that grows in acidic materials; also: **acidophile.** adj. **acidophilic**

ACIDOPHILUS MILK n. a preparation of milk that has been acted on (fermented) by a bacterium (*Lactobacillus acidophilus*), used in treating some intestinal disorders.

ACIDOSIS n. a disturbance in the normal *acid-base balance* of the body in which the blood and body tissues are more acidic than normal. It may result from retention of carbon dioxide, as in drowning or lung malfunction; from prolonged or severe diarrhea or vomiting; from impaired kidney function; or as a complication of *diabetes mellitus* (compare: *alkalosis*). adj. **acidotic**

ACID POISONING n. poisoning resulting from the ingestion of a toxic acidic compound, such as hydrochloric acid, sulfuric acid, or nitric acid, many of which are found in cleaning products. Emergency treatment includes giving copious amounts of water or milk to dilute the acid; vomiting should not be induced.

ACINIFORM adj. grape-shaped, as some tumors.

ACINUS n. general term for a small saclike structure, esp. that found in a gland. pl. **acini** adj. **acinar, acinic, acinose, acinous**

ACNE n. an inflammatory disease of the *sebaceous glands* of the skin, usually on the face and upper body, characterized by papules, pustules, comedones (blackheads) and in severe cases by cysts, nodules and scarring. The most common form—acne vulgaris—usually affects persons from puberty to young adulthood. Treatment includes topical and oral antibiotics, topical vitamin A derivatives, *dermabrasion,* and *cryosurgery* (see also *acne rosacea*). adj. **acneiform,** like acne

ACNE ROSACEA n. chronic *acne* of the cheek and nose area, seen in adults and characterized by red coloring due to dilated blood vessels; also: **rosacea.**

ACOREA n. the absence of the pupil in an eye.

ACOU- comb. form indicating an association with hearing (e.g., **acousma**, a hallucination that strange sounds are heard).

ACOUSTIC NERVE n. an older term for *auditory nerve* (the VIIIth *cranial nerve*).

ACQUIRED adj. resulting from outside factors; not inherited or *congenital*; for example, dislikes for some odors and foods are acquired.

ACQUIRED IMMUNE DEFICIENCY SYNDROME (AIDS) n. a serious and often fatal condition in which the *immune system* breaks down and does not respond normally to infection. The victims commonly develop *Kaposi's sarcoma* and recurrent and intractable infections, often caused by organisms that do not normally present a serious threat to humans (e.g., *Pneumocystis carinii* parasite, *Aspergillus* fungi). The disease became epidemic in the early 1980's, affecting almost exclusively male homosexuals, intravenous drug users, Haitians, and hemophiliacs. The cause is unknown, but a virus is suspected.

ACQUIRED IMMUNITY n. any form of immunity (insusceptibility to a particular disease) not innate but obtained during life. It may be natural, actively acquired by the development of *antibodies* after an attack of an infectious disease (e.g., chickenpox) or passively acquired, as when a mother passes antibodies against a specific disease to a fetus through the *placenta* or to an infant through *colostrum*; or it be may be artificial, acquired through *vaccination*.

ACQUIRED REFLEX n. see *conditioned reflex*.

ACRITICAL adj. without a crisis, as of some diseases; not critical.

ACRO- comb. form indicating an association with a limb (an extremity) or an extreme state (e.g., **acroanesthesia**, loss of sensation in the extremities).

ACROCYANOSIS n. an abnormal condition characterized by bluish discoloration and coldness of the extremities, esp. the hands, caused by spasm of the blood vessels brought about by exposure to cold, emotional stress, or other factors; also called **Raynaud's sign**.

ACROMEGALY n. a hormonal disorder occurring in middle-aged people and characterized by progressive enlargement and elongation of the hands, feet, and face, often accompanied by headache, muscle pain, and visual and emotional disturbances. It is caused by an overproduction of *growth hormone* by the *anterior pituitary gland* (due to a tumor) and is treated by radiation or surgery of the pituitary; also: **acromegalia**. adj. **acromegalic**

ACROMICRIA n. a condition of having underdeveloped fingers and toes and other parts; also: **acromikria**.

ACROMION n. the high point of the shoulder; an extension of the spinous part of the *scapula*. adj. **acromial**

ACROMPHALUS n. abnormal protrusion of the navel, sometimes marking the start of umbilical hernia.

ACROMYOTONIA n. an abnormal pulling of the muscles that move the hand or foot, causing a contraction deformity; also: **acromyotonus**.

ACROPHOBIA n. an abnormal fear or dread of high places.

ACTH see *adrenocorticotropic hormone*.

ACTIFED n. trade name for a fixed-combination drug containing a *bronchodilator*, *antihistamine*, and *vasoconstrictor*; it is used in the treatment of upper respiratory infections and hypersensitivity reactions involving the bronchi.

ACTING OUT v. 1. in psychiatry, indulging or manifesting some forbidden or detrimental behavior by a patient in treatment who experiences trouble in talking about a conflict in a therapeutic session; 2. more broadly, unconsciously showing feelings, not in words but in actions (as in impulsively breaking something without admitting anger).

ACTINO- prefix indicating an association with a ray or radiation (e.g., **actinotherapy**, treatment of disease by means of special rays, such as ultraviolet radiation).

ACTINOMYCOSIS n. a disease of cattle and humans (in humans, caused by the bacteria *Actinomyces israeli*) characterized by the appearance of lumpy abscesses that exude pus through long sinuses. The most common and least severe form of the disease (cervicofacial actinomycosis) affects the face and neck region and is often called "lumpy jaw". Less common, more serious forms affect the chest (thoracic actinomycosis) and abdomen (abdominal actinomycosis). Fever, chills and sweats, and weakness may occur in all forms of the disease. Treatment includes incision and drainage of the abscesses and administration of penicillin. adj. **actinomycotic**

ACTION POTENTIAL n. the electrical charge (microvoltage) on a nerve cell that causes it to give off its impulse.

ACTIVATED CHARCOAL n. a general antidote used to treat some forms of acute poisoning.

ACTIVATION n. 1. stimulation of the brain by way of the *brain stem* (*reticular activating system*); 2. the stimulating of activity in an organism, body part, or chemical.

ACTIVE IMMUNITY n. a form of *acquired immunity* in which the body produces its own *antibodies* against disease-causing *antigens*. It can occur naturally after infection or artificially after *vaccination* (compare *passive immunity*).

ACTIVE TRANSPORT n. the carrying of a substance (e.g., drug, amino acid) across a cell membrane against the concentration or pressure gradient and requiring the expenditure of energy (compare *osmosis*; *passive transport*).

ACUPUNCTURE n. a method of producing analgesia or treating disease by inserting very thin needles into specific sites on the body along channels, called meridians, and twirling, energizing, or warming the needles; it is used by practitioners of traditional medicine in China.

ACUTE adj. 1. coming on suddenly and severely; 2. sharp, as an acute pain (compare *chronic*).

ACUTE CHILDHOOD LEUKEMIA n. progressive, *malignant* disease of the blood-forming tissues that is the most common type of *cancer* in children. See also *acute lymphoid leukemia*.

ACUTE LYMPHOID LEUKEMIA (ALL) n. a rapidly progressive malignancy of the blood-forming tissues, characterized by proliferation of immature lymphoblastlike cells in the bone marrow, spleen, lymph nodes and circulating blood. Most common in children, particularly from ages two to ten, it has a sudden onset with fever, pallor, loss of appetite, fatigue, hemorrhage, and recurrent infections. Treatment involves *chemotherapy*, blood transfusions, and treatment of secondary infections. Since the mid-1970's there have been improved survival rates; also called **acute lymphoblastic leukemia**.

ACUTE MYELOCYTIC LEUKEMIA (AML) n. a malignant disease of blood-forming tissues characterized by uncontrolled proliferation of granular leukocytes (a type of white blood cell). It may occur at any age but is most frequent in adolescents and young adults. Onset, which often is gradual, is marked by spongy bleeding gums, anemia, fatigue, bone pain, and recurrent infection. Treatment includes *chemotherapy*, repeated transfusions, *immunotherapy*, and bone marrow transplants.

ACUTE ORGANIC BRAIN SYNDROME n. sudden confusion and disorientation in an otherwise mentally normal person, resulting from drugs, infections, head injury, or other factors.

AD- prefix meaning ''toward'' (e.g., *adduction*), ''sticking to'' (e.g., *adhesion*), ''increase of'' (e.g., *adjunct*).

-AD suffix meaning ''toward a given part'' (e.g., **cephalad**, toward the head).

ADACTYLY n. an absence of fingers and/or toes; also: **adactylia, adactylism**.   adj. **adactylous**

ADAMANTINE adj. 1. pert. to tooth enamel; 2. hard-surfaced.

ADAM'S APPLE n. bulge at the front of the neck formed by the thyroid cartilage of the *larynx*.

ADAMS-STOKES SYNDROME n. condition characterized by recurrent sudden attacks of *unconsciousness*, with or without *convulsions*, caused by transient heart block; also: **Stokes-Adams syndrome**

ADAPTATION n. the ability of an organism or body part to adjust to changes in its environment; 2. the adjustment of the eye to changing light in the surroundings (see *light adaptation*); 3. decrease in the frequency of nerve response under conditions of constant stimulation (compare: *habituation*).

ADDICT n. a person whose use of a particular substance (e.g., heroin, alcohol) is such that abrupt deprivation of the substance produces characteristic withdrawal symptoms.

ADDICTION n. a condition of strong or irresistible dependence on the use of a particular substance (e.g., heroin, alcohol) such that abrupt deprivation of the substance produces characteristic withdrawal symptoms.

ADDISON'S DISEASE n. a disease caused by failure of function of the cortex of the *adrenal gland*, resulting in deficiency of *adrenocortical hormones* and disturbance of the normal levels of glucose and minerals in the body. Symptoms, often gradual in onset, include weakness, anorexia, fatigue, increased pigmentation, weight loss, and reduced tolerance to cold. Treatment includes administration of adrenocortical hormones and maintenance of normal levels of glucose and *electrolytes* in the blood. Many people with Addison's disease wear a MedicAlert ID; also called **Addison's syndrome**.

ADDITIVE n. something added, as a flavoring or dye to food, either natural or artificial (a recent Food and Drug Administration review of 415 additives showed that nearly all were harmless).   adj. pert. to an added substance or action.

ADDUCT v. to pull toward the body or a part (compare *abduct*).

ADDUCTION n. the moving of a part toward the body (esp. toward a line that would pass through the body's center, from head to foot); for example, returning an outstretched arm to the side of the trunk.

ADDUCTOR n. a muscle that, when flexed, pulls a part toward the body or the body's vertical midline.

ADEN-, ADENI-, ADENO- comb. form indicating an association with a *gland* or glands (e.g., **adenectomy**, surgical removal of a gland: **adenalgia**, pain in a gland).

ADENINE a chemical (a *purine*) contained in *DNA* and *RNA* (also found in tea) and important in carrying genetic information in cells.

ADENITIS n. inflammation of a *lymph node* or gland, often associated with infection, as in neck adenitis in cases of throat infection.

ADENOCARCINOMA n. a *malignant epithelial* cell-tumor of a gland or tumor in which the cells form a glandular structure.

ADENOHYPOPHYSIS n. the anterior lobe of the pituitary gland (see *anterior pituitary gland*).

ADENOID n. lymphatic tissue in the back of the nasal passage, on the wall of the *nasopharynx*. Adenoids may become enlarged and cause difficulty in breathing through the nose after repeated infection. adj. **adenoid**, glandlike.

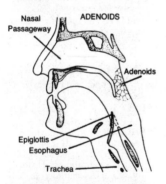

Nasal Passageway   ADENOIDS

Adenoids

Epiglottis
Esophagus

Trachea

ADENOIDECTOMY n. surgical removal of the adenoids. This operation was once commonly performed along with *tonsillectomy* (removal of the tonsils) but is now much less common, usually performed only when pharyngeal complications are present.

ADENOMA n. a *benign* epithelial tumor in which the cells are derived from glandular tissue or have a glandular structure. An adenoma may cause the affected gland to become overactive.

ADENOMALACIA n. a condition in which a gland or glands become soft.

ADENOMATOSIS n. a condition in which many glandlike growths develop.

ADENOMEGALY n. gland enlargement.

ADENOMYOMATOSIS n. an abnormal condition in which many nodules develop in the tissues of or around the *uterus*.

ADENOMYOSIS n. a condition in which the *endometrium* (lining of the uterus) grows into the uterine muscle tissue; also: **adenomyometritis**.

ADENOPATHY n. a general term for gland disease and enlargement, esp. of the *lymph* glands.

ADENOSCLEROSIS n. glandular hardening.

ADENOSINE n. a compound that is a major constituent of many biologically important molecules, including the hereditary material DNA and RNA, the energy-storage compounds ATP and AMP, and many enzymes.

ADENOSIS n. a general term for a disease of the glands, esp. the lymph glands.

ADENOVIRUS n. any of a large group of viruses, many of which are responsible for upper respiratory infections (e.g., the common cold) and other common infections.

ADH see *antidiuretic hormone*.

ADHESION n. a band of fibrous tissue that causes normally separate structures to stick together. Adhesions are most common in the abdomen, where they frequently follow surgery, injury, or inflammation. If they cause pain or other symptoms or interfere with normal functioning, surgical intervention is necessary.

ADIENT adj. having a tendency to move toward a *stimulation* source, e.g., light or warmth.

ADIPO- comb. form indicating an association with *fat* or fatness (see also terms beginning with *lipo-*) (e.g., **adipogenesis**, fat formation).

ADIPONECROSIS n. the death of fat cells or fatty tissue in the body.

ADIPOSE adj. fatty, composed of fat.

ADIPOSE TISSUE n. a type of *connective tissue* containing many fat cells. It forms a layer under the skin and serves as an insulating layer and as an energy reserve.

ADIPOSIS n. 1. a condition in which there is an abnormal amount of fat present in the body because of overeating, a metabolic disorder, or glandular malfunction; 2. corpulence, obesity.

ADJUNCT n. something that is added, as an accessory agent or procedure. adj. **adjunctive**

ADJUSTMENT n. 1. a change to a more satisfactory condition, as in overcoming emotional problems; 2. in chiropractic, correction of a displaced vertebra.

ADJUVANT n. something that helps or reinforces a process, as in enhancing an immune response (see *adjunct*, *buffer*, *catalyst*).

ADNEXA n. pl. accessory parts that enable an organ to function; for example, the adnexa of the eye are the eyelids, tear glands and tear ducts and the fallopian tubes are adnexa of the uterus. adj. **adnexal**

ADOLESCENCE n. the period between puberty and adulthood (see *age*), marked by extensive physical, psychological and emotional changes.

ADRENAL adj. 1. pert. to the *adrenal gland*; 2. near the *kidney*(s).

ADRENAL GLAND n. either of a pair of triangular-shaped endocrine, or ductless, *hormone*-secreting, glands, situated atop a kidney. The gland is composed of two major parts: an outer cortex and inner medulla. The cortex secretes androgens (precursors of the sex hormones *testosterone* and *estrogen*), aldosterone and other *mineralocorticoids* (essential for the maintenance of normal saltwater balance in the body) and cortisol and many other glucocorticoids essential for protein and carbohydrate metabolism and the functioning of the cardiovascular system, the kidneys, and other organs. The medulla secretes *epinephrine* and *norepinephrine*, hormones involved in the body's response to stress. Also, sometimes called **suprarenal gland**.

ADRENALINE   see *epinephrine*.

ADRENARCHE, n. an increase in the activity of the adrenal glands that occurs before puberty.

ADRENERGIC adj. indicating a relationship to *epinephrine*, its release, or its actions, esp. in association with the *sympathetic autonomic nervous system*; called also **sympathomimetic** (compare: *cholinergic*).

ADRENO- comb. form indicating an association with the adrenal glands (e.g., **adrenomegaly**, enlargement of one or both of the adrenal glands; **adrenocortical**, pert. to the cortex of the adrenal gland).

ADRENOCORTICOTROPIC HORMONE (ACTH) n. a hormone secreted by the *anterior pi-*

tuitary gland that is essential for the development of the cortex of the *adrenal gland* and its secretion of *corticosteroids* (mineralocorticoids and glucocorticoids). ACTH secretion is stimulated by stress, trauma, major surgery, fever, and other conditions. An ACTH preparation is a widely used drug in the treatment of *rheumatoid arthritis*, certain allergic conditions, and many other disorders. Also called: **corticotropin**.

ADSORPTION n. the adherence of a thin layer of a gas, liquid, or dissolved substance to the surface of another. For example, in some gas masks, *activated charcoal* acts as an adsorbent, picking up gases on its surface (compare *absorption*). adj. **adsorbent**

ADULT n. a fully grown and developed organism.

ADULTERANT n. added matter that lessens the purity, effectiveness, or reliability of a substance.

ADVANCEMENT n. the act of freeing a part, as a tendon, and reattaching it surgically at another (advanced) place.

ADVENTITIA n. the outer connective tissue layer of an organ (see *tunic*). adj. **adventitial**

ADVENTITIOUS adj. not inherited; accidental; acquired from outside the organism (e.g., a scar on the arm).

AER-, AERO- comb. form indicating an association with air, oxygen, or gas (see also *pneumo-*) (e.g., **aerocele**, an air-filled swelling).

AERATE v. to charge with air or *oxygen*.

AEREMIA n. a painful condition in which a sudden drop in outside pressure (as in coming up from a deep dive or ascending rapidly to a high altitude) causes nitrogen bubbles to form in the blood; also called **aeroembolism**, the **bends**,

caisson disease, **nitrogen narcosis**.

AEROBE n. an organism that thrives in air or more particularly oxygen (compare *anaerobe*). adj. **aerobic**

AEROBIC EXERCISE n. an exercise system based on continuous action movements, as in swimming, dancing, or bicycling. designed to increase oxygen consumption and improve functioning of the *lungs* and *cardiovascular system*.

AERODONTALGIA n. pain in the teeth resulting from change in air pressure, as in flying or climbing a mountain.

AEROEMBOLISM n. 1. air-caused blockage in an artery 2. *aeremia*. (See also *embolism*.)

AEROPHAGIA n. swallowing of air, usually followed by belching, flatulence and discomfort; also: **aerophagy**.

AFEBRILE adj. having no *fever*.

AFFECT n. 1. the emotional reactions associated with an experience; 2. in psychiatry, the emotional tone behind an expressed emotion or behavior (e.g., some schizophrenics have flattened affect).

AFFERENT adj. carrying inward, toward the center, as a nerve carrying a sensory impulse (e.g., cold, texture) to the brain (compare *efferent*).

AFFLUX n. a sudden filling of a body part with blood or other liquid.

AFTERBIRTH n. the fetus-supporting material (*placenta* and fetal membranes) expelled from the mother's *uterus* after a baby is born.

AFTERBRAIN n. the back and lower parts of the brain that include the *pons* and *cerebellum*.

AFTERHEARING n. the continuing sensation of hearing a sound that has actually stopped.

AFTERIMAGE n. the continuing sensation of seeing an image that is no longer visible.

AFTERPAINS n. pains from uterine contractions felt by a woman after her baby is born.

AGALACTIA n. a condition in which *milk* is not secreted or is not contained in a mother's breasts after she has delivered a child; also: **agalactosis**.

AGALORRHEA n. a stopping or limiting of *milk* flow from the breasts.

AGAMMAGLOBULINEMIA n. a rare immunological disorder characterized by the virtual absence of *gamma globulins* from the blood serum and resultant heightened susceptibility to infection. It may be *congenital* (sex-linked and persistent and transient during the first few weeks of life) or *acquired* (often as result of a cancer and/or its treatment) (compare *hypogammaglobulinemia*).

AGE n. lifetime, from birth to the present (or to *death*), generally given in calendar years for these common groups: **neonate**—birth to four weeks; **infant**—birth to age 1 year; **child**—birth to puberty; **adolescent**—*puberty* to adulthood; **adult**—maturity onward; **aged**—a nonspecific term, generally meaning of retirement age and beyond. (See also *bone age, chronological age, developmental age, mental age.*)

AGENESIS n. nondevelopment of a part or organ; *impotence*; also: **agenesia**.

AGENT ORANGE n. a chemical used to kill plants, esp. during the Vietnam War as a means of removing underbrush, and containing a poison that can adversely affect the skin, liver, kidneys, and nervous system.

AGERASIA n. an appearance of youthfulness in an old person. ˇ

AGGLUTINATION n. the clumping together of *antigen*-carrying cells or microorganisms as a result of their interaction with specific antibodies.

AGGLUTINATION TEST n. a blood test used to identify unknown *antigens*. A sample with the unknown antigen is mixed with a known *antibody*; whether or not *agglutination* occurs helps in identifying the unknown antigen. The test is useful in determining susceptibility to certain diseases, in blood typing, and in tissue matching (e.g., for transplants).

AGGLUTININ n. a substance—an *antibody*—that causes clumping of a specific *antigen* (e.g., the Rh factor).

AGGLUTINOGEN n. a substance that causes *agglutinin* production.

AGGRESSION n. hostile behavior directed against oneself or others, arising from frustration or inner drives.

AGING n. the process of growing old. Generally during aging a person's height decreases, bone tissue diminishes, hair becomes gray and/or is thinned or lost, nose and ears lengthen, eye lenses become more rigid, and other physical changes occur. The process seems to relate to an "internal clock" that is specific for each type of organism, the human maximum being about 105 years. Aging is believed to be influenced by genetics and life-style and possibly inhibited by exercise and mental activity, a "positive attitude," and a balanced and restricted diet.

AGNOSIA n. inability to recognize things because of loss in sensory perception.

AGONADAL adj. lacking gonads, or sex glands.

AGONIST n. 1. one of a pair of muscles (e.g., the triceps) that

contracts during the relaxing phase
of the other, the *antagonist*; 2. a
drug or other substance that aids
another drug or a bodily process.

AGORAPHOBIA n. an abnormal
fear or dread of open or public
places.

-AGRA suffix indicating sharp pain
or seizure (e.g., **melagra**, muscle pain in the arms or legs).

AGRANULOCYTOSIS n. an
acute blood disorder, often resulting from radiation or drug
therapy, characterized by a severe decrease in granulocytes (a
type of white blood cells), and
manifested by fever, prostration,
and ulcers of the mucous membranes of the mouth, rectum and
vagina area; also: **agranulosis**,
granulocytopenia. adj. **agranulocytic**

AGRAPHIA n. loss of ability to
write one's thoughts, caused by a
lesion in the *cerebral cortex* of
the brain. adj. **agraphic**

AGROMANIA n. a strong desire
to be alone or out in open space.

AGUE n. an old term for chill or
fever, esp. during *malaria*.

AID abbreviation for *artificial insemination* by a *donor*.

AIDS see *acquired immune deficiency syndrome*.

AIR EMBOLISM n. abnormal
presence of air in the bloodstream; the air blocks the normal
flow of blood through the vessels.
It can occur accidentally during
surgery, hypodermic injection, or
intravenous administration, or can
result from *puncture* injury.

AIR SICKNESS n. nausea, vomiting, and headache caused by
airplane motion and the changes
in gravity experienced during
flight, esp. in turbulence. Symptomatic relief is provided by *antihistamines* (compare *car sickness*; *motion sickness*; *seasickness*).

AKARYOCYTE see *prokaryote*.

AKINESIA n. motionlessness;
temporary paralysis; also: **akine-
sis**.

ALA n. structure that resembles a
bird's wing (e.g., *ala nasi*, flared
walls of the nose). pl. **alae**
adj. **alar**, **alate**.

ALALIA n.inability to speak, e.g.,
in paralysis of the *vocal cords*.
adj. **alalic**

ALBA adj. general term, meaning
"white," for some structures,
tissues, or diseases (e.g., linea
alba, the "white line" of the front
of the abdomen, between two
muscles); also: **albicans**.

ALBEDO RETINAE n. a fluid
swelling of the *retina*.

ALBINISM n. an abnormal *congenital* condition characterized by
lack of normal pigment in the skin,
eyes, and hair. An albino person
has pale skin, white hair, and pink
eyes and is susceptible to eye and
skin disorders.

ALBINO n. a person with *albinism*.

ALBRIGHT'S DISEASE n. a
disorder of bone and cartilage that
causes skeletal lesions, sometimes skin lesions, and, in girls,
precocious *puberty*; also **polyos-
totic fibrous dysplasia**.

ALBUGINEA n. a whitish cover,
as of the *testicle* (also called tunica albuginea testes) or of the eyeball (*sclera*).

ALBUMIN n. a water-soluble protein found in most animal tissues.
Determination of the types and
levels of albumin in blood, urine,
and other body tissues and fluids
is the basis of many diagnostic
tests. The constant presence of
albumin in the urine usually indicates kidney disease.

ALBUMINEMIA n. the presence
of albumin in the blood, specifically in the serum or plasma.

ALBUMINURIA n. the presence
of excessive albumin in the urine,
usually indicative of kidney im-

pairment but sometimes due to vigorous exercise; also: **proteinuria**.

ALCOHOL n. a general term for liquids that are volatile organic compounds made from hydrocarbons by distillation. Most often refers to ethyl alcohol (C_2H_5OH), which is used as a rubbing compound and topical antiseptic, as a solvent and preservative in many drugs and biological preparations; and is drunk in alcoholic beverages. When ingested, alcohol acts as a central nervous system depressant and has many physiological effects (see also *alcoholism*).

ALCOHOL WITHDRAWAL SYNDROME see *withdrawal*.

ALCOHOLIC n. a person with alcoholism; one who uses alcohol to such an extent or in such a way as to interfere with his/her health or efficient functioning.

ALCOHOLICS ANONYMOUS n. an international organization established in 1934 as a support group for persons who want to free themselves by means of self-help and other programs from their dependence on or addiction to alcohol. A member is expected to acknowledge his/her drinking problem, to attend meetings regularly, to share experiences and difficulties, and to try to maintain sobriety "one day at a time."

ALCOHOLISM n. a chronic condition in which alcoholic drinks are taken to excess, leading to a breakdown in health and inability to function properly; dependence on or addiction to alcoholic beverages such that abrupt deprivation leads to withdrawal symptoms. Alcoholism may occur at any age; its cause is unknown but hereditary and biochemical as well as cultural and psychosocial factors are believed to play important roles. The consequences of alcoholism include impaired in-tellectual functioning, physical skills, memory, and judgment; peripheral abnormalities in nerve function; esophageal and gastrointestinal problems; impaired liver function, sometimes leading to cirrhosis of the liver; and damage to the heart muscle. Impaired emotional, social, and often economic/professional functioning also affects the self, family, and community. Alcoholism in pregnant women is also thought to damage the growth and development of the fetus (*fetal alcohol syndrome*). Acute withdrawal symptoms include tremor, anxiety, hallucinations, and in severe cases *delirium tremens*. Treatment includes psychotherapy, often in groups such as *Alcoholics Anonymous*, and the use of certain drugs like *Antabuse* that cause vomiting if alcohol is ingested. adj. **alcoholic**

ALDOSTERONE n. a hormone (one of the *mineralocorticoids*) released by the cortex of the adrenal gland; it regulates salt (sodium and potassium) and water balance in the body.

ALDOSTERONISM n. a condition characterized by an overproduction of *aldosterone* from the adrenal cortex. It may result from disease of the adrenal cortex (*Conn's syndrome*) or secondarily as a result of kidney or liver disease or other disorders. Symptoms include sodium retention, increased blood pressure, *alkalosis*, muscular weakness, and cardiac abnormalities; also **hyperaldosteronism**.

ALEXIA n. loss of reading ability; also called **word blindness**. adj. **alexic**

ALEXITHYMIA n. inability to express one's feelings; inability to identify particular bodily reactions (e.g., sweating, fast heartbeat) occurring with emotional excitement.

ALGE-, ALGESI-, ALGO- comb. form indicating an association with pain (e.g., **algesia**, sensitivity to pain).

-ALGIA suffix indicating an association with pain (e.g., *neuralgia*).

ALIMENTARY CANAL n. the digestive tube through which food passes and is digested and absorbed. It extends from the mouth to the anus and includes the mouth, pharynx, esophagus, stomach, small intestine, and large intestine; also **alimentary tract** (see also *digestive system*).

ALIMENTATION n. the act or process of providing or receiving nourishment.

ALKALEMIA n. a state of higher than normal alkalinity in the blood (representing a lower concentration of hydrogen ions); state in which the *pH* of the blood is higher than the normal range (7.35 to 7.45).

ALKALI n. a general term for a compound (e.g., potassium hydroxide) that has the properties of a *base* (vs. *acid*); it contains the hydroxyl ion (OH^-), forms a salt when combined with an acid, and forms a soap when combined with a fatty acid.   adj. **alkaline**

ALKALINURIA n. a condition in which the normally slightly acid urine is alkaline.

ALKALI POISONING n. poisoning resulting from the ingestion of an alkali compound (e.g., amnonia, lye). Emergency treatment includes giving copious amounts of water or milk; vomiting should not be induced.

ALKALOSIS n. a disturbance in the normal *acid-base balance* of the body in which the blood and body tissues are more alkaline than normal; it may result from *hyperventilation*, vomiting, or other conditions that cause an increase in base ions or a decrease in acid ions (compare *acidosis*).   adj. **alkalotic**

ALKYLATING AGENT n. any of a group of drugs used in the chemotherapeutic treatment of cancer. Antineoplastic drugs, alkylating agents interfere with the proliferation of cells.

ALLANTOIS n. one of the extraembryonic membranes surrounding the developing *fetus*. Lying between the inner *amnion* and outer *chorion*, it carries blood from the embryo to the placenta and forms umbilical blood vessels.

ALLELE n. one of two or more alternative forms of a hereditary unit (*gene*) situated in the same site on paired (homologous) chromosomes and determining a given characteristic of an organism. For example, the gene for blue eye color and the gene for brown eye color are two alleles of the gene for eye color; also: **allelomorph**   adj. **allelic**

ALLERGEN n. a substance (e.g., ragweed pollen or the proteins of milk, egg, or wheat) that can cause an *allergy*.   adj. **allergenic**

ALLERGOLOGY n. The medical specialty dealing with allergies, their causes and treatment.

ALLERGY n. a *hypersensitivity reaction* to the presence of an agent (*allergen*) that is intrinsically harmless such as animal hairs, dust, pollen, or substances in certain foods. Symptoms vary widely but may include bronchial congestion, the appearance of a rash (often itchy), vomiting, edema, conjunctivitis, runny nose or serious systemic reactions leading to *anaphylactic shock* and possibly death. Allergies are very common, affecting probably more than 15% of the U.S. population. Allergies are diagnosed through skin tests (patch test, scratch test) and other laboratory procedures. Treatment is avoidance of the allergen, if possible; the use of *antihistamine* drugs to relieve the symptoms; desensitizing injections in some cases (e.g., hay fever); and other measures (see also *hay fever*, *hives*). adj. **allergic**

ALLO- comb. form indicating an association with another or a condition of abnormality or reversal (e.g., **alloploidy**, a condition of having inherited two or more sets of *chromosomes* from different species).

ALLOGRAFT n. a tissue segment from one member to be applied as a graft to another member of the same species (but of a different genetic makeup).

ALLOPATHY n. a system of medicine that aims to produce (e.g., through drugs, compresses) a condition opposite to or antagonistic to that affecting the ill person, as for example, applying cold for a fever (compare *homeopathy*). adj. **allopathic**

ALLOPURINOL n. a drug, known under the trade name Zyloprim, used to treat gout and other conditions in which there is a buildup of uric acid. Adverse effects include blood abnormalities, gastrointestinal upsets, and allergic reactions.

ALL-OR-NONE LAW n. principle describing the characteristic response of a nerve fiber or a muscle, esp. the heart muscle, whereby any stimulus above threshold level causes the nerve or muscle to respond to its fullest extent or not at all.

ALOGIA n. loss of speaking ability, resulting from brain defect or injury.

ALOPECIA n. loss of hair; baldness. It may be partial or complete; permanent or temporary. It often results from normal aging, hereditary factors, hormonal imbalances, certain diseases, and certain drugs and treatments (e.g., *chemotherapy*). There is no treatment, and attempts to use transplants with artificial materials have generally proved unsuccessful and

in some cases dangerous. adj. **alopecic**

ALPHA FETOPROTEIN (AFP) n. a protein normally synthesized by a *fetus*. Determination of the AFP levels in amniotic fluid (through *amniocentesis*) or in the blood of pregnant women during a certain time in pregnancy can be used to detect the presence of neural tube defects such as *spina bifida* and *anencephaly* in the fetus. Elevated AFP levels in the serum of adults may indicate certain cancers and other diseases.

ALPHA RHYTHM n. a brain-wave frequency of moderate voltage that is characteristic of a person who is awake but relaxed. It is one of four brain wave patterns (compare *beta rhythm*, *delta rhythm*, *theta rhythm*); also called **alpha wave**.

ALS see *amyotrophic lateral sclerosis*.

ALTITUDE SICKNESS n. syndrome caused by low oxygen concentration at high altitudes associated with mountain climbing or air travel in unpressurized aircraft. Symptoms include rapid breathing, headache, dizziness, anxiety or euphoria; also sometimes called **mountain sickness**.

ALUMINUM n. a common metallic element. Aluminum preparations are widely used in astringents, deodorants, antiperspirants, antiseptics, and antacids (see Table of Elements).

ALUPENT n. trade name for a *bronchodilator* (metaproterenol sulfate) used in the treatment of asthma; side effects include hypertension and heart irregularities.

ALVEOLI n. pl. of *alveolus*.

ALVEOLITIS n. 1. inflammation of the small saclike structures (*alveoli*) in the lungs, caused by inhaling dusts and marked by shortness of breath, cough, fever, and joint pain. With repeated exposure to the source of irritation, the condition may become chronic (see also *bagassosis* and *farmer's lung*); 2. inflammation of the socket of a tooth, sometimes occurring after tooth extraction (see also *dry socket*).

ALVEOLO- comb. form indicating an association with an *alveolus* or of alveoli (e.g., **alveolo-capillary**, pert. to the alveoli and capillaries of the lungs).

ALVEOLUS n. any tiny saclike structure, esp. the tiny air sacs of the lungs where the exchange of oxygen and carbon dioxide takes place; 2. the socket in the jaw that retains the root of a tooth; 3. a small depression or pit. pl. **alveoli** adj. **alveolar**

ALVEOLUS

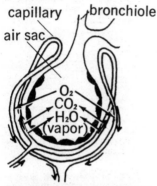

Gas exchange in an alveolus. Oxygen (O_2) enters the capillaries; carbon dioxide (CO_2) and water (H_2O) vapor pass from capillaries to alveoli for excretion.

ALZHEIMER'S DISEASE n. a progressive loss of mental ability and function, often accompanied by personality changes and emotional instability. It is a common disorder, affecting both men and women; it usually starts between ages 50 and 60, often with memory lapses and changes in behavior; it progresses to include symptoms of confusion, restlessness, inability to plan and carry out activities and sometimes hallucinations and

loss of sphincter (e.g., bladder) control. The cause is unknown but plaques and *neurofibrillary tangles* are commonly found in the brain tissue. There is no cure, with treatment aimed at alleviating the symptoms. Also called **presenile dementia**.

AMALGAM n. in psychology, the effort to overcome *anxiety* by acting on it through a combination of different approaches, as denial and counteraction; also called **emotional amalgam**.

AMASTIA n. absence of one or both breasts, either from developmental fault or surgery.

AMAUROSIS n. blindness, esp. in the absence of an obvious eye lesion (e.g., that due to disease of the spine or brain). adj. **amaurotic**

AMAUROTIC FAMILY IDIOCY see *Tay-Sachs disease*.

AMB-, AMBI-, comb. form indicating an association with both sides (e.g., **ambidexterity**, the ability to use both hands with equal skill, as in writing).

AMBIENT adj. pert. to a surrounding or environmental quality (e.g., ambient air).

AMBLYOPIA n. dimness of vision without detectable organic lesion of the eye.

AMBULATION n. the act of walking or moving about.

AMBULATORY adj. able to walk, thus descriptive of a patient not confined to bed.

AMEBA n. a one-celled jellylike organism whose shape changes. Some amebas cause disease in humans (see *amebiasis*).

AMEBIASIS n. an infection with an ameba that is *pathogenic*, esp. *Entamoeba histolytica*, the cause of *amebic dysentery*; also: **amebiosis, amebosis**.

AMEBIC adj. pert. to or caused by an ameba (e.g., *amebic dysentery*).

AMEBIC DYSENTERY n. an inflammation of the intestine caused by *Entamoeba histolytica*, usually acquired through feces-contaminated food or water, and characterized by frequent, loose, usually blood-tinged stools and sometimes liver involvement. Treatment usually includes metronidazole.

AMELIA n. *congenital* absence of an arm or leg (compare *phocomelia*).

AMELOBLAST n. an *enamel*-forming cell (of teeth).

AMENORRHEA n. abnormal stoppage or absence of the *menstrual flow*. It may be caused by *congenital* abnormality of the reproductive tract or by endocrine (hormonal) dysfunction, malnutrition, marked change in the amount of body fat (as in loss of body fat in strenuous exercise programs), severe trauma, or emotional upset. Treatment involves correction of the underlying cause and hormone therapy if necessary; also: **amenia.**   adj. **amenorrheal**

AMETRIA n. *congenital* absence of the *uterus*.

AMETROPIA n. an abnormal eye condition marked by failure of the image to focus properly on the retina; common types of ametropia are *astigmatism*, *myopia* (nearsightedness), and *hyperopia* (farsightedness).   adj. **ametropic**

AMINE n. an organic compound that contains nitrogen.

AMINO ACID n. an organic compound, containing an amino group (NH_2) and a carboxyl group (COOH), that is the end product of protein digestion and the basic building blocks from which proteins are synthesized in the cell. Ten amino acids, termed essential amino acids, cannot be synthesized in adequate amounts and at the necessary rate by the body

and must be supplied in foods; they are: isoleucine, leucine, lysine, methionine, phenylalanine, threonine, tryptophan, valine, histidine (essential for children), and arginine (essential in early life). Other amino acids necessary for growth and metabolism of the body, including alanine, glycine, cystine, tyrosine, glutamic acid and serine, can be synthesized in the body. Protein-rich foods (e.g., milk, meat, cheese, eggs) supply the body with essential amino acids.

AMINOACIDURIA n. the abnormal presence of amino acids in the urine, usually a result of a metabolic defect.

AMINOPHYLLINE n. a bronchodilator used to treat asthma, bronchitis, and emphysema; among the adverse side effects are gastrointestinal upset and central nervous system stimulation.

AMITRIPTYLINE n. a drug, commonly known under its trade name Elavil, used to treat depression. Adverse side effects include sedation and various cardiovascular, neurologic, and gastrointestinal problems; it also interacts with many other drugs and is used with caution in combination with any other agents.

AMMONIURIA n. the presence of excessive ammonia in the urine.

AMNESIA n. loss of memory, due to injury to the brain or severe emotional trauma. There are several kinds of amnesia, including *anterograde amnesia*, *retrograde amnesia*, and *transient global amnesia*.   adj. **amnesic**

AMNIOCENTESIS n. the taking of *amniotic fluid* by needle puncture through the abdominal wall of the pregnant woman to aid in the diagnosis of fetal abnormalities (e.g., *Down's syndrome*, *Tay-Sachs disease*). The test cannot be performed until about the 15th

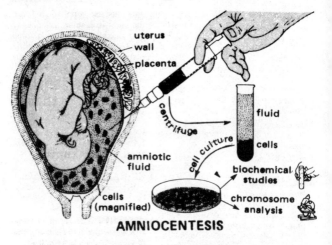

uterus
wall

placenta

centrifuge

fluid

cells

cell culture

amniotic
fluid

cells
(magnified)

biochemical
studies

chromosome
analysis

AMNIOCENTESIS

or 16th week of pregnancy and is recommended when a hereditary pattern in the family or the mother's age (over 35) increases the chance of fetal defects.

AMNION n. the inner membrane sac around the developing *fetus* (the outer membrane sac being the *chorion*) (compare *placenta*). adj. **amnionic, amniotic**

AMNIOTIC FLUID n. liquid that surrounds the *fetus* during pregnancy, serving as protection for the developing fetus, as a shock absorber, and as medium for the exchange of materials between fetus and mother.

AMNIOTIC SAC n. thin-walled bag that contains the fetus and *amniotic fluid* during pregnancy.

AMOBARBITAL n. a barbiturate drug with sedative-hypnotic effects used for the relief of *insomnia* and as an *anticonvulsant*; commonly known as **truth serum**.

AMORPHOUS adj. lacking a specific shape or form (e.g., the *ameba*).

AMOXICILLIN n. an antibiotic, specifically a semisynthetic oral penicillin, used in the treatment of several bacterial infections.

AMOXIL n. trade name for *amoxicillin*.

AMP (ADENOSINE MONO-PHOSPHATE) n. a body chemical found in muscle and important in metabolism; cyclic AMP (cAMP) is involved in nervous system, hormone, and cell functions.

AMPHETAMINE n. a *central nervous system* stimulant used to treat *narcolepsy* and some forms of *depression* and childhood *attention-deficit disorders*. It alleviates fatigue, promotes alertness and decreases appetite. Overdosage causes gastrointestinal complaints, rapid heart rate, restlessness, sleeplessness, and in very high doses hallucinations and feelings of panic. It has a high potential for abuse, resulting in *tolerance* and *dependence*; slang: **speed**.

AMPHI- comb. form indicating a doubling, affecting both sides, of both kinds (e.g., **amphigonadism**, a state of having tissues for both ovaries and testes; true *hermaphroditism*).

AMPHORIC BREATH SOUND n. an abnormal hollow sound heard with a *stethoscope* that indicates a cavity in the lung.

AMPHOTERICIN B n. a drug, used topically and systemically, to treat certain fungal infections; adverse side effects with systemic use include *thrombophlebitis*, nausea, and fever; with topical use, local *hypersensitivity reactions*.

AMPICILLIN n. an *antibiotic* (semisynthetic penicillin) used to treat a wide variety of infections; adverse side effects include nausea, diarrhea, and *anaphylaxis*.

AMPULE n. a sealable sterile glass tube used to contain medicines, usually for injection by needle; also: **ampul**.

AMPULLA n. a dilated flasklike part or structure, esp. the widened portion of a tube.   pl. **anpullae** adj. **ampullar, ampullary**

AMPUTATION n. the surgical removal of a limb, part of a limb or other body part by surgery (e.g., to treat *gangrene* or recurrent infection, severe trauma, or malignancy) or by trauma.

AMPUTEE n. one who has had a limb removed through surgery, trauma, or congenital malformation.

AMYGDALA n. an almond-shaped part or structure, specifically the two rounded bulges on the bottom sides of the *cerebellum*, part of the brain's *limbic system*. Destruction of the amygdala can result in rage and peculiar sexual behavior.

AMYLASE n. an enzyme that catalyzes part of the reactions by which starch is broken down into simpler carbohydrates. It is present in saliva, pancreatic juices, certain microorganisms, and certain foods.

AMYL NITRATE n. a *vasodilator* drug sometimes used to treat *angina pectoris*; adverse side effects include *hypotension*, nausea, headache, dizziness, and allergic reactions.

AMYLOIDOSIS n. a disorder in which starchlike glycoproteins (amyloids) accumulate in body tissues, impairing their function. The condition usually results from chronic infections or inflammatory diseases or from certain malignancies.

AMYOPLASIA n. deficiency in muscular development.

AMYOTONIA n. lack of muscle tone, weakness.

AMYOTROPHIA n. a progressive wasting of a muscle or group of muscles; also: **amyotrophy**.

AMYOTROPHIC LATERAL SCLEROSIS (ALS) n. a degenerative disease of the central nervous system characterized by progressive muscle *atrophy*, starting in the limbs and spreading to the rest of the body, often accompanied by hyperreflexia. Of unknown cause, it usually manifests itself after age 40, affecting more men than women, and progresses rapidly. There is no known treatment; also called **Lou Gehrig's disease**.

AMYXIA n. a condition in which no mucus is produced.

AN-, ANA- 1. prefix meaning "upward," "backward," "duplicate" (e.g., **anastalsis**, the reversed muscular action of the intestine, opposite to *peristalsis*); 2. prefix meaning "not" (e.g., *anaerobe*, an organism not needing air or oxygen).

ANABOLIC STEROID n. any of a group of compounds, derived from *testosterone* or prepared synthetically, which aid in constructive metabolism, including the building of cell components such as proteins and fats. They are used to treat certain anemias and malignancies, to promote body growth and weight gain, to strengthen bones in *osteoporosis*, to counter the effects of *estrogen*, or to promote masculinizing characteristics. Anabolic steroids are sometimes used—illegally—by athletes in an attempt to improve their strength and performance.

ANABOLISM n. a phase of *metabolism* involving the conversion, in cells, of simple structures into the complex molecular forms of living material.

ANACLISIS n. in psychoanalysis, the state of needing someone for support, as an infant's dependence on the mother.

ANAEROBE n. an organism that thrives without oxygen (compare *aerobe*). adj. **anaerobic**

ANAL adj. pert. to the *anus*.

ANALOGUE n. a part having a function like that of another but of a different source or species (e.g., the crop of an earthworm is analogous to the human stomach); also: **analog**.

ANAL PHASE n. the second period in *psychosexual* development of the person, as defined by Freud. The phase occurs in early childhood (1 to 3 years) and involves conflicts of autonomy with shame and doubt (compare *genital*, *latency*, *oral*, and *phallic* *phases*).

ANALBUMINEMIA n. an abnormally low level of *albumin* in the blood serum.

ANALEPTIC n. a drug that stimulates (e.g., *caffeine*) the central nervous system or strengthens or invigorates the body.

ANALGESIA n. absence of sensibility to pain, while remaining conscious, due to nerve damage (as in *leprosy*), *hypnosis*, *acupuncture*, the use of pain-relieving drugs (analgesics), or anything that activates the body's natural pain-relieving system (*endorphins*) (compare *anesthesia*). adj. **analgesic**

ANALGESIC n. a pain-relieving substance (e.g., *aspirin*, *acetaminophen*).

ANALYSIS n. the division of a thing into its elements (as a chemical) or fundamental parts (as in a procedure); a shortened form for *psychoanalysis*. pl. **analyses** adj. **analytic**

ANAMNESIS n. 1. *memory*; the faculty of remembering, of recollecting; 2. the detailed data collected about a patient and used in analyzing the case.

ANAMNESTIC adj. pert. to the *antibody* production that occurs rapidly the second time a given substance (*antigen*) is put into the body.

ANAPHASE n. a stage in cell division in which the *chromosomes* move from the center plane of the cell toward the poles (see *mitosis*).

ANAPHORESIS n. condition marked by lack of function of the sweat glands.

ANAPLASIA n. regression of fully developed cells into a more primitive (embryonic) form, occurring in some tumors.

ANAPHRODISIA n. loss or absence of sexual feeling. adj. **anaphrodisiac**

ANAPHYLACTIC SHOCK n. a severe and sometimes fatal *hypersensitivity reaction* to the injection or ingestion of a substance (e.g., penicillin, shellfish, insect venom, vaccine) to which the organism has become sensitized by a previous exposure. Symptoms, including anxiety, weakness, shortness of breath, laryngeal edema, cardiac and respiratory abnormalities, hypotension, and shock, may occur within minutes of exposure. Treatment must be prompt and usually involves the use of *epinephrine*, the maintenance of an open airway, and the treatment of cardiac and other problems. Persons with known hypersensitivity reactions are advised to avoid the offending agent and, if that is not always possible (e.g., insect venom), to carry an emergency kit with epinephrine and other necessary first-aid items.

ANAPHYLAXIS n. a strong hypersensitivity reaction to the ingestion or injection of a substance (e.g., penicillin, shellfish) to which the organism has become sensitized by a previous exposure. Symptoms may include a localized wheal and itching and swelling or in severe cases *anaphylactic shock* and even death. adj. **anaphylactic**

ANASTOMOSIS n. 1. a communication between two blood vessels, lymph vessels, or nerves; 2. an opening or passage, made by surgery, trauma, or pathology, between two normally separate tubular and hollow parts (e.g., two parts of the intestine) (compare *fistula*). pl. **anastomoses** adj. **anastomotic**

ANATOMY n. the study and science of the structure of an organism and its parts (compare *physiology*) (see also *gross anatomy*; *microscopic anatomy*). adj. **anatomic, anatomical**

ANDR-, ANDRO- comb. form indicating an association with the male sex (e.g., **androglossia**, a male-quality voice in a woman).

ANDROGEN n. a general term for substances that produce secondary masculine characteristics (e.g., deep voice, facial hair); a male hormone (e.g., *testosterone*). adj. **androgenous, androgenic**

ANDROGYNE n. a person with both ovaries and testes, underdeveloped external male and female sex organs but a predominantly female aspect (compare *pseudohermaphroditism*). adj. **androgynous**

ANDROSTERONE n. a male sex hormone.

ANEMIA n. a condition in which the *hemoglobin* content of the blood is below normal limits. It may be hereditary, congenital, or acquired. Basically anemia results from a defect in the production of hemoglobin and its carrier, the red blood cell (e.g., production of abnormal hemoglobin, misshapen red blood cells, or inadequate levels of hemoglobin); increased destruction of red blood cells; or blood loss (e.g., in hemorrhage after injury or in excessive menstrual flow), the most common cause is a deficiency in *iron*, an element necessary for the formation of hemoglobin. Symptoms vary with the severity and cause of the anemia but may include fatigue, weakness, pallor, headache, dizziness, and anorexia. Treatment also depends on the cause and severity and may include an iron-rich diet, iron supplements, blood transfusions, and the correction or elimination of any pathological conditions causing the anemia. There are several types of anemia, including *aplastic anemia, pernicious anemia, sickle-cell anemia,* and *thalassemia*. adj. **anemic**

ANENCEPHALY n. a defect in the development of the brain and skull, resulting in small or missing brain hemispheres; also: **anencephalia**. adj. **anencephalic, anencephalous**

ANERGIC adj. 1. characterized by inactivity, lack of energy; 2. pert. to *anergy*.

ANERGY n. lack or reduction of immune response to a specific *antigen*; also: **anergia**. adj. **anergic**

ANESTHESIA n. absence of sensation, esp. that of *pain*. In *general anesthesia*, which is administered before a major operation (e.g., removal of a lung), total unconsciousness results from injection or inhalation of anesthetic drugs. In *local anesthesia* loss of sensation is confined to a given small part or area of the body (e.g., the tissues surrounding a tooth to be extracted). In *regional anesthesia* loss of sensation is produced in a specific area of the body (e.g., in the pelvic area during childbirth by an *epidural* anesthetic). In *topical anesthesia* loss of sensation is confined to the surface skin or mucous membranes (e.g., benzocaine solution sprayed on the skin). Anesthesia may also be produced by *hypnosis*, *acupuncture*, and nerve damage (as in leprosy). adj. **anesthetic**

ANESTHESIOLOGY n. 1. the science and study of the use of *anesthesia* and of anesthetic drugs; 2. a medical specialty in the use of drugs and other means to avert or reduce pain in patients, esp. during surgery.

ANESTHETIC n. a drug (e.g., procaine hydrochloride [Novocain]) that causes temporary loss of sensation.

ANEUPLOIDY n. a condition in which the number of *chromosomes* is either more or fewer than normal. adj. **aneuploid**

ANEURYSM n. a saclike widening in a blood vessel; it occurs most often in the *aorta* but can also occur in other blood vessels. Aneurysms are usually caused by *atherosclerosis* or *hypertension*, sometimes by trauma, infection, or other factor. An aneurysm may rupture, causing hemorrhage, or it may lead to the formation of *thrombi* and/or *emboli* that may block an important blood vessel. Common types of aneurysms include aortic aneurysm and cerebral aneurysm. Treatment includes use of drugs to reduce the force of cardiac contraction, analgesic and antihypertensive drugs if indicated, and, in some cases, surgical resection of the aorta or affected artery. adj. **aneurysmal**

ANGI-, ANGIO- comb. form indicating an association with blood vessels or *lymph* vessels (e.g., **angiectasis**, abnormal widening and sometimes lengthening of an artery or vein).

ANGIITIS n. inflammation of a blood or lymph vessel.

ANGINA n. a severe pain, often spasmodic and with a choking feeling, esp. choking pain in the chest (*angina pectoris*); also: **angor**.

ANGINA PECTORIS n. chest pain, often accompanied by a feeling of choking or impending death; the pain typically radiates down the left arm. It is usually caused by lack of oxygen to the heart muscle, resulting from atherosclerosis of the coronary arteries; attacks are precipitated by exertion, exposure to cold, or stress. Pain is relieved by rest and use of drugs (e.g., nitroglycerine) to dilate the coronary arteries.

ANGIOCARDIOGRAM n. an X-ray of the heart obtained by following with a rapid series of X-ray films the passage of a contrast medium through the heart and its associated vessels. It is useful in diagnosing heart defects and disorders.

ANGIOLOGY n. the medical specialty dealing with diseases of the blood and lymph vessels and their treatment; the science of vessels.

ANGIOMA n. a benign tumor made up primarily of blood vessels (hemangioma) or lymph vessels (lymphangioma).

ANGIOPATHY n. any abnormality affecting the blood vessels.

ANGIOPLASTY n. surgery done on arteries, veins, or capillaries; a technique in which a balloon is inflated inside a blood vessel to flatten any *plaque* (patch) that obstructs it and causes it to become narrowed (used esp. to open coronary arteries).

ANGIOTELECTASIA n. a condition characterized by dilatation and enlargement of capillaries.

ANGIOTENSIN n. a chemical in the blood that causes blood vessels to become narrowed; also: **angiotonin**.

ANGLE n. the shape formed by the joining of two lines or parts (e.g., the costovertebral angle formed by the attachment of the lowest rib to the spinal column at the *lumbar* region); also: **angulus**. pl. **anguli** adj. **angular**

ANGSTROM n. a unit of measure of wavelength (as of ultraviolet radiation or X-rays) equal to one ten-millionth of a meter, or 0.1 nanometer.

ANHIDROSIS n. failure of sweat gland function.

ANHYDROUS adj. having no water (e.g., the waterless form of a chemical compound, as anhydrous ammonia).

ANICTERIC adj. without *jaundice*.

ANILE adj. imbecilic; acting like a feeble, trembling old person.

ANIMA n. the inner self (compare *persona*).

ANKLE n. the joint at which the foot attaches to the leg, formed by the ends of the lower leg bones (*tibia* and *fibula*) and the *talus*, the topmost of the bones in the foot.

ANKYLOGLOSSIA n. the condition in which the band of tissue (*frenum*) connecting the lower surface of the tongue to the floor of the mouth is abnormally short, limiting the normal movement of the tongue; also called **tongue-tied**.

ANKYLOSING SPONDYLITIS n. a chronic disease, affecting primarily males under the age of 30, characterized by inflammation and stiffening of the spine and joints, sometimes leading to *ankylosis*, or fusion, of the involved joints. Treatment includes anti-inflammatory agents and pain-relievers; also **Marie-Strumpell disease** (compare *rheumatoid arthritis*).

ANKYLOSIS n. rigidity of a joint, often in an abnormal position, resulting from disease (e.g., *rheumatoid arthritis*) or injury, or produced intentionally as a surgical treatment. pl. **ankyloses**

ANLAGE n. in the developing embryo, a structure or part on which some later development depends; *rudiment; primordium*.

ANODYNE n. a pain-relieving drug.

ANOMALY n. a marked abnormality, as of an organ or part, esp. a congenital or inherited defect. adj. **anomalous**

ANOMIE n. feeling of isolation, anxiety, or disorientation from any norms (considered by some as a major cause of suicide).

ANOPERINEAL adj. pert. to the *anus* and surrounding area (*perineum*).

ANORCHISM n. absence of one *testis* or both testes; also: **anorchia, anorchidism**. adj. **anorchidic**

ANORECTAL adj. pert. to the *anus* and *rectum* considered together.

ANORECTIC adj. pert. to *anorexia*; lacking appetite.

ANOREXIA n. state in which a person has a lack or loss of appetite, resulting in an inability to eat (see also *anorexia nervosa*). adj. **anorectic, anorexic**

ANOREXIA NERVOSA n. an emotional disorder, occurring most commonly in adolescent females, characterized by abnormal body image and fear of obesity and prolonged refusal to eat, leading to emaciation, *amenorrhea*, and other symptoms and sometimes resulting in death. Treatment includes psychotherapy and nourishment.

ANORGASMIA n. absence of a *climax* (*orgasm*) in sexual relations.

ANOSMIA n. absence of the sense of smell. It may be temporary, as from a cold or respiratory infection, or permanent, resulting from damage to olfactory nasal tissue or the *olfactory nerve*. adj. **anosmatic, anosmic**

ANOVULATION n. absence of egg production or release from the *ovary*. It may be caused by ovarian immaturity or post-maturity; pregnancy or lactation; dysfunction of the ovary; hormonal imbalance; oral contraceptive pills; or as a side effect of other medication; also: **anovulia**. adj. **anovular, anovulatory**

ANOVULATORY adj. not associated with ovulation, the development and release of a mature ovum (egg) from the ovary, as in anovulatory menstruation.

ANOVULATORY DRUG n. a drug that inhibits ovulation, as an *oral contraceptive pill*.

ANOXIA n. an abnormally low amount of *oxygen* in the body (see *hypoxia*), as can occur at high altitudes or in certain diseases (e.g., anemia, heart failure, impaired respiration). adj. **anoxic**

ANTABUSE n. trade name for *disulfiram*, a drug used in the treatment of *alcoholism*,

ANTACID n. a chemical that reduces acidity (e.g., sodium bicarbonate), esp. one taken to relieve "upset stomach."

ANTAGONIST n. 1. one of a pair of muscles (e.g., the *biceps*) that relaxes during the contraction of the other muscle (the *agonist*, e.g., the *triceps*); 2. any chemical that works against the action of another.

ANTE- comb. form referring to a preceding time, place, or condition (e.g., **antenatal**, before birth).

ANTECUBITAL adj. pert. to region of the arm in front of the elbow; it is the site often used for drawing blood for examination.

ANTEMORTEM adj. before death.

ANTEPARTUM adj. occurring during pregnancy, before childbirth.

ANTERIOR adj. at or toward the front of a part, organ, or structure, or toward the head in four-legged animals (compare *posterior*).

ANTERIOR PITUITARY GLAND n. the anterior lobe of the pituitary gland, the *endocrine gland* situated at the base of the brain. Under the control of the *hypothalamus*, it secretes hormones that control other endocrine glands throughout the body as well as hormones that have a direct effect on body growth and metabolism. Important anterior pituitary hormones are: *growth hormone*, *follicle-stimulating hormone* (FSH), *thyroid-stimulating hormone* (TSH), *adrenocorticotropic hormone* (ACTH), *luteinizing hormone* (LH), and *prolactin* (*luteotropic hormone*, or LTH). Also called **adenohypophysis**.

ANTERO- comb. form indicating a position to the front of, or placement before, a part or reference point (compare *retro-*, *postero-*) (e.g., **anteroinferior**, at or toward the front and below).

ANTEROGRADE AMNESIA n. the inability to recall long-ago events with recall of recent happenings (compare *anterograde memory*).

ANTEROGRADE MEMORY n. inability to recall recent events but with normal recall of events long past; also called **senile memory**.

ANTHELMINTIC n. a drug (e.g., piperazine) or chemical that kills intestinal worms.

ANTHRACOSIS n. a chronic lung disease, occurring in coal miners and others exposed to coal dust and soot, characterized by black deposits on the lungs and bronchi and impaired lung function; also: **black lung, miner's lung** (see also: *pneumoconiosis*).

ANTHRAX n. a bacterial (*Bacillus anthracis*) disease of cattle and other farm animals that can be transmitted to humans from infected animals and animal products. The disease causes skin lesions, fever, muscle pain, nausea, and internal hemorrhage; in a serious, often fatal, form, it also attacks the lungs. Treatment is by penicillin or tetracycline. adj. **anthracic**

ANTI- prefix meaning ''counter,'' ''against,'' ''opposite'' (e.g., **antibacterial**, pert. to a substance that destroys bacteria).

ANTIADRENERGIC adj. pert. to blocking or countering the effects of impulses conveyed by the adrenergic postganglionic fibers of the *sympathetic nervous system*.

ANTIBIOTIC n. a drug (e.g., penicillin), derived from a microorganism or produced synthetically, that destroys or limits the growth of a living organism, esp. a disease-producing bacteria (e.g., *Streptococcus*) or fungus.

ANTIBODY n. a complex molecule (*immunoglobulin*) produced by lymph tissue in response to the presence of an *antigen* (such as a protein of bacteria or other infecting organism) and that neutralizes the effect of that foreign substance (see also *monoclonal antibody*).

ANTICANCER adj. used in the treatment of cancer, esp. anticancer drugs (e.g., vincristine sulfate).

ANTICHOLINERGIC adj. pert. to the blocking of acetylcholine receptors; this results in the inhibition of nerve impulse transmission in the *parasympathetic nervous system*.

ANTICOAGULANT n. a substance that delays blood clotting (*coagulation*) (e.g., coumarin, heparin). Anticoagulants are used to prevent clotting in blood used for transfusions and in blood vessels (e.g., in patients with *phlebitis*). adj. **anticoagulative**

ANTICONVULSANT n. a drug (e.g., Dilantin) effective in preventing or treating *convulsions* (e.g., in *epilepsy*).

ANTIDIABETIC n. a drug used to treat or prevent *diabetes mellitus*.

ANTIDIARRHEAL n. a drug or other substance used to control or stop diarrhea (e.g., Lomotil).

ANTIDEPRESSANT n. drug used to prevent or treat *depression*.

ANTIDIURETIC n. a drug that limits the formation of urine.

ANTIDIURETIC HORMONE (ADH) n. a hormone that inhibits the production of *urine* by increasing the reabsorption of water in the kidney. It is secreted by the *hypothalamus* and stored and released by the *posterior pituitary gland* in response to stress, pain, and certain changes in electrolyte balance and blood volume; also called **vasopressin**.

ANTIDOTE n. a drug that neutralizes or minimizes the effects of a poison (e.g., pralidoxine chloride, an antidote against poisoning by intake of an organophosphate pesticide) (compare *antitoxin*).

ANTIEMETIC n. a drug or other substance that prevents or alleviates vomiting and nausea or limits their effects, sometimes used to treat motion sickness (e.g., Emetrol, a mint-flavored solution of glucose, fructose, and orthophosphoric acid).

ANTIENZYME n. a chemical used to inactivate an enzyme, esp. an enzyme that itself inactivates a substance or process in the body (e.g., the amino acid D-phenyl-alanine has been tested for use against enkephalinase enzymes, which block the action of body-manufactured pain relievers known as *enkephalins*).

ANTIEPILEPTIC see *anti-convulsant*.

ANTIFLATULENT n. an agent that reduces intestinal gas (*fla-tus*).

ANTIFUNGAL n. an agent that destroys or prevents the growth of fungi (e.g., Griseofulvin).

ANTIGEN n. a substance (e.g., a *toxin*) or organism (e.g., an *ameba*) that, when entering the body, causes the production of an *antibody* that reacts specifically with the antigen to neutralize, destroy, or weaken it. The presence of certain antigens is the criterion for typing in the *ABO blood grouping system* and is important in tissue cross-matching for transplants (e.g., the HLA antigen in kidney transplants). adj. **antigenic**

ANTIGEN-ANTIBODY REACTION n. the process by which the immune system recognizes an *antigen* and causes the production of *antibodies* specific against that antigen.

ANTIHISTAMINE n. a drug, used to treat allergies, hypersensitivity reactions, and colds, that works to reduce the effects of *histamine* (e.g., chlorpheniramine maleate [Coricidin]). adj. **antihistaminic**

ANTIHYPERTENSIVE n. a drug that reduces *hypertension* (high blood pressure).

ANTI-INFLAMMATORY n. a drug that counteracts or reduces *inflammation* (e.g., *aspirin*).

ANTIMALARIAL adj. pert. to destruction or suppression of the causes and carriers of malaria; n. drug used to treat malaria.

ANTIMICROBIAL n. an agent that destroys or limits the growth of a microscopic organism.

ANTIMYCOTIC n. an agent that destroys or limits the growth of a *fungus*.

ANTINEOPLASTIC n. a drug that controls or kills cancer cells, used in the treatment of cancer by *chemotherapy*. There are several types of antineoplastic drugs, including alkylating agents (e.g., chlorambucil), antimetabolites (e.g., fluorouracil), periwinkle plant derivatives (e.g., vinblastine, vincristine), and antineoplastic antibiotics (e.g., adramycin, actinomycin-D, mithramycin). All are associated with unpleasant and sometimes serious side effects, which may include nausea and vomiting, hair loss, and suppression of bone marrow function.

ANTIPRURITIC n. a substance that prevents or relieves itching (e.g., topical anesthetic).

ANTIPSYCHOTIC n. a drug used to treat a *psychosis* (e.g., *schizophrenia*).

ANTIPYRETIC n. a drug that reduces *fever* (e.g., aspirin).

ANTISEPSIS n. the destruction or inhibition of infection-producing microorganisms, thus preventing *infection*.

ANTISEPTIC n. an agent (e.g., soap) that slows or stops the continuing growth of microorganisms but may not actually kill them. adj. **antiseptic**

ANTISERUM n. serum that contains antibodies against a specific disease; it is used to confer *passive immunity* (compare *vaccine*).

ANTISOCIAL PERSONALITY see *sociopathic personality*.

ANTISPASMODIC n. an agent that relieves or prevents *spasm*.

ANTITOXIN n. a drug or other agent (e.g., *antivenin*) that prevents or limits the effect of a mi-

croorganism's poison (*toxin*).
adj. **antitoxic**

ANTITUSSIVE n. a substance that relieves coughing (e.g., syrup that promotes the action of *cilia* in the respiratory tract and helps remove *mucus*).

ANTIVENIN n. a drug (*antitoxin*) used to counteract the effects of venom from the bite of an insect, a snake, or other animal.

ANTIVERT n. tradename for an antihistamine (meclizine hydrochloride) used in the prevention and treatment of motion sickness.

ANTIVIRAL n. a drug that destroys viruses (e.g., *interferon*).

ANTRUM n. in anatomy, a cavity or cavelike structure. pl. **antra** adj. **antral**

ANULUS n. a ringlike part; also: **annulus**. pl. **anuli**

ANURESIS see anuria.

ANURIA n. the inability to urinate, the cessation of urine production and excretion. It can be caused by diseases of the kidney and bladder or by serious decline in blood pressure. Untreated, it leads to *uremia* and fatal consequences. adj. **anuretic**

ANUS n. the opening of the *rectum*, at which the passing of *feces* is controlled by a circular muscle system (*sphincter* ani). adj. **anal**

ANXIETY n. a state of mild-to-severe apprehension, often without specific cause, resulting in body changes such as quickened heartbeat and sweat. Natural body chemicals (e.g., inosine) help to reduce anxiety and its effects.

ANXIETY ATTACK n. an acute episode of intense anxiety and feelings of panic, accompanied by symptoms such as palpitations, breathlessness, sweating, gastrointestinal complaints and feelings of imminent disaster. The attacks usually occur suddenly, may last from a few seconds to an hour or more, and may occur infrequently or several times a day. Treatment includes reassurance; the use of anxiolytic and ataraxic drugs; sedation, if necessary; and often psychotherapy to alleviate the underlying causes.

ANXIOLYTIC n. a drug that relieves anxiety. adj. anxiety-relieving

AORTA n. the main trunk of the arterial blood circulatory system from which all other arteries (except the pulmonary) branch. This large artery stems from the heart at the *left ventricle*, passes upward (ascending aorta) toward the neck, arches (aortic arch) and loops and descends downward (descending aorta) along the left side of the vertebral column through the chest region (thoracic aorta), through the *diaphragm* to the abdomen (abdominal aorta) where it divides into two iliac arteries. Major arteries (e.g., carotid, coronary) branch from the aorta, transporting the aorta's freshly oxygenated blood to the various organs of the body. The aortic valve, situated between the left ventricle and the aorta, prevents blood from flowing back from the aorta into the heart. adj. **aortal, aortic**

AORTIC ANEURYSM see *aneurysm*.

AORTIC ARCH see *aorta*.

AORTIC STENOSIS n. a narrowing or stricture of the *aortic valve*, due to *congenital* malformation or the result of disease (e.g., *rheumatic fever*), that obstructs the flow of blood from the heart's left ventricle into the *aorta*, leading to decreased cardiac output. Symptoms include faint pulse in the extremities, systolic murmur, and exercise intolerance. Children with aortic stenosis are usually restricted from strenuous sports activities (e.g., football). Treatment involves surgical repair of the valve.

AORTIC VALVE n. valve in the heart between the left ventricle and the aorta that prevents blood from flowing from the aorta back into the heart.

AORTITIS n. inflammation of the aorta, usually due to advanced *syphilis*, sometimes to *rheumatic fever*.

APATHY n. absence or suppression of feeling, concern, passion; indifference to things generally found exciting. adj. **apathetic**

APC abbreviation for *aspirin*, *phenacetin*, and *caffeine*, a drug combination found in some over-the-counter remedies for headache and other mild pain.

APERTURE n. a hole or opening (see also *orifice*, *pupil*).

APEX n. the top or pointed end of a structure, as the apex, or tip, of the tongue. pl. **apices** adj. **apical**

APGAR SCORE n. an evaluation of an infant's physical condition usually made one minute after birth and then repeated five minutes after birth. Five factors: heart rate, muscle tone, respiratory effort, color, and reflex irritability are scored from a low of zero to a normal of 2 and the five scores combined to give a total score of 0 to 10. In general a total score below seven indicates distress.

APHAGIA n. inability to swallow, due to pain or paralysis, as in *myasthenia gravis*.

APHAKIA n. absence of the natural *lens* of the eye, as when a *cataract* has been surgically removed. adj. **aphakic**

APHASIA n. inability to speak or express oneself in writing or to comprehend spoken or written language because of a brain lesion (e.g., the result of a stroke). adj. **aphasic**

APHERESIS n. a procedure, similar to *dialysis*, for cleansing the blood through filters; used experimentally to treat persons with certain disorders (see *plasmaphoresis*).

APHRODISIA n. sexual desire, esp. if extreme.

APLASIA n. failure of an organ or part to develop (compare *hyperplasia*; *hypoplasia*; *phocomelia*) (see also *aplastic anemia*). adj. **aplastic**

APLASTIC ANEMIA n. a deficiency of the formed elements (e.g., red blood cells, white blood cells) of the blood due to a failure of the cell-producing machinery of the bone marrow, caused by a neoplasm or, most commonly, by exposure to toxic chemicals, radiation, or certain drugs.

APNEA n. a state of not breathing; an arrest of respiration. Attacks of apnea occur in some people during sleep (see *sleep apnea*) and in some newborn babies (see *periodic apnea of the newborn*). adj. **apneic**

APOCRINE GLAND n. any of several large, deep exocrine glands found in the axillary (armpit), genital, anal, and mammary regions, that secrete a strong sweat with a characteristic odor.

APOENZYME n. a protein that combines with a *coenzyme* (nonprotein, e.g., some *vitamins*) to form an active *enzyme*.

APOMORPHINE n. a *morphine*-derivative used to induce vomiting in some types of poisoning and sometimes used in low doses as an expectorant and sedative. Adverse side effects include respiratory and central nervous system depression.

APONEUROSIS n. the tendon-like expansion with which a flat muscle attaches to other parts. pl. **aponeuroses** adj. **aponeurotic**

APOPLEXY n. a long-used (now obsolete) term for a cerebral *stroke*, in which the brain's blood system becomes impaired and muscle control and other nerve function may be affected.   adj. **apoplectic**

APPARATUS n. in anatomy, a group of parts that work together in performing a given function (e.g., auditory apparatus, all the components of the organ of hearing—the ear, including outer, inner, and middle parts).   pl. **apparatuses**

APPENDAGE n. something attached or appended; the cecal appendage is the *appendix vermiformis*, commonly called simply the appendix (see also *adnexa*); also: **appendix·**

APPENDECTOMY n. surgical removal of the *appendix*. When a patient has *appendicitis*, the operation is performed to prevent the appendix from rupturing.

APPENDICITIS n. inflammation of the vermiform *appendix*. Symptoms are pain in the abdomen, generally but not exclusively on the right side, nausea, vomiting, low-grade fever, and elevated white blood cell counts. Treatment is *appendectomy*.

APPENDIX n. an appendage, esp. the vermiform appendix, the apparently functionless wormlike (vermiform) or fingerlike attachment to the first part of the large intestine (*cecum*) in the lower right abdomen (see *appendicitis*).

APPERCEPTION n. the whole perception process, receiving, recognizing, appreciating, assimilating, and interpreting stimuli taken in by the senses (e.g., hearing the roar of a wave on the beach and appreciating the contribution of the separate drops of water that cause the roar) (compare *gestaltism*).   adj. **apperceptive**

APPETITE n. normal desire, esp. for food, but also for other needs, including sex.

APRAXIA n. loss or impairment

of the ability to make purposeful movements, usually caused by a neurological disorder.   adj. **apraxic**

AQUEOUS adj. 1. made with water (e.g., a chemical compound); 2. like water (e.g., the *aqueous humor* of the eye).

AQUEOUS HUMOR n. the clear, watery fluid circulating in the anterior and posterior chambers of the eye.

ARACHNODACTYLY n. a congenital condition in which the fingers and/or toes are long, thin, and spiderlike.

ARACHNOID MEMBRANE n. the thin, delicate membrane that is the middle of the three membranes (*meninges*) enclosing the brain and spinal cord; the outer membrane is the *dura mater*, the inner the *pia mater*.

ARC n. a structure or pathway shaped like a bow or loop (see also *arch*); also: **arcus**

ARCH n. a bowlike structure or part (e.g., *maxillary arch*, the structure that forms the *palate*).

ARCH SUPPORT n. an artificial support for the arch of the foot, generally inserted in shoes, helping, in some cases, to relieve back pain.

AREA n. a general anatomical region (e.g., the *aortic* area, that portion of the chest surface over the *cartilage* of the right second rib where it attaches to the breastbone, the site at which aortic sounds are best heard through a *stethoscope*).

AREATA adj. developing or showing as patches (e.g., **alopecia areata**, patchy baldness); also: **areatus**

AREFLEXIA n. absence or loss of reflexes, a sign of possible nerve damage.

AREOLA n. 1. a small space, as that in tissue (see *interstice*); 2. the circle around a pimple, the *iris*, or the *nipple*.   pl. **areolae**   adj. **areolar**

ARM n. the upper extremity or limb, esp. from the shoulder to the hand and including the upper arm (see *humerus*), *forearm* (*ulna* and *radius*), and wrist (*carpus*).

ARISTOCORT n. trade name for a glucocorticoid (triamcinolone) used as an anti-inflammatory agent.

AROUSAL n. increased responsiveness to stimulation; increased desire for sexual activity.

ARRECTOR PILI n. the small muscle of a *hair follicle* that, when contracted, causes a *goose bump*.

ARREST n. a stopping, as of a rhythm or muscle function (e.g., *cardiac arrest*, a sudden stopping of the heart).

ARRHYTHMIA n. abnormal heartbeat rhythm, caused by drugs, disease, the body's physiology, or a combination of factors. adj. **arrhythmic**

ARSENIC n. a chemical element used in some medicines (e.g., arsenic trioxide, for treating skin diseases) and poisons.

ARSENIC POISONING n. poisoning caused by the ingestion or inhalation of arsenic, an ingredient in some pesticides, dyes, and medicinal products. Small amounts absorbed over a long period may cause headache, nausea, coloring of the skin, and the appearance of white lines on the nails. Ingestion of large amounts leads to severe gastrointestinal problems, swelling of the arms and legs, and possibly renal failure, shock, and death.

ARTERIAL adj. pert. to an artery or arteries.

ARTERIAL BLEEDING n. bleeding from an artery, with the blood bright red and coming in spurts. It can be stopped by applying pressure to the artery between the wound and the heart.

ARTERIAL BLOOD n. blood found in the arteries. Except in the pulmonary artery, arterial blood is rich in oxygen to be transported to the tissues of the body.

ARTERIAL BLOOD GASES n. the oxygen and carbon dioxide in arterial blood. Determination of the levels of these gases is important in the diagnosis of many diseases (e.g., *emphysema*, chronic obstructive lung disease, *polycythemia*) (see also *blood gases*).

ARTERIAL PRESSURE n. the stress exerted by the circulating blood on the arteries. It is a result of the product of cardiac output and vascular resistance (see also *blood pressure*).

ARTERIECTASIS n. abnormal distension of an artery; also: **arteriectasia**.

ARTERIO- comb. form indicating an association with an artery or arteries (e.g., **arteriocapillary**. pert. to arteries and capillaries; **arteriovenous**, pert. to arteries and veins).

ARTERIOGRAM n. an X-ray of an artery filled with a contrast medium.

ARTERIOLE n. the smallest branch of an artery, leading to a capillary network. adj. **arteriolar**

ARTERIOSCLEROSIS n. a disorder of the arteries, common with advancing age and in certain diseases (e.g., *hypertension*), characterized by calcification, loss of elasticity and hardening of the walls of the arteries, resulting in decreased blood flow, especially to the brain and extremities. Symptoms include intermittent limping, memory deficits, headache, and dizziness. There is no specific treatment, but moderate exercise, a low-fat diet, and avoidance of stress are generally recommended.

ARTERITIS n. inflammation of an *artery* or arteries, occurring alone or accompanying another disorder (e.g., *rheumatic fever*).

ARTERY n. a vessel that carries blood away from the heart to the other tissues throughout the body. Except for the pulmonary artery (which carries blood to the lungs), arteries carry oxygen-rich blood.

Most arteries are named for the body part they traverse or reach (e.g., the **femoral artery** courses along the *femur*) (see also *aorta*). adj. **arterial**

MAJOR ARTERIES

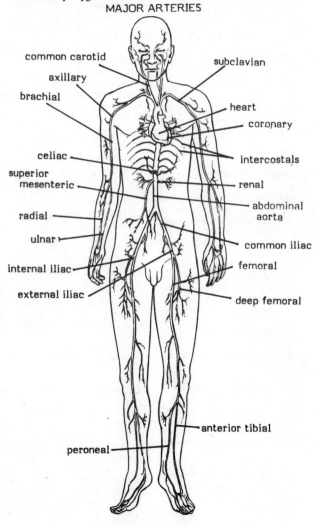

- common carotid
- subclavian
- axillary
- brachial
- heart
- coronary
- celiac
- intercostals
- superior mesenteric
- renal
- radial
- abdominal aorta
- ulnar
- common iliac
- internal iliac
- femoral
- external iliac
- deep femoral
- anterior tibial
- peroneal

ARTH-, ARTHRO- comb. form indicating an association with a joint or joints (e.g., **arthrodysplasia**, joint abnormality or deformity).

ARTHRALGIA n. pain in a joint or joints.

ARTHRITIS n. inflammation of a joint that may cause swelling, redness, and pain. There are several types of arthritis, the most common of which are *gout* (gouty arthritis), *osteoarthritis*, and *rheumatoid arthritis*. adj. **arthritic**

ARTHROCENTESIS n. introduction of a needle into a joint and the removal of fluid from it (e.g., to determine what chemicals or microorganisms may be present).

ARTHROGRAPHY n. X-ray of a joint.

ARTHROPLASTY n. the surgical reconstruction or replacement of a joint that is congenitally malformed or that has degenerated as a result of injury or disease (e.g., *osteoarthritis*).

ARTICULATION n. a joint; the place at which two or more bones join (e.g., the knee or shoulder). adj. **articular**

ARTIFACT n. a synthetic object found in a body part, esp. something (as a clip or thread) seen on an X-ray film or in a microscopic field that does not normally belong there.

ARTIFICIAL BLOOD n. a fluid that can carry large amounts of oxygen and is being tested as a temporary substitute for blood. The most common so far tested is known as Fluosol-DA; it is similar to Teflon and made up of inert perfluorochemicals. Most clinical studies have involved those seriously in need of blood but who refuse blood transfusions (e.g., on religious grounds, such as Jehovah's Witnesses).

ARTIFICIAL HEART n. a device designed to replace the heart and pump blood throughout the body. An artificial heart was implanted in a human for the first time in late 1982 and worked in the patient for over 110 days, before he died of complications. Further work on the device is continuing.

ARTIFICIAL INSEMINATION (AI) n. introduction of *sperm* into the female birth canal by means of an instrument (e.g., a slender tube and syringe) to increase the likelihood of *conception*. The sperm specimen may be provided by the woman's husband (AIH) or partner or by an anonymous donor (AID).

ARTIFICIAL JOINT n. metal and/or plastic parts surgically inserted (commonly the hip or the knee) to replace a natural *joint* (see also *prosthesis*).

ARTIFICIAL ORGAN n. a synthetic device to replace a natural organ or to assist its function (e.g., *artificial heart*, artificial kidney, artificial pancreas).

ARTIFICIAL RESPIRATION n. an emergency procedure for maintaining a flow of air through the pulmonary system, using mechanical means or hand pressure, to aid a person whose breathing has stopped (e.g., because of drowning, injury, or drugs) or is otherwise not controlled (see *cardiopulmonary resuscitation*; *iron lung*).

ARTIFICIAL SKIN n. a synthetic (e.g., plastic, cowhide collagen, shark cartilage) two-layer covering now used experimentally to treat burn victims.

ASBESTOS n. a fiberlike, fire-resistant mineral commonly used as an insulator and roofing material, it is now implicated in causing lung disease (*asbestosis*) (even when inhaled in small amounts and for a limited time) and as a *carcinogen*.

ASBESTOSIS n. a chronic, progressive lung disease, resulting from breathing in the mineral asbestos and common among asbestos miners and roofers; it is marked by *fibrosis* of lung tissue. Symptoms include shortness of breath and cough, often leading to respiratory failure; lung cancer is a frequent complication (see also *pneumonoconiosis*).

ASCARIASIS n. infection with *Ascaris* worms, acquired through feces-contaminated water or food. Symptoms may involve coughing, wheezing, and fever or gastrointestinal complaints. Treatment is by piperazine and other drugs.

ASCITES n. abnormal accumulation of protein-and-electrolyte rich fluid in the abdomen (peritoneal cavity), often a complication of another serious disease (e.g., *cirrhosis*, *nephrosis*, *congestive heart failure*); (also called **abdominal dropsy**). adj. **ascitic**

ASCORBIC ACID n. water-soluble vitamin C (see Table of Vitamins), essential for normal connective tissue, bone and skin development, for fighting bacterial infection, and to prevent *scurvy*. Found esp. in citrus fruits, potatoes, and leafy vegetables.

-ASE a suffix that identifies an *enzyme* (e.g., *cholinesterase*).

ASEPSIS n. the state of being without infection or contamination; *sterile*. adj. **aseptic**

ASEXUAL adj. lacking sexual involvement; having no sex.

ASIATIC FLU n. *influenza* caused by the Asian virus, first isolated in 1957.

-ASIS comb. form denoting a condition (e.g., *elephantiasis*) (compare *-osis*).

ASPERGILLOSIS n. an uncommon and serious infection with a fungus of the genus *Aspergillus*, most often occurring in those weakened by another disease or with impaired immunological responses (e.g., those undergoing chemotherapy, receiving immunosuppressive drugs following a transplant, or having *AIDS*) and characterized by inflammation and lesions of the ear and other organs.

ASPHYXIA n. a condition in which insufficient or no oxygen reaches the tissues, thereby threatening the life of the organism. Common causes are drowning, electric shock, inhaling poison gas, and choking. v. **asphyxiate** adj. **asphyxiated**

ASPIRATION n. 1. the action of breathing in, esp. inhaling an unwanted substance or foreign object; 2. the use of suction to take liquids or gases from a body cavity or area, as in aspiration biopsy.

ASPIRATION PNEUMONIA n. an inflammation of the lungs and bronchi caused by inhaling *vomitus*; it most often occurs during anesthesia or recovery from anesthesia or during an acute episode of alcoholism. Treatment includes suctioning and the administration of oxygen and drugs to reduce inflammation.

ASPIRIN n. acetylsalicylic acid, a drug commonly used to relieve pain (analgesic) and reduce fever (antipyretic) and inflammation (anti-inflammatory); it may also prevent blood clotting and help prevent strokes, heart attacks, and cataracts. Side effects include stomach discomfort and gastrointestinal bleeding (which may be small in amount and occult); for these reasons buffered aspirins are available (see *buffered aspirin*). Accidental overdosage of aspirin is a common form of poisoning, esp. among children (see *salicylate poisoning*).

ASSAY n. a test to determine the amount of a given chemical in a mixture, the potency of a drug, or the purity of a compound. v. to analyze a substance

ASSERTIVENESS TRAINING n. a method used in psychological *therapy* in which one is taught to state negative and positive feelings directly and frankly.

ASSOCIATION n. a connection of two or more things or events (see *free association*).

ASTHENIA n. a weakened state; lack or loss of physical strength (see *neuresthenia*).   adj. **asthenic**

ASTHMA n. a respiratory disorder characterized by recurrent episodes of difficulty in breathing, wheezing (esp. on expiration), cough, and thick mucus production, usually caused by a spasm or inflammation of the bronchial airways. Attacks are precipitated by exposure to an *allergen* (e.g., pollen, dust, food), strenuous exercise, stress, or infection. Asthma is most common in childhood (occurring more often in boys) and has a strong hereditary factor. Treatment involves the use of *bronchodilators* and elimination of the causative agent (also called **bronchial asthma**). adj. **asthmatic**

ASTIGMATISM n. a defect in vision in which the light rays cannot be focused properly on the *retina* because of abnormal curvature of the *cornea* or *lens* of the eye; corrective lenses improve vision.   adj. **astigmatic**

ASTIGMATISM

Irregular cornea

Irregular lens

In astigmatism light rays cannot be focused clearly on the retina because the curvature of the cornea or lens is irregular.

ASTRAGALUS n. an ankle bone (now better known as the *talus*).

ASTRINGENT adj. causing the skin to draw tight; also styptic (as styptic pencil, containing the astringent alum, to stop bleeding in minor cuts from shaving).   n. a substance that, when applied to the skin, draws it tight.

ASYMMETRY n. lack of mirror-image correspondence between paired parts or normally similar sides of a body or organ (e.g., having one hand or a side of the face that is not the mirror image of the other). adj. **asymmetrical**

ASYMPTOMATIC adj. without *symptoms*.

ASYNCLITISM n. in *labor*, presentation of the head of the *fetus* at an abnormal angle.

ASYNERGY n. discoordination of body parts or organs that normally work together harmoniously; also: **asynergia**.   adj. **asynergic**

ASYSTOLE n. absence of heart beat; failure of the ventricles of the heart to contract; *cardiac arrest*.   adj. **asystolic**.

ATABRINE n. trade name for a drug (quinacrine hydrochloride) used to treat *malaria*.

ATARAX n. trade name for a minor *tranquilizer* (hydroxyzine hydrochloride) used to treat anxiety and motion sickness.

ATARAXIS n. mental calm, esp. when consciousness is unimpaired.   adj. **ataractic, ataraxic**

ATARAXIC DRUG n. a *tranquilizer*; a *sedative* drug that does not produce sleep (see *neuroleptic*).

ATAVISM n. a throwback; development of a characteristic or disease known to have occurred in an earlier ancestor rather than in the parents.   adj. **atavistic**

ATAXIA n. lack of coordination in muscle action manifested as unsteady movements and staggering gait and caused by brain or spinal cord lesion (see *degenerative disorders*).   adj. **ataxic**

ATELECTASIS n. incomplete expansion of all or part of the lung in a newborn or collapse of lung tissue in the adult. Collapse, caused by obstruction of the airways or compression on the lung (e.g., by tumor or enlarged lymph glands), produces increasing difficulty in breathing and fever, and often leads to pneumonia and serious complications.   adj. **atelectatic**.

ATHEROGENESIS n. formation of fatty (*lipid*) deposits (*atheromas*), on the walls of the arteries, as in *atherosclerosis*.

ATHEROMA n. a clump of material, a fatty deposit, from the lining (*intima*) of an artery.

ATHEROSCLEROSIS n. a common disorder of the arteries in which plaques of material (mostly *cholesterol* and lipids) form on the inner arterial walls, making them thick and nonelastic and narrowing the opening of the vessel, thus causing decreased flow of blood to those organs supplied by the artery. Common with aging, a frequent complication of *hypertension*, obesity and diabetes, and associated with some hereditary metabolic disorders, atherosclerosis is an important cause of heart disease. In some cases segments of occluded arteries may be replaced (as in *coronary bypass surgery*). Preventive measures include a low-fat diet, exercise, and avoidance of smoking and stress.   adj. **atherosclerotic**

ATHETOSIS n. a condition characterized by slow, continuous, involuntary position changes of the hands and feet and other parts of the body, as sometimes seen in *cerebral palsy*.

ATHLETE'S FOOT n. a fungal infection (*ringworm*) of the foot, generally starting between the toes, causing itching. Later, *bacteria* may replace the *fungus* and cause the skin between the toes to turn white, crack, and peel off. Treatment is by antifungal preparations.

ATHLETE'S HEART n. the oversized heart commonly found in professional athletes and those trained for endurance; it is believed to result from overexertion for an extended period. The heart's increased pumping capacity delivers more oxygen to the skeletal muscles.

ATLAS n. the first cervical vertebra; the first *vertebra* in the neck, hinging with the skull at the *occipital* bone (compare *axis*).

ATONY n. lack of normal *tone*, usually of a muscle, muscle system, or the bladder; also: **atonia**, **atonicity**.   adj. **atonic**

ATOPOGNOSIA n. inability to locate correctly a pinprick, point of touch, or other sensation; also: **atopognosis**.

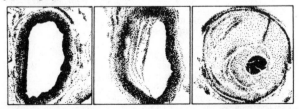

In atherosclerosis fatty deposits form on the walls of an artery, gradually narrowing the opening.

ATLAS

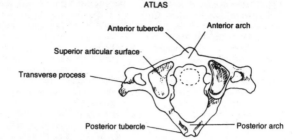

Anterior tubercle · Anterior arch · Superior articular surface · Transverse process · Posterior tubercle · Posterior arch

Courtesy Carolina Biological Supply Co.

ATOPY n. *allergy* to which one has an inherited tendency.

ATOXIC adj. not producing or resulting from poison; also **nontoxic**.

ATP (ADENOSINE TRIPHOSPHATE) n. a compound consisting of adenosine, ribose, and three phosphate groups and involved in the storage and transfer of energy in cells, esp. in muscle.

ATRESIA n. a condition in which a normal opening or tube in the body is closed or absent (e.g., the *urethra*). adj. **atresic, atretic**

ATRIAL adj. pert. to the *atrium* or atria of the heart.

ATRIAL FIBRILLATION n. condition characterized by rapid and random contraction of the atria of the heart, causing irregular beats of the ventricles and resulting in decreased heart output and frequently clot formation in the atria. A type of cardiac arrhythmia, atrial fibrillation occurs in rheumatic heart disease, mitral stenosis, and other heart disorders. Treatment is by drugs (e.g., digitalis) or electroshock to retore normal heart rhythm.

ATRIO- comb. form indicating an association with the *atrium* of the heart (e.g., **atrioventricular**, pert. to an atrium and a ventricle of the heart, considered together).

ATRIOVENTRICULAR BUNDLE see *bundle of His*.

ATRIOVENTRICULAR (AV) NODE n. area of specialized heart muscle, located in the septal wall of the right atrium, that receives impulses from the *sino-atrial node* (pacemaker) and transmits them to the *bundle of His* and thus to the walls of the ventricles, causing them to contract.

ATRIOVENTRICULAR VALVE n. either of two valves in the heart through which blood flows from the atria to the ventricles. The left atrioventricular valve is the *mitral valve*; the right the *tricuspid valve*.

ATRIUM n. 1. either of the two upper chambers of the heart. The right atrium receives deoxygenated blood from the *vena cava* and then passes it into the *right ventricle*, which pumps it to the *lungs*, where it gives off waste products and receives oxygen. The freshly oxygenated blood then passes through the *pulmonary vein* to the *left atrium* and from there to the *left ventricle* and then the rest of the body; 2. the main section of the middle ear; 3. chamber serving as an entrance to another organ (e.g., atrium of the *larynx*). pl. **atria** adj. **atrial**

ATROMID-S n. trade name for the drug *clofibrate*, which reduces lipids in the blood serum and is used to treat some cardiovascular diseases.

ATROPHY n. a decrease in size of a part or organ, resulting from a wasting away of tissue, as may occur, e.g., in disease or from lack of use.   adj. **atrophic**

ATROPINE n. a antispasmodic drug commonly obtained from belladonna and related plants and used to calm gastrointestinal motility, to dilate the pupils of the eye, and to treat certain eye and other disorders.

ATTACHMENT n. the dependence of a person on an object or another human being. Personality problems can result if the relationship is broken, as by separation, before the person is fully mature.

ATTENTION DEFICIT DISORDER n. a syndrome, affecting mostly children and more common among boys, characterized by various learning and behavioral problems, including short attention span, impulsivity, and sometimes *hyperactivity* and impairments in perceptual, language, and motor skills, without any major physical or psychiatric cause. Various treatments (e.g., *Ritalin*, certain amphetamines, restricted diet) have been tried (see also *hyperactivity*, *minimal brain dysfunction*).

ATTENTION SPAN n. length of time that one can concentrate on a given object or activity (compare *autism*). Some disturbed patients have extremely short attention spans, e.g., less than a few minutes.

ATTENUATION n. the process of weakening, esp. of the potency of a drug or other agent or of the virulence of a disease-causing germ.

AUDIO- comb. form indicating an association with sound or hearing (e.g., **audiovisual**, pert. to sound and sight).

AUDIOGRAM n. a record of an individual's hearing sensitivity.

AUDIOMETRY n. measurement of the sense of hearing. Originally it included only measures of pure-tone thresholds but now the hearing of different speech sounds and the processing of sound stimuli in the brain are also measured.

AUDITION n. the act of hearing; the ability to hear (see also *ear*). adj. **auditory**

AUDITORY CANAL n. the tubelike structure that leads from the outside of the ear to the *eardrum*; also called **auditory meatus**.

AUDITORY CENTER n. the part of the brain that receives impulses from the ear by way of the *auditory nerve* for interpretation as hearing. The center is at the side of each brain hemisphere (temporal lobe) in a fold of the *cerebral cortex*.

AUDITORY NERVE n. one of a pair of major sensory nerves, the VIIIth *cranial nerves*, that carry impulses from the inner ear to the brain for interpretation as hearing; also called the **auditory vestibular nerve** or, less commonly, the **acoustic nerve**.

AURA n. a sensation, as light, halos, or warmth, that may signal the start of a *migraine* or an epileptic attack. pl. **aurae** adj. **aural**

AURAL adj. pert. to the ear.

AUREOMYCIN n. a trade name for a yellow-powder *antibiotic* drug (chlor*tetracycline*) used in treating infections caused by certain bacteria or other microorganisms.

AURICLE n. 1. the outer visible part of the ear; also **pinna**. 2. *atrium*, either of the two upper chambers of the heart.   adj. **auricular**, pert. to the ear.

AURUM n. the element *gold* (see Table of Elements), used in some medications (e.g., for arthritis) and, because of its stability and noncorrosiveness, in dentistry.

AUSCULTATION n. the act of listening to body sounds, including those of the lungs, heart, and abdomen, as an aid to diagnosis (see *stethoscope*). adj. **auscultatory**

AUT-, AUTO- comb. form meaning "self" (e.g., **autoagglutination**, clumping of blood cells caused by factors in one's own blood serum).

AUTISM n. abnormal withdrawal into oneself, marked by severe communication problems, short *attention span*, inability to interact socially, and extreme resistance to change. Children with autism are extremely difficult to teach. adj. **autistic**

AUTOCLAVE n. a tanklike device that securely seals itself (hence the name) and can withstand high internal temperatures and pressures, used in sterilizing, with steam, surgical instruments and research materials.

AUTOEROTICISM n. sexual gratification through self-stimulation, without regard for another person; sensual gratification through *masturbation*, fantasy, or visual experience.

AUTOGRAFT n. tissue that is removed from one site and then attached to another site on the same person (e.g., skin from the thigh to replace burned skin on the arm).

AUTOIMMUNE DISEASE n. any of a large group of diseases marked by an abnormality of the functioning of the *immune system* that causes the production of *antibodies* against one's own tissues and other body materials. Autoimmune diseases include *systemic lupus erythematosus*, *rheumatoid arthritis*, and other collagen diseases; and idiopathic thrombocytopenic purpura, autoimmune leukopenia, and other hemolytic disorders.

AUTOIMMUNITY n. production of antibodies against the tissues of one's own body, producing *autoimmune disease* or *hypersensitivity reactions*.

AUTONOMIC adj. regulated or controlled by the mechanisms within oneself, specifically referring to the *autonomic nervous system*, which maintains many of the body's involuntary functions (e.g., breathing, digestion).

AUTONOMIC NERVOUS SYSTEM n. that part of the nervous system that regulates involuntary vital functions, such as the activity of the heart and smooth muscle. It is divided into two parts: the *sympathetic nervous system*, which, when stimulated, constricts blood vessels, raises blood pressure, and increases heart rate; and the *parasympathetic nervous system*, which, when stimulated, increases intestinal and gland activity, slows heart rate and relaxes sphincter muscles.

AUTONOMIC REFLEX n. any of a number of reflexes that control the activity of body parts, as, for example, urination, sweating, heart rate.

AUTOPSY n. examination, using dissection and other methods, of a body after death to determine the cause of death, the extent of injuries, or other factors.

AUTOREGULATION n. the process of maintaining a generally constant physiological state of a cell or organism.

AUTOSOMAL DOMINANT DISEASE n. a disorder (e.g., *Huntington's chorea*) caused by a dominant *mutant* (abnormal) *gene* on an *autosome* (non-sex *chromosome*). Evidence of the disorder may not occur for several decades. The mutant gene is inherited from one or both parents or is the result of a fresh mutation. If both parents have the mutant dominant gene, all offspring will be affected; if one parent is affected, 50% of the off-

AUTONOMIC NERVOUS SYSTEM ----parasympathetic division
— sympathetic division

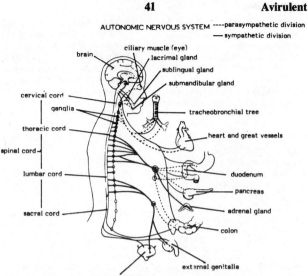

ciliary muscle (eye)
lacrimal gland
sublingual gland
submandibular gland
brain
cervical cord
ganglia
tracheobronchial tree
thoracic cord
heart and great vessels
spinal cord
lumbar cord
duodenum
pancreas
sacral cord
adrenal gland
colon
external genitalia
ureters and bladder

spring will be affected; the normal children of an affected parent do not carry the trait.

AUTOSOMAL RECESSIVE DISEASE n. a disorder caused by the presence of two recessive (homozygous) *mutant* (abnormal) genes on an *autosome*. If only one mutant recessive (heterozygous) gene is present, the person is not affected with the disease but is a carrier of it. One fourth of the children of two heterozygous (carrier) parents will be affected, and another one half will be carriers. All of the children of two homozygous affected persons will be affected. The children of one normal and one affected with the disease will all be carriers. When close relatives (e.g., first cousins) marry, the chance that an offspring will inherit an abnormal recessive gene from both parents is increased, as it is among persons marrying within certain ethnic groups (e.g., *Tay-Sachs disease* among Ashkenazic Jews).

AUTOSOME n. n. a *chromosome* (other than a sex chromosome), usually appearing in pairs in body cells but as single chromosomes in *sperm* or *ovum* (*gametes*, or sex cells).

AVASCULAR n. adj. without blood vessels.

AVERSION n. extreme dislike and desire to move away from the source of antagonism (e.g., wanting to run away from a snake).

AVERSION THERAPY n. a process in which undesirable behavior is treated by accompanying the behavior with a disagreeable experience, such as extreme nausea (the treatment has been used to help persons stop smoking cigarettes or drinking alcohol).

AVERSIVE adj. repelling; noxious, as a stimulus used in avoidance training or aversion therapy.

AVIRULENT adj. unable to produce disease or its effects.

AVITAMINOSIS n. vitamin deficiency.

AVOIDANCE n. a noninvolvement, as a psychological defense to free oneself from fear, anxiety, or other adverse feelings.

AVULSION n. the tearing or forcible separation of one body part from another.

AXILLA n. the armpit. pl. **axillae** adj. **axillary**

AXILLARY NODE n. any of the lymph glands of the armpit that help to fight infection in the neck, chest, and arm area.

AXIS n. 1. the second cervical vertebra; the second bone of the vertebral column, located in the neck region (compare *atlas*); 2. an imaginary line used as a reference for the relationship of parts or actions (e.g., the body axis being the imaginary line from the head to the feet). pl. **axes** adj. **axial**

AXOLEMMA n. the outer membrane cover of an *axon*.

AXON n. the nerve cell process that carries the impulse away from the cell body to the site of action or response, the *effector* (e.g., muscle); some axons are sheathed in *myelin* (compare *dendrite*). adj. **axonal**

AZATHIOPRINE n. an *immunosuppressive* drug (trade name Imuran) used to prevent rejection following organ transplants and in the treatment of certain inflammatory conditions.

AZOTEMIA n. the presence of an abnormally high level of nitrogen-bearing materials (e.g., *urea*) in the blood. adj. **azotemic**

AZOTURIA n. excess of *urea* or other nitrogen-containing compounds in the urine. adj. **azoturic**

AZYGOUS adj. not paired, as some organs (e.g., the heart).

AZYMIA n. absence of an *enzyme*.

b

B: BLOOD TYPE n. one of the four blood groups (the others being A, AB, and O) in the *ABO blood group system* for classifying human blood based on the presence or absence of two *antigens*—A and B—on the surface of *red blood cells*. A person with type B blood produces antibodies against A antigens that cause the blood cells to agglutinate, or clump together. A person with type B blood must receive blood transfusions only from others with type B blood or from those with type O blood (see also *blood typing*).

B CELL n. a lymphocyte (a type of white blood cell) important in the body's *immune system* and response to infection, esp. by bacteria, or to invasion by other foreign substance (*antigen*). B cells develop in the bone marrow and circulate through the body until,

Neuron showing an axon with a myelin sheath.

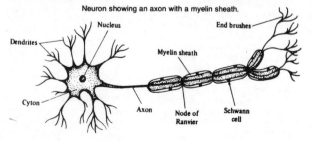

when confronted by an *antigen*, they greatly increase in number and produce *antibodies* specific against that antigen.

B: VITAMINS n. a series of water-soluble vitamins (e.g., *thiamine*, *riboflavin*, *niacin*, *pyridoxine*, *folic acid*, *cobalamin*) essential for normal metabolism and first believed to be a single vitamin (see *vitamin*; Table of Vitamins).

BABESIOSIS n. an infection caused by a protozoan (*Babesia*), transmitted by the bite of certain ticks; it is characterized by headache, fever, muscle pain, and nausea; also **babesiasis**.

BABINSKI REFLEX n. an extension or moving of the big toe upward or toward the head with the other toes fanned out and extended when the sole of that foot is stroked from below the heel toward the toes on its lateral side (outside). The *reflex* is normal in infants, but in others usually indicates brain or spinal cord disease; also: **Babinski sign**.

BABY n. an infant; a child not yet able to walk.

BACILLARY adj. 1. pert. to or caused by a *bacillus*; 2. rod-shaped, like a bacillus; also: **bacillar, bacilliform**.

BACILLI n. pl. of *bacillus*.

BACILLEMIA n. the presence of bacilli in the blood.

BACILLURIA n. the presence of bacilli in the *urine*, usually due to bladder or kidney infection.

BACILLUS n. a common rod-shaped bacterium (genus *Bacillus*) that normally lives in soil, water, and organic materials and helps in the process of decay. Only a few species (e.g., *Bacillus anthracis*, the cause of anthrax) cause human disease. pl. **bacilli**

BACITRACIN n. an antibiotic used to treat many bacterial infections, esp. those involving the skin.

BACK n. the posterior part of the body trunk from the nape of the neck to the buttocks.

BACKACHE n. pain in the back. Backache is a common complaint; it may be caused by muscle strain or other muscle injury or disorder, by pressure on a nerve, resulting from vertebral disk injury or other injury, or as a symptom of many other disorders. Treatment depends on the cause; it may include bed rest, heat, and the use of drugs to relieve pain and muscle spasms.

BACKBONE see *vertebral column*.

BACTEREMIA n. the presence of bacteria in the blood.

BACTERIA n. pl. of *bacterium*.

BACTERIAL adj. pert. to or caused by bacteria, as in bacterial endocarditis.

BACTERIAL RESISTANCE n. the development of resistance to a drug (e.g., penicillin) by bacteria previously susceptible to its destructive effects.

BACTERICIDE n. a drug or other chemical that kills bacteria (compare *bacteriostasis*). adj. **bactericidal**

BACTERIOGENIC adj. caused by, or producing, *bacteria*.

BACTERIOLOGY n. the science and study of *bacteria*, their development, and their effects on human tissue; today generally included in *microbiology*. adj. **bacteriologic, bacteriological**

BACTERIOLYSIN n. an antibody, produced against *bacteria*, that causes the microorganisms to break down (*lyse*).

BACTERIOLYSIS n. the breakdown of microorganisms, specifically *bacteria*. adj. **bacteriolytic**

BACTERIOPHAGE n. a *virus*, sometimes called a bacterial virus but more generally simply *phage*, that causes bacteria to break down (*lyse*).

BACTERIOSTASIS n. a condition in which the growth and multiplication of bacteria are inhibited but the bacteria are not killed, by the use of biological or chemical agents (compare *bactericide*). adj. **bacteriostatic**

BACTERIOTOXIC adj. 1. having the effect of poison (*toxin*) on bacteria; 2. caused by poisons produced by bacteria.

BACTERIUM n. any of a large group of small, unicellular microorganisms (class Schizomycetes) found in the soil, water, and air, some of which cause disease in humans and other animals. Bacteria are generally classified as rod-shaped (*bacillus*), spherical (*coccus*), comma-shaped (*vibrio*), or spiral (*spirochete*). pl. **bacteria** adj. **bacterial**

Types of bacteria

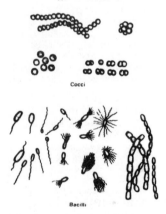

Cocci

Bacilli

Spirilla

BAG n. a pocketlike container for fluids or other substances, esp. a plastic or rubber container attached to the body to receive the contents (*urine* or *feces*) emitted from an artificial opening created in an *ileostomy* or other operation.

BAG OF WATERS n. the sac of *amniotic fluid* surrounding the *fetus* during pregnancy.

BAGASSOSIS n. a lung disease caused by inhaling bagasse (sugarcane dust) and marked by fever, malaise, and difficulty in breathing; also: **bagasscosis**.

BALANCE n. 1. a coordinated, harmonious working of parts or systems (see *acid-base balance*); 2. an instrument for weighing.

BALANCED DIET n. a diet containing adequate amounts of all essential nutrients (vitamins and minerals, proteins, fats, and carbohydrates) needed for growth and the maintenance of normal health and energy levels.

BALANITIS n. inflammation of the head (*glans*) of the *penis*, usually accompanied by a discharge and tightening of the *foreskin*.

BALANOPOSTHITIS n. inflammation of the head (*glans*) of the *penis* and of the foreskin (*prepuce*), often the result of bacterial or fungal (frequently *venereal*) infection; it is characterized by soreness and discharge.

BALDNESS n. loss or absence of hair, commonly of the scalp; *alopecia*. In **male-patterned baldness** the hairline recedes at the forehead and hair is lost at the back and top of the head.

BALL-AND-SOCKET JOINT n. a *joint* in which the globular head of an articulating bone fits into a cuplike cavity of another to allow the distal bone to rotate, as in the shoulder joint and hip joint.

BALLOTTEMENT n. checking for the correctness of position or the size of a floating part or organ or a fetus by gently flicking or bouncing it with the hand or finger(s) and feeling its response (e.g., an unborn child felt through the birth canal or the abdominal wall).

BALNEOTHERAPY n. the use of baths to treat disease, esp. to relieve pain and improve circulation.

BANK n. in medicine, the storage of human materials for later use, usually by other persons (e.g., *blood bank*, *eye bank*, *sperm bank*).

BANTI'S SYNDROME n. a progressive disorder characterized by enlargement of the spleen, anemia, gastrointestinal bleeding, and other symptoms and often occurring as a complication of alcoholic cirrhosis of the liver; also called **Banti's disease**.

BARAGNOSIS n. inability to determine weight differences.

BARBER'S ITCH n. inflammation of the hair follicles of the face, caused by bacterial or fungal infection.

BARBITURATE n. a drug (e.g., phenobarbital) that depresses brain and spinal cord activity and was once widely used to treat *convulsions* and produce *sedation*. Barbiturates are potentially habit-forming and have largely been replaced by safer drugs.

BARBITURISM n. a poisoning resulting from the use of barbiturates, marked by slurred speech, sleepiness, loss of memory, disorientation, and, in serious cases, depressed respiration, coma, and death.

BARIATRICS n. the study of body weight, esp. the causes and treatment of *obesity*; the medical specialty for treatment of overweight.

BARIUM n. a chemical element, compounds of which have several uses in medicine, esp. barium sulfate, which when swallowed (barium meal) or given in an *enema*, presents a contrast on X-ray film (see Table of Elements).

BARORECEPTOR n. a nerve ending that senses changes in pressure.

BARREL CHEST n. a large, rounded chest that is normal in some stocky persons and in some persons living in high-altitude areas where the oxygen content of the air is low, but is abnormal in others, often a sign of *emphysema*.

BARREN adj. unable to produce young; *sterile*.

BARRIER n. an object or structure that blocks an action or flow or separates parts from one another.

BARTHOLIN'S GLAND n. either of two small, mucus-secreting glands located on the posterior and lateral parts of the vestibule of the *vagina*.

BARTHOLINITIS n. inflammation of one or both *Bartholin's glands*, usually caused by bacteria, and characterized by swelling, pain, and abscess formation.

BASAL adj. pert. to the fundamental, basic, or lowest, as in **basal anesthesia**, the first stage of unconsciousness.

BASAL BODY TEMPERATURE n. temperature of the body taken in the morning before rising or moving about or eating or drinking anything; changes in the basal body temperature are used in the basal body temperature method of family planning to determine the fertile time in a woman's *menstrual cycle*.

BASAL BODY TEMPERATURE METHOD OF FAMILY PLANNING n. a method of family planning based on the identification of the fertile period (the time when *conception* is most likely to occur) in a woman's *menstrual cycle* obtained by not-

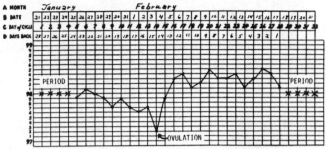

A basal temperature chart can be used for family planning.

ing the rise in basal body temperature that typically occurs with *ovulation*. The fertile period is calculated to start six days before ovulation is expected (from the data of previous cycles) and to continue until the temperature is elevated for five days (compare *calendar method of family planning*) (see also *contraception*).

BASAL GANGLIA n. masses of *gray matter* lying in the brain's *cerebral cortex* and involved in the control of body movements.

BASAL METABOLISM n. the basic rate of energy flow needed to maintain the body.

BASAL METABOLISM TEST n. the measurement of oxygen intake by a person about 14 hours after eating as an indication of the amount of energy required to maintain vital body functions (e.g., circulation, respiration, digestion). Breathing into a tube that leads to a measuring apparatus, the person remains at rest (but does not sleep) during the test. For each interval of time, the more oxygen consumed, the more oxidation is occurring and the higher is the basal metabolic rate (BMR). The test has largely been replaced by newer techniques.

BASE n. 1. the bottom or supporting structure; 2. the main part of a chemical compound; 3. a sub-stance that has a hydroxyl (OH) ion, tastes bitter, turns litmus paper blue, and, when combined with an acid, forms a salt. adj. **basic, basilar**

BASHFULNESS n. a chronic behavior response of self-consciousness, timidity, and avoidance of personal attention in public; a withdrawing, self-conscious temperament.

BASI-, BASIO-, BASO- comb. forms indicating an association with a chemical *base* (e.g., **basophilic**, easily stained with dyes that are chemical *bases*) or with a structural *base* (**basicranial**, pert. to the base of the skull).

BASILAR MEMBRANE n. cellular structure in the ear that forms a floor of the *cochlear duct* and provides a base for the *organ of Corti*, the main organ of hearing.

BASOPHIL n. a type of *white blood cell*, with coarse granules that stain blue when exposed to a basic dye. Basophils normally constitute 1% or less of the total white blood cell count but may increase or decrease in certain diseases.

BATHO-, BATHY- comb. form indicating an association with depth (e.g., **bathypnea**, deep breathing).

BATHYCARDIA n. unusually low placement of the heart, not caused by disease.

BATHYESTHESIA n. sensation in the deeper parts of the body (e.g., the muscles and joints), as opposed to the skin.

BATTERED CHILD n. an infant, child, or adolescent who has been seriously injured, generally many times, by one or more adults, frequently the parent(s), whose mistreatment of the victim shows a pattern of abnormal, abusive behavior (see *child abuse*).

BATTERED WOMAN n. a woman who is the victim of repeated episodes of physical violence, usually accompanied by verbal abuse and often leading to serious physical and psychological damage, inflicted by the man with whom she lives.

BCG VACCINE n. an immunizing agent, prepared from Calmette-Guérin bacillus, against tuberculosis.

BEARING DOWN n. the sensation and effort by a pregnant woman to expel the baby; it is characteristic of the second stage of *labor*.

BEAT n. a single *pulse* or throb, esp. of the heart; the apical (*apex*) beat is heard over the left side of the chest, between the fourth and fifth ribs.

BED n. 1. in anatomy, a general term for a structure or tissue that provides support, as a *nail* bed, the skin over which a nail extends as the fingernail or toenail grows; 2. a hydrostatic bed, of rubber, filled with water and used to avert bedsores (*decubitus ulcers*).

BEDBUG n. an arthropod (*Cimex lectularius*) that feeds on humans and other animals, sucking blood and causing redness, pain, and itching at the site of the bite. Bedbugs can be removed when covered with a jellylike preparation and the bite site treated with topical anti-inflammatory and *analgesic* preparations.

BEDRIDDEN n. unable to leave the bed; not *ambulatory*.

BEDSORE see *decubitus ulcer*.

BEDWETTING see *enuresis*.

BEE STING n. injury caused by the venom of a bee, marked by pain and swelling at the site of the bite and often by the presence of a bee stinger, which should be removed. Ice or cold applications relieve pain. Multiple stings or stings to certain parts of the body can cause serious reactions. A single sting can cause *anaphylactic shock* and even death in a person hypersensitive to bee venom; such persons should carry emergency medical supplies if they expect to be exposed to the possibility of bee stings.

BEHAVIOR MODIFICATION n. a technique for changing undesirable behavior into acceptable behavior, generally by rewarding (see *reinforcement*) appropriate responses and ignoring or punishing inappropriate behavior (compare *biofeedback*).

BEHAVIORISM n. a branch of psychology concerned with objective observations of behavior, as evidence of such processes as intent and *drive*, without influence from personally biased (*subjective*) statements.

BEJEL n. a chronic, non-venereal form of *syphilis*, caused by the spirochete *Treponema pallidum*, widespread in the Middle East and northern Africa, most commonly among children and their family members. Lesions in the mouth region spread to other areas of the body. Treatment is by penicillin.

BELCHING see *eructation*.

BELLADONNA n. a plant (*Atopa belladonna*) from which certain medicines (alkaloids, e.g., *atropine*) are derived.

BELL'S PALSY n. a feature-distorting paralysis of one side (or infrequently both sides) of the face, often affecting the eye or mouth, and resulting from injury, disease of the facial nerve, or an unknown cause. If permanent deformity occurs, cosmetic surgery may be helpful.

BELLY n. 1. a common term for the *abdomen*; 2. a general term for the full and rounded part of a structure, as of a voluntary muscle (e.g., the *biceps*).

BENADRYL n. trade name for an antihistamine (diphenhydramine hydrochloride) used to treat hypersensitivity reactions and sometimes to produce sedation.

BENDS n. a painful, sometimes fatal condition in which, because of a rapid drop in outside pressure, nitrogen bubbles form in the body and cause pain, disorientation, and faintness, as when a diver ascends too quickly. Treatment is by return to a higher pressure environment and gradual decompression in a special chamber; also called **caisson disease, decompression sickness**.

BENEDICT'S SOLUTION n. copper sulfate dissolved in water containing sodium citrate and sodium carbonate; it is used to test for sugar (*glucose*) in the urine.

BENEDICT'S TEST n. a test for sugar in the urine. After adding 8 drops of urine to 5 milliliters of Benedict's solution, the liquid is boiled for 2 minutes and then cooled. Sugar (*glucose*) is present if the residue is red, yellow, or green, and indicates that the person may have *diabetes mellitus*. Red represents a greater amount of sugar than yellow; yellow, a greater amount of sugar than green.

BENIGN adj. mild, noncancerous, and/or not spreading (compare *malignant*), as of a disease or growth, esp. a benign tumor.

BENZEDRINE n. a trade name for *amphetamine*, a central nervous system stimulant.

BENZOCAINE n. a local anesthetic agent found in many over-the-counter preparations for pain and itching.

BENZODIAZEPINE n. a chemical from which several mind-affecting (psychoactive) drugs are prepared; included are the tranquilizers diazepam (Valium) and chlordiazepoxide (Librium) and the sedative-hypnotic flurazepam (Dalmane). Tolerance and dependence can occur with prolonged use of benzodiazepines.

BERIBERI n. a disease, resulting from a deficiency of vitamin B_1 (*thiamine*), characterized by appetite and weight loss, disturbed nerve function, fluid retention, and heart failure. The disease is common in parts of Asia, particularly in areas where the diet is limited to highly milled rice, but is rare in the United States.

BERYLLIOSIS n. poisoning, resulting from the inhalation of *beryllium*, marked by cough, chest pain, shortness of breath, and damage to lung tissue.

BERYLLIUM n. a metallic element (see Table of Elements).

BESTIALITY n. sexual involvement of a human with an animal.

BETA BLOCKER n. any of a group of drugs (e.g., propranolol) widely used in the treatment of some forms of *hypertension* and *heart disease*. The drugs decrease the rate and force of heart contraction and help to lower blood pressure by blocking the beta-adrenergic receptors of the *autonomic nervous system*.

BETA CELLS n. *insulin*-producing cells found in the islands of Langerhans of the *pancreas*.

BETA RHYTHM n. a brain-wave frequency of low voltage, the "busy waves" of the brain, characteristic of a person who is awake and alert. It is one of four brain-wave patterns (compare *alpha rhythm, delta rhythm, theta rhythm*); also called **beta wave**.

BI- a prefix meaning "two," "twice," "using both" (e.g., **bicapsular**, pert. to two capsules).

BICEPS n. a muscle having two heads, esp. the one at the front of the upper part of the arm, which flexes the arm and draws the hand toward the shoulder.

BISCUSPID n. a tooth (or other part) having two blunt points on its top. Such teeth are located between the *canines* and the *molars*.

BICUSPID VALVE see *mitral valve*.

B.I.D. in prescriptions, an abbreviation meaning "twice a day".

BIFOCAL GLASSES n. lenses that include curvatures of two focal lengths, to improve both near vision and distant vision (compare *trifocal glasses*).

BILATERAL adj. having or occurring on two sides, as in bilateral hearing loss; having two layers.

BILE n. a thick, yellow-green-brown fluid made by the *liver*, stored in the *gallbladder*, and discharged into the upper part of the digestive tract (*duodenum*), where it breaks down fats, preparing them for further digestion; also called **gall**.

BILHARZIASIS see *schistosomiasis*.

BILIARY adj. pert. to *bile* or the *gall bladder* and its ducts.

BILIARY TRACT n. the *gall bladder* and its ducts, which transport *bile*; also: **biliary system**.

BILIOUS adj. 1. pert. to *bile*; 2. having the feeling of general irritability, loss of appetite, indigestion, constipation, and vomiting that can result from a liver disorder.

BILIRUBIN n. an orange-yellow pigment in *bile*. The abnormal accumulation of bilirubin in the blood and skin causes *jaundice*, and testing for bilirubin levels in the blood helps in the diagnosis of several diseases.

BINOCULAR adj. pert. to both eyes; using both eyes; made for use by both eyes (e.g., a binocular microscope).

BIO- comb. form indicating an association with life (e.g., **biometrics**,the application of statistical methods to data on living organisms).

BIOASSAY n. a test, usually involving living organisms, of the effect or potency of a drug.

BIOCHEMISTRY n. the study of chemical processes in living organisms.

BIODEGRADABLE adj. able to be broken down by living organisms, esp. with reference to the action of microorganisms on organic wastes and refuse.

BIOENGINEERING n. a branch of *biology* dealing 1. with the processing or artificial production of plant and animal materials, esp. in the fermentation of organic products; 2. the application of engineering principles to medical problems (e.g., manufacture of artificial limbs and other organs).

BIOFEEDBACK n. a technique, apparently learnable, that enables a person to manipulate ordinarily involuntary processes, such as heartbeat and blood pressure, through concentration and knowledge (feedback) of bodily effects or responses as they occur and are monitored by special machines that provide visual and or auditory data.

BIOFLAVONOID n. any of a group of chemicals (flavonoids) found in many plants and essential for the health of *capillary* walls and the metabolism of *ascorbic acid*; rich sources include cherries, grapes, lemons, plums, and many other fruits; also called **vitamin P**.

BIOHAZARD n. something that endangers life or living things (e.g., a radiation overdose, an oil spill, insecticide overuse).

BIOLOGICAL n. medicinal preparation made from living organisms and their products, as *serums*, *vaccines*, *antitoxins*.

BIOLOGICAL CLOCK see *circadian rhythm*.

BIOLOGY n. the science of life and living things, including the study of microorganisms (*microbiology*), plants (botany) and animals (zoology). adj. **biological**, **biologic**

BIOMEDICAL adj. pert. to the activities and applications of the basic sciences (e.g., *biochemistry*, *anatomy*) to the diagnosis and treatment of patients (clinical medicine).

BIONICS n. the study of the applicability of machines and devices to resolving medical problems, as in the replacement of natural parts (e.g., the bionic arm).

BIOPHYSICS n. the science that applies physics to biological problems (e.g., applying the laws of hydraulics to development of an artificial heart).

BIOPSY n. the removal of a small amount of tissue and/or fluid from a living body and its examination by microscopic and/or other analytical methods to establish or confirm the presence of a disease, to follow its course, and/or to estimate its outcome. The specimen is usually obtained by suction through a needle, but other methods and instruments, including surgery, are also used.

BIORHYTHM n. a supposed regular pattern of changes in a person's energy level, responsiveness, and attitude, as determined by genetic, physiologic, or other internal individual factors, or by external factors such as atmospheric pressure, ion content of the air, or amount of stress accumulated (see also *circadian rhythm*).

BIOTIN n. a B-complex vitamin (see Table of Vitamins) that aids in body growth and helps fix carbon dioxide in microorganisms and humans; found in liver, egg yolk, and yeast (formerly called **vitamin H**).

BIPOLAR DISORDER n. a mental disorder characterized by episodes of *mania* and *depression*. One or the other phase may be dominant at a given time; the phases may alternate; or aspects of both phases may be present at the same time. Treatment is by psychotherapy and the use of antidepressants and tranquilizers; also called **manic-depressive disease**.

BIRTH n. the act of being born; the emergence of the *fetus* from the *uterus*, its separation from the mother, and the start of its independent life (usually after about 266 days of *gestation*); also **parturition**.

BIRTH CANAL n. the passage (uterus and vagina) through which an infant passes during vaginal birth.

BIRTH CONTROL see *contraception*.

BIRTH CONTROL PILL see *oral contraceptive*.

BIRTH DEFECT n. an abnormality that is present at birth. It may be the result of a genetic abnormality or of an abnormality during pregnancy or the birth process. A *cleft palate*, resulting from incomplete development and union of the parts forming the palate is an example of a birth defect; also: **congenital defect**.

BIRTH INJURY n. harm to an infant's body or to his/her ability to function as a result of instruments used or actions taken during the birth process.

BIRTHMARK n. a discoloration or other blemish present at birth (see also *nevus*).

BIRTH ORDER n. the sequence of births among siblings; one's position in the sequence is believed by some psychologists to affect learning ability, intelligence, and the development of personality.

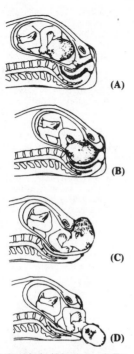

Major stages in the birth process. (A) The fetus is low in the uterus as labor contractions begin. (B) The cervix widens as the baby's head moves through the vagina, now called the birth canal. (C) The crown of the head becomes visible in the vaginal opening. (D) The baby's body turns and one shoulder emerges, after which the remainder of the body is born rapidly. (From *Human Sexuality*, third ed. by James Leslie McCary, copyright 1978 by Litton Educational Publishing, Inc. Reprinted by permission of D. Van Nostrand Company.)

BIRTH RATE n. the number of live babies born during a given period for a stipulated population (e.g., the 1981 birth rate for the United States was 15.9 per 1,000 population).

BIRTH WEIGHT n. the weight of a baby at birth; in the United States average birth weight is about 7.5 lbs (3,500 grams). Babies weighing less than 5.5 lbs (2,500 grams) at term are considered small-for-gestational age;

those over 10 lbs (4,500 grams) large-for-gestational age.

BIRTHING CHAIR n. a chair specially designed to aid and provide comfort for a woman during *labor* and *childbirth*, It may be a stool with a straight back and hole in the center of the seat or a specially contoured chair. The woman's upright position is thought by many to allow gravity to help shorten labor and aid in the expulsion of the baby. The chair cannot be used if the woman is anesthesized. (See also *natural childbirth*).

BIRTHING ROOM n. a room, usually in a hospital or other health facility, set aside for childbirth. The room is usually designed to be warm, friendly, and familial and not cold as a hospital delivery or operating room often is. (See also *natural childbirth*).

BISECT v. to divide into two parts or to separate one part from another.

BISEXUAL adj. having both male and female *gonads* (see *hermaphrodite*); having the drives and characteristics of both sexes. n. **bisexuality**

BISMUTH n. a metallic element, the salts of which are sometimes used in drugs (see Table of Elements).

BITE n. 1. the wound or puncture resulting from a bite, as from an insect or other animal; 2. the position of the jaws and teeth when biting, referred to as *occlusion*; in a closed bite, the lower jaw protrudes, and in an open bite, some opposing teeth do not touch (compare *malocclusion*).

BLACK DEATH n. bubonic plague, esp. the 14th century epidemic that killed many people.

BLACK EYE n. a bluish discoloration around the eye resulting from damage to the tissues and clotting of blood under the skin; a bruise about the eye socket (see also *hematoma*).

BLACKHEAD n. the common name for a *comedo*.

BLACK LUNG DISEASE n. abnormal condition marked by increasing loss of lung function (*pneumoconiosis*), resulting from continuous inhalation of coal dust or other substances; it is prevalent among coal miners. Evidence shows that smoking tobacco may seriously aggravate the condition; also called **coal miner's lung**.

BLACKOUT n. 1. temporary loss of consciousness, sometimes preceded by *tunnel vision* and then full loss of vision, as when the body is under excessive gravitational pull (or force) during flying; 2. lapse of memory of occurrences and the passage of time during a period of heavy alcohol consumption, sometimes occurring after bouts of heavy drinking.

BLADDER n. 1. the **urinary bladder**, a muscular and membranous sac that stores *urine*. Urine produced in the kidneys passes through the *ureters* into the bladder; sphincters control the release of urine from the bladder through the *urethra* and out of the body; 2. any saclike, fibrous and membranous organ that holds liquids secreted into it for later passage to another part of the body or out of the body, as in the *gallbladder*, which stores bile.

BLAND DIET n. a diet that is chemically and mechanically nonirritating, often prescribed in cases of *peptic ulcer*, *colitis*, and other intestinal disorders and after abdominal surgery. Spicy and highly seasoned foods, raw fruits and vegetables, and carbonated beverages are usually avoided.

-BLAST suffix indicating a development (embryonic) stage that precedes the mature cell (e.g., **erythroblast**, stage before the mature *erythrocyte*).

BLASTO- prefix indicating an association with early embryonic development (e.g., **blastomere**, one of the two cells resulting from the cleavage of a fertilized *ovum*).

BLASTOCELE n. the liquid-filled cavity of the early ball-shaped embryo (*blastula*). By increasing the embryo's surface area, the blastocele assists in the absorption of oxygen and nutrients; also **blastocoele, blastocoel**.

BLASTOCYST n. an embryonic stage, following the *morula* stage in human development, characterized by a spherical ball of cells with a central fluid-filled cavity (*blastocele*) and during which time, usually about the eighth day after *fertilization*, implantation in the wall of the *uterus* occurs.

BLASTULA n. the ball-like, one cell-layer thick stage of development of an embryo.

Blastula

BLASTOMYCOSIS n. an infection, caused by the fungus of *Blastomyces dermatitidis*, that produces lesions on the skin, especially in exposed areas, or the lungs and other internal organs. Treatment is by antifungal agents.

BLEB n. a blisterlike collection of fluid under the skin, varying from bean to egg-sized.

BLEEDER n. 1. a common term for a person who has a tendency to bleed (e.g., a *hemophiliac*) because the ability of the blood to clot is deficient or absent; 2. a bleeding blood vessel, as during surgery.

BLENN-, BLENNO- comb. form indicating an association with *mucus* (e.g., **blennadenitis**, mucous gland inflammation).

BLENOXANE n. trade name for an *antineoplastic* (bleomycin sulfate) drug used in the chemotherapeutic treatment of some cancers.

BLENNORRHAGIA n. excessive discharge of mucus.

BLENNURIA n. presence of mucus in the urine.

BLEPHAR-, BLEPHARO- comb. form indicating an association with an eyelid (e.g., **blepharoplegia**, paralysis of the eyelid).

BLEPHARITIS n. inflammation of the eyelids, characterized by redness, swelling, and dried crusts of mucus and caused by infection, allergic reaction, or other factors.

BLEPHAROSPASM n. eyelid muscle spasm, resulting in near closure of the eye, usually due to pain in the eye.

BLEPHARISM n. a condition in which the person blinks continuously (compare *tic*).

BLEPHAROPTOSIS n. drooping of the upper eyelid due to paralysis.

BLINDNESS n. 1. inability to see; 2. inability to perceive correctly information received by the eyes.

BLIND SPOT n. a normal gap in the visual field, the result of a spot on the *retina* insensitive to light and located where the *optic nerve* enters the eye.

BLISTER n. a *vesicle* filled with *serum*; a collection of fluid below the skin, usually resulting from a burn.

BLOAT n. swelling or filling with gas, as in abdominal distension.

BLOCK n. 1. anything that stops, interrupts, or obstructs a flow, as of a nerve impulse, conscious ability, or blood passage (see *bundle-branch block*; *mental*

block); 2. *anesthesia* of a particular region of the body (see *caudal block*; *saddle block*).

BLOOD n. a fluid tissue that is pumped by the heart through arteries, capillaries and veins carrying oxygen and nutrients to body cells and carbon dioxide and other waste products away from body cells. Human blood is composed of a pale yellow fluid called *plasma* in which are suspended *red blood cells*, *white blood cells*, *platelets*, and a variety of chemicals, including hormones, proteins, carbohydrates, and fats. Adult males have about 70 ml/kg of body weight, women about 65 ml/kg.

BLOOD BANK n. a unit or department, usually associated with a hospital or laboratory, that collects, processes and stores blood for use in *blood transfusions* and other purposes.

BLOOD-BRAIN BARRIER n. a barrier that exists between circulating blood and brain tissue, due presumably to a property of the blood vessels or covering tissues of the brain, whereby large molecules in the blood (e.g., a virus) are prevented from entering the brain and its surrounding fluid. The barrier serves to protect the *central nervous system*.

BLOOD CELL n. any of two types of cells—*red blood cells* (erythrocytes) and *white blood cells* (leukocytes)—found in human blood. *Platelets*, though not true cells, are also sometimes included; also: *blood corpuscles*.

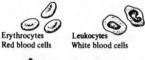

Erythrocytes
Red blood cells

Leukocytes
White blood cells

Platelets

The two major types of blood cells: erythrocytes and leukocytes. Platelets, necessary for blood coagulation, are sometimes considered blood cells.

BLOOD CLOT n. a gelatinous mass made up of *red blood cells* (erythrocytes, *white blood cells* (leukocytes) and *platelets* in a meshwork of the protein *fibrin*; it results from the process of *blood coagulation*.

BLOOD CLOTTING see *blood coagulation*.

BLOOD COAGULATION n. the process by which liquid blood is changed into a semi-solid mass, a *blood clot*. It can occur in an intact *blood vessel*, but usually starts with an injury and the exposure of blood. Platelets clump at the wound site and chemical changes in the blood lead to the formation of a fibrin meshwork and the trapping of *blood cells* into a clot; also: **blood clotting**.

BLOOD COUNT n. the enumeration of *red blood cells* (erythrocytes), *white blood cells* (leukocytes) and sometimes *platelets* found in an accurately diluted one cubic millimeter-sample of blood. Erythrocytes normally number 4.5 million (women) to 5 million (men), leukocytes 5,000 to 10,000, and platelets 150,000 to 450,000. Changes from the normal numbers usually indicate disease and are used as an aid to diagnosis (see also *differential blood count*).

BLOOD CORPUSCLE n. see *blood cell*.

BLOOD CROSSMATCHING n. the mixing of the *red blood cells* of a donor with the blood serum of a potential recipient to determine whether the blood is compatible and can be used for transfusion.

BLOOD DONOR n. one who gives blood for transfusion purposes. Persons with type O blood are considered universal donors because their blood can be given to those not only with type O blood but also to those with type A, AB, or B blood.

BLOOD GASES n. the gases, including oxygen, nitrogen, and carbon dioxide, dissolved in the blood. Changes from the normal levels of these gases usually indicate disease (e.g., *emphysema*, *polycythemia*) and determination of blood gas levels is an important aid to the diagnosis of some diseases.

BLOOD GROUP n. the classification of blood, based on the presence or absence of certain antigens on the surface of red blood cells, used to determine compatibility for transfusions. There are many systems for classifying blood; the most commonly used is the *ABO blood group system*.

BLOOD-LETTING n. the process of removing blood from the body. An ancient practice, generally discarded for centuries, it has recently stirred renewed interest, esp. in the form of *plasmapheresis*, the removal of the fluid *plasma* from the blood.

BLOOD PLASMA see *plasma*.

BLOOD PLATELET see *platelet*.

BLOOD POISONING see *septicemia*.

BLOOD PRESSURE n. the force of blood on the walls of the arteries resulting from the squeezing effect of the heart's left ventricle (*systole*), with residual maintenance (*diastole*) as the heart chambers relax and expand. Abbreviated **BP**, blood pressure is usually measured, using a sphygmomanometer placed at the brachial artery in the arm, as the force needed to raise a column of mercury and expressed in millimeters (mm) of mercury (Hg) as a fraction, the upper number representing the systolic pressure, the lower number the diastolic pressure. Blood presure varies with age, sex, condition of the arteries, force of the heart muscle contraction, emotional state and general health of the arteries and heart. Adult blood pressure is usually considered normal at about 120/80 mm Hg; in children it is lower. High blood pressure is termed *hypertension*, low blood pressure *hypotension*.

BLOOD SERUM see *serum*.

BLOOD SUBSTITUTE n. a substance (e.g., *plasma*, packed blood cells) used to replace or expand the volume of blood (see also *artificial blood*).

BLOOD SUGAR see *glucose*.

BLOOD TEST n. 1. any of several techniques used to determine if the cellular makeup (e.g., *blood count*), chemical levels (e.g., amount of glucose), or other factors (e.g., capillary blood coagulation time) are within normal limits or to ascertain if disease-producing organisms or their products, alcohol, drugs, or poisons are present. 2. Informally, a test for *syphilis* (*Wasserman test*) required in many states before a marriage license can be obtained.

BLOOD TRANSFUSION n. the administration of whole blood or its components to replace blood lost through surgery, disease, or injury. *Blood typing* is the first step to ensure that donor and recipient's blood match in the transfusion of whole blood.

BLOOD TYPING n. a technique for determining a person's blood type or group. In typing for the commonly used *ABO blood group system*, blood cells are matched with serum known to be type A or type B; and whether or not *agglutination* (clumping) of the cells occurs determines the type.

BLOOD UREA NITROGEN (BUN) n. the amount of nitrogenous material present in the blood as urea; it is an indicator of kidney function. Higher-than-normal levels occur in kidney failure, shock, gastrointestinal bleeding, *diabetes mellitus*, and some other disorders; lower-than-normal values are found in malnutrition and liver disease and are normal during pregnancy.

BLOOD VESSEL n. any of the network of tubes that transport blood throughout the body, including arteries, veins, arterioles, and venules.

BLOODY SHOW n. vaginal bleeding, often an early sign of *labor*.

BLUE BABY n. an infant born with a *heart defect* that limits blood flow to the lungs, causes *arterial blood* to mix with *venous blood*, and causes the skin to be bluish because of limited oxygen in the blood. Some of the heart defects can be corrected by surgery, usually performed in the first weeks or months of life.

BLUSH n. a reddening of the face resulting from expansion and filling of the facial blood vessels, occurring in times of embarrassment, extreme self-consciousness, or heat exposure.

BOARD n. in medical specialties, a certifying body (e.g., the National Board of Medical Examiners, whose examinations must be passed for licensure in certain states, or the American Board of Neurosurgery, whose examinations lead to certification in that specialty).

BODY n. 1. the torso of an animal; the trunk; 2. a *cadaver*; 3. a specialized part within a larger structure (e.g., the polar bodies at the ends of certain microorganisms).

BODY IMAGE n. one's concept of his/her own body, which may be realistic or unrealistic in terms of the way one is seen by others.

BODY LANGUAGE n. the conveying of meaning, intent, or motive—directly (e.g., making a fist) or subtly (e.g., changing stance or position)—with the body, distinct from verbal communication.

BODY TEMPERATURE n. the level of heat produced and sustained by body processes. In adults, oral (taken by mouth) temperatures range from 96.5° to 99°F, with 98.6°F generally being regarded as normal; axillary (armpit) temperatures are typically lower, rectal temperatures higher. Body temperature normally varies during the day, depending on the level of activity, ambient temperature, and other factors; the normal range is greater for children than for adults. Marked changes in body temperature (e.g., *fever*) are generally indicative of disease.

BOIL n. an inflammation of the skin and underlying tissue in which pus forms, usually at the site where a hair projects from the skin (see also *furuncle*; *sebaceous cyst*).

BONDING n. the attachment that occurs between infants and their parents, esp. the mother, considered significant for the child's psychological development and the child-parent relationship. With natural childbirth, the mother not anesthetized and the father often present, opportunities for bonding activities (e.g., eye-to-eye contact, fondling) immediately after birth, when the infant is in an alert and reactive state, are increased.

BOLUS n. a chewed mass of food in the mouth ready to be swallowed.

BONE n. 1. the hard, dense specialized form of *connective tissue* that forms most of the *skeleton*. In addition to providing shape and structure to the body, bone stores mineral salts and aids in the formation of blood cells. Under an outer *periosteum* layer, *compact bone*, a hard mass made up of layers of bone cell (*osteocyte*) tissue in concentric layers (*Haversian system*), forms the outer shell of most bones, surrounding inner *spongy bone* with its net-

work of bony bars, bone marrow, blood vessels, and nerves. Bones are classified as long (e.g., femur), short (e.g., those in the wrist), flat (e.g., skull bones), or irregular (e.g., spinal column bones); 2. an individual part of the skeleton, one of the 206 bones of the human body (e.g., *rib*, *sternum*, *tibia*).　　adj. **bony**

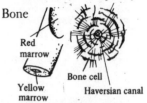

Bone

Red marrow

Yellow marrow

Bone cell

Haversian canal

Bone contains a network of Haversian canals through which blood vessels pass.

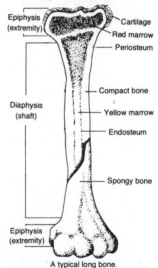

Epiphysis (extremity) — Cartilage

Red marrow

Periosteum

Compact bone

Diaphysis (shaft) — Yellow marrow

Endosteum

Spongy bone

Epiphysis (extremity)

A typical long bone.

BONE AGE n. age determined by comparison of a person's bone development, as shown on X rays, with that of normal persons of the same chronological age.

BONE MARROW n. specialized soft tissue found within bone. **Red bone marrow**, widespread in the bones of children and found in some adult bones (e.g., sternum, ribs), is essential for the formation of mature *red blood cells*. Fat laden **yellow bone marrow**, more common in adults, is found primarily at the ends of long bones.

BONE MARROW ASPIRATION n. withdrawal through a special needle of a sample of bone marrow tissue for examination, esp. in the diagnosis of certain blood disorders and malignancies.

BONE POWDER n. bone tissue (usually from *cadavers*), which is reduced to a powder, treated with hydrochloric acid to remove minerals, dried, and sterilized, for implanting into areas where original bone has been injured and removed. New bone growth is stimulated by the bone powder through *osteoinduction*.

BOOSTER INJECTION n. a supplementary dose ("booster shot") of a *vaccine* or other immunizing substance, given to raise or restore the presumably waning effectiveness of a previous dose.

BORDER n. a common term for the margin of a part (e.g., the *vermilion* border, the deeper colored portion of the lip).

BORIC ACID n. a white, odorless powder once commonly used as an eye wash and topical antiseptic.

BOTULISM n. severe and often fatal form of *food poisoning* resulting from eating food (usually canned or otherwise preserved) containing the microorganism *Clostridium botulinum*, which produces a *toxin* (botulin) that causes fatigue followed by marked disturbances in vision, muscle weakness, and often fatal respiratory complications. Hospitalization and use of *antitoxin* is required.

BOWEL n. the intestines, esp. the large intestine.

BOWLEG n. abnormal bending outward of the leg from the knee downward, with a gap between the knees; it is most often the result of disease or nutritional disorder but is sometimes caused by arthritis; also **bandy leg**.

BOWMAN'S CAPSULE n. any of numerous cup-shaped structures in the kidney each of which contains a *glomerulus* that filters wastes from the blood.

BP see *blood pressure*.

BRACE n. a device, usually of metal, plastic, wood, or leather, or a combination of these, used to support an injured or paralyzed part in the correct position (see also *dropfoot brace*).

BRACHI-, BRACHIO- comb. form indicating an association with the arm (e.g., **brachiocrural**, pert. to the arm and leg).

BRACHIAL adj. pert. to the arm.

BRACHIAL ARTERY n. main artery of the upper arm.

BRACHIAL PLEXUS n. network of nerves arising from the spine in the neck region and supplying the arm, hand, and parts of the shoulder.

BRACHIALGIA n. pain in the arm.

BRACHY- comb. form meaning "shortness" (e.g., **brachydactyly**, shortness of the fingers and/ or toes).

BRACHYCEPHALY n. a congenital malformation of the skull in which the skull is abnormally short and broad; also: **brachycephalia**.

BRADLEY METHOD OF CHILDBIRTH n. a method of psychophysical preparation for natural childbirth that includes education about the physiology of pregnancy, exercises and nutrition during pregnancy, and techniques of breathing and relaxation, with the assistance of the husband, for labor and childbirth (compare *Lamaze method*; *Read method*).

BRADY- comb. form meaning "slowness" (e.g., **bradyrhythmia**, slowness of pulse or heart rate).

BRADYCARDIA n. unusually slow heartbeat (pulse rate lower than 60 in an adult). Some healthy people, esp. athletes, have low pulse rates, but bradycardia usually indicates a disorder of some kind that can, if untreated, lead to seriously decreased cardiac output and circulatory problems.

BRADYKINESIS n. abnormal slowness of all voluntary activity, including speech, caused by disease or sometimes tranquilizer use.

BRADYLALIA n. extremely slow speech due to brain lesion.

BRADYPNEA n. abnormally slow breathing.

BRAIN n. the mass of nervous tissue in the skull (*cranium*); the main part of the central nervous system, the primary center for regulating body activities. The brain includes the two hemispheres of the *cerebrum*, the *cerebellum*, the *pons*, and the *medulla oblongata*, each part with specialized functions. The brain is covered by protective membranes (*meninges*) and contains cavities (*ventricles*) containing *cerebrospinal fluid*.

BRAIN DEATH n. irreversible unconsciousness with total loss of brain function, usually determined by loss of reflex activity and respiration and fixed, dilated pupils while the heart continues to beat. In the United States, legal definitions of brain death vary from state to state, but usually electrical activity of the brain must be shown to be absent on at least two *electroencephalograms* taken 12 to 14 hours apart (see also *death*).

BRAIN RHYTHM n. a characteristic pattern of electrical activity (voltage) in the brain, recordable as a wave-form tracing (*electroencephalogram*). There are four basic brain rhythms: *alpha rhythm*, *beta rhythm*, *delta rhythm*, and *theta rhythm*.

THE BRAIN

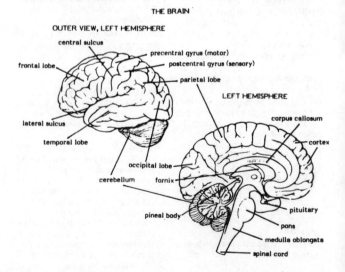

OUTER VIEW, LEFT HEMISPHERE

central sulcus
precentral gyrus (motor)
postcentral gyrus (sensory)
frontal lobe
parietal lobe
LEFT HEMISPHERE
lateral sulcus
corpus callosum
temporal lobe
cortex
occipital lobe
cerebellum
fornix
pituitary
pineal body
pons
medulla oblongata
spinal cord

BRAIN SCAN n. a painless diagnostic procedure using radioactive isotopes to examine the brain and localize and identify possible lesions or other abnormalities (see also *CAT scan*, *PETT*).

BRAIN STEM n. portion of the brain that connects with the *spinal cord* and includes all parts of the brain (e.g., *pons*, *medulla*) except the *cerebrum* and *cerebellum*.

BRAIN WAVE   see *brain rhythm*.

BRAN n. the outer covering of a cereal grain that provides roughage when used as food. Bran is recommended by some specialists as effective in promoting the elimination of solid wastes from the bowel and in helping to avoid certain diseases (e.g., *diverticulosis*).

BRAXTON-HICKS CONTRACTIONS n. irregular contractions of the muscles of the pregnant uterus that increase in intensity and frequency as pregnancy progresses so that near term they may be hard to distinguish from true labor: also called **false labor**.

BREAST n. the front of the chest, esp. either of the two masses of tissue—*mammary glands*—that include and surround the nipples. In females the mammary glands produce milk after the birth of a baby. Each breast is made up of glandular lobules that secrete milk. The milk passes into ducts (lactiferous ducts), is stored in dilations of the ducts (ampullae), and is discharged through tiny openings in the nipple area (see also *lactation*).

BREASTBONE   see *sternum*.

BREAST CANCER n. one of the most common malignancies in women in the United States, with several known risk factors, including a family history of breast cancer, early *menarche*, late

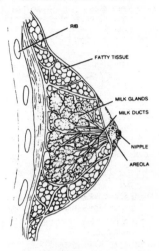
Cross section of a female breast.

menopause, having no children or having them late in life, exposure to ionizing radiation, obesity, hypertension, chronic cystic disease of breast, and possibly a high-fat diet. Early symptoms are usually detected by the woman during breast self-examination and include a small, painless lump; thick or dimpled skin; or a change in the nipple; later symptoms include nipple discharge, pain and swollen lymph glands in the armpit area. Diagnosis is made by physical examination, *mammography*, and laboratory examination of tumor cells obtained through biopsy. Treatment depends on the location and size of the tumor and whether or not it has spread to other areas and may be *lumpectomy* or some type (e.g., radical or simple) of *mastectomy*, often followed by *chemotherapy* and/or *radiotherapy*. Since early diagnosis and treatment greatly improve the rate of cure, women are advised to practice regular *breast self-examination*.

How to examine your breasts

In the shower:

Examine your breasts during bath or shower; hands glide easier over wet skin. Fingers flat, move gently over every part of each breast. Use right hand to examine left breast, left hand for right breast. Check for any lump, hard knot or thickening.

Before a mirror:

Inspect your breasts with arms at your sides. Next, raise your arms high overhead. Look for any changes in contour of each breast, a swelling, dimpling of skin or changes in the nipple.

Then, rest palms on hips and press down firmly to flex your chest muscles. Left and right breast will not exactly match—few women's breasts do.

Regular inspection shows what is normal for you and will give you confidence in your examination.

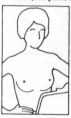

Lying down:

To examine your right breast, put a pillow or folded towel under your right shoulder. Place right hand behind your head—this distributes breast tissue more evenly on the chest. With left hand, fingers flat, press gently in small circular motions around an imaginary clock face. Begin at outermost top of your right breast for 12 o'clock, then move to 1 o'clock, and so on around the circle back to 12. A ridge of firm tissue in the lower curve of each breast is normal. Then move in an inch, toward the nipple, keep circling to examine *every part of your breast*, including nipple. This requires at least three more circles. Now slowly repeat procedure on your left breast with a pillow under your left shoulder and left hand behind head. Notice how your breast structure feels.

Finally, squeeze the nipple of each breast gently between thumb and index finger. Any discharge, clear or bloody, should be reported to your doctor immediately.

American Cancer Society

BREAST-FEEDING n. the suckling (nursing) of an infant at a mother's breast (*mamma*) (as contrasted with bottle-feeding). Many authorities recommend breast-feeding as a means for establishing a bond between mother and infant and giving the infant the natural benefits of mother's milk for nutrition and immunity.

BREAST MILK n. milk-like fluid secreted by female breasts after childbirth and believed to be excellent food for newborns, providing necessary nutrients and some level of immunity against certain diseases.

BREAST PUMP n. a device for extracting milk from the breast of a woman who is nursing or has recently given birth.

BREAST SELF-EXAMINATION n. the process of observing (in front of a mirror) and palpating the breast and surrounding area to detect any lumps or other changes that may indicate disease (e.g., breast cyst or breast cancer); many authorities recommend that women examine their breasts monthly.

BREATH n. air that is taken into and let out from the lungs through the nose or mouth; one inhalation of air; one exhalation of air.

BREATHING n. the action of taking air into the lungs and then letting it out, a process normally done without thinking and controlled by the *autonomic nervous system* (compare *expiration*, *inhalation*, *respiration*).

BREECH PRESENTATION n. situation at birth in which the feet, knees, or buttocks of the infant appear first; occurs in about 3% of all births and is sometimes hazardous; also called: **breech birth**.

BREGMA n. the junction point at the top of the skull at which two bone seams (coronal and sagittal sutures) meet.   adj. **bregmatic**

BRIGHT'S DISEASE   see *nephritis*.

BRILL'S DISEASE n. a mild form of *typhus*.

BROCA'S AREA n. an area of the cerebral cortex involved in speech production.

BRODIE'S ABSCESS n. a form of *osteomyelitis*, with chronic abscess at the head of a bone. Treatment is by antibiotics and excision and drainage of the abscesses.

BRODMANN AREAS n. numbered (1-47) areas of the cerebral cortex, each distinguished by different cellular components and each involved in a specific function (e.g., area 17 is involved in vision, area 4 in motor function).

BROMHIDROSIS n. bad-smelling body odor resulting from bacterial action on sweat from armpits, groin, and/or feet.

BROMIDE n. a salt containing bromine, once formerly used as a sedative but now replaced by safer drugs.

BROMIDE POISONING n. poisoning caused by excessive intake of bromides; symptoms include vomiting, confusion, hallucinations, irritability, a skin rash, and sometimes coma; also: **brominism**

BROMINISM n. bromide poisoning.

BRONCHI n. pl. of *bronchus*.

BRONCHI-, BRONCHO- comb. form indicating an association with one (*bronchus*) or more (*bronchi*) passages leading to the lungs (e.g., **bronchoesophageal**, pert. to the bronchi and esophagus).

BRONCHIAL adj. pert. to the *bronchi*.

BRONCHIAL ASTHMA   see *asthma*.

BRONCHIECTASIS n. persistent, abnormal widening of the bronchi, with an associated cough and the spitting up of pus-filled mucus. The condition may be *congenital* or may result from infection (e.g., *whooping cough*) or obstruction due to a tumor or an inhaled foreign body. Treatment is by antibiotics, physiotherapy, or (less often) surgery.

BRONCHIOLE n. a small branch in the bronchial system, leading toward and ending in the *alveoli* of the lung.

BRONCHIOLITIS n. a viral infection of the lower respiratory tract, occurring most often in children under one or two years of age and characterized by respiratory distress, wheezing on expiration, low-grade fever, cough, and nasal discharge. The disease usually disappears within a week or ten days. Antibiotics and bronchodilators are not generally used, treatment being mainly symptomatic (e.g., vaporizer, suctioning if necessary).

BRONCHITIS n. inflammation of a *bronchus* or of the bronchi. Acute bronchitis, a common disorder often following an *upper respiratory infection*, is characterized by cough, fever, and chest pain. Treatment is by pain and fever reducers, steam inhalation and antibiotics, if indicated. Chronic bronchitis, bronchial inflammation that is persistent, often caused by cigarette smoking, exposure to other irritants, or recurrent infections, is characterized by mucus secretions, cough, and frequently increasing difficulty in breathing.

BRONCHODILATOR n. a drug that relaxes and dilates bronchial passageways to improve the passage of air to the lungs.

BRONCHOPNEUMONIA n. acute inflammation of the bronchi and of the alveoli of the lungs, characterized by fever, chills, shallow breathing, cough, and chest pain. It usually follows an earlier infection, starting at the smallest, most remote air chan-

nels (bronchioles) and resulting in the formation of pus and the clogging of those channels. Treatment is by bedrest, and antibiotics and oxygen, if necessary.

BRONCHOSCOPY n. examination of the bronchi through a special device (bronchoscope). Sometimes samples of tissue or fluid are taken for examination and small foreign bodies can sometimes be removed. adj. **bronchoscopic**

BRONCHOSPASM n. spasm of the bronchi, causing them to narrow, making exhalation difficult and noisy; it is commonly associated with *asthma* and *bronchitis*.

BRONCHUS n. one of the two large channels that lead from the *trachea* to smaller branches (*bronchioles*) and ultimately to the air sacs (*alveoli*) of the lung. pl. **bronchi** adj. **bronchial**

BRONKOSOL n. trade name for a *bronchodilator* (isoetharine hydrochloride) used in the treatment of asthma, emphysema, and bronchitis.

BRUCELLOSIS n. a disease caused by infection with a bacteria (*Brucella* species) obtained by association with infected livestock or their products and causing chills, weakness, headache, and recurring fever. Treatment includes bedrest and tetracyclines; also called **Malta fever; Mediterranean fever; undulant fever**.

BRUISE n. an injury that does not cause the skin to break or bleed but usually results in discoloration because of clotted blood below the skin's surface.

BRUIT n. an abnormal sound, as a murmur, heard on listening with a *stethoscope*.

BRUXISM n. rhythmic or spasmodic grinding of the teeth, esp. during sleep; often caused by emotional tension.

BUBO n. a *lymph node*, esp. in the armpit or groin, that is inflamed and enlarged because of *tuberculosis*, *gonorrhea*, *plague*, or other infection. adj. **bubonic**

BUBONIC PLAGUE n. a serious, sometimes fatal infection, caused by toxin of the bacteria *Yersinia pestis* and transmitted by the bite of fleas from infected rats or squirrels; it is characterized by high fever, prostration, painful swollen lymph glands (buboes) in the groin and armpits, delirium, and bleeding from superficial blood vessels. Treatment is by antibiotics and drainage of buboes if necessary. The Black Death of the Middle Ages, bubonic plague can become epidemic in areas with large populations of infected rats.

BUCCA n. the cheek. adj. **buccal**

BUERGER'S DISEASE n. a disease of unknown cause, affecting primarily men who are heavy tobacco users, in which arteries, most often in the legs and feet, become inflamed and occluded, causing burning, numbness, tingling, and, if inadequate blood supply continues, *phlebitis*, tissue damage and possibly *gangrene*; also **thromboangiitis obliterans**.

BUFFER n. a chemical that is added to another to avert a radical change in concentration or *pH* in the second; a device or system that tends to prevent change, as in body temperature or blood pressure.

BUFFERED ASPIRIN n. *aspirin* that has been combined with one or more other chemicals to prevent change in the aspirin's composition under certain circumstances, as in passing through the stomach. Buffered aspirin was formulated to help persons who become ill as the result of the action of gastric juice on ordinary aspirin.

BULB n. a knoblike structure, mass,

or part (e.g., the bulb of a hair, the bulbus pili); 2. old term for the *medulla oblongata* part of the brain; also: bulbus. pl. **bulbi** adj. **bulbar**

BULBOURETHRAL GLAND n. either of two small glands located on each side of the *prostate* and secreting a fluid component of *semen*.

BULIMIA n. condition marked by insatiable craving for food, leading to episodes of continuous eating, often followed by vomiting, purging, depression, and self-deprivation. It is sometimes seen in emotionally disturbed persons, often alternating with bouts of *anorexia nervosa*. adj. **bulemic**

BULK n. the part of a food (e.g., fiber) that, when eaten, forms a mass that promotes intestinal movement (*peristalsis*) (see *roughage*).

BULK CATHARTIC n. a *laxative* that acts by softening and increasing the mass of fecal matter.

BULLA n. a blister (*vesicle*); a large *bleb* in the skin that contains fluid (*serum*). pl. **bullae** adj. **bullous**

BUN see *blood urea nitrogen*.

BUNDLE n. a cluster (*fascicle*) of filaments or elongated parts, specifically muscle fibers or nerves (e.g., the *bundle of His*, a group of heart muscle fibers that conduct impulses to the ventricles).

BUNDLE BRANCH BLOCK n. an abnormality in the conductive tissues of the heart (*bundle of His*) that may cause a reduced heart rate. It may occur after *myocardial infarction* or as a result of other heart or neurological disease. A *pacemaker* may be required in severe cases.

BUNDLE OF HIS n. a band of fibers in the heart through which the cardiac impulse is transmitted from the *atrioventricular node* to the ventricles; also: **atrioventricular bundle**.

BUNION n. a swelling and thickening of the joint where the big toe joins the foot, displacing the big toe toward the other toes. Caused by chronic irritation from ill-fitting shoes, bunions may become painful and require surgery.

BURKITT'S LYMPHOMA n. a malignancy of the lymphatic system, seen mostly in central Africa, characterized by lesions of the jaw or abdomen (esp. in children) often followed by central nervous system involvement. The *Epstein-Barr virus* (EBV) is believed to be the cause; *chemotherapy* is usually effective treatment.

BURN n. tissue injury resulting from exposure to excessive sun, heat, radiation (e.g., overexposure to X rays or radioactive elements), a caustic, or electricity. Tissue changes include reddening and pain (first degree), blistering (second degree), and destruction of tissue (third degree). Treatment involves alleviation of pain, careful cleaning of injuries, prevention of infection, maintenance of normal fluid and *electrolyte* balances in the body, care of wounds, and, in cases of severe burn, prevention or care of *shock*. In severe burns skin grafts and plastic surgery may be necessary.

BURN CENTER n. a facility designed, with sophisticated equipment, for the care of persons severely burned. A network of burn centers has been established throughout the United States.

BURNOUT n. a condition marked by physical and emotional exhaustion, often described as "having no energy," being apathetic, not caring anymore; it typically occurs in people who are overworked, frustrated by lack of accomplishments and/or subject to continued job stress, particularly those in service professions (e.g., teacher, nurse, social worker).

BURSA n. a fluid-containing, membrane-lined cavity located in connecting tissues, usually in the vicinity of joints, where friction would otherwise occur, the bursa serving as a lubricating and protective system between *tendon* and *bone*, *tendon* and *ligament*, or other structures.

BURSITIS n. inflammation of a *bursa*, often precipitated by injury, infection, excessive trauma or effort, or arthritis or similar condition and characterized by pain and often limited mobility. Treatment is by analgesics, anti-inflammatory agents, immobilization of the affected area, and in some cases the use of corticosteroid injections at the affected site.

BUTAZOLIDIN n. tradename for anti-inflammatory agent *phenylbutazone*.

BUTTERFLY RASH n. a red, scaly eruption on both cheeks with a narrow band across the nose, characteristic of certain diseases (e.g., *lupus erythematosus, rosacea*).

BUTTOCK n. one of the two masses of muscle and fat tissue, divided by a cleft, that is prominent at the lower back of the torso, both masses forming the seat; a *gluteal* prominence; the *nates*.

BYPASS n. any surgically created, temporary or permanent channel or route around a part, esp. a part that has been damaged (e.g., a *coronary bypass*); a *shunt*.

BYSSINOSIS n. a lung disease caused by breathing in the dust of cotton, flax, or hemp. Symptoms, which are typically more pronounced when the patient returns to work after the weekend rest, are tightness of the chest, shortness of breath, and wheezing.

C

C: VITAMIN n. a vitamin (*ascorbic acid*) essential for general metabolism, the health of capillary walls, and wound healing, and believed by some to help guard against certain infections. Rich sources are citrus fruits, tomatoes and potatoes (see *vitamin*; Table of Vitamins).

C symbol for the element *carbon*.

C abbreviation for *Celsius* (centigrade) *temperature scale*.

CA symbol for *cancer*; symbol for element *calcium*.

CACHEXIA n. a severe state of wasting, malnutrition, and poor health, as occurs, e.g., in certain advanced cancers and advanced tuberculosis; also: **cachexy**. adj. **cachectic**

CADAVER n. a dead body, a corpse, esp. one used for the study of *anatomy*. adj. **cadaveric**

CAESAREAN see *Cesarean section*.

CAFFEINE n. a central nervous system stimulant that is an alkaloid derived from the dried leaves of tea plants and the beans of coffee plants, found in coffee, tea, cola drinks, and some medicines. It is used to counter drowsiness and mental fatigue; it also acts as a *diuretic*. Excessive intake of caffeine frequently causes restlessness, insomnia, and gastrointestinal complaints (see also *caffeinism*).

CAFFEINISM n. poisoning from excessive intake of coffee or other caffeine-containing products, resulting in upset stomach, restlessness, nervousness, and increased heartbeat.

CAISSON DISEASE see *bends*; *air embolism*.

CALAMINE n. a chemical (zinc oxide with added iron oxide) used in the form of a pink powder or lotion to treat itching and mild skin irritations.

CALAMUS n. a reed-shaped part, particularly the calamus scriptorius, a pen-shaped structure in the brain cavity.

CALCANEUS n. the heelbone, the largest of the tarsals; also **calcaneum**. adj. **calcaneal**

CALCAR n. a spurlike projection, as that of the femur neck (calcar femorale).

CALCAREOUS adj. chalky, containing *calcium* or lime.

CALCIFEROL n. one of the *D vitamins*; a chemical found in milk and fish liver oils and used to prevent and treat *rickets*, *osteomalacia*, and other disorders of calcium metabolism; also called **vitamin D$_2$**; **ergocalciferol**.

CALCIFICATION n. hardening of tissue resulting from the formation of calcium salts within it; the abnormal hardening (calcinosis) leads to impaired organ function (e.g., in the kidneys or arteries). The process can result from a disturbance in the normal balance of hormones, vitamin D, and calcium and other minerals in the body.

CALCITONIN n. a hormone secreted by the *thyroid gland* that regulates the level of calcium in the blood and stimulates bone formation.

CALCIUM n. an element, the fifth most abundant in the human body, found primarily in bone but also present in body fluids and soft-tissue cells. It is important for nerve impulse transmission, muscle function, blood coagulation, teeth and bone formation, and heart function. (See also Table of Elements).

CALCULUS n. a stone that forms in the body, usually in hollow organs or ducts, where it may cause obstruction and inflammation (see also *gallstone*; *kidney stone*). pl. **calculi**

CALEFACIENT adj. producing warmth or the sensation of warmth (e.g., a hot-water bottle or a commercial ointment for muscle soreness).

CALENDAR METHOD OF FAMILY PLANNING n. a method of family planning in which the fertile days (the days during which *conception* is most likely to occur) in a woman's *menstrual cycle* are determined by examining the timing of six or more consecutive menstrual cycles on a calendar, determining the average length of the menstrual cycle, and then applying the fact that ovulation typically occurs 14 days before the onset of a period and that sperm and ovum are each viable for a few days in the female reproductive tract. The fertile period therefore extends from a few days before ovulation to a few days after. If, for example, a woman has an average menstrual cycle of 28 days, she would be expected to ovulate on day 14 and her fertile days to extend from approximately day 10 through day 18 of her cycle. During these fertile, or "unsafe," days, coitus should be avoided if pregnancy is not desired, should be practiced if pregnancy is desired. Since a woman's menstrual cycle is often not regular and may be affected by illness, emotional upset, change in climate, and other factors, the calendar method is not considered one of the most effective means of family planning; also called **rhythm method** (compare *basal body temperature method of family planning*) (see also contraception).

CALF n. the thick part at the back of the leg below the knee that contains the gastrocnemius muscle, which flexes when one stands on the toes.

CALIBER n. the diameter of a tube or vessel (e.g., a blood vessel).

CALISTHENICS n. exercises usually done as a group, with provided cadence or rhythm and under the direction of a leader, as a means for developing or retaining

flexibility, strength, and muscle tone (compare *aerobic exercise*).

CALLOSUM see *corpus*.

CALLUS n. 1. a hardened area of skin as on the bottom of the foot; 2. the tissue formed around a bone fracture. adj. **callous**

CALORIE n. 1. the amount of heat needed to raise one gram of water one degree on the *Celsius scale*; also: **small calorie**. 2. amount of heat equal to 1,000 small calories: also: **large calorie**. 3. unit equal to one large calorie, denoting the heat expenditure of an organism and the energy or fuel value of a food. adj. **caloric**

CALVARIA n. the dome of the skull which varies in shape (e.g., oval, circular) from one individual to another. adj. **calvarial**

CAMBIUM n. the inner layer of the tissue covering a bone (*periosteum*).

CAMPHOR n. a chemical, derived from the plant *Cinnamomum camphora* or made artificially, having a penetrating smell and sometimes used for the treatment of skin conditions (although the effectiveness of such treatment is in question). Camphor is poisonous if swallowed and can be life-threatening.

CANAL n. a relatively narrow tube, generally for conducting materials other than blood or lymph (e.g., the *alimentary canal*, for carrying food from the mouth to the stomach and intestines for digestion and for expelling wastes through the canal's end, the *anus*).

CANALIZATION n. the formation of channels or passages through tissue.

CANCER n. an abnormal, *malignant* growth of cells that invade nearby tissues and often spread (*metastasize*) to other sites in the body, interfering with the normal function of the affected sites. Although the basic cause of cancer remains unknown, most forms of cancer can be traced to a specific causal or precipitating factor, as, e.g., cigarette smoking, exposure to cancer-producing chemicals or ionizing radiation, or overexposure to the sun; viruses are associated with some cancers and genetic (familial) susceptibility plays a role in certain forms of the disease. The incidence of different types of cancer varies greatly with age, sex, ethnic group and geographic location. In the United States cancer is second to heart disease as a cause of death with breast cancer and lung cancer leading the statistics. The parts of the body most often affected by cancer are the breast, lungs, colon, uterus, oral cavity, and bone marrow. Major signs of cancer include a change in bladder or bowel habits; a sore that does not heal; a persistent cough or hoarseness; unusual bleeding or discharge; thickening or lump in the breast or other part of the body; indigestion or difficulty in swallowing; and change in a wart or mole. The treatment of cancer may involve surgery, the irradiation of affected parts, and/or the use of *chemotherapy*. The prognosis depends on the type and site of the cancer, the promptness of initial treatment, and other factors; about one-third of those patients with newly diagnosed cancers are ultimately permanently cured (see also *breast cancer*, *carcinoma*, *leukemia*, *lymphoma*, *metastasis*, *neoplasm*, *sarcoma*).

CANDIDIASIS n. an infection caused by a *Candida* species of fungus (e.g., *Candida albicans*), affecting most often the skin, mouth, and vagina, and causing itching, peeling, whitish exudate, and sometimes easy bleeding. Common forms of candidiasis include *thrush* and some types of *vaginitis* and *diaper rash*. Treatment is by oral and topical antifungal drugs (e.g., nystatin) and sometimes use of *gentian violet*.

CANINE n. any of the four teeth, two in each jaw, flanking the *incisors* and projecting beyond the level of the other teeth.

CANKER n. an ulcerlike sore, esp. of the mouth.

CANNABIS n. a *psychoactive* substance derived from the leaves of the plant *Cannabis sativa* and related *Cannabis* species and found in marihuana and other hallucinogens (street drugs); it is sometimes used in the care of some cancer patients as an antiemetic to counter nausea and vomiting associated with *chemotherapy*.

CANNULA n. a flexible tube inserted into a cavity for transferring fluids or other materials into or out of it (e.g., as in *amniocentesis* to withdraw *amniotic fluid*).

CANNULATION n. insertion of a cannula into a body cavity or duct (e.g., trachea); also: **cannulization**.

CANTHUS n. angle formed by the upper eyelid with the lower eyelid, one being inner (nasal) and the other outer (temporal).   pl. **canthi**   adj. **canthal**

CAPACITY n. 1. the amount of material an organ or other part can hold when filled (e.g., lung capacity); 2. the ability to perform an action (capability).

CAPILLARY n. 1. a tiny blood vessel connecting arterioles and venules. Through the one-cell-layer-thick walls (approx. 0.008 mm diameter) of capillaries oxygen and nutrients are passed from arterioles to body tissues and carbon dioxide and other wastes are passed from body tissues to venules; 2. any other small, hairlike tube for carrying *lymph* or other material.

CAPITATE n. one of the eight bones of the wrist (os capitatum). adj. shaped like a head.

CAPSID n. the cover (a protein) of a simple *virus* particle (*virion*).

CAPSULE n. 1. an envelopelike structure enclosing an organ or part (e.g., Bowman's capsule, which encloses the glomerulus in the kidney); 2. a membrane that surrounds a microorganism (e.g., covering around a bacterium); 3. a medicine-containing shell of gelatin or other material that can dissolve in the stomach, releasing the capsule's contents. adj. **capsular**

CAPUT n. 1. the head; 2. the enlarged or headlike part of an organ (e.g., caput humeri, head of the humerus that fits into a cavity in the scapula).

CARBOHYDRATE n. any of a group of organic compounds (containing the elements carbon, hydrogen, and oxygen), including starches and sugars, that are the chief energy sources of the body. They are synthesized by green plants (through the process of photosynthesis), consumed by humans in the forms of cereals, flour products, fruits, and vegetables, and either absorbed immediately or stored in the form of *glycogen*.

CARBON n. a nonmetallic element present in virtually all living things and all organic matter (see Table of Elements).

CARBON DIOXIDE n. a colorless, odorless gas (CO_2) given off from the lungs as a waste product of *respiration*. Carbon dioxide levels in the blood regulate the breathing rate, and the acid-base balance of the blood and other body fluids is influenced by the levels of carbon dioxide and its compounds (see *apnea*, *hyperventilation*).

CARBON MONOXIDE n. a colorless, odorless gas (CO), formed by the incomplete burning of organic materials (e.g., automobile fuel). Carbon monoxide is extremely toxic; by combining with *hemoglobin* carbon monoxide can cause loss of oxygen transport to tissues, paralysis, and death.

CARBON MONOXIDE POISONING n. a toxic condition caused by the inhalation and absorption of carbon monoxide gas. The carbon monoxide combines with *hemoglobin*, displacing oxygen, and causes loss of oxygen to body tissues. Symptoms include headache, shortness of breath, confusion, drowsiness, unconsciousness, and if continued, death. Treatment involves removal of the carbon monoxide environment and the administration of oxygen.

CARBUNCLE n. a cluster of boils or abscesses (resulting from infection with *Staphylococcus bacteria*) deep under the skin from which pus escapes to the skin surface. Treatment is by surgical drainage, antibiotics, and compresses.

CARCIN-, CARCINO- comb. form indicating an association with *cancer*, specifically a *carcinoma* (e.g., **carcinolysis**, the breakdown of cancer cells, as by a drug).

CARCINOGEN n. a specific substance or chemical that gives rise to a cancer; a cancer-forming agent.

CARCINOGENIC adj. pert. to a carcinogen.

CARCINOMA n. a malignant growth of cells (*epithelial cells*) that arises in the coverings and linings of the body parts (e.g., skin and mucous membranes) and in glands; these cells tend to invade adjacent tissues and to spread (*metastasize*) to other parts of the body via the lymphatic channels and/or bloodstream (compare *leukemia*, *lymphoma*, *sarcoma*).

CARCINOMA IN SITU n. a small cluster or nest of malignant cells that has not yet invaded the deeper epithelial tissue layers or spread to other parts of the body; preinvasive cancer (e.g., carcinoma in situ of the uterine cervix). Treatment at this early stage is often successful.

CARD-, CARDIO- comb. form indicating an association with the *heart* (e.g., **cardioaortic**, pert. to the heart and *aorta*).

CARDIA n. 1. that part of the stomach that connects with the esophagus; 2. obsolete term for heart.

CARDIAC adj. pert. to the heart (e.g., a cardiac disorder such as mitral valve prolapse); to the cardiac, or upper, part of the stomach; or, colloquially, to someone with a heart condition.

CARDIAC ARREST n. a sudden cessation of cardiac output and blood circulation, usually caused by *ventricular fibrillation* or other serious abnormality in function of the ventricles of the heart, and leading to oxygen lack, buildup of carbon dioxide, acidosis, and, if untreated, to kidney, lung, and brain damage and death. Treatment is by immediate *cardiopulmonary resuscitation (CPR)*; also: **cardiopulmonary arrest**.

CARDIAC ARRHYTHMIA n. an abnormal rate of muscle contraction in the heart, caused by malfunction of impulse-conducting fibers in the heart or inability of the heart to respond to stress (e.g., fever, excessive exercise, altered metabolic balance). Types of arrhythmia include *bradycardia*, *heart block*, and *tachycardia*.

CARDIAC CYCLE n. the cycle of events during which an electrical impulse is conducted through special fibers in the heart muscle, causing contraction of the atria followed by contraction of the ventricles, which action pumps blood through the body. The cycle can be shown on an *electrocardiogram* as a series of waves, termed P, Q, R, S, and T waves; changes in wave patterns indicate abnormalities in the cardiac cycle.

CARDIAC MASSAGE n. repeated, rhythmic compression of the heart through the chest wall or during surgery directly to the heart in an effort to maintain circulation after *cardiac arrest* or other serious cardiac malfunction.

CARDIAC MONITOR n. a device for continual observation of the function of the heart. It may include electrocardiograph, oscilloscope, and other recordings of heart function; there may be an alarm to alert medical personnel to abnormal changes.

CARDIAC MURMUR n. see *heart murmur*.

CARDIAC MUSCLE n. special striated muscle of the heart, involuntary in function. (It is unusual because involuntary muscle is usually smooth, not striated.)

CARDIAC OUTPUT n. the amount of blood expelled by the ventricles of the heart in a given period of time. A normal resting adult has a cardiac output of 2.5 to 3.6 liters per minute.

CARDIAC RESUSCITATION see *cardiopulmonary resuscitation*.

CARDIECTASIS n. expansion of the heart.

CARDIOGRAM n. electronic recording of the rhythm and changes in the heart; also: *electrocardiogram*.

CARDIOGRAPHY n. technique of electronically recording the activity of the heart to produce a *cardiogram*; also: *electrocardiography*.

CARDIOHEPATOMEGALY n. enlargement of both the heart and the liver.

CARDIOLOGY n. a medical specialty that involves the study of the heart and the diagnosis and treatment of its diseases.

CARDIOMEGALY n. enlargement of the heart, in athletes a normal finding but in others an indication of disease (e.g., hypertension).

CARDIOPULMONARY RE-SUSCITATION (CPR) n. an emergency procedure, consisting of external cardiac massage and artificial respiration, used to revive a person who has collapsed, has no apparent pulse and has stopped breathing in an effort to restore blood circulation and prevent death or brain damage due to lack of oxygen. The technique, best if performed by two people, is as follows: (person 1) place the victim on his/her back; pull the chin upward away from the chest; clear the mouth of any objects; lightly pinch the nostrils closed; and, after sealing your mouth over the victim's mouth, blow forcefully into his/her lungs; repeat every four seconds. (person 2) place the heel of one hand, with the other hand over it, on the center of the victim's chest and straight upward from it; shift your weight to apply pressure on your hands to move the chest down about 1½ inches; then remove the pressure while holding hands in place; repeat every second. Infants and children need less pressure exerted, and only one hand should be used to apply it. (See also *Heimlich maneuver*).

CARDIOSPASM n. spasm of the cardiac sphincter (the valve between the distal end of the esophagus and the stomach), which prevents the normal passage of food into the stomach.

CARDIOVASCULAR SYSTEM n. body parts, including the heart and blood vessels, involved in the pumping of blood and transport of nutrients, oxygen and waste products throughout the body.

CARDIOVERSION n. reestablishment of heart rhythm by means of electric shock.

CARDITIS n. inflammation of the heart, usually resulting from infection (e.g., rheumatic fever or streptococcal sore throat), which causes pain, impaired circula-tion, and possibly damage to the heart muscle (see also: *endocarditis*, *myocarditis*, *pericarditis*).

CARIES n. the breakdown and death of tooth tissue, resulting in soft, discolored areas. Studies suggest that eating sugary foods tends to produce tooth decay as does failure to brush the teeth and remove food particles, whereas fluoridation (e.g., in water, toothpaste) tends to prevent it; also: **cavity**.

CARMINATIVE n. a chemical (e.g., simethicone) that prevents the formation of stomach gas (*flatus*) or eases its passing.

CAROTENE n. a red or orange pigment (a hydrocarbon), common to such foods as carrots, yams, and egg yolks, which is converted to vitamin A in the body; also used as a food coloring. An excess of carotene in the blood (carotinemia) may cause the skin to turn yellow.

CAROTID adj. pert. to the *carotid artery*.

CAROTID ARTERY n. either of two main arteries of the neck, supplying the head and neck.

CARPAL TUNNEL SYNDROME n. a common disorder of the wrist and hand, caused by compression of the median nerve in the wrist area and manifested by pain, tingling, burning, and muscular weakness, sometimes spreading to the arm and shoulder. It is more common in women, esp. during pregnancy and menopause, but may also occur in both sexes as a result of trauma, rheumatoid arthritis, diabetes mellitus, or other disorder. Treatment involves pain relief (sometimes by the use of corticosteroids), the splinting and support of the wrist (esp. at night), and surgery if the condition persists.

CARPUS n. the wrist, composed of eight bones between the forearm and the hand. adj. **carpal**

CARRIER n. a person, generally in apparent good health, who harbors organisms that can infect and cause disease in others (compare *vector*). Probably the most notorious carrier was Typhoid Mary.

CAR SICKNESS n. nausea from acceleration, deceleration, and other motions experienced while riding in a car (compare *airsickness; motion sickness; seasickness*).

CARTILAGE n. tough supporting connective tissue serving to protect and connect body parts; it is found chiefly in body tubes (e.g., trachea) and joints. (In the embryo the parts of the skeleton that develop into bone.) Cartilage has no nerves or blood supply of its own. adj. **cartilaginous**

CARTILAGINIFICATION n. the abnormal formation of *cartilage* from other tissues (a tendency in some Orientals).

CASEIN n. the chief protein of milk, the basis of curds and cheese.

CAST n. 1. a firm covering or bandage, often made with plaster of Paris or similar substance, used to stabilize an injured body part during healing (e.g., a fractured leg); 2. a mold used to copy a body part (e.g., a mold of teeth and jaws for fitting *dentures*).

CASTRATION n. surgical removal of the *testes* or *ovaries*, usually done to inhibit hormone secretion in cases of breast cancer in women, prostate cancer in men. Bilateral castration produces *sterility*.

CASTRATION ANXIETY n. an unrealistic fear of injury to or loss of the sexual organs, sometimes the result of guilt over forbidden sexual desires or some threatening experience; in children the fear often involves being hurt by a parent (for boys, the father; for girls, the mother) because of one's sexual feelings toward the parent of the opposite sex (compare *Oedipus*).

CAT, CAT SCAN see *computed tomography*.

CATA- comb. form meaning "downward," "under," or "against" (e.g., **catabasis**, the decline of a disease).

CATABIOSIS n. the normal aging of cells.

CATABOLISM n. a phase of metabolism in which complex chemicals are reduced to simpler forms (compare *anabolism*). adj. **catabolic**

CATALEPSY n. a trancelike state in which the voluntary muscles become rigid and the body does not react to stimuli or change in position; occurs in phychotic patients and occasionally in persons under hypnosis. adj. **cataleptic**

CATALYST n. a chemical (e.g., an enzyme) that speeds up the rate of a chemical reaction but is itself not permanently changed in the process. adj. **catalytic**

CATAPHASIA n. a speech disorder characterized by repetition of the same word several times in succession.

CATARACT n. an eye disorder in which the *lens* becomes less transparent (more opaque) so that light rays cannot reach the *retina* and there is progressive painless loss of vision. Most cataracts are caused by degenerative changes after age 50, but some may be caused by trauma to the eye or exposure to certain chemicals; some are hereditary and some congenital (due perhaps to viral infection during pregnancy). Treatment is removal of the lens and use of special *contact lenses* or eyeglasses or the implantation of an intraocular lens (IOL); in children soft cataracts may be removed by fragmentation (via ultrasound) and drainage (see *epikeratophakia*).

CATARRH n. mucous membrane infection, esp. of the nose. adj. **catarrhal**

CATATONIA n. a syndrome in which motor behavior is disturbed, usually characterized by body rigidity and stupor but sometimes by impulsive and purposeless activity. It is usually associated with mental illness, esp. schizophrenia, but occasionally occurs in other disorders (e.g. *encephalitis*). adj. **catatonic**

CATECHOLAMINE n. any of a group of chemicals, including *epinephrine* and *norepinephrine*, produced in the medulla of the *adrenal gland* and also synthetically for use as drugs. They function in the body's response to stress and affect many physiological and metabolic activities (e.g., heartbeat, nerve responses, muscle activity).

CATGUT n. a chemically treated *suture* (sewing) material made from the tissues of mammals and used in surgery.

CATHARSIS n. 1. purging the body of chemical or other material (e.g., by the use of a *cathartic* to stimulate bowel evacuation); 2. in psychology, communicating one's thoughts to relieve the mind of anxiety (see *abreaction*). adj. **cathartic**

CATHARTIC n. an agent that promotes evacuation of the bowel, esp. fluid evacuation by stimulating *peristalsis* (e.g., senna, aloe products); by increasing the bulk or fluidity of the *feces* (e.g., magnesium sulfate, magnesium hydroxide); or by lubricating the intestinal wall (e.g., mineral oil) (compare *laxative*).

CATHETER n. a flexible, usually rubber or soft plastic, tube inserted into the body for removing or instilling fluids for diagnosis or treatment purposes. In its most common use a catheter is inserted through the urethra into the bladder to withdraw urine and empty (e.g., before surgery) or irrigate the bladder. v. **catheterize**

CATHEXIS n. emotional attachment to an idea, object, or person. adj. **cathectic.**

CAT-SCRATCH DISEASE n. a disease, caused by the scratch or bite of a healthy cat or by a horn or splinter, characterized by inflammation and pustule formation of the affected skin, followed by lymph node swelling and sometimes by fever and malaise. No treatment is usually necessary, the disease spontaneously abating; also called **cat scratch fever**.

CAUDA n. a taillike structure (e.g., cauda equina, the bundle of nerves in the lower part of the spinal cord). pl. **caudae** adj. **caudal,** pert. to the lower part of the spine.

CAUDAL ANESTHESIA n. a type of regional anesthesia involving the injection of an anesthetic into the tail end (the small-of-the-back part) of the spinal canal to prevent pain in that region, as during the delivery of a baby or during anal or genitourinary surgery; now largely replaced by other forms of regional anesthesia, esp. *epidural anesthesia*.

CAUDAL BLOCK n. see *caudal anesthesia*.

CAUL n. intact amniotic sac surrounding the fetus at birth that must be broken to allow the baby to breathe.

CAUSALGIA n. a burning feeling in a limb, usually associated with skin changes and resulting from nerve injury.

CAUSTIC n. an agent that produces a burn or destroys tissue by chemical action (e.g., silver nitrate).

CAUTERIZE v. to destroy tissue for medical reasons (e.g., the removal of a wart) by burning with a hot iron, electron current, or chemical.

CAVERNA n. a cavity or cavern-like structure.

CAVITY n. 1. a hollow; a cavelike structure (e.g., the cranial cavity, the inside of the skull); 2. a general term for dental *caries*.

CECUM n. any part ending in a cul-de-sac; specifically, the closed pocketlike beginning of the large intestine in the lower right part of the abdomen; the appendix is an offshoot of the cecum. adj. **cecal**

-CELE suffix indicating a swelling or tumor (e.g., **cystocele**, a protusion of the *bladder* through the wall or the *vagina*).

CELIAC DISEASE n. a disorder of children and adults caused by an inability to tolerate gluten and wheat protein and characterized by diarrhea (stools are pale, frothy, and foul-smelling), loss of weight, abdominal distension, and lethargy. It is often accompanied by lactose (milk sugar) intolerance. Treatment is a high-protein, gluten-free, and, if necessary, milk-free, diet.

CELIO- comb. form indicating an association with the abdomen (e.g., **celioma**, an abdominal tumor).

CELIOCENTESIS n. hollow needle puncture into the abdomen to remove materials for diagnostic examination.

CELIOSCOPY n. examination of the abdomen by means of an instrument (*endoscope*) inserted through an incision in the abdominal wall.

CELL n. an individual living unit, the basic structure for tissues and organs, made up of an outer membrane (cell membrane), the main mass (cytoplasm), and the nucleus, which controls the cell's metabolism and reproduction; a single living part (e.g., a red blood cell) or organism (e.g., a protozoan). adj. **cellular**

CELL DIVISION see *meiosis*; *mitosis*.

CELLULITIS n. inflammation of tissue, esp. that below the skin, characterized by redness, pain, and swelling. Treatment is by antibiotics.

CELLULOSE n. the basic constituent (a polysaccharide) of plant fiber, providing bulk necessary for proper intestinal function. Fruit, bran, and green vegetables provide cellulose.

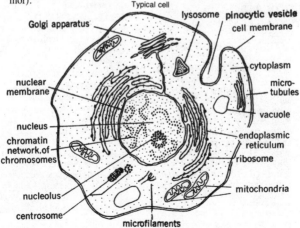

Typical cell

Golgi apparatus · lysosome · pinocytic vesicle · cell membrane · cytoplasm · micro-tubules · vacuole · endoplasmic reticulum · ribosome · mitochondria · nuclear membrane · nucleus · chromatin network of chromosomes · nucleolus · centrosome · microfilaments

CELSIUS adj. pert. to a temperature scale in which the freezing point of water is 0° and the boiling point is 100°, as compared with 32° and 212° respectively on the *Fahrenheit* scale. The name honors Anders Celsius who devised it; also called **centigrade.**

CEMENTUM n. a layer of specialized tissue (modified bone) in a tooth, covering the root and neck.

CENTER n. 1. midpoint; 2. a group of cells that have a special function (e.g., the speech center in the left brain hemisphere); also: **centrum.**

CENTER FOR DISEASE CONTROL (CDC) n. a U.S. government agency, centered in Atlanta, Georgia, concerned with the investigation, diagnosis and control of disease. New and unusual diseases (e.g., *toxic shock syndrome*, *AIDS*) are often intensively investigated by the CDC in cooperation with state and local health departments and private researchers and clinicians.

CENTESIS n. puncture (by hollow needle) of a cavity or organ to draw out fluid (e.g., *amniocentesis*).

CENTIGRADE see *Celsius*.

CENTRALIS adj. toward or at the center.

CENTRAL NERVOUS SYSTEM n. one of the two main divisions of the human nervous system (the other being the *peripheral nervous system*), consisting of the *brain* and the *spinal cord*. The main coordinating and controlling center of the body, the central nervous system processes information to and from the peripheral nervous system. The system is made up of *gray matter* (mostly nerve cells and associated parts) and *white matter* (mostly nerve fibers) and contains protective *cerebrospinal fluid*.

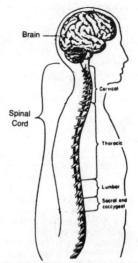

The central nervous system consists of the brain and spinal cord.

CENTRIFUGATION n. separation of media or particles by spinning them in suspension, the heavier materials being whirled to the outer part of the container; used, e.g., to separate blood cells from plasma in unclotted blood. adj. **centrifugal**

CEPHAL-, CEPHALO- comb. form indicating an association with the head (e.g., **cephalocaudal**, pert. to head and tail, or along that axis).

CEPHALALGIA n. *headache*.

CEPHALHEMATOMA n. a collection of blood beneath the scalp of a newborn caused by pressure during birth.

CEPHALIC INDEX n. a measurement used to determine whether the head is of normal shape. The index is a ratio of the width of the head (measured where the width is greatest) multiplied by 100 and divided by the length of the head (measured where it is greatest). A number of 74.9 or less indicates a head much longer than it is wide; 75 to 80, one that has a medium length; and more than 80, one that is disproportionately short.

CEPHALOSPORIN n. any of several antibiotics obtained from microorganisms (including fungi of the genus *Cephalosporium*) and used for treating infections caused by *aerobes*.

CEREBELLUM n. that part of the brain located behind the *cerebrum* and above the *pons* and concerned with the coordination and control of voluntary muscular activity. adj. **cerebellar**

CEREBRAL adj. pert. to the *cerebrum* of the brain (e.g., **cerebral hemisphere**, one of the halves of the cerebrum).

CEREBRAL CORTEX n. the thin layer of *gray matter*, with many folds on the surface of the *cerebrum*, that is the center for higher mental functions, perception, behavioral responses, and other functions. It is classified into many areas, each with specific functions (e.g., speech center).

CEREBRAL HEMORRHAGE n. flow of blood from a ruptured blood vessel in the brain; causes include high blood pressure, head injuries, and *aneurysm*. Symptoms, which depend on the site of the bleeding and the type of blood vessel involved, may include numbness and diminished mental function, or, if severe, coma and death (see also *cerebrovascular accident*).

CEREBRAL PALSY n. loss or deficiency of muscle control due to permanent, nonprogressive brain damage occurring before or at the time of birth. Symptoms include difficulty in walking, poor coordination of the limbs, lack of balance, speech or other sense organ difficulties, and sometimes mental retardation. Treatment depends on the difficulties present

and may include leg braces, speech therapy, and antispasmodic or muscle-relaxing drugs.

CEREBRAL THROMBOSIS n. a blood clot in a cerebral vessel.

CEREBRATION n. mental activity, thinking.

CEREBRI-, CEREBRO- comb. form indicating an association with the *cerebrum*, specifically the cerebral hemispheres (e.g., *cerebrovascular*).

CEREBROSPINAL adj. pert. to the brain and spinal cord.

CEREBROSPINAL FLUID (CSF) n. normally clear liquid, produced in the *ventricles* of the brain, that fills and protects the cavities in the *brain* and *spinal cord*. In the adult there is normally about 140 milliliters of cerebrospinal fluid. Samples of the fluid, obtained by *lumbar puncture*, may be used to diagnose certain diseases.

CEREBROVASCULAR adj. pert. to the blood vessels of the brain.

CEREBROVASCULAR ACCIDENT (CVA) n. an abnormal condition in which hemorrhage or blockage of the blood vessels of the brain leads to oxygen lack and resulting symptoms—sudden loss of ability to move a body part (as an arm or parts of the face) or to speak, paralysis, weakness, or, if severe, death. Usually only one side of the body is affected. Physical therapy and speech therapy can result in some degree of recovery; also called **stroke**.

CEREBRUM n. the main mass of the human brain; the two cerebral hemispheres that control conscious activity. adj. **cerebral**

CERUMEN n. earwax.

CERVICAL adj. 1. pert. to the neck area (e.g., one of the cervical vertebrae); 2. pert. to the cervix of the *uterus* ("cervical cancer" usually means cancer of the cervix of the uterus) or to a constricted necklike part of another organ.

CERVIC-, CERVICO- comb. form indicating an association with the neck (e.g., **cervicofacial**, pert. to the neck and face) or with the *cervix* of the uterus (e.g., **cervicovesical**, pert. to the uterine cervix and the bladder).

CERVICAL CAP n. a *contraceptive* device consisting of a small rubber cap fitted over the cervix to block the entrance of sperm into the uterus. It may be left in place days or weeks at a time and is reported to be similar to the *diaphragm* in contraceptive efficacy.

CERVICAL DISC SYNDROME n. an abnormal condition caused by compression of cervical (neck region) nerve roots, resulting from trauma or degenerative disease or other factors, that produces pain in the neck region, often radiating to the shoulder, arm and hand, *paresthesia*, and some muscular weakness. Treatment may involve analgesics, immobilization of the area to allow rest, traction, and, if severe, surgery; also called **cervical root syndrome**.

CERVICAL SMEAR n. a small amount of the secretions and superficial cells of the cervix of the *uterus*, which are examined microscopically to detect the presence of any abnormal cells; the smear is taken with a special instrument inserted through the vagina (see also *Papanicolaou test*).

CERVICAL VERTEBRAE n. any of the first seven segments of the *vertebral column*, located in the neck region (see also *atlas, axis*).

CERVICITIS n. inflammation of the cervix of the *uterus*, often caused by fungal or bacterial infection, characterized by redness, vaginal discharge, pelvic pain, slight bleeding on intercourse, itching, and burning. Treatment is by antibiotics, topical ointments, or *cautery*.

CERVIX n. the neck or necklike part of an organ, esp. the neck of the uterus, that part of the uterus that extends into the *vagina;* dilation of the cervix permits the passage of the fetus in childbirth. adj. **cervical**

CESAREAN SECTION n. surgical incision through the abdomen and uterus for removal of a fetus, performed when conditions (e.g., maternal hemorrhage, premature separation of the *placenta*, fetal distress, baby too large for passage through mother's pelvis) for normal vaginal delivery are deemed hazardous for mother or baby. The rate of Cesarean deliveries in the United States has recently increased. Hazards include those of major surgery for the mother and the possibility of too-early birth of the baby; also: **Caesarean, C-section**.

CESIUM n. a metallic element, sometimes used in medical radiology (see Table of Elements).

CESTODE see *tapeworm*.

CHAFING n. irritation of the skin by friction, from clothing or from one sweaty body part rubbing against another.

CHAGAS DISEASE n. a disease, caused by a parasite (usually *Trypanosoma cruzi*) transmitted by the bite of an insect, characterized by a lesion at the site of the bite, fever, enlarged lymph glands, rapid heart beat, and, in chronic form, by abnormalities of the heart muscle, esophagus, or colon. The acute form usually resolves itself without treatment.

CHALASIA n. abnormal relaxation of a muscle or opening, esp. abnormal relaxation of the sphincter muscle between the esophagus and stomach, resulting in reflux of stomach contents into the esophagus and regurgitation. Treatment involves a diet of frequent small meals, and, in infants, feeding in the upright position.

CHALAZION n. a nonmalignant small swelling on the eyelid that often requires surgical removal.

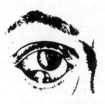

Chalazion

CHALLENGE v. injecting an *antigen* into the body to determine the immunological result.   n. an immunological test of *antigen* reactivity.

CHAMBER n. an enclosed area, e.g., the aqueous chamber, the *humor*-filled part of the eyeball; the heart chambers (auricles and ventricles).

CHANCRE n. a painless sore, esp. that associated with *syphilis*, which has the appearance of a hard ulceration (compare *canker*).

CHANCROID n. a contagious venereal ulcer; it usually appears as a papule on the skin of the genitalia that then ulcerates and, if untreated, produces *buboes* in the groin. Caused by the bacteria *Haemophilus ducreyi*, it is usually treated with sulfa drugs.

CHANGE OF LIFE n. colloquial for *menopause*.

CHARACTERISTIC n. a distinguishing feature of an organism (e.g., a Mendelian, or inherited, characteristic).

CHARLEYHORSE n. colloquial for muscle cramp or soreness, esp. in the thigh or calf, usually after strenuous activity. Treatment is by heat application and a gradual stretching of the affected muscle.

CHECKUP n. colloquialism for a thorough physical examination, which may include an *electrocardiogram*, blood and urine tests, and other special procedures and laboratory tests, depending on the age, sex, and general health of the person.

CHEIL-, CHEILO- comb. form indicating an association with the lip (e.g., **cheiloplasty**, surgical correction of a lip defect).

CHEILITIS n. inflammation and cracking of the skin of the lips due to overexposure to the sun, vitamin deficiency, or allergic reaction to cosmetics (see also *cheilosis*).

CHEILOSCHISIS   see *harelip*.

CHEILOSIS n. disorder of the lips and mouth marked by fissures and scales and caused by a deficiency of riboflavin.

CHEIR-, CHEIRO- comb. form indicating an association with the hand (e.g., **cheiroplasty**, surgical correction of a hand defect).

CHEIROMEGALY n. a condition in which the hands are abnormally large.

CHELATION n. a chemical bonding that is used to remove some substances (e.g., metallic poisons) from tissues.

CHEM-, CHEMO- comb. form indicating an association with chemicals or chemistry (e.g., **chemocautery**, tissue destruction by chemicals).

CHEMOSIS n. *edema* of the mucous membrane of the eyeball and eyelid lining, resulting from injury, infection, or certain systemic diseases (e.g, anemia, kidney disease).

CHEMOSURGERY n. destruction of malignant or otherwise diseased tissue by use of chemicals (e.g., in the treatment of skin cancer).

CHEMOTAXIS n. movement by a cell or organism toward (positive) or away from (negative) a chemical stimulus.

CHEMOTHERAPY n. the treatment of disease by chemical agents. The term includes the use of drugs (e.g., antibacterials, antifungals) to harm or kill disease-causing microorganisms but is most commonly used to refer to the use of drugs to treat cancer. Anti-cancer (antineoplastic) drugs generally inhibit the proliferation of cells and include alkylating agents (e.g., chlorambucil), antimetabolites (e.g., fluorouracil), periwinkle plant derivatives (e.g., vincristine), antineoplastic antibiotics (e.g., adramycin, mithramycin), and radioactive isotopes (e.g., iodine-131, phosphorus-32, gold-198). All these agents are associated with side effects, the most common of which are nausea and vomiting, suppression of bone marrow function, and loss of hair.

CHEST n. the upper part of the torso, the thorax.

CHEYNE-STOKES RESPIRATION n. an abnormal pattern of respiration with slow and shallow breathing (apnea) alternating with periods of deep rapid breathing; it is sometimes seen in *congestive heart failure*, certain respiratory diseases (esp., in the elderly), and as a result of narcotic drug overdose.

CHIASM n. an X-shaped structure; the crossing of two lines or tracts, esp. the crossed fibers of the *optic nerve* (chiasma opticum).

CHICKENPOX n. an acute contagious disease, caused by herpes varicella zoster virus, characterized by a rash of *vesicles* on the face and body. Chickenpox is a common chidhood disease; it is usually mild in otherwise healthy children but may be serious in babies, children weakened by other diseases, and in adults. After an incubation period of two to three weeks, the disease usually begins with slight fever and malaise, after which itchy macules develop, often first on the back and chest; followed by fluid-containing vesicles that break easily and become encrusted. Treatment consists of fever-reducing drugs, lotions to relieve itching, and rest. No vaccine against chickenpox is available; one attack usually confers life-long *immunity*, but the virus lays dormant in nerve cells, sometimes to be reactivated, causing *shingles*; also called **varicella** (see also *herpes zoster*).

CHILBLAIN n. redness and swelling, sometimes accompanied by burning and itching, of the skin due to exposure to cold (compare *frostbite*).

CHILD ABUSE n. physical, emotional or sexual maltreatment of a child, often resulting in serious and often permanent injury or impairment and sometimes in death. It may be overt, as in severely beating a child, or covert, as in depriving the child of needed affection and emotional support. Child abuse occurs in all socioeconomic levels (though it is probably reported more among the poor who visit hospital clinics or social agencies) and among children and parents of all ages, but certain factors are thought to increase the risk of child abuse; among these are parents who were themselves abused as children; parents involved in marital strife; emotionally unstable parents or those undergoing extreme stress (e.g., unemployment); and children who are very young (particularly in cases of beatings and physical abuse), difficult by temperament, or have emotional or physical handicaps (see also *child neglect*).

CHILD NEGLECT n. failure of parents or others entrusted with the care of the child to provide adequate physical and emotional care, so that the child's health and development is endangered (see also *child abuse*).

CHILL n. 1. a feeling of cold due to cold environment; 2. shivering and sensation of cold, often marking the start of an infection and development of a fever.

CHINESE RESTAURANT SYNDROME n. headache, feeling of tingling and burning, and sometimes feeling of facial pressure, caused by eating food containing monosodium glutamate (MSG), which is commonly used in Chinese cooking.

CHIRALGIA n. pain in the hand, esp. of nontraumatic origin.

CHIROPODY n. study of the foot, including its structure and the treatment of minor foot disorders. The preferred term is *podiatry*.

CHIROPRACTIC n. a system of diagnosis and treatment based on the belief that many diseases are caused by pressure on nerves due to misalignments (*subluxations*) of the *spinal column* and that such diseases can be treated by correction (e.g., by massage) of the misalignment.

CHLOASMA n. permanent or transient tan or brownish pigmentation, esp. of the face, associated with pregnancy or the use of oral contraceptives; also called **mask of pregnancy**.

CHLOR-, CHLORO- comb. form indicating greenness (e.g., *chlorophyll*) or an association with *chlorine* (e.g., *chloroform*).

CHLORAL HYDRATE n. a sedative and sleep-inducing drug now seldom used in medicine because of its irritating (to skin and mucous membranes, esp. the stomach) and potentially addictive properties. (Combined with alcohol, it is known colloquially as "knock-out drops" or a "Mickey Finn".)

CHLORAMBUCIL n. a drug, known under the trade name Leukeran, used to treat some forms of cancer.

CHLORAMPHENICOL n. an antibacterial and antirickettsial agent, commonly known by its trade name Chloromycetin, effective in treating many serious infections (esp. typhoid fever) but associated with some serious reactions (e.g., bone marrow depression) and now used with caution.

CHLORDIAZEPOXIDE n. a minor *tranquilizer*, commonly known under the trade name Librium, used to treat anxiety.

CHLORINATION n. the addition of small amounts of a compound of chlorine (e.g., chlorine dioxide) into a water supply to kill organisms that might otherwise cause disease (see *chlorine* in Table of Elements).

CHLORINE n. an element important in certain body processes (e.g., in *hydrochloric acid*, a stomach secretion essential for digestion) and used as a disinfectant (e.g., in swimming pools). It has a strong odor and is irritating to the respiratory tract and poisonous if ingested (see Table of Elements).

CHLOROFORM n. a chloride-containing liquid used as a solvent, sedative and anesthetic. Although widely used as a general anesthetic (the first inhalation anesthetic) in earlier times and still used in some Third World countries (largely because no sophisticated equipment is needed), chloroform is now recognized as a dangerous drug (e.g., it can cause liver damage and low blood pressure) and has been largely replaced by safer anesthetics.

CHLOROPHYLL n. the pigment of green plants that absorbs light and converts it into energy for the synthesis of *carbohydrates*.

CHLOROSIS n. old term for iron-deficiency *anemia*, esp. in women.

CHLOROTHIAZIDE n. a diuretic and antihypertensive drug, widely known under the trade name Diuril, used in the treatment of high blood pressure and edema. Adverse side effects include electrolyte imbalances.

CHLORPROMAZINE n. a major *tranquilizer* and antiemetic, widely known under the trade name Thorazine, used in the treatment of certain psychotic disorders and severe nausea and vomiting.

CHOKING n. a condition due to the blocking of the airway to the lungs, as with food or other swallowed object or with swelling of the larynx. The affected person is unable to speak, tries to cough, becomes red and then purplish in the face, and becomes increasingly desperate to breathe, usually pointing to the throat, and, if unrelieved, collapses. Emergency treatment involves removal of the obstruction if possible and resuscitation if necessary (see *Heimlich maneuver*).

CHOL-, CHOLE-, CHOLO- comb. form indicating an association with *bile* or the bile ducts (e.g., **cholangiolitis**, inflammation of the smallest bile ducts).

CHOLANGIOGRAPHY n. X-ray examination of the bile ducts, after a special contrast medium has been injected.

CHOLANGITIS n. inflammation of the bile ducts marked by pain in the upper right quadrant of the abdomen, intermittent fever, and sometimes *jaundice*. Caused by bacterial infection or an obstruction (e.g., calculi or tumor), it is treated by antibiotics or surgery.

CHOLECYSTECTOMY n. surgical removal of the *gall bladder* to treat inflammation (*cholecystitis*) and/or presence of stones in the gall bladder (*cholelithiasis*).

CHOLECYSTITIS n. inflammation of the *gall bladder*. In acute form, usually caused by a gallstone that cannot pass through the *cystic duct*, there is upper right quadrant pain, vomiting, and flatulence. In the chronic form, pain is often felt after a fatty meal. Surgery is the usual treatment.

CHOLELITHIASIS n. the presence of gallstones in the *gall bladder*, which may cause no symptoms or cause vague abdominal discomfort, flatulence, and intolerance to certain foods. If severe pain or obstruction and inflammation occur, *cholecystectomy* is recommended.

CHOLELITHOTOMY n. removal of gallstones through an incision in the *gall bladder*.

CHOLEMESIS n. the vomiting of *bile*.

CHOLERA n. acute infection with the bacteria *Vibrio cholerae*, characterized by severe diarrhea and vomiting, often leading to dehydration, electrolyte imbalances and, if untreated, death. Spread by water and food contaminated with the feces of infected persons, it is endemic in some parts of the world and frequently occurs at times of natural disasters (e.g., earthquake, floods). Treatment is by antibiotics and electrolyte replacement; a vaccine is available.

CHOLESTASIS n. interruption in bile flow, caused by *hepatitis*, or other liver disorder, alcohol or drug use or obstruction (e.g., by calculi or tumor) in bile ducts, and marked by pale fatty stools, itching, and *jaundice*.

CHOLESTEROL n. a complex chemical present in all animal fats and widespread in the body, esp. in bile, the brain, blood, adrenal glands and nerve-fiber sheaths. It also forms deposits in blood vessels (*atherosclerosis*) and forms *gallstones*. In the body, cholesterol is involved in the synthesis of certain hormones (e.g., cortisone, estrogen) and vitamin D and in the absorption of fatty acids. Many studies indicate that excessive cholesterol levels in the blood can clog arteries and predispose to heart attacks and strokes, but whether the level of cholesterol can be controlled by avoiding *saturated fats* in the diet is still in dispute.

CHOLINE n. a *vitamin* of the B complex, found in most tissues of animals and important (as part of *acetylcholine*) in nerve impulse transmission and in liver function. Some recent evidence indicates that it may also be important in retaining mental function in the elderly.

CHOLINERGIC adj. having effects similar to those resulting from the action of *acetylcholine* (e.g., in nerve transmission) compare *adrenergic*).

CHONDROMA n. a benign, fairly common tumor of cartilage cells.

CHONDROMALACIA n. a softening of cartilage, esp. of the knee, causing pain, swelling, and degenerative changes.

CHONDROSARCOMA n. a *malignant neoplasm* of cartilage cells, most often occurring in long bones, the scapula or the pelvic girdle.

CHORDA n. a cordlike structure; a tendon. adj. **chordal**

CHORDITIS n. inflammation of the *spermatic cords* or of the *vocal cords*.

CHOREA n. a disease of the nervous system characterized by involuntary, rapid and spastic jerks, esp. of the shoulders, hips, and face (see *Huntington's chorea*).

CHORION n. the outer membrane of the embryo sac, which gives rise to the *placenta* (the inner membrane is the *amnion*). adj. **chorionic**

CHORIORETINITIS n. inflammation of the cell layer (*choroid*)

behind the *retina* and of the retina itself, resulting in blurred vision.

CHOROID n. a membrane in the eye, between the *retina* and the *sclera*, having many blood vessels. adj. **choroidal**

CHRISTMAS DISEASE see *hemophilia*.

CHROM-, CHROMO- comb. form indicating color (e.g., **chromatic**, pert. to color and its production).

CHROMATID n. one of the two identical strands of a *chromosome*, occurring as a result of the replication of the chromosome during cell division.

CHROMATIN n. the easily stained, *gene*-carrying part of the cell nucleus. It consists of *DNA* (deoxyribonucleic acid, the basic hereditary material) and protein (usually histone).

CHROMATISM n. 1. abnormal coloring or pigmentation; 2. hallucinatory perception of colored lights.

CHROMATOGRAPHY n. any of several techniques for analyzing compounds and mixtures by virtue of the differences in absorbency of the various components of the compound or mixture.

CHROMESTHESIA n. 1. the color sense; 2. the confusion of actual sensation (e.g., of taste or smell) with imaginary sensations of color.

CHROMOBLASTOMYCOSIS n. a skin disease, caused by infection with a fungus, characterized by itchy warty nodules in a break in the skin that sometimes spread and ulcerate. Treatment is by excision of the nodules and topical antibiotics.

CHROMOSOMAL ABERRATION n. any change in the normal structure or number of chromosomes, often causing physical and mental abnormalities (e.g., *Down's syndrome*, *Kleinfelter's syndrome*).

CHROMOSOMES n. threadlike structures in every cell nucleus that carry the inheritance factors (genes); they are composed of *DNA* (deoxyribonucleic acid, the gene material) and a protein (usually histone). A human cell normally contains 46 chromosomes, or 22 homologous pairs and 1 pair of sex chromosomes; one member of each pair of chromosomes is derived from each parent. (See also *diploid*, *haploid karyotype*). adj. **chromosomal**

CHRONIC adj. long-lasting or frequently recurring (e.g., pain) (compare *acute*).

CHRONIC LYMPHOCYTIC LEUKEMIA (CLL) n. a *neoplasm* of blood-forming tissue, more common in men and with advancing age, with an insidious start, progressing to fatiguability, anorexia, weight loss, and swelling of the lymph glands, spleen, and liver. Normal activities may be continued for many years and remissions may be induced by *chemotherapy* or *irradiation*.

CHRONIC MYELOCYTIC LEUKEMIA (CML) n. a *malignant neoplasm* of blood-forming tissues, occurring most often in older people, with an insidious start and progressing to malaise, bleeding gums, heat intolerance, skin lesions, abdominal discomfort, and spleen enlargement.

CHRONOLOGICAL AGE n. the age of a person expressed as the period of time (e.g. months, years) that has elapsed since birth.

CHRYSOTHERAPY n. treatment of disease (e.g. *rheumatoid arthritis*) with chemicals containing gold; possible side effects include blood, skin, kidney, and liver disorders.

CHYLE n. the cloudy fluid product of digestion in the small intestines, made up of emulsified fats; it is absorbed through *lacteals* into the *lymphatic system* and from there passes into the blood.

CHYME n. the thick, semifluid mixture, consisting of partly digested food and digestive juices, that passes from the stomach to the *duodenum* of the small intestine.

CICATRIX n. a *scar*.

-CIDE suffix meaning "killing" (e.g., **amebicide**, a substance that is fatal to amebae).

CILIA n. 1. eyelashes; 2. hairlike projections from a cell, esp. in the upper respiratory tract, where cilia move particles of dust or other materials. sing. **cilium**

CILIARY BODY n. thick part of a vascular membrane joining the *iris* and *choroid* of the eye.

CILIARY MOVEMENT n. the rhythmic action of hairlike structures (*cilia*) in certain body parts (e.g., the lining of the bronchial tubes); the sweeping action helps to move *mucus* or remove foreign particles (e.g., dust) from the tissue.

CIMETIDINE n. drug, known under the trade name Tagamet, used to treat peptic ulcers and certain other conditions in which decreased acid secretion in the stomach is desired. Adverse effects include diarrhea, dizziness, and skin reactions.

CINGULUM n. an encircling structure or part (e.g., the beltlike band at the base of a tooth). pl. **cingula**

CIRCADIAN RHYTHM n. the biological "clock" or rhythm of an organism, such as the natural sleep-wake cycle in a person's 24-hour schedule. Changing that rhythm can affect biological, mental, and behavioral functions (e.g., suffering "jet lag").

General scheme of blood circulation in the body.

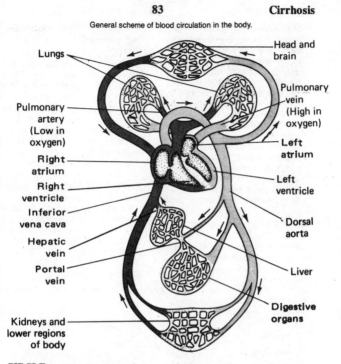

CIRCLE n. a structure or part having closed, ringlike shape (e.g., the circle of Willis, consisting of communicating arteries in the brain).

CIRCULATION n. a general term for the movement of the blood, lymph, or other fluids in a continuous path through the body, as in blood moving through the network of arteries and veins. adj. **circulatory**

CIRCULATORY FAILURE n. failure of the *cardiovascular system* to supply adequate levels of blood to body tissues, as a result of hemorrhage, heart malfunction, or collapse of the peripheral vascular system.

CIRCULATORY SYSTEM n. network of channels through which a fluid passes around the body, esp., the network of arteries and veins transporting blood in the body.

CIRCUM- comb. form meaning "around" (e.g., **circumanal**, pert. to the area around the *anus*).

CIRCUMCISION n. surgical removal of the foreskin (*prepuce*) of the *penis* widely performed on newborn boys (required in the Jewish and certain other religions) though its medical benefit is not proved and some risks (e.g., injury to the *urethra*, hemorrhage) are associated with the procedure. In adult males it is sometimes done to treat *balanitis* or *phimosis*.

CIRCUMDUCTION n. a circular movement of a limb or eye.

CIRRHOSIS n. a chronic diseased condition of the *liver* in which fibrous tissue and nodules replace normal tissue, interfering with blood flow and normal functions of the organ, including gastrointestinal functions, hormone metabolism, and drug detoxification. A chief cause of cirrhosis is chronic *alcoholism*, and *hepatitis* and other infections may also be responsible. Symptoms include nausea, flatulence, light-colored stools, and abdominal discomfort. Treatment is by rest, a protein-rich diet, and abstinence from alcohol. If untreated, liver and kidney failure and gastrointestinal hemorrhage can occur, leading to death.

CISTERNA n. a reservoir, esp. for holding lymph or spinal fluid (e.g., cisterna chyli, the chyle cistern). pl. **cisternae** adj. **cisternal**

CITRIC ACID n. a compound, derived from citrus fruits and fermented cane sugar, used to flavor foods and beverages and certain drugs, esp. laxatives.

CLAUDICATION n. limping or lameness. In **intermittent claudication** pain, esp. in the leg muscles, occurs with walking because the blood supply to these muscles is inadequate; the pain disappears with rest.

CLAUSTROPHOBIA n. an abnormal dread of being confined in closed rooms or small spaces; it is more common in women, can often be traced to an earlier traumatic experience, and is treated by psychotherapy and sometimes *desensitization therapy*.

GREAT VESSELS

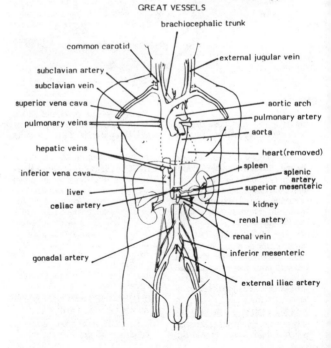

CLAUSTRUM n. an anatomical part that serves as a barrier, esp. a particular gray matter layer in the brain. pl. **claustra** adj. **claustral**

CLAVICLE n. the collarbone; the long, curved horizontal bone just above the first rib that connects the *scapula* (shoulder blade) with the *sternum* (breastbone). adj. **clavicular**

CLAVICLE

Sternal extremity   Acromonial extremity

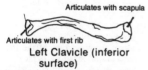

Left Clavicle (superior surface)

Articulates with scapula

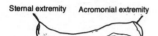

Articulates with first rib

Left Clavicle (inferior surface)

Courtesy Carolina Biological Supply Co.

CLEARANCE n. removal of something, as of wastes, from the blood by the kidney.

CLEAR LIQUID DIET n. a diet that supplies fluid with minimal residue and includes clear and flavored drinks (e.g., ginger ale), fat-free broth, strained fruit juices, and gelatin desserts. It is not nutritionally adequate and can be used for only a limited time (e.g., one day postoperative).

CLEAVAGE n. 1. the process of dividing, as of the fertilized egg into successive multiples of cells, from the single cell; 2. a line formed by a groove between two parts.

CLEFT n. a division, fissure, or cleavage, esp. one resulting in the nonunion of parts in the developing *fetus* (e.g., a *cleft palate*).

CLEFT FOOT n. an abnormal condition in which the separation between the third and fourth toes extends into the foot.

CLEFT LIP see *harelip*.

CLEFT PALATE n. a congenital defect in which there is a fissure in the midline of the *palate*, either partial or through both hard and soft palates and into the nasal cavities, often associated with cleft in the upper lip. A common birth defect (occurring in about 1 in 2,500 births and more frequently in females), it is treated by special feeding techniques, reconstructive surgery, care of any associated speech, hearing, and oral problems, and emotional support.

CLIMACTERIC n. a time in a woman's life associated with changes in her endocrine system and other body systems, often accompanied by emotional changes; it ends with *menopause* when reproductive capability ceases. Colloquially called **change of life**.

CLIMAX n. 1. the severest stage of a disease; 2. the height of sexual excitement; orgasm.

CLINIC n. a health-care facility, part of an institution or hospital, designed to treat walk-in patients and/or for training medical personnel.

CLINICAL adj. pert. to bedside patient care (e.g., clinical medicine) in contrast to basic-science studies (e.g., experimental medicine).

CLINOCEPHALY n. a congenital defect in which the top of the head appears to be pushed in (is concave); also: **clinocephalism**.

CLINODACTYLY n. congenital defect in which one or more fingers or toes are abnormally positioned or bent.

CLINORIL n. trade name for antiinflammatory agent (*sulindac*) used in the treatment of *rheumatoid arthritis* and *ankylosing spondylitis*.

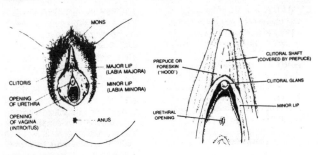

(left) Position of clitoris in relation to other structures of the vulva; (right) shaft of clitoris covered by foreskin.

CLITORIS n. a small erogenous part made up of erectile tissue at the front of the female external genital organs between the *labia minora*.   adj. **clitoral**

CLOFIBRATE n. a drug, known under the trade name Atromid-S, used to lower high blood levels of cholesterol and triglycerides.

CLOMID n. trade name for a fertility drug (clomiphene citrate), the use of which has been associated with *multiple births*.

CLONE n. a group of genetically identical cells or organisms reproduced asexually from a single cell or individual.   adj. **clonal**

CLONUS n. an abnormal condition in which a skeletal muscle alternately contracts and relaxes; a rhythmical spasm; often indicative of central nervous system disease.   adj. **clonic** (as a clonic *convulsion*)

CLOT n. a clump of material formed out of the contents of a fluid, as of blood (see *blood coagulation*).   v. to coagulate

CLOTTING TIME n. the time required for blood to clot, usually determined by observing clot formation in a small sample of blood; used to diagnose some clotting disorders and to monitor *anticoagulant* drug therapy.

CLUBBING n. a condition of the fingers and toes in which their ends become wide and thickened; clubbing is often a symptom of disease, esp. heart or lung disease.

CLUBFOOT n. a congenital abnormality of the foot, esp. one in which the front part of the foot turns toward the inside of the heel. Less severe conditions can be treated by splinters or casts applied during infancy; more severe conditions require surgery (see also *talipes*)

CLUSTER HEADACHE   see *histamine headache*.

COAGULATION n. the clotting process (see *blood coagulation*).

COAGULATION FACTOR n. any of thirteen factors in the blood including *fibrinogen* and *prothrombin*, the actions of which are essential for *blood coagulation*.

COALESCENCE n. fusion, as when the edges of a wound grow together.

COARCTATION n. a constricting or narrowing, esp. with reference to a congenital defect of the aorta, which is usually repaired surgically.

COAT n. a covering, esp. a membrane that forms a wall.

COBALT n. a metallic element, the radioactive *isotope* of which (^{60}Co) is used in the treatment of cancer. Cobalt is contained in vitamin B$_{12}$ (see Table of Elements).

COCAINE n. a white, crystalline powder, derived from the leaves of the coca plant (*Erythroxylon coca*) or prepared synthetically, once used as a topical *anesthetic*, esp. for eye, ear, nose and throat examination, but now a *drug of abuse*, used for its stimulating and anesthetic properties. Adverse reactions include restlessness, euphoria, and tremors; it is *addictive*.

COCCIDIOMYCOSIS n. an infection caused by the fungus *Coccidioides immitis*, largely confined to the southwestern United States and Central and South America, where it is sometimes called desert rheumatism. At first the symptoms resemble those of the common cold or influenza, but the disease may later recur, after apparent recovery, in more serious form, with fever, weight loss, and arthritic pains. Treatment is by antibiotics.

COCCIDIOSIS n. a disease of tropical and subtropical areas, caused by the protozoan parasite *Isospora belli* or closely related species, characterized by watery diarrhea, fever, and malaise. It usually subsides within two weeks, rarely persisting to cause serious complications.

COCCUS n. a round or generally round *bacterium*. pl. **cocci** adj. **coccal**

COCCYX n. the four fused, partly developed *vertebrae* forming the tailbone in humans. adj. **coccygeal**

COCHLEA n. the snail-shaped part of the *inner ear* (see *labyrinth*) whose sensory cells are stimulated by sound waves during hearing. adj. **cochlear**

CODEINE n. a chemical (alkaloid), derived from *opium* or *morphine*, used as a pain reliever and cough suppressant. Side effects include nausea, constipation, and drowsiness; if taken in large amounts or for a long period, it is potentially addictive.

COD LIVER OIL n. oil from the liver of codfish and other fishes used to treat calcium and phosphorus deficiency and as a supplementary source of vitamins A and D.

CODON n. a code for a specific *amino acid*, formed of three successive bases in a *DNA* molecule.

COELOM n. the body cavity of an embryo that gives rise in humans to the pleural, pericardial, and peritoneal cavities.

COENZYME n. a nonprotein substance (sometimes a *vitamin*) that functions to aid the action of an *enzyme*.

COFACTOR n. a substance (e.g., a coenzyme) that must join with another to produce a given result.

COFFEE n. a *caffeine*-containing beverage made from the seeds of the coffee plant, sometimes useful in medicine as a *stimulant* to counter the effects of drowsiness (sometimes drug-induced) or as a treatment for some types of headache.

COGNITION n. the mental faculty of knowing, including perceiving, thinking, recognizing, and remembering. adj. **cognitive**

COHESION n. the force of molecular attraction. adj. **cohesive**

COITUS n. the sexual union of a man and a woman in which the *penis* is inserted into the *vagina*, usually accompanied by excitement and often *orgasm* and *ejaculation*. adj. **coital**

COITUS INTERRUPTUS n. a *contraceptive* method during *coitus* in which the penis is removed from the vagina before ejaculation in an effort to prevent *sperm* from entering the female's body. It is not considered a reliable method of contraception, however, because sperm are often released without sensation before ejaculation; also called **withdrawal method**.

COLCHICINE n. a pain-relieving drug, derived from the saffron plant, used to treat *gout*; common side effects include nausea, vomiting, and diarrhea.

COLD n. an infection involving the nasal passages and upper part of the breathing system (not including the lungs) and including such symptoms as a runny nose, watery eyes, and a sore throat. Caused by one of many different *viruses* (mainly rhinoviruses), a cold may be treated with rest, decongestants, and increased fluids, but usually not with *antibiotics*, which do not affect viruses (compare *coryza*, *influenza*, *rhinitis*); also called **common cold**.

COLD SORE n. a "fever blister" caused by *herpes simplex virus*, occurring on the skin or mucous membranes (e.g., at the corner of the mouth).

COLIC n. 1. acute pain in the gut, esp. intestinal pains with spasms (*cramps*); acute pain associated with passage of a stone or spasm of smooth-muscle tube or other organ, as in the passage of gallstones (biliary colic) or kidney stones (renal colic); 2. in infants, recurrent (usually daily, often at the same time of day) episodes of persistent crying, usually accompanied by signs of abdominal distress; it may be caused by intestinal gas (from air swallowed with food), though other explanations (e.g., neurological immaturity) have also been proposed. adj. **colicky**

COLITIS n. inflammation of the *colon*, either episodic and functional (*irritable bowel syndrome*, *spastic colon*) or more serious, chronic and progressive bowel disease (e.g., *Crohn's disease*, *ulcerative colitis*). Irritable bowel attacks, often precipitated by stress, are characterized by colicky pain and constipation or diarrhea; they are treated by stress avoidance and a bland diet. Chronic diseases lead to ulceration of intestinal tissue, bleeding, severe diarrhea, and other complications.

COLLAGEN n. a protein of connective and other tissues (e.g., *bone*, *cartilage*). adj. **collagenous**

COLLAGEN DISEASE n. any of several disorders (e.g., *ankylosing spondylitis*, *disseminated lupus erythematosus*, *polyarteritis nodosa*, *scleroderma*) marked by disruption of connective tissue.

COLLAPSE n. 1. general prostration; 2. a state of extreme depression or exhaustion; 3. deflation, as of a lung.

COLLARBONE see *clavicle*.

COLO- comb. form indicating an association with the *colon* (e.g., **colorectal**, pert. to the *colon* and *rectum*).

COLON n. the segment of large intestine from the *cecum* to the *rectum*. adj. **colonic**

COLONIC IRRIGATION n. washing out of the lower part of the bowel by forcing large amounts of water or another cleaning medium into it.

COLONY n. in microbiology, a group of organisms grown from a single parent cell.

COLORADO TICK FEVER n. a generally mild viral infection, transmitted by the bite of a tick and common in the Rocky Mountain area of the United States; it is characterized by headache; pains in the legs, eyes and back; and fever and chills, with the symptoms usually occurring in two episodes before final remission.

COLOR BLINDNESS n. any of various abnormal conditions characterized by an inability to distinguish colors. The most common form is *daltonism*, occurring mostly in males (approx. 8% of Caucasian males) as a sex-linked inherited trait characterized by an inability to distinguish red from green. Total color blindness, or achromatic vision, is rare and due to a defect of the *retina*.

COLOSTOMY n. the surgical creation of an opening (*stoma*) in the abdominal wall to allow material to pass from the bowel through that opening rather than through the *anus*. A colostomy may be temporary, to allow an inflamed area of the intestine to heal, or it may be permanent, as in cancer of the colon or rectum.

COLOSTRUM n. the first fluid given off by the mother's breasts just before or after the birth of her baby; it contains white blood cells, protective antibodies, protein, and fat in a thin, yellow fluid.

COLP-, COLPO- comb. form indicating an association with the *vagina* (e.g., colpitis, inflammation of the *vagina*).

COLPOCELE n. hernia into the *vagina*.

COLPOCYSTITIS n. inflammation of the *vagina* and *bladder*.

COLPOHYSTERECTOMY n. vaginal *hysterectomy*.

COLPOSCOPY n. visual examination of the upper *vagina* through an instrument (colposcope).

COLPOXEROSIS n. a condition in which the *vagina* is unusually dry.

COLUMN n. a pillarlike anatomical structure, esp. the spinal column and brain structures in the embryo.

COMA n. a state of profound unconsciousness, from which one cannot be aroused, resulting from drug action, toxicity (as in *nephritis*), brain injury, or disease. adj. **comatose**

COMBAT FATIGUE n. any of various mental disorders, resulting from fatigue and the stress of combat, characterized by depression, anxiety, and often memory and sleep disorders; it is usually temporary but may occasionally lead to long-term emotional disorders; also called **combat neurosis, shell shock**.

COMEDO n. commonly called a *blackhead*; an accumulation, in a hair follicle or oil gland, of dead cells and oily substance; it is the basic lesion in *acne* vulgaris. pl. **comedones**

COMMINUTED FRACTURE see under *fracture*.

COMMON BILE DUCT n. the duct, formed by junction of the hepatic and cystic ducts, that carries *bile* into the *duodenum*.

COMMON COLD see *cold*.

COMMUNICABLE DISEASE n. any disease transmitted from one person or animal to another, either directly through body discharges (e.g., nasal droplets, sputum, feces) or indirectly through substances or objects (e.g., contaminated drinking glasses, toys, bed linens) or *vectors* (e.g., flies, mosquitoes, ticks). Communicable diseases include those caused by viruses, bacteria, fungi, and parasites; also called **contagious diseases** (compare *infectious disease*).

COMPENSATION n. 1. adjustment after a change, to reattain balance or specific status for a part or function, as when the eye compensates for a change in light intensity by a corresponding change in *pupil* size; 2. making up for a physical injury or loss; as when a kidney enlarges after the other one is removed; 3. a defense mechanism for adjusting to real or imagined inadequacies, as when a student who cannot master a foreign language works very hard for good science grades. adj. **compensatory**

COMPLEMENT n. one of a series of enzymes, part of the immune-response mechanism in the blood serum, that works to break down invading microorganisms.

COMPLEMENT FIXATION n. an immunologic response in which an *antigen* combines with an *antibody* and its *complement* causing the complement to become inactive. This phenomenon is the basis of certain blood tests to determine the presence of antibodies against specific diseases.

COMPLEMENT FIXATION TEST n. blood test in which a sample of serum is exposed to a particular antigen and complement to determine whether antibodies to that particular antigen are present; used as a diagnostic aid (e.g., *Wasserman test* for syphilis).

COMPLETE BLOOD COUNT (CBC) n. determination of the number of red and white blood cells (and sometimes platelets) in a cubic milliliter sample of blood. One of the most common laboratory tests, it is an important aid to diagnosis (e.g., anemia, presence of infection). *Hemoglobin* levels may also be included in the test, as can determination of the percentages of the various types of white blood cells (*differential blood count*).

COMPLEX n. 1. in psychology, the related mental processes that interact to affect a person's behavior (e.g., inferiority complex); 2. a group of chemicals or materials, related structurally or functionally as in the immune system; 3. a group of symptoms (see *syndrome*).

COMPLEX FRACTURE n. see under *fracture*.

COMPLICATION n. any disease or other unwanted effect that occurs during the course of or because of another physical disorder (e.g., *bedsores* resulting from *paralysis*).

COMPOUND n. a substance composed of two or more elements chemically combined in definite proportions and usually differing in properties from the elements considered separately (e.g., table salt, nonpoisonous at normal levels, consists of two highly poisonous elements—sodium and chloride); generally, any combination of several things.

COMPOUND FRACTURE n. see under *fracture*.

COMPRESS n. a pad, usually of cloth or gauze (sometimes hot, cold, or medicated), applied with pressure to an inflamed part or to a wound to help control bleeding or to keep parts from protruding through a wound.

COMPRESSION BANDAGE n. a strip of cloth wrapped around a part to stop hemorrhage, immobilize the part, or keep fluid from collecting in a limb.

COMPRESSION FRACTURE see under *fracture*.

COMPULSION n. a persistent, irresistible urge to do something that is usually contrary to one's own standards or wishes; a compelling impulse (compare *obsession*).

COMPUTED TOMOGRAPHY (CT) n. a method for examining the body's soft tissues (e.g., the *brain*) using X rays, with the beam passing repeatedly (scanning) through a body part, and a computer calculating tissue absorption at each point scanned, from which a visualization of the tissue is developed. Formerly called computed (or computerized) axial tomography (CAT), the technique enables the radiologist to study normal structures as well as detect tumors, fluid buildup, dead tissue, and other abnormalities.

CONCAVE LENS n. a *lens* of glass or hard plastic that has one or both surfaces curved so the outer rim is thicker and the hollowed (caved) center is thinner; used to improve the vision of persons with nearsightedness (*myopia*).

CONCEPTION n. 1. fertilization of the female egg cell (*ovum*) by a male *sperm* cell; the beginning of pregnancy; 2. the originating of a new idea; 3. a concept.

CONCEPTUS n. the product of conception, the fertilized egg with its enclosing membranes in the *uterus* (see also *embryo, fetus*).

CONCHA n. a shell-shaped structure (e.g., the concha auriculae, in the ear) (compare *cochlea*). pl. **conchae**

CONCRETION n. 1. a stonelike formation within an organ (e.g., the kidney); 2. abnormal joining of two parts; solidification.

CONCUSSION n. a violent jarring or shaking, as from a severe blow or shock, esp. one to the head. A concussion may cause a limited period of *unconsciousness*.

CONDITION n. 1. a general term for the state of a patient; 2. a health *disorder*. v. to undergo physical training.

CONDITIONED RELFEX n. a *reflex* developed by training with a specific repeated stimulus, as in Pavlov's experiment in which a dog salivates at the sound of a bell after a period in which each feeding was preceded by the ringing of a bell.

CONDITIONING n. a psychological term for any of several types of learning that lead to specific responses to particular stimuli (see also *operant conditioning*).

CONDOM n. a thin sheath, usually of rubber or plastic, placed over the *penis* and used during *coitus* as a protection against venereal disease and as a reasonably effective *contraceptive*.

CONDUCTION n. the transport of energy through a system, as

impulses through the nerves or as sound waves to the inner ear.

CONDUCTION ANESTHESIA n. type of *anesthesia* produced by an anesthetic agent along the course of a nerve to inhibit the conduction of pain impulses to the area supplied by that nerve; also called *nerve block anesthesia*.

CONDUCTIVE HEARING LOSS n. type of hearing loss caused by inadequate conduction of sound through the external and middle ear to the inner ear; an increase in volume usually compensates for this defect (compare *sensorineural hearing loss*).

CONDYLE n. a rounded bump on a bone where it forms a joint with another bone or bones (as the rounded head of the *femur* into the cup-shaped *acetabulum*). adj. **condylar**

CONE n. a light-sensitive cell in the *retina* of the eye; the cones are responsible for color vision and visual sharpness. adj. **conic, conical**

CONFINEMENT n. 1. state of being restrained to a particular place to limit activity; 2. *labor* and childbirth.

CONFLICT n. a state of mental struggle and frustration caused by the simultaneous presence of equally desirable, undesirable or otherwise opposing or incompatible thoughts, drives, desires, or wishes.

CONFLUENT adj. merging, as tissues, *pustules,* or lesions.

CONFUSION n. state of mind in which one is unsure of the present time, place or self-identity, causing bewilderment and inability to act decisively; it usually indicates organic mental disorder but may also occur in times of severe stress.

CONGENITAL adj. present at birth. A congenital anomaly (abnormality) may be inherited, acquired during pregnancy, or inflicted as the result of the birth process; two examples are *cleft palate* and *Down's syndrome*.

CONGENITAL ANOMALY n. an abnormality, esp. a structural one, present at birth; also called **birth defect**.

CONGESTION n. an abnormal collection of blood or other fluid (e.g., mucus, bile), as in the lungs (pulmonary congestion).   adj. **congestive**

CONGESTIVE HEART FAILURE n. an abnormal condition characterized by circulatory congestion usually caused by a heart disorder and retention of salt and water by the kidneys; it usually develops chronically with shortness of breath, prolonged circulation time, and *edema* of the extremities. Treatment includes rest, *diuretics*, and oxygen and *digitalis*, if necessary.

CONJUNCTIVITIS n. inflammation of the mucous membrane lining of the eyelids and the front of the eye, caused by bacterial or viral infection, allergy, or irritation. The eyes look pink; the eyelids are stuck together in the morning, and there is discomfort, but usually not pain. Treatment depends on the cause; also called **pinkeye**.

CONNECTIVE TISSUE n. material that supports and binds other tissues and parts of the body; it includes *skin*, *bone*, *tendons*, *ligaments*, and interlacing fibrils. Many diseases of connective tissue are difficult to cure, e.g., *lupus erythematosus*, *rheumatoid arthritis*, and *sarcoidosis*.

CONN'S SYNDROME n. a disorder of the cortex of the *adrenal gland* (most often due to a benign tumor, rarely to another cause), in which excess secretion of *aldosterone* leads to disturbances in salt-water balance and symptoms of weakness, convulsions, muscular cramps and twitching, abnormal skin sensations (e.g., burning, itching), and sometimes paralysis.

CONSANGUINITY n. relationship by common ancestry (bloodline); blood relationship.

CONSCIOUS adj. alert, aware, or attentive; able to perceive and respond.

CONSTIPATION n. difficulty in having bowel movements because of loss of muscle tone in the intestine, very hard stools, or other causes (e.g., *diverticulitis*, intestinal obstruction). An increase in roughage (fruits, vegetables, bran) in the diet along with plenty of water often helps this condition.

CONSTITUTION n. a person's physical and mental makeup, including inherited qualities and general physique.

CONSULT v. to discuss with or seek advice from, esp. in deciding on diagnosis or treatment of a medical problem.   n. **consultation**

Types of connective tissue

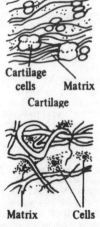

Cartilage
cells   Matrix
Cartilage

Matrix   Cells
Fibrous connective tissue

CONTACT DERMATITIS n. skin rash resulting from exposure to an irritant such as an alkali or acid (in, e.g., a cleaning product) or to a substance to which one has an allergic response (e.g., *poison ivy*).

CONTACT LENS n. a small, curved, glass or plastic lens placed on the eye to correct vision or deliver medication. The lens is fitted to the individual's eye and made to float on a tear film. Contact lenses must be inserted carefully and periodically removed and cleaned. Soft contact lenses, made of a hydrophilic plastic, are more comfortable and can be worn for longer periods than the earlier glass contact lenses.

CONTAGION n. the passing of disease from a sick person to others (see *communicable diseases*).

CONTAMINATION n. the inclusion, intentionally or accidentally, of unwanted substances or factors; pollution.

CONTINENCE n. 1. self-restraint or moderation, as in eating or in sexual activity; 2. the ability to hold urine and feces and to voluntarily control their passage from the body.

CONTRA- a prefix meaning "against" (e.g., *contraindication*) or "opposite" (e.g., *contrafissure* a fracture opposite the site of the blow).

CONTRACEPTION n. a process or technique for the prevention of pregnancy. Methods include total abstinence from *coitus*; *coitus interruptus* (withdrawal); periodic abstinence or *rhythm* (refraining from coitus during a woman's fertile time, the time around *ovulation*, which is determined by the *calendar method* or by determination of *basal temperature*); the use of mechanical devices to block sperm from moving up the female genital tract (including the *condom, diaphragm, intrauterine device* [IUD], *cervical cap,*

sponge); biochemical methods (birth control pill or *oral contraceptive,* hormonal injections); chemical means (*spermicidal* creams, jellies, foams and suppositories); and sterilization (*vasectomy* in men, *tubal ligation* in women).

CONTRACEPTIVE n. a means of preventing fertilization mechanically (e.g., by *condom, diaphragm, IUD, sponge, cervical cap*) by blocking the passage of sperm in the female reproductive tract; chemically by killing or immobilizing the sperm with spermicidal jellies, foams, creams, or suppositories; or biochemically by creating hormonal conditions in the female that make pregnancy impossible (e.g., *oral contraceptive pill*).

CONTRACTION n. 1. a shortening, or tension increase, as in muscle action; a persistent abnormal shortening; 2. in *labor,* rhythmic tightening of the upper uterine musculature that decreases the size of the uterus and pushes the fetus through the birth canal; uterine contractions typically begin mildly and then increase in severity and frequency, sometimes coming at a rate of one every two minutes and lasting about one minute.

CONTRACTURE n. abnormal, usually permanent contraction of a muscle due to atrophy of muscle fibers, extensive scar tissue over a joint, or other factors (see also *Dupuytren's contracture*).

CONTRAINDICATION n. any factor prohibiting the use of a particular procedure or drug for a specific patient because of the likelihood of unwanted results. For example, the administration of penicillin is contraindicated if the person has had a severe allergic reaction to the drug.

CONTRECOUP n. an injury to one side that results from a blow to the opposite side (as a blow to the forehead causing damage to the back of the skull or rear part of the brain).

CONTROL n. in experimental design, the standard used for comparison, as a *placebo*-receiving group of subjects in a drug-efficacy study.

CONTUSION n. a *bruise*; a superficial, nonlacerating injury from a blow.   adj. **contusive**

CONVALESCENCE n. a period of recovery from injury, illness, or surgery, generally the time after the crisis has passed until health is regained.

CONVERSION n. unconscious defense mechanism by which emotional conflicts are repressed and turned into physical symptoms having no organic base (e.g., pain, numbness).

CONVERSION HYSTERIA n. emotional disorder in which emotional conflicts are converted into physical symptoms (e.g., blindness, paralysis, pain). Treatment is by psychotherapy; also called **conversion disorder, conversion reaction**.

CONVULSION n. a sudden, involuntary and violent contraction of a group of muscles, sometimes with loss of consciousness; sometimes caused by high fever in otherwise healthy infants and young children, or it may occur in a seizure disorder (e.g., *epilepsy*) or following head injury.

COOLEY'S ANEMIA n. see *thalassemia*.

COORDINATION n. the working together of parts in performing a function, esp. of the muscles in body movements.

COPING n. an adjustment of one's activities to overcome stress in the environment without change in goals.

COPPER n. a metallic element essential to normal body function (see Table of Elements).

COPROLALIA n. repetitive use of obscenities in speech, as may occur involuntarily in *Gilles de la Tourette syndrome*.

COPULATION see *coitus*.

CORD n. an elongated, flexible part (e.g., the umbilical cord, vocal cords, and the spinal cord). adj. **cordal**

CORDITIS n. inflammation of the spermatic cord, caused by infection, hydrocele, tumor, or injury to the groin and characterized by pain and sometimes swelling and tenderness in the *testes*.

CORECTOPIA n. unnatural placement of the *pupil* of the eye toward one side, rather than the center, of the *iris*.

CORIUM n. the layer of skin below the *epidermis*; it consists of several layers and contains blood vessels, lymph vessels, hair follicles, glands, and nerves; also called **dermis**.

CORN n. horny mass of epithelial cells overlying a bone, usually on the toes and resulting from chronic pressure (e.g., from ill-fitting shoes). Treatment includes paring or peeling of the hard tissue and relief of the pressure.

CORNEA n. the outer, transparent portion of the eye, consisting of five layers through which light passes to the *retina*.   adj. **corneal**

CORNEAL TRANSPLANT (GRAFT) n. replacement of a diseased or damaged *cornea* with one taken from a donor eye, usually from a person who recently died.

CORNEUM n. the outermost, horny layer (stratum corneum) of the skin; the upper layer of the *epidermis*.

CORNU n. a hornlike part (e.g., the ethmoid cornu of the nose). adj. **cornual**

CORONA n. a crown or crownlike structure or part, as the enamel covering of a tooth (dental crown). pl. **coronae** adj. **coronal** (as the coronal suture of the skull).

CORONARY adj. surrounding, as a crown, esp. the **coronary arteries** surrounding the heart.

CORONARY ARTERY n. one of a pair of arteries that branch from the *aorta* and supply the heart. Any malfunction or disease of these arteries (coronary artery disease such as coronary *atherosclerosis*) can seriously affect the heart (e.g., depriving it of necessary oxygen and nutrients).

CORONARY BYPASS n. a type of open-heart surgery in which a prosthesis or section of a blood vessel (e.g., the saphenous vein) is grafted onto a *coronary artery* and connected to the *aorta* to bypass a diseased or blocked section of the coronary artery in an effort to improve the blood supply to the heart, decrease the work load of the heart, and relieve *angina*. The operation was introduced in the 1960's and has been widely used since, but the possible risks of *thrombosis* or closure of the graft and the benefits of alternate methods of treatment have recently made the operation somewhat controversial.

CORONARY CARE UNIT (CCU) n. a hospital area specialy equipped to treat patients with serious, life-threatening cardiac problems.

CORONARY INSUFFICIENCY n. abnormally limited blood flow through the arteries supplying the heart muscle, which can cause chest pain (*angina*).

CORONARY OCCLUSION n. an obstruction of a *coronary artery*, caused by a blood clot or progressive *atherosclerosis*.

CORONARY THROMBOSIS n. the presence of a blood clot in any of the arteries supplying the heart muscle, thereby obstructing the flow of blood to the heart (see also *thrombus*).

COR PULMONALE n. enlargement of the heart's right ventricle due to disease of the lungs (e.g., chronic obstructive lung disease, emphysema) or pulmonary vascular system. Symptoms include chronic cough, shortness of breath on exertion, fatigue, and other signs of oxygen lack to the body tissues.

CORPUS n. a specialized part that can be distinguished from the surrounding tissues (e.g., the corpus callosum, a white-matter bridge between the two hemispheres of the brain). pl. **corpora** adj. **corporeal**

CORPUS LUTEUM n. the so-called yellow body in the *ovary*; it is endocrine tissue that fills the space left by a released egg and is shed in menstruation if the egg (*ovum*) is not fertilized but remains to produce *progesterone* if *fertilization* occurs. pl. **corpora lutea**

CORPUSCLE n. any small body, esp. a red blood cell (*erythrocyte*) or a white blood cell (*leukocyte*). adj. **corpuscular**

CORRELATION n. the degree or extent to which two measures (variables) occur together. Statisticians report a correlation (symbol r) as ranging from $+1.0$ (absolute direct agreement) to -1.0 (absolute inverse relationship), with .0 being an uncorrelated, fully random relationship.

CORTEX n. the outer part of an organ, esp. that of the *brain* (*cerebral cortex*), *kidney* (renal cortex), or *adrenal gland* (adrenal cortex) (compare *medulla*) adj. **cortical**.

CORTIC-, CORTICO- comb. form indicating an association with an outer covering (cortex) (e.g., **corticospinal**, pert. to the brain's *cortex* and the *spinal cord*).

CORTICOSTEROID n. any of a group of hormones, including *cortisol* and *corticosterone* and other glucocorticoids as well as mineralocorticoids, produced in the adrenal cortex and important for the metabolism of carbohydrates and proteins, for water and salt balance, and for the function of the *cardiovascular system*, the kidneys, and other organs. These hormones are also produced synthetically, for use as drugs in the treatment of a very large variety of diseases, including deficiency of natural adrenal production and many inflammatory conditions (e.g., *rheumatoid arthritis*). Large doses and/or prolonged use of the drugs is associated with many side effects, including increased susceptibility to infection, fluid retention, emotional changes, and *peptic ulcer*.

CORTISOL n. the adrenal cortex hormone hydrocortisone, used in the treatment of *rheumatoid arthritis* and other inflammatory conditions.

CORTICOSTERONE n. a hormone of the adrenal cortex that promotes sodium (salt) retention.

CORTISONE n. a hormone of the adrenal cortex that functions in carbohydrate metabolism and which as a drug, is used to treat inflammatory conditions.

CORYZA n. inflammation of the mucous membranes of the nose, causing the nose to run (e.g., in allergic coryza, hay fever, common cold).

COSMETIC SURGERY n. any surgical procedure to improve the appearance of a part, esp. to remove scar tissue or a birthmark or excessive tissue, as on the face (face-lifting) or the nose (rhinoplasty) (see also *plastic surgery*).

COST-, COSTI-, COSTO- comb. form indicating an association with a *rib* (e.g., **costochondral**, pert. to a rib and its cartilage).

COSTA n. one of the 12 pairs of *ribs* forming the general shape of the chest (*thorax*). pl. **costae** adj. **costal**

COUGH n. a sudden, forceful and audible expulsion of air from the lungs that clears the air passages of irritants and helps to prevent aspiration of foreign particles into the lungs. It is a common symptom of a cold or other upper respiratory infection, of bronchitis, pneumonia, tuberculosis, or other lung disease, and of some forms of heart disease. Treatment depends on the cause; it may include use of *antitussive* drugs.

COUMADIN n. trade name for anticoagulant *warfarin*.

COUMARIN n. an *anticoagulant* drug used to prevent and treat a *thrombus* or *embolus*.

COUNT n. numerical indication of the number of items (e.g., blood cells, bacteria) in a particular unit or sample (see *blood count*).

COWPOX n. a mild disease characterized by a pustular rash and caused by vaccinia virus transmitted to humans from infected cattle. Cowpox infection confers immunity to *smallpox*, which is caused by a similar virus.

COXA n. the *hip*, the hip joint. pl. **coxae**

COXSACKIEVIRUS n. any of a group of viruses that infect the intestinal tract, producing a variety of symptoms, primarily affecting children in the summer months.

CPR see *cardiopulmonary resuscitation*.

CRAB LOUSE n. a body louse (*Phthirus pubis*) that infects the hair of the genital region and is often transmitted venereally.

CRADLE CAP n. a common *dermatitis* of infants characterized by thick, yellow, greasy scales on the scalp. Treatment is by oils and ointments to soften the scalp and by frequent shampoos.

CRAMP n. painful, often spasmodic, uncontrollable tightening of a muscle (e.g., in the calf) usually relieved by pulling the end of the affected part (the foot) in the opposite direction, stretching the involved muscle; pain resembling a muscular cramp.

CRANI-, CRANIO- comb. form indicating an association with the *cranium* or skull (e.g., **craniocerebral**, pert. to the skull and cerebrum).

CRANIAL NERVES n. the 12 pairs of nerves, each pair having sensory or motor functions, or both, that extend from the brain without passing through the spinal cord. (The XIth pair arise from both the brain and the upper spinal cord.) The 12 pairs of nerves are:

CRANIAL NERVES

Number	Name	Type	Function
I	olfactory	sensory	sense of smell
II	optic	sensory	sense of sight
III	oculomotor	motor	eye movements; pupil contraction
IV	trochlear	motor	eye movements
V	trigeminal	motor and sensory	facial sensation; jaw motions
VI	abducens	motor	eye movements
VII	facial	motor and sensory	facial expression; taste
VIII	vestibulocochlear (acoustic)	sensory	balance; hearing
IX	glossopharyngeal	motor and sensory	swallowing; taste
X	vagus	motor and sensory	swallowing; speech; taste
XI	(spinal) accessory	motor	swallowing; speech; head/shoulder movements
XII	hypoglossal	motor	tongue movements; proprioceptors

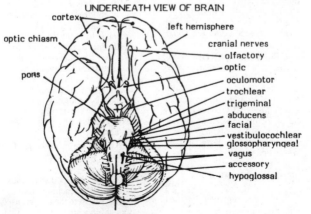

UNDERNEATH VIEW OF BRAIN

cortex
left hemisphere
optic chiasm
cranial nerves
olfactory
pons
optic
oculomotor
trochlear
trigeminal
abducens
facial
vestibulocochlear
glossopharyngeal
vagus
accessory
hypoglossal

medulla oblongata

Cranial nerves as they enter the underside of the brain.

CRANIOTOMY n. a surgical opening into the skull, performed to control bleeding, remove tumors, or relieve pressure inside the *cranium*.

CRANIUM n. the skull; specifically the bony enclosure of the brain; it is composed of eight bones (frontal, occipital, sphenoid, ethmoid, 2 temporal and 2 parietal).

CREATINE n. a compound produced in the body and found in muscle and blood, the phosphate form of which is an energy source for muscle flexion.

CREPITATION n. 1. a grating sound, as made by the rubbing of the ends of a fractured bone; 2. a crackling chest sound heard with the stethoscope. adj. **crepitant**

CREPITUS n. 1. the noisy release of bowel gas (*flatus*) from the intestine; 2. a grating or crackling sound (*crepitation*).

CRETINISM n. severe, congenital *hypothyroidism* characterized by *dwarfism*, mental retardation, coarse dry skin and features, and muscular incoordination. It results from thyroid deficiency or inadequate iodine intake by the mother while the fetus is developing. Relatively rare in the United States, the disorder occurs mainly in areas where the diet lacks sufficient iodine and *goiter* is prevalent.

CREUTZFELDT-JAKOB DISEASE n. a rare, fatal abnormality of the brain, caused by an unidentified *slow virus*; it typically occurs in middle age, producing symptoms of progressive *dementia*, difficulty in speech, muscle wasting, and involuntary movements, leading to death, usually within one year.

CRIB DEATH n. see *sudden infant death syndrome*.

CRISIS n. 1. the turning point in a disease, after which the patient either improves or gets worse; 2. the turning point in events affecting a person emotionally. pl. **crises**

CRISIS INTERVENTION n. in psychiatry, treatment to help resolve an immediate problem or reduce an emotional trauma, the aim being to restore the person to the precrisis level of functioning.

CRITICAL adj. being in or approaching a state of crisis in a disease; being at risk or in uncertain condition.

CROHN'S DISEASE n. a chronic inflammatory condition affecting the colon and/or terminal part of the small intestine and producing symptoms of frequent episodes of diarrhea (the feces are nonbloody and semisoft), abdominal pain, nausea, fever, weakness and weight loss. Treatment is by antiinflammatory agents; antibiotics, if necessary, to control infection; and adequate provisions for nutrition (compare *ulcerative colitis*).

CROSSED EYE see *strabismus*.

CROSSMATCHING n. procedure used by blood banks to determine the compatibility of donor's blood with that of a potential transfusion recipient after initial typing has been done.

CROUP n. a disease of infants and young children, characterized by harsh coughing, hoarseness, fever, and difficulty in breathing, usually due to viral infection. Mild cases can be relieved by the use of vaporizers, humidifiers, or steam from hot running water (to relieve spasm of muscles in the larynx), but children with high fever or severe respiratory distress should be hospitalized. adj. **croupy**

CRUS n. the leg from the knee to the foot. pl. **crura** adj. **crural**

CRUTCH n. a wooden or metal staff, usually reaching from the ground almost to the armpit, used as an aid in walking (e.g., with a broken leg).

CRY-, CRYO- comb. form indicating an association with cold (e.g., **cryogen**, a chemical that freezes and destroys diseased tissue).

CRYESTHESIA n. hypersensitivity to cold.

CRYOANESTHESIA n. insensibility resulting from deep cold.

CRYOCAUTERY n. 1. an instrument for destroying tissue by freezing it; 2. the application of a substance (e.g., carbon dioxide) that freezes and destroys tissue.

CRYOSURGERY n. the use of extreme cold (e.g., liquid nitrogen) to destroy unwanted tissue (e.g., warts, cataracts, skin cancer). The cooling agent is applied by means of a metal probe; temperatures as low as $-160°$ C can be achieved.

CRYPT n. a pocketlike structure, as in a part with deep indentations.   adj. **cryptic**

CRYPTORCHIDISM n. failure of one or both testes to move into the *scrotum* as the male fetus develops; also **cryptorchidy**, **cryptorchism**.   adj. **cryptorchid**

CRYPTOCOCCOSIS n. a disease, caused by the fungus *Cryptococcus neoformans*, in which jellylike nodules develop in internal tissues, often first in the lungs, causing symptoms of cough; and then spreading to the nervous system, causing headache and visual and speech difficulties. In North America, middle-aged men in the southeastern states are the prime victims. Treatment is by antifungal agents.

C-SECTION   see *Cesarean section*.

CT   see *computed tomography*.

CUBITUS n. 1. the elbow; 2. the arm from the elbow to the fingertips.   adj. **cubital**

CUBOID BONE n. a tarsal (ankle) bone on the lateral side of the foot.

CUL-DE-SAC n. a one-entry, pouchlike structure; a blind pouch (e.g., the *appendix*).

CULDOSCOPY n. a technique for visually examining the pelvic organs of a woman by insertion of a culdoscope (special instrument) through the vagina; the technique is incidentally used as a means of sterilization by the sealing of the uterine (Fallopian) tubes, making fertilization impossible.

CULTURE n. a deliberate growing of microorganisms in a solid or liquid medium (e.g., agar, gelatin), as of bacteria in a Petri dish.

CUNEUS n. wedge-shaped part of the back lobe of the brain.

CUPULA n. a part shaped like a small inverted cup (e.g., cupula pleurae, the roof of the pleural cavity).

CURARE n. a substance, derived from the tropical *Strychnos* plant, that is a powerful muscle relaxant used as an adjunct to *anesthesia*; in large doses it may cause paralysis and death.

CURET n. a scoop-shaped instrument used to remove material from a surface or cavity (e.g., the uterus) by scraping; also: **curette**.

CURETTAGE n. the scraping of a cavity, esp. the inside of the uterus or other surface, either to remove a tumor or other unwanted material or to obtain a sample of tissue for analysis.

CURIUM n. a radioactive metallic element.

CURVATURE n. outline of a part of structure, esp. the spinal column, that is not in a straight line.

CUSHING'S DISEASE n. disorder in which excessive secretion of ACTH by the pituitary (due, e.g., to a tumor) causes increased secretion of hormones by the adrenal cortex, leading to fat deposition on the face, back, and chest; edema; high blood sugar levels; muscle weakness; and increased susceptibility to infection. Treatment involves removal of ACTH-secreting tissue in the pituitary or if this is not possible, removal of the adrenal glands; also called **hyperadrenalism** (compare *Cushing's syndrome*).

CUSHING'S SYNDROME n. a disorder caused by excessive *cortisol*; symptoms include a moon face, mental or emotional disturbances, high blood pressure, weight gain, and, in women, abnormal growth of facial and body hair. The syndrome may be due to overproduction of cortisol by the adrenal glands or by prolonged administration of certain drugs (compare *Cushing's disease*).

CUSP n. 1. a tapered point, esp. those on the tops of the teeth; 2. any of the small flaps or leaflike divisions of the valves of the heart. adj. **cuspid**

CUTANEOUS adj. pert. to the *skin*.

CUTICLE n. 1. layer of skin at the base of the nail; 2. the *epidermis*.

CUTIS n. the pliable protective organ that covers the body; the *skin*.

CVA abbreviation for *cerebrovascular accident*.

CYAN-, CYANO- comb. form indicating blueness (e.g., **cyanoderma**, bluish discoloration of the skin).

CYANIDE POISONING n. poisoning from the ingestion of cyanide (found in bitter almond oil and wild cherry syrup) which causes rapid heart rate, drowsiness, convulsions, and frequently death within 15 minutes. Treatment involves *gastric lavage*, oxygen, and the use of certain drugs.

CYANOSIS n. bluish discoloration of the skin and mucous membranes, occurring when the oxygen in the blood is sharply diminished, as in carbon monoxide poisoning. adj. **cyanotic**

CYANOCOBALAMIN n. a vitamin of the B-complex group essential for normal metabolism, nerve function, and blood formation; rich sources are liver, kidney, and other meats and dairy products. Also used to prevent and treat *pernicious anemia* and certain other anemias; also called **vitamin B$_{12}$**; *antipernicious anemia factor*.

CYCLE n. a series of steps or events that occur regularly (e.g., the *menstrual cycle*, the monthly series of changes in a woman's body when pregnancy does not occur). adj. **cyclic**

CYCLOPIA n. developmental abnormality in which there is only one eye.

CYCLOPROPANE n. a flammable *anesthetic* gas that provides good anesthesia and skeletal muscle relaxation with minimal side effects, but has been largely replaced by safer nonflammable anesthetic agents.

CYPROHEPTADINE n. an antihistamine, known under the trade name Periactin, used to treat some allergic reactions. Adverse effects include drowsiness, dry mouth, rapid heart rate, and hypersensitivity reactions.

CYST n. 1. a closed, fluid-filled sac embedded in tissue (as in the breast) that is abnormal or results from disease; 2. an anatomically normal sac (e.g., the gallbladder or the **dacrocyst**, the tear sac in the eye).

CYST-, CYSTI-, CYSTO- comb. forms indicating an association with a cyst or with the bladder (e.g., **cystolith**, a stone in the bladder).

CYSTIC FIBROSIS n. an inherited disease, usually recognized in infancy or early childhood, in which the glands, esp. those of the *pancreas*, *lungs*, and *intestines*, become clogged with thick mucus. The sweat is typically salty, containing high levels of sodium and chloride. Respiratory infections are common and can lead to death. Life expectancy has improved markedly and many victims now reach adulthood; also called **fibrocystic disease of the pancreas; mucoviscidosis.**

CYSTITIS n. inflammation of the *urinary bladder* and *ureters*, characterized by pain, urgency and frequency of urination, and blood in the urine. More common in women, it may be caused by bacterial infection, stones, tumor, or trauma. Treatment depends on the cause and may include increased fluid intake and antibiotics.

CYSTOCELE n. a condition, sometimes occurring after childbirth, in which the urinary bladder bulges through the wall of the vagina.

CYSTOPLEGIA n. bladder paralysis.

CYSTOSCOPY n. examination of the *urinary bladder* by means of an instrument (cytoscope) inserted into it through the *urethra*.

CYT-, CYTO- comb. form indicating an association with a cell (e.g., **cytocide**, a substance that destroys cells).

CYTOGENESIS n. the developmental process in cell formation.

CYTOLOGY n. the science of cells, their development and functions.   adj. **cytologic**

CYTOLYSIS n. the breakdown of cells, esp. by the destruction of the cell's outer membrane.

CYTOMEGALOVIRUS (CMV) n. any of a group of herpes viruses that normally produce disease only in humans with impaired or immature immunological systems, including newborns, those being treated with immunosuppressive drugs (e.g., transplant patients), and those with *AIDS*.

CYTOPLASM n. all of the substance of a cell outside the *nucleus*.   adj. **cytoplasmic**

CYTOTOXIC adj. pert. to the destruction of cells.

CYTOTOXIC DRUG n. drug commonly used in chemotherapeutic treatment of cancer to inhibit the proliferation of cells.

d

D: VITAMIN n. a collective term for several chemicals (e.g., *calciferol*, *ergosterol*), contained naturally in fish liver oil and egg yolk, and essential to health, esp. the absorption of calcium and phosphorus (see Table of Vitamins).

DACRY-, DACRYO- comb. form indicating an association with tears (e.g., **dacryorrhea**, an excessive flow of tears).

DACRYOCYSTITIS n. inflammation of the lacrimal (tear) sac, due to obstruction of the tube draining the tears into the nose and characterized by tearing and discharge from the eye. Treatment is by antibiotics.

DACRYOPYOSIS n. a condition in which pus is present in the tear duct or gland.

DACTYL n. a finger or toe.

DACTYL-, DACTYLO- comb. form indicating an association with the fingers or toes (e.g., **dactyledema**, excessive fluid in a finger, causing it to puff up).

DACTYLOMEGALY n. abnormally large fingers and/or toes.

DALMANE n. trade name for sedative-hypnotic (*flurazepam* hydrochloride) used to treat sleep disturbances.

DALTONISM n. a sex-linked inherited form of color blindness characterized by the inability to distinguish the color red.

D AND C n. see *dilatation and curettage*.

DANDER n. scales from animal skins or hair or bird feathers, which may cause an allergic reaction in some persons.

DANDRUFF n. a condition in which scales of white flaky or grayish waxy material (dead skin) are shed by the scalp. Treatment involves regular use of a detergent shampoo.

DAPSONE n. drug used to treat *leprosy* and certain skin disorders.

DARK ADAPTATION reflex changes in the eye to allow vision in decreased light (e.g., in dim light after being in normal light); it involves a dilation of the pupil so that more light enters the eye (compare *light adaptation*).

DARVOCET n. trade name for a fixed combination drug containing the pain-reliever and fever-reducer *acetaminophen* and the pain reliever propoxyphene (*Darvon*).

DARVON n. trade name for a widely used prescription *analgesic* (*propoxyphene* hydrochloride); it is used to treat mild-to-moderate pain.

DARVON COMPOUND n. trade name for a fixed-combination prescription analgesic drug, containing *Darvon* (propoxyphene hydrochloride) and aspirin, phenacetin, and caffeine (APC); it is used to treat mild-to-moderate pain.

DATRIL n. trade name for nonprescription drug *acetaminophen*.

DDT n. abbreviation for dichlorodiphenyltrichloroethane, an insecticide once widely used in agriculture but now largely replaced by safer chemicals in many parts of the world. Inhalation or accidental ingestion of DDT may cause acute poisoning with symptoms of vomiting, malaise, tremors, convulsions, and abnor-

malities of heart and lung function and of the nervous system, leading to coma and death. Treatment is by gastric lavage, if necessary, and careful monitoring and response to specific symptoms.

DEAF adj. unable to hear.

DEAFNESS n. partial or complete loss of hearing in one or both ears, caused by the absence or incomplete development of the ear, the auditory nerve, or parts of the brain; by damage to the hearing apparatus (e.g., from infection or injury); or by degeneration (from aging) of the hearing apparatus. In assessing deafness, the degree of hearing loss, the types of sounds that can be discriminated, and the cause of the impairment—generally classified as *conductive hearing losses* or *sensorineural hearing loss*—are determined; treatment depends on these findings and may involve the use of a *hearing aid*.

DEATH n. a state of the body in which brain function ceases and heart function can be maintained only artificially; the state at which loss of brain and heart function is not reversible. In *brain death*, which has recently become of legal importance, normal reflexes (e.g., respiration) are absent and consciousness cannot be recovered; organs may then be removed for *transplantation* before the heartbeat has stopped.

DEATH INSTINCT n. in psychoanalytic (Freudian) theory, an unconscious urge to die.

DEATH RATTLE n. the gurgling sound that a dying person may produce as air is forced through fluid collected in the trachea and lungs.

DEATH WISH n. a desire, conscious or unconscious, for oneself or another to die.

DEBILITY n. weakness, lack of strength.

DEBRIDEMENT n. the removal of nonhealthy tissue and foreign material from a wound or burn to prevent infection and permit healing.

DECADRON n. trade name for a corticosteroid drug (*dexamethasone*) used to treat some inflammatory conditions.

DECALCIFICATION n. the loss of calcium from tissues, esp. bone.

DECAY n. 1. the gradual breakdown of dead tissue or other dead organic material, due to the action of microorganisms; 2. a process of decline or aging.

DECIDUA n. the epithelial tissue of the *endometrium*, the lining of the uterus, that is shed in *menstruation* and after the birth of a baby.   adj. **decidual**, **deciduous**

DECIDUOUS TOOTH n. any of the 20 teeth that appear during infancy and early childhood and are later shed, generally between the ages of 6 and 13, to be replaced by the permanent teeth; also called **milk tooth**; **primary tooth**.

DECLOMYCIN n. trade name for an antibacterial drug (the *tetracycline* demeclocycline hydrochloride) effective in the treatment of many bacterial, rickettsial, and other infections.

DECOAGULANT n. an agent that inhibits clot formation in the blood; also: **anticoagulant**.

DECOMPRESSION SICKNESS see *bends*.

DECONGESTANT n. a drug (e.g., epinephrine) that reduces *congestion*; decongestants may be applied as nasal sprays or drops or taken by mouth.

DECORTICATION n. removal of all or part of the outer layer (*cortex*) of an organ or structure, e.g., the kidney.

DECRUDESCENCE n. the lessening of severity of symptoms.

DECUBITUS n. the reclining position, as in a bed.

DECUBITUS ULCER n. inflammation or sore on the skin over a bony prominence (e.g., shoulder blade, elbow, hip, buttocks, heel), resulting from prolonged pressure on the area, usually from being confined to bed. Most frequently seen in elderly and immobilized persons, decubitus ulcers may be prevented by frequent change of position, cleanliness, and use of skin lubricants; once present, the ulcers must be washed and dried carefully, and a sterile dressing with moisturizing oil applied; if severe, debridement and drainage may be necessary; also called **bedsore**.

DECUSSATION n. a natural crossing over of fibers, esp. nerve fibers, or other parts, from opposite sides of the body, to form an X shape.

DEFECATION n. the passage of *feces* out of the body; bowel movement.

DEFECT n. an abnormality, either the absence of a part, ability, or function or its imperfect presence. A **congenital defect** is an imperfection, not necessarily inherited, present at birth.

DEFENSE n. the ability to resist or impede an attack of disease, infection, or other phenomenon.

DEFENSE MECHANISM n. a psychological, unconscious reaction or process for avoiding or controlling anxiety and emotional conflict (see *compensation*).

DEFERVESCENCE n. the time of fever decline.   adj. **defervescent**

DEFIBRILLATION n. the stopping, usually by electric shock, of heart muscle contractions that are out of normal rhythm (fibrillating). In this common emergency procedure, a defibrillator delivers an electric shock (of preset voltage) to the heart through the chest wall in an attempt to restore normal heart rhythm.

DEFICIENCY DISEASE n. any disease resulting from lack of a vitamin, mineral, or other essential nutrient. *Scurvy*, *rickets*, and *night blindness* are examples of deficiency diseases (see Table of Elements; Table of Vitamins).

DEFICIT n. a reduction, from the normal level, in the amount of a substance or in a level of function (e.g., oxygen deficit, a condition that exists in cells during temporary oxygen shortage caused by strenuous exercise).

DEFORMITY n. condition in which the body in general or any part of it (e.g., the hand) is misshapen, distorted, or malformed. A deformity may result from injury, disease, or birth defect (e.g., Arnold-Chiari deformity in which part of the brain protrudes through the skull).

DEGENERATION n. physical and/or mental decline that involves tissue and cellular changes and the loss of specialized function; the extreme result is death of the parts involved and loss of their function. adj. **degenerative**

DEGENERATIVE DISORDER n. any of several conditions that lead to progressive loss of function (e.g., *chorea*, *parkinsonism*).

DEGLUTITION n. the process of *swallowing*.

DEGUSTATION n. the act of tasting; the tasting sense (compare *gustation*).

DEHISCENCE n. the splitting open of an organ, part, or surgical wound.

DEHYDRATION n. extreme loss of water from the body tissues, often accompanied by imbalance of sodium, potassium, chloride, and other *electrolytes* in the body. Dehydration may occur in prolonged diarrhea, vomiting, or perspiration and is of more concern in infants and young children. Symptoms include thirst, dry skin, cracked lips, and dry mouth. Treatment involves restoring the fluid and electrolyte balance either by having the person drink liquids or by the intravenous administration of water and salts.

DÉJÀ VU n. a sense that what one is seeing or experiencing has been encountered before, when actually it has not. Déjà vu occurs in normal persons but is more frequent in certain disorders (e.g., some forms of *epilepsy*).

DELIRIUM n. a usually brief state of incoherent excitement, confused speech, restlessness, and hallucinations. It may occur in high fever, ingestion of certain toxic substances and drugs, nutritional deficiencies, endocrine imbalance, or severe stress (e.g., postoperative) or mental illness. Treatment includes bed rest, quiet, the use of drugs to quiet the patient, and treatment of the underlying cause (compare *dementia*). adj. **delirious**

DELIRIUM TREMENS (DTs) n. acute and severe (sometimes fatal) mental disturbance caused by prolonged and excessive alcohol intake or by withdrawal from alcohol use after prolonged drinking. Symptoms include loss of appetite and restlessness, followed by excitement, disorientation, sweating, shaking, anxiety, extreme perspiration, and terrifying hallucinations. The acute episode, a medical emergency, is followed by sleep and convalescence, sometimes plagued by complications such as respiratory infections, heart failure, and extreme fatigue. Treatment includes use of sedative drugs and adequate nutrition (usually including vitamin supplements) (see also *Korsakoff's psychosis*).

DELIVERY n. in obstetrics, the birth of a child.

DELTA RHYTHM n. a brain-wave frequency of high voltage that is characteristic of dreamless, deep sleep from which an individual is not easily aroused. It is the slowest of the four brain-wave patterns (compare *alpha rhythm, beta rhythm, theta rhythm*); also called **delta wave**.

DELTOID MUSCLE n. the large, thick triangular muscle that covers the shoulder and is involved in arm movements.

DELUSION n. a false belief; a continuing irrational idea that cannot be changed by logical argument. Delusions common in mental illness include delusion of grandeur, of persecution by others, and of affliction with disease. adj. **delusional**

DEMAND FEEDING n. giving food to a baby or animal whenever it shows a need, in contrast to schedule feeding, in which feedings are given according to a fixed, preset schedule (e.g., every four hours).

DEMENTIA n. a progressive state of mental decline, esp. of memory function and judgment, often accompanied by disorientation, stupor, and disintegration of the personality. It may be caused by certain metabolic diseases, drug intoxication, or injury, in which cases it is often reversible once the underlying cause is treated. In other cases it is caused by a disease (e.g., *Alzheimer's disease*), brain injury, or degeneration brought about by aging (*senile dementia*) that causes changes that are irreversible (compare *delirium*).

DEMENTIA PRAECOX n. obsolete for *schizophrenia*.

DEMEROL n. a trade name for a prescription *narcotic analgesic* (*meperidine*) used to treat moderate-to-severe pain.

DEMINERALIZATION n. loss of mineral salts, esp. from bone, as can occur in *hyperparathyroidism* and *osteomalacia*.

DEMULCENT n. an oil, salve, or other agent that soothes and relieves skin discomfort.

DEMULEN n. trade name for an *oral contraceptive*.

DEMYELINATION n. process of destruction or removal of the *myelin* covering of some nerve fibers, resulting in their impaired function; it occurs in *multiple sclerosis* and some other disorders.

DENDRITE n. one of the branching processes or treelike parts of a nerve cell that conveys impulses to the nerve cell body (compare *axon*). adj. **dendritic**

DENGUE n. a virus-caused disease, rare in the United States, that is transmitted by the Aëdes mosquito mostly in tropical and subtropical areas; it is marked by fever, muscle and joint pain, headache, and rash. Symptoms recur after a brief interval and the patient may require some time to recover.

DENT-, DENTA-, DENTI-, DENTO- comb. form indicating an association with the teeth (e.g., **dentalgia**, toothache).

DENTAL adj. pert. to a tooth or teeth.

DENTAL CARIES see *caries*.

DENTIN n. the bonelike major tissue found in a tooth, covering the *pulp* and being itself covered by the *enamel* above the gums; also: **dentine**.

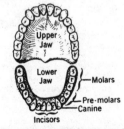

The arrangement of teeth in the upper and lower jaws.

DENTITION n. 1. the development and eruption of teeth (see *teething*); 2. the number, type, and arrangement of teeth in the mouth.

DENTURE n. a manufactured, removable replacement for one or more natural teeth.

DEOSSIFICATION n. loss or removal of the mineral content of bone tissue.

DEOXYRIBONUCLEIC ACID (DNA) n. a large molecule, shaped like a double helix and found primarily in the *chromosomes* of the cell nucleus, that contains the genetic information of the cell. The genetic information is coded in the sequence of subunits making up the DNA molecule (see also *gene*).

DEPENDENCE n. a state in the habitual use of a drug (e.g., her-oin) or other product (e.g., alcohol or tobacco) at which point adverse symptoms result upon withdrawal from use. adj. **dependent**

DEPERSONALIZATION n. a sense of dreamlike unreality and a loss of the sense of one's own identity, often resulting from stress or anxiety.

DEPILATORY n. a chemical or other agent that removes hair. adj. able to remove hair.

DEPOLARIZATION n. a loss, reduction, or change in the chemical or electrical polarity of a part such as occurs in the transmission of an impulse along a nerve fiber.

DEPRESSANT n. a drug that decreases or slows the function or activity of a body part or system (e.g., a cardiac depressant slows the heartbeat).

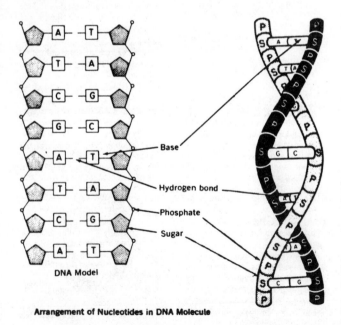

DNA Model

Base
Hydrogen bond
Phosphate
Sugar

Arrangement of Nucleotides in DNA Molecule

DEPRESSION n. 1. in anatomy, a hollow or depressed area, a downward placement; 2. in physiology, a decrease in function or activity; 3. in psychology, a dejected state of mind with feelings of sadness, discouragement and hopelessness, often accompanied by reduced activity and ability to function, unresponsiveness, apathy, and sleep disturbances. The condition may be mild and temporary, a sign of emotional disorder, or severe and long-lasting and a sign of serious *psychosis*. Treatment depends on the severity of the condition and may include psychotherapy, use of *antidepressant* drugs, and occasionally the use of electroshock therapy. Evidence indicates that a tendency toward some forms of depression may be inherited.

DEREISM n. a fantasy state in which thinking is removed from reality and logic, sometimes manifested in severe form in *schizophrenia*. adj. **dereistic**

DERM-, DERMA-, DERMO-, DERMATO- comb form indicating an association with the skin (e.g., **dermovascular**, pert. to blood vessels of the skin). adj. **dermal**

DERMA n. the skin. adj. **dermal**

DERMABRASION n. removal of scars, tattoos, and other marks by sanding or wire-brushing off some of the outer skin layer while the skin surface is frozen.

DERMATITIS n. acute or chronic inflammation of the skin, which becomes red and itchy and may develop blisters or other eruptions. There are many causes, including allergy, disease (e.g., *eczema*), and infection. Treatment depends on the cause.

DERMATOGLYPHICS n. the study of the patterns of lines (as whorls, loops, and arches in the fingertips, forming the fingerprints) on the hands and feet, which are unique to each person. Of interest to criminologists, these patterns are also significant in the study of genetic disorders.

DERMATOLOGY n. the medical specialty concerned with the skin and its development, function, diseases, and treatment. adj. **dermatologic, dermatological**

DERMATOME n. a surgical instrument for cutting thin slices of tissue for grafting.

DERMATOMYCOSIS n. a fungus infection of the skin, esp. on moist parts protected by clothing, as the groin or feet (e.g., athlete's foot); also: **dermatophytosis**.

DERMATOSIS n. a disorder of the skin, esp. one in which there is no inflammation (e.g., occupational dermatosis, skin disease caused by exposure to irritants on the job).

DERMIS see *corium*.

DERMOID CYST n. a tumor, with an epithelium-lined wall and a cavity containing fatty material or bits of bone, hair, and cartilage; most are benign.

DESCENDING AORTA n. main part of the *aorta* that runs from the aortic arch into the trunk of the body, consists of the thoracic and abdominal aortas, and from which arteries supplying many parts of the body (e.g., esophagus, ribs, stomach) branch.

DESCENDING COLON n. part of the *colon* extending from the end of the transverse colon on the left side of the abdomen in the region of the spleen downward to the *sigmoid colon* in the pelvis.

DESCENSUS n. a fall or drop, as of an organ from its original or normal position (e.g., descensus uteri, a dropping of the uterus until it protrudes from the vagina).

DESENSITIZATION n. 1. removal of the sensation of pain, as by cutting a nerve; 2. in immunology, relief from an allergic reaction to a specific foreign material (allergen or immunogen), as in desensitizing injections for hay fever sufferers; 3. in psychology, a treatment method for modifying fear-induced behavior, involving a gradual facing of the cause (e.g., being among animals) until it fails to induce fear or anxiety (compare *reciprocal inhibition*).

DESQUAMATION n. normal loss of bits of outer skin in the form of scales.

DETACHED RETINA n. separation of the *retina* from the *choroid* in the back of the eye, usually resulting from internal changes in the eye, sometimes from severe injury. Symptoms include the sensation of flashing lights as the eye is moved and the appearance of floating spots in front of the eye. Treatment is by *cauterization* or other surgery.

DETOXIFICATION n. process of removing a poison (*toxin*) or neutralizing its effect, normally a function of the *liver*.

DEVELOPMENT n. the gradual change from a simple to a more complex level; the physical, mental, and emotional changes an individual organism undergoes from its earliest form through its adult form. adj. **developmental**

DEVELOPMENTAL AGE n. a measure of a child's developmental progress in, e.g., body size, motor skills, or psychological functioning, expressed as an age (see also *bone age*, *chronological age*, *mental age*).

DEVIANT adj. varying from a normal state, esp. in behavior (see also *sexual deviant*).

DEVIATED SEPTUM n. an abnormal shift in position of any wall-like part that separates two chambers, most often referring to the nasal cavity. **Deviated nasal septum** is a common condition, causing symptoms of obstructed nasal passages, *sinusitis*, recurrent infection, nosebleeds, and difficulty in breathing. Treatment is by surgery.

DEVIATION n. 1. a movement away from a normal course or activity, as an abnormal deflection of the line of sight; 2. in ophthalmology, an abnormal position of an eye or the eyes.

DEXAMETHASONE n. a corticosteroid drug, known under the trade names Decadron and Oradexon, used to treat allergic reactions and inflammatory conditions. Adverse side effects include electrolyte and hormonal imbalances.

DEXEDRINE n. trade name for a central nervous system stimulant (dextroamphetamine sulfate) used in the treatment of *narcolepsy* and some hyperkinetic and attention-deficit syndromes in children; it was formerly used to reduce appetite in the treatment of obesity. Adverse side effects include restlessness, increased blood pressure, and other signs of central nervous system excitation; and nausea and loss of appetite. It must be used with caution in those with hypertension, cardiovascular disease, and many other disorders. It is potentially addictive.

DEXTR-, DEXTRO-, comb. form indicating a position to the right or a right-hand direction, motion, tendency, or relationship (e.g., **dextrocerebral**, pert. to right brain hemisphere-dominance) (compare *levo-*).

DEXTROCARDIA n. a condition in which the heart is positioned toward the right side of the chest. This may be a *congenital* defect, sometimes accompanied by reversal of the arrangement of other body parts (transposition) or it may be caused by disease.

DEXTROSE n. a simple sugar, also called *glucose*, used in intravenous feeding; table sugar (sucrose) is broken down to dextrose in the body.

DHOBIE ITCH n. a skin infection, caused by the fungus *Tinea cruris*, marked by ringed lesions in folds of the skin of the thigh region; it is aggravated by obesity, tight clothing, and warmth. Treatment is by antifungal agents and cold compresses (also called **jockstrap itch**).

DI- prefix meaning "two" (e.g., **diphasic**, having two phases).

DIABETES n. either of two disorders—*diabetes insipidus* and *diabetes mellitus*—in which a great amount of urine is passed. Used alone the term usually refers to diabetes mellitus.

DIABETES INSIPIDUS n. an uncommon metabolic disorder characterized by extreme thirst and the passing of very large amounts of urine; it is caused by failure of the pituitary gland to produce or secrete sufficient amounts of antidiuretic hormone (ADH) or less often by failure of the kidneys to respond to ADH; the pituitary (or kidney) malfunction may be due to trauma, surgery, or lesion, but in many cases the cause is unknown. Treatment is by removal of the underlying cause, if possible, and by administration of vasopressin (ADH) and careful monitoring to prevent dehydration and electrolyte imbalance, esp. in the young. Diabetes insipidus differs from diabetes mellitus in that in the former excessive sugar is not present in the blood or urine.

DIABETES MELLITUS n. a complex and chronic disorder of metabolism due to total or partial lack of *insulin* secretion by the *pancreas* (specifically by the beta cells of the islands of Langerhans in the pancreas) or to the inability of insulin to function normally in the body. Symptoms include excessive thirst and urination, weight loss, and the presence of excessive sugar in the urine and the blood. The disease is common and evidence suggests that the incidence is increasing. There are two major forms: generally more severe, inherited, juvenile diabetes and usually less severe adult, or late-onset, diabetes, which usually appears between the ages of 40 and 60; in adult diabetes a hereditary predisposition may be triggered by obesity, severe stress, pregnancy, menopause, or other factors. There is no cure for diabetes mellitus. Treatment depends on the severity of the disease; mild forms may be managed with diet alone, but other cases require the use of drugs to lower blood sugar levels (oral antidiabetics) or injections of insulin. Severe and/or untreated cases frequently lead to serious complications, including premature *atherosclerosis*, often affecting the legs and leading to ulcers of the feet; kidney disorders; and eye disorders, sometimes leading to blindness. (See also *diabetic coma*; *insulin shock*.)   adj. **diabetic** (as in *diabetic diet*).

DIABETIC COMA n. a loss of consciousness that can occur in *diabetes mellitus* as a result of failure to take prescribed *insulin* or the presence of some stress (e.g., infection, surgery) that increases the need for insulin. Warning signs include great thirst, headache, nausea, and vomiting. If left untreated, the condition can lead to death. Treatment includes the administration of insulin and steps to correct dehydration and electrolyte imbalances (compare *insulin shock*).

DIABETIC DIET n. a diet designed to help maintain normal levels of sugar in the blood in cases of *diabetes mellitus*. It may be used alone or in combination with drugs.

DIAGNOSIS n. identification of a disease or other condition by evaluating the patient's appearance, symptoms, and history; by physical examination; and, if needed, by analyzing the results of laboratory tests (e.g. urinalysis, blood count) and other procedures (e.g., X rays) (see also *differential diagnosis*). adj. **diagnostic**

DIALYSIS n. 1. a method, involving a semipermeable membrane, used to separate smaller particles from larger ones; 2. a medical procedure for filtering waste products from the blood of some kidney-disease patients or for removing poisons or drugs.

DIAPEDESIS n. the passage of blood cells through the intact walls of the vessels that contain them.

DIAPER RASH n. a reddening of the skin and eruption of spots and raised lesions in the diaper area of infants, caused by irritation from ammonia produced by the breakdown of urine or by irritation from feces or warmth. Treatment includes frequent diaper changes, careful washing, drying and ventilation of the affected area, and the use of antimicrobial agents.

DIAPHORESIS n. perspiration, esp. profuse perspiration associated with fever, stress, physical exertion or exposure to heat. adj. **diaphoretic**

DIAPHRAGM n. 1. the muscular partition that divides the chest from the abdomen and functions in respiration, moving downward during inspiration (breathing in) to increase the volume of the thoracic (chest) cavity and moving upward during expiration (breathing out) to decrease the volume; 2. a rubber or plastic dome-shaped cup that fits over the cervix of the *uterus* and that is used, with *spermicidal* jelly, as a *contraceptive*; it acts as a barrier to the passage of *sperm* upward in the female reproductive tract.

DIAPHRAGMATIC HERNIA see *hiatus hernia*.

DIAPHYSIS n. the shaft of a long bone (compare *epiphysis*). pl. **diaphyses**

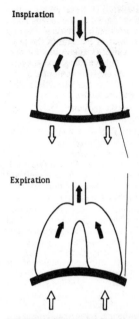

Inspiration

Expiration

During inspiration the diaphragm moves downward, the ribs move forward and outward, enlarging the chest cavity. Air then rushes in. During expiration the diaphragm rises, the chest cavity becomes smaller and air is forced out of the lungs.

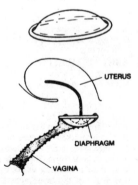

UTERUS

DIAPHRAGM

VAGINA

A diaphragm placed over the cervix

DIARRHEA n. the frequent passage of loose, watery stools (the stools may contain mucus, blood or excessive fat), sometimes accompanied by nausea, vomiting, abdominal cramps, and feelings of malaise and weakness. Diarrhea may be a symptom of a viral or bacterial infection (mild or severe), food poisoning, disorder of the colon (e.g., *colitis*), gastrointestinal tumor, metabolic disorder, or other disease. Untreated, it can lead to dehydration, electrolyte imbalance, and weakness. Treatment depends on the cause, but the symptom itself may be treated with an antidiarrheal drug (e.g., Lomotil).

DIASTOLE n. the period between two contractions of the heart, when the chambers widen and fill with blood. On heart muscle contraction (*systole*), the blood is pumped through the heart and into the arteries. (In blood pressure readings, diastole is the second [or lower] number given). adj. **diastolic**

DIATHERMY n. the use of high-frequency, ultrasound or microwaves to raise the temperature of a part of the body (e.g., the arm); sometimes used to treat deep-seated pain.

DIAZEPAM n. a minor tranquilizer, commonly known under the trade name Valium, used to treat anxiety and tension, and as a skeletal muscle relaxant in cases of muscle spasm, and as an anticonvulsant in some cases of epilepsy; it is commonly prescribed for many conditions. The drug may cause drowsiness and fatigue, and withdrawal symptoms may occur after discontinuance of prolonged or high-dosage use.

DICK TEST n. a skin test for determining susceptibility to *scarlet fever*. The toxin responsible for scarlet fever is injected through the skin; if an inflammation appears, the person is not immune to the disease.

DICLOXACILLIN n. antibacterial drug used to treat staphylococcal infections, esp. those resistant to penicillin.

DICUMAROL n. an *anticoagulant* prescribed to prevent and treat *embolism* and *thrombosis*; adverse side effects include gastrointestinal disturbances such as nausea and diarrhea; its use has been largely replaced by newer, safer drugs (e.g., warfarin preparation [Coumadin]); also: **dicoumarol.**

DIET n. 1. the food and drink one normally takes; 2. a special schedule of food and drink to meet particular needs (as in the treatment of *diabetes mellitus*). See also *high-protein diet.*

DIETHYLSTILBESTEROL (DES) n. a nonsteroid manufactured (synthetic) chemical that has the properties of *estrogen*, a female sex hormone. It is used to treat problems of *menopause* and *menstruation* and to limit milk production in the breasts. It was formerly used in cases of threatened abortion and has now been found to be associated with a higher-than-normal incidence of vaginal cancer (and other cancers of the reproductive tract) in the daughters of women so treated during pregnancy.

DIFFERENTIAL BLOOD COUNT n. enumeration (numbers or percentages) of the specific types of *white blood cells* found in a given volume (usually 1 cubic milliliter) of blood; used as an aid to *diagnosis.*

DIFFERENTIAL DIAGNOSIS n. a systematic method for diagnosing a disorder that lacks unique signs or symptoms; for example, headache may have many causes and the patient's other symptoms as well as the results of laboratory tests and other procedures must be considered in arriving at a correct diagnosis.

DIFFERENTIATION n. the process of changing from an original unspecialized form to a different, more specialized, form or function, e.g., cell differentiation in the developing *embryo*.

DIFFUSION n. the movement of particles from an area of high concentration to an area of low concentration to produce an even distribution in the available space.

DIGESTION n. the process of breaking down food, by mechanical (e.g., chewing, churning) and chemical (e.g., the action of enzymes) means, into substances that can be absorbed and used by the body.

DIGESTIVE SYSTEM n. those parts of the body that function in a coordinated manner for the digestion and absorption of food. It includes the *digestive tube* and accessory organs (e.g., *gall bladder*, *liver*) that secrete enzymes used in the digestion of foods.

DIGESTIVE TUBE n. tube, of mucous membrane and muscle tissue, about 8.3 meters (27 feet) long in the adult, extending from the *mouth* through the *pharynx*, *esophagus*, *stomach*, *small intestine* and *large intestine* to the *anus*; also called **alimentary canal** (see also *digestive system*).

DIGITALIS n. any of several drugs (e.g., *digoxin*, *digitoxin*) derived from foxglove plants (*Digitalis* genera) and sold under various trade names, used to strengthen heart muscle contraction and regulate the beat of poorly functioning hearts.

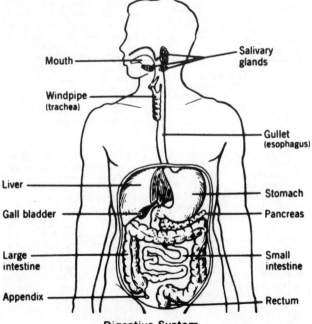

Digestive System

DIGITATE adj. having fingers or fingerlike projections.

DIGITOXIN n. a drug—a digitalis preparation, sold under various trade names (e.g., Crystodigin)—used to treat congestive heart failure and other abnormalities of heart rhythm.

DIGOXIN n. a drug—a digitalis preparation sold under various trade names (e.g., Lanoxin)—used to treat congestive heart failure and certain heart rhythm abnormalities.

DILANTIN n. trade name for a nonsedative *anticonvulsant* drug (diphenylhydantoin) used in the treatment of epilepsy.

DILATATION n. enlargement of an organ or an opening, either as a normal physiologic response (e.g., widening of the *pupil* of the eye as a response to decreased light, widening of the uterine *cervix* during labor to allow passage of the baby) or done deliberately as in the use of drugs to widen the pupil of the eye or the use of a dilator to open the cervix.

DILATATION AND CURETTAGE (D & C) n. dilatation of the *cervix* of the uterus and scraping of the *endometrium* (lining) of the uterus. It is a common procedure, usually performed using local anesthetic, to remove uterine tissue for examination and diagnosis, to stop prolonged or heavy bleeding, to remove the products of conception (a method of *abortion*), to remove retained fragments of the placenta after childbirth or abortion, and to remove small tumors.

DILAUDID n. trade name for a narcotic pain reliever (*hydromorphone* hydrochloride) used to treat moderate-to-severe pain.

DILUTION n. decrease in the amount of a substance in a solution for each unit of volume, usually the result of adding water to increase the volume.

DIMETANE n. trade name for an *antihistamine* (brompheniramine maleate) used to treat hypersensitivity reactions, including rhinitis, itching, and skin reactions. Adverse side effects include drowsiness, dry mouth, and rapid heartbeat.

DIMETAPP n. trade name for a fixed-combination drug containing two decongestants (phenylephrine hydrochloride and phenylpropanolamine hydrochloride) and an antihistamine (brompheniramine maleate [Dimetane]); it is used to relieve nasal congestion and to treat certain hypersensitivity reactions such as rhinitis.

DIMETHYL SULFOXIDE (DMSO) n. an anti-inflammatory agent used topically to treat some injuries.

DIPHENHYDRAMINE n. an *antihistamine* drug, commonly known under the trade name Benadryl, used to treat hay fever and other allergic reactions involving the nasal passages. It is also sometimes used to treat motion sickness and to produce sedation.

DIPHTHERIA n. an acute, contagious infection caused by the bacterium *Corynebacterium diphtheriae*, which produces a toxin affecting the whole body and characterized by severe inflammation of the throat and larynx with production of a membrane lining the throat, along with fever, chills, malaise, brassy cough, and, in some cases (esp. if untreated or unusually severe) by impaired function of the heart muscle and peripheral nerves. More common in children and once epidemic in many parts of the world, it is now rare in the United States because of routine immunization (*DPT*) against the disease. Treatment is by diphtheria antitoxin, antibiotics, rest, increased fluid intake, and *tracheostomy*, if necessary (see also *Schick test*).

DIPLOID adj. pert. to an individual or cell that has two complete sets of homologous chromosomes, one set from each parent; the diploid chromosome number is found in somatic (body) cells, not in gametes (sex cells), and is characteristic for each species, being 46 in normal human body cells (compare *haploid*).

DIPLOMATE n. a specialist whose competence has been certified by the appropriate professional group (e.g., the American Board of Internal Medicine).

DIPLOPIA n. double vision, in which a single object is seen as two objects. If one eye is covered, diplopia often disappears.

DIPSOMANIA n. an intense, persistent desire to drink alcoholic beverages to excess; alcoholism.

DIS- prefix meaning "reversal," "removal," "exclusion," or "separation" (e.g., **disarticulation**, separation of two bones in a joint).

DISABILITY n. a weakness, defect, disorder, or other impairment that results in reduction or loss of mental or physical function; an incapacity.

DISC n. a flattened, rounded part, esp. referring to the cushioning tissues between the *vertebrae*; also: **disk.**

DISCHARGE n. 1. a substance that is excreted from an organ or part; 2. the electrical action of a nerve cell.

DISCOID LUPUS ERYTHEMATOSUS (DLE) n. a chronic, recurrent disease, thought to be an *autoimmune disease* and occurring primarily in women between 20 and 40 years of age, characterized by a butterfly-shaped eruption of scale-covered red lesions over the cheeks and bridge of the nose (sometimes in other areas). Treatment includes avoidance of the sun or use of a sunscreen and use of steroid and antimalarial drugs (compare *systemic lupus erythematosus* [SLE]).

DISEASE n. 1. an impairment of health or a condition of abnormal functioning; 2. a disorder with recognizable symptoms (e.g., fever, inflammation) that result from infection, improper diet, or other cause.

DISEQUILIBRIUM n. loss or weakness of balance.

DISINFECT v. to kill germs that may cause infection.

DISK see **disc.**

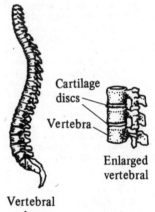

Cartilage discs

Vertebra

Enlarged vertebral

Vertebral column

Discs separate and cushion the vertebrae.

DISLOCATION n. the displacement of a part, esp. a bone, from its normal position, as in a shoulder or the *vertebral column*.

DISORIENTATION n. mental confusion, characterized by a loss of awareness of space, time or personal identity; it may be caused by drugs, severe stress, or organic disease.

DISPENSARY n. 1. a place, such as a physician's office or pharmacy, where medicines and other curative materials are given to patients; 2. a free clinic for outpatients.

DISPLACEMENT n. 1. the shifting of something out of its normal position; 2. unconscious transfer of feeling from an originally experienced object to another, more acceptable one (a *defense mechanism*).

DISSECTION n. separation of body tissues, usually along natural divisions, by cutting or probing, for visual or microscopic examination.

DISSEMINATED LUPUS ERYTHEMATOSUS see *systemic lupus erythematosus*.

DISSOCIATION n. 1. the reversible separation of chemical molecules into simpler forms; 2. in psychiatry, separation of certain ideas, thoughts or emotions from the consciousness, often as a *defense mechanism*.

DISSOCIATIVE DISORDER n. neurosis in which repressed emotional conflict causes a separation in the personality with confusion in identity. Marked by symptoms of amnesia, dream state, or multiple personality, it is treated with psychotherapy, hypnosis, and antianxiety drugs (compare *conversion disorder*).

DISTAL adj. 1. away from the center; toward the far end of something; 2. farthest from the point of origin (compare *proximal*).

DISTENSION n. a state of being stretched out or enlarged, as abdominal distension from gas (*flatus*).

DISTILLED WATER n. water cleansed of impurities and microorganisms by converting it into steam and then condensing it again (usually several times) as a liquid. It has many uses, as for mixing chemicals and irrigating body parts.

DISULFIRAM n. an alcohol deterrent, commonly known under the trade name Antabuse, used in the treatment of alcoholism. It causes nausea, abdominal cramping, and sweating if alcohol is ingested. Adverse reactions include optic neuritis and polyneuritis; drowsiness and skin eruptions occur in some patients. The drug interacts with many other drugs and must be used with caution in those taking drugs for many disorders.

DIUCARDIN n. trade name for a *diuretic* and *antihypertensive* agent used to treat edema, congestive heart failure, and high blood pressure.

DIUPRES n. trade name for a fixed-combination drug, containing a *diuretic* (Diuril) and antihypertensive agent *reserpine*, sometimes used to treat high blood pressure.

DIURESIS n. increased secretion of urine, usually due to drinking large amounts of liquid or the action of a diuretic drug (e.g., Diuril, Lasix) or occurring as a symptom of disease (e.g., *diabetes mellitus*).

DIURETIC n. a drug that promotes the production and excretion of urine; it is commonly used in the treatment of edema, hypertension, and congestive heart failure. There are several types of diuretics, including thiazides (e.g., *chlorothiazide* [Diuril] and hydrochlorothiazide [Esidrix]), loop diuretics (furosemide [Lasix]), and others (spironolactone [Aldactone]). Several adverse reactions are common to diuretics, chiefly electrolyte (esp. sodium and potassium) imbalances.

DIURIL n. trade name for a diuretic (*chlorothiazide*) used to treat edema and hypertension.

DIVERTICULITIS n. inflammation of an abnormal sac (*diverticulum*) at a weakened point in the digestive tract, esp. the colon. Symptoms include cramplike abdominal pain, fever, and diarrhea or constipation. Treatment is by rest, antibiotics; severe cases may require surgery.

DIVERTICULOSIS n. the presence of abnormal pouchlike sacs through the muscular layers of the colon. The condition, increasingly common in persons over the age of 50, produces few or no symptoms, except occasional rectal bleeding (compare *diverticulitis*).

DIVERTICULUM n. a pouchlike herniation through the muscular wall of a tubular organ, esp. the colon.   pl. **diverticula**

DIZYGOTIC TWINS   n. see *fraternal twins*.

DIZZINESS n. a sensation of unsteadiness, faintness or whirling in space, often with inability to maintain balance; it has many causes, including middle-ear disorder, drug (including alcohol) intoxication, and hypertension. A dizzy person is in danger of falling and therefore should be placed on a bed or the floor.

DMSO n. see *dimethyl sulfoxide*.

DNA n. see *deoxyribonucleic acid*.

D.O.A. n. abbreviation for "dead on arrival," a term used by physicians, ambulance personnel, and others to signify that the patient was dead on arrival at the hospital or other health-care facility.

DOLOR n. pain, adj. **dolorific**

DOMINANCE n. the ability of a specific genetic characteristic to appear at the expense of another (compare *recessive*).

DONNATAL n. a fixed-combination drug, containing a sedative (*phenobarbital*) and several other agents, used to decrease gastrointestinal spasm.

DONOR n. a person who gives living tissue (e.g., eye, blood) to be used in another person.

DOPAMINE n. a chemical found in the brain and elsewhere in the body that functions as a *neurotransmitter*. As a drug, also known under the trade names Dopastat and Intropin, it is used to treat shock and hypotension.

DORIDEN n. a trade name for a sedative (*glutethimide*) used to treat anxiety and insomnia.

DORSAL adj. pert. to the back or posterior (compare *ventral*).

DORSI-, DORSO- comb. form indicating an association with the back (dorsum) (e.g., **dorsolateral**, pert. to the back and sides).

DORSIFLEXION n. the bending of a part backward.

DORSUM n. 1. the back; 2. the back surface of any part, e.g., the dorsum of the hand. pl. **dorsa** adj. **dorsal, dorsalis**

DOSAGE n. the schedule of how much and how frequently a drug or other therapeutic agent (e.g., vitamins) is to be administered.

DOSE n. the amount of a medication or other substance, or of radiation, to be given at one time (see also *lethal dose*).

DOSIMETRY n. 1. measurement of the dose of radiation emitted by a radioactive source; 2. calculation of the appropriate dose of radiation to treat a particular condition in a particular patient.

DOUBLE-BLIND STUDY n. an experiment in which neither the investigator nor the subject knows whether the subject received the experimental variable (e.g., a drug) or a *placebo*, thus reducing any influence such knowledge might have on the reactions of the subject and the expectations or interpretations of the investigator.

DOUBLE PNEUMONIA n. pneumonia of both lungs at the same time.

DOUBLE VISION n. see *diplopia*.

DOUCHE n. introduction of a jet of water or special fluid into or around a given part, esp. the vagina, to cleanse or free the part from odor-causing contents, or to treat pelvic or vaginal infection.

DOWN'S SYNDROME n. a congenital defect, usually caused by the presence of an extra No. 21 chromosome (trisomy) and characterized by mental retardation (the I.Q. averages 50–60); oblique placement of the eyes; a small head flattened at the back; a large, furrowed tongue; short stature; bowel defects; and heart abnormalities. The syndrome, the most common of the chromosomal abnormalities, is associated with advanced maternal age, esp. over age 35 (1 in 80 offspring of women over age 40 will be affected); it can be detected through *amniocentesis*. Care of a Down's syndrome child involves both the prevention of physical problems (e.g., respiratory infections to which these children are especially prone) and long-range programs to promote mental and motor skills. (A less common form of the disease, caused by a translocation of a chromosome, is an inherited [genetic] defect, not associated with maternal age).

DOXEPIN n. a tricyclic *antidepressant* drug, known under the trade names Sinequan and Adapin, used to treat depression. Side effects include sedation, dry mouth, and gastrointestinal, cardiovascular, and neurologic disturbances.

DOXYCYCLINE n. a *tetracycline antibiotic*, also known under the trade name Vibramycin, effective against many infections.

DPT VACCINE n. abbreviation for diphtheria and tetanus toxoids and pertussis (whooping cough) vaccine. The combination vaccine is usually given in a series of injections during infancy and early childhood.

DRAIN n. a tube inserted into a body cavity, sometimes during surgery, to remove unwanted material.

DRAINAGE n. the drawing off of fluid from a body cavity, usually fluid that has accumulated abnormally.

DRAMAMINE n. trade name for a drug (dimenhydrinate) used to prevent and treat nausea, esp. that due to motion sickness.

DRIVE n. the natural force that compels one to an action, as the hunger drive directs one to eat. The basic drives are sex, hunger, and thirst. A secondary drive is a learned or acquired drive, not directly related to satisfying a physical need (e.g., a striving for recognition).

DRIXORAL n. trade name for a fixed-combination drug containing an antihistamine, a bronchodilator, and a vasoconstrictor; it is used to treat upper respiratory congestion.

DROP FOOT n. a condition in which the foot is flexed toward the sole (plantar surface) or droops and cannot be voluntarily flexed toward a normal position.

DRUG n. 1. substance taken by mouth, injection, or applied locally to prevent or treat a disorder (e.g., to ease pain); 2. a chemical substance introduced into the body to cause pleasure or a sense of changed awareness, as in the nonmedical use of *lysergic acid diethylamide* (LSD).

DRUG ABUSE n. use of a drug for nontherapeutic purposes (e.g., to alter one's sense of awareness, as with LSD). Commonly abused substances include barbiturates, alcohol, sedatives, and amphetamines. Drug abuse can lead to physical and mental damage and, with some substances, to drug dependence and addiction.

DRUG ADDICTION n. a condition marked by an overwhelming desire to ingest or otherwise take a drug to which one has become habituated because of long-term use and by the development of withdrawal symptoms (mental and/or physical) if the drug is not taken. Heroin and barbiturates are common addictive drugs.

DRUG DEPENDENCE n. a condition in which one craves or depends on a particular drug that one is accustomed to taking.

DRY SOCKET n. inflammation at the site of an extracted tooth, characterized by pain, pus and frequently infection.

DUCHENNE'S MUSCULAR DYSTROPHY see *muscular dystrophy*.

DUCT n. a tubelike channel for carrying fluids or other materials from one organ or part to another (e.g., the *bile duct*, which carries bile to the *duodenum*).

DUCTLESS GLANDS n. see *endocrine glands*.

DUCTULE n. a small duct, e.g., one of the small tubes found in the tear glands.

DUCTUS ARTERIOSUS n. a blood vessel in the fetus connecting the pulmonary artery directly to the ascending aorta, thus bypassing the pulmonary circulation. It normally closes at birth; failure to close—**patent ductus arteriosus**—often requires surgical correction.

DUCTUS DEFERENS n. duct, about 45 centimeters (18 inches) long, leading from *testis*, looping around the bladder, and ending in the *ejaculatory duct*; also **vas deferens**.

DUMPING SYNDROME n. a group of symptoms, including nausea, dizziness, sweating, and faintness, occurring after a meal, particularly a meal rich in carbohydrates, in patients who have had stomach surgery; it is due to a too-rapid emptying of the stomach contents and the development of low sugar levels in the blood.

DUODENO- comb. form indicating an association with the *duodenum* (e.g., **duodenocholan-**

geitis, inflammation of both the duodenum and the common *bile duct*).

DUODENAL ULCER n. an ulcer in the *duodenum*; it is the most common type of *peptic ulcer*.

DUODENUM n. the first part of the small intestine; it receives material from the stomach (through the pyloric valve) and passes it to the jejunum, the medial part of the small intestine. The duodenum plays a vital role in digestion, receiving acid chyme from the stomach, bile from the bile duct, pancreatic juices from the pancreas, and intestinal juices—all of which function in the chemical breakdown of food molecules.   adj. **duodenal**

DUPUYTREN'S CONTRACTURE n. a painless condition in which the fourth and fifth fingers bend into the palm of the hand and resist extension due to a progressive thickening of tissue beneath the skin in the palm. Of unknown cause, it primarily affects middle-aged men. Treatment involves surgical excision of the excess tissue.

DURA MATER n. thickest and outermost of the three membranes (*meninges*) that enclose the brain and spinal cord (the others being the *pia mater* and the *arachnoid*).

DWARFISM n. underdevelopment of the body, characterized primarily by abnormally short stature, often with underdeveloped limbs and with other defects. Causes include genetic defects, pituitary or thyroid malfunctioning, kidney disease, and certain other disorders.

DYADIC adj. pert. to a relationship involving two persons, e.g., that of doctor and patient in therapy, esp. psychotherapy.

DYAZIDE n. trade name for fixed-combination drug containing two *diuretics* (hydrochlorothiazide and triamterene); it is used to treat *hypertension* and *edema*.

DYNAMO- comb. form indicating force or strength (e.g., **dynamogenesis**, energy development).

DYS- comb. form meaning "bad," "abnormal," "difficult," "adverse" (e.g., dysesthesia, distorted sense, esp. of touch).

DYSAPHIA n. defect in the sense of touch.

DYSARTHRIA n. difficulty in pronouncing words clearly or correctly, usually because of poor control over the speech muscles.

DYSCHEZIA n. difficulty in passing stools, usually from long-continued, voluntary suppression of the urge to defecate.

DYSCRASIA n. any diseased or imbalanced state of the body or its systems (e.g., blood dyscrasia, any abnormal condition of the blood). adj. **dyscratic**

DYSENTERY n. intestinal inflammation caused by bacteria, protozoa, parasites, or chemical irritants and marked by abdominal pain; frequent, bloody stools; and rectal spasms. Treatment includes replacement of lost fluids and sometimes antibiotics. adj. **dysenteric**

DYSEQUILIBRIUM n. any abnormality in the sense of balance.

DYSFUNCTION n. a state in which the proper response or activity of a part (e.g., a muscle) or organ is weak, absent, or otherwise abnormal. adj. **dysfunctional**

DYSFUNCTIONAL UTERINE BLEEDING n. uterine bleeding due to hormonal imbalance, not diseased condition (e.g., uterine tumor).

DYSGENESIS n. abnormal development of an organ or part, esp. in the embryo stage. adj. **dysgenic**

DYSGRAPHIA n. an impairment of the ability to write correctly, due to a brain or motor disorder.

DYSKINESIA n. difficulty in carrying out voluntary movements (see also *tardive dyskinesia*). adj. **dyskinetic**

DYSLEXIA n. an impairment of the ability to read in which letters and words are reversed. Dyslexia, which affects more boys than girls, is usually linked to a central nervous system disorder, although some experts believe that it represents a complex of problems, possibly including visual defects, impaired hearing, stress, and inadequate instruction. adj. **dyslexic**

DYSLOGIA n. impairment of the power to think logically and rationally.

DYSMENORRHEA n. painful menstruation. Primary dysmenorrhea, intrinsic to the process of menstruation and not the result of any other disease or condition, is very common. Typically, cramplike pain in the lower abdomen, sometimes accompanied by nausea, vomiting, intestinal cramps and other discomfort begins just before or with the onset of menstrual flow; oral contraceptives and antiprostaglandins lessen the discomfort but for some women in whom the pain is severe potent analgesics may be needed. Secondary dysmenorrhea, caused by a specific disorder (e.g., uterine tumor, pelvic infection, *endometriosis*), is usually marked by pain that lasts longer and is often accompanied by bladder or bowel discomfort; treatment depends on the underlying cause.

DYSOSMIA n. a condition in which the sense of smell is impaired.

DYSPAREUNIA n. an abnormal condition in women in which sexual intercourse is painful; it may be caused by abnormality of the genitalia, psychophysiological reactions, inadequate sexual arousal, or other factors.

DYSPEPSIA n. stomach upset; a disorder of the digestive function, marked by vague discomfort, heartburn, or nausea. adj. **dyspeptic**

DYSPHAGIA n. a condition in which swallowing is difficult or painful, due to obstruction of the esophagus or muscular abnormalities of the esophagus or pharynx.

DYSPHASIA n. speech impairment, usually due to brain injury, stroke, or tumor.

DYSPHONIA n. difficulty in speaking due to impairment of the voice.   adj. **dysphonic**

DYSPLASIA n. a general term for any abnormal change or development, as in the shape or size of cells.   adj. **dysplastic**

DYSPNEA n. shortness of breath or labored, difficult breathing; causes include strenuous activity, lung disorders, heart disease, and extreme stress or tension.

DYSPRAXIA n. a decrease in proper function (as of an organ) or of ability to coordinate muscular actions.

DYSTOCIA n. abnormal *labor*, due to abnormal position of the fetus, contracted or obstructed *birth canal*, or other factor.

DYSTONIA n. abnormal muscle tone, esp. sudden muscle spasms due to a rare inherited disease (dystonia musculorum deformans) or sometimes to drug reaction.

DYSTROPHY n. degeneration or defective development of a tissue, esp. muscles, which lose strength and decrease in size (see also *muscular dystrophy*). adj. **dystrophic**

DYSURIA n. painful or difficult urination; it may be caused by inflammation of the bladder (*cystitis*) or urethra (*urethritis*) or other disorders.

e

E: VITAMIN n. any of a group of fat-soluble *vitamins* (*tocopherols*) important in reproductive function and blood cell production; rich sources are vegetable oils, nuts, soybeans, and eggs (see *vitamin*; Table of Vitamins).

EAR n. the hearing organ, including three general structures: the outer (external) ear; the middle ear, including the eardrum cavity and the three tiny bones that transmit the hearing vibrations; and the inner (internal) ear, including the main organ of hearing

EAR

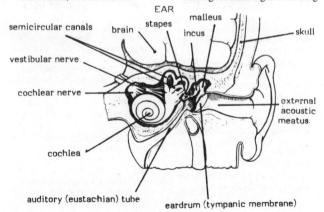

semicircular canals   brain   stapes   malleus   incus   skull

vestibular nerve

cochlear nerve   external acoustic meatus

cochlea

auditory (eustachian) tube   eardrum (tympanic membrane)

(the organ of Corti), the balance mechanism, and other parts.

EARACHE n. pain in the ear; it may be caused by ear disease or by infection or disease of the nose, mouth region, throat, and other nearby areas; also called **otalgia**.

EARDRUM n. the *tympanic membrane*, a thin membrane separating the outer ear from the middle ear. Sound waves entering the outer ear cause the membrane to vibrate; these vibrations are transmitted by three tiny *ossicles* (bones) in the middle ear to the inner ear and the main organ of hearing (the *organ of Corti*).

EARWAX see *cerumen*.

ECCHYMOSIS n. a bruise; a discolored (purplish) spot resulting from an accumulation of blood under the skin's surface, by injury or fragility of the blood vessel walls (see also *petechia*).

ECCRINE adj. pert. to sweating or sweat glands.

ECCRINE GLAND n. a type of sweat gland distributed over much of the body; its secretion is clear, has only a slight odor, and functions in cooling the body (compare *apocrine gland*).

ECCYESIS n. development of an embryo outside of the uterus (see also *ectopic pregnancy*).

ECG abbreviation for *electrocardiogram*.

ECHINO- comb. form indicating an association with spines or spinyness (e.g., **echinosis**, a state in which the red blood cells have an irregular appearance).

ECHINOCOCCOSIS n. an infection with a larval tapeworm (*Echinococcus*), usually transmitted through contact with infected dogs (esp. their stool). It is characterized by cyst formation in tissue, esp. the liver; symptoms depend on the tissue affected. Treatment involves surgical excision of the cysts; also called **hydatid disease**.

ECHOCARDIOGRAPHY n. a diagnostic procedure using ultrasound waves to study the heart, its structure and motions; also called **ultrasonic cardiography**.

ECHOENCEPHALOGRAPHY n. a diagnostic procedure using ultrasound waves to study the brain; it may reveal expanding lesions or expansion of brain ventricles.

ECHOLALIA n. in psychiatry, automatic and meaningless repetition of another's words, sometimes occurring in schizophrenia and other neurological and mental disorders.

ECHOVIRUS n. any of a group of small viruses, some of which are responsible for human illnesses.

ECLAMPSIA n. a rare (approx. 0.2% of all pregnancies in the United States) and serious pregnancy disorder. Eclampsia is characterized by convulsions, coma, high blood pressure, protein in the urine, and edema; signs of impending convulsions include headache, blurred vision, epigastric pain, and anxiety. Once the convulsions are controlled and emergency treatment of the pregnant woman completed, delivery of the infant is usually necessary (infant mortality is 25%) (see also *toxemia*). adj. **eclamptic**

ECSTASY n. emotional state marked by exalted delight, exhilaration, extreme joy. adj. **ecstatic**

ECT abbreviation for *electroconvulsive therapy*.

ECTASIA n. dilatation or distension of a part or organ, e.g., alveolar ectasia, abnormal expansion of the air sacs in the lungs; also: **ectasis** (compare *atelectasis*).

ECTO- comb. form meaning "outer," "outside," (e.g., **ectogenous**, coming from the outside, as disease-causing germs) (compare *endo-*).

ECTODERM n. in the embryo, the outside layer of cells from which the nervous system, skin, special sense organs (e.g., eyes, ears), and certain other body parts arise. (The two other cell layers are the *endoderm* and *mesoderm*.) adj. **ectodermal**, **ectodermic**

ECTOMORPH n. a person whose physique is thin, fragile, and generally nonmuscular (compare *endomorph*, *mesomorph*). adj. **ectomorphic**

-ECTOMY suffix indicating surgical removal of a part or organ (e.g., appendectomy, removal of the appendix).

ECTOPIA n. an abnormal positioning of a part or organ, esp. at the time of birth. adj. **ectopic**

ECTOPIC PREGNANCY n. an abnormal pregnancy, occurring in about 2% of all pregnancies, in which the fertilized egg (conceptus, embryo) implants outside of the uterus, most often (90%) in the Fallopian tube (*tubal pregnancy*) but occasionally in the ovary (ovarian pregnancy) or abdominal cavity (abdominal pregnancy). As the embryo develops the tube ruptures or other complications arise, usually causing hemorrhage and requiring immediate surgery; also called **extrauterine pregnancy**.

ECTRO- comb. form indicating *congenital* absence (e.g., **ectromelia**, congenital absence or marked shortening of the long bones of one or more limbs).

ECTRODACTYLY n. congenital absence of some fingers or toes.

ECTROGENY n. congenital absence of any body part or organ.

ECTROPION n. turning outward (eversion) of an edge or margin, esp. of the eyelid (which may occur from injury, facial nerve paralysis, or atrophy of eye tissue).

ECZEMA n. an inflammation of the skin that usually produces itching and the development of small blisterlike formations that release fluid and then form a crust. It may be caused by contact with a specific irritant or occur without apparent cause. adj. **eczematous**

EDECRIN n. trade name for the *diuretic* ethacrynic acid used to treat *edema*.

EDEMA n. the abnormal collection of fluid in spaces between cells, esp. just under the skin or in a given cavity (e.g., peritoneal cavity) or organ (e.g., the lungs [pulmonary edema]). Causes include injury, heart disease, kidney failure, *cirrhosis*, and *allergy*. Treatment depends on the cause. adj. **edematous**

EDENTULOUS adj. without teeth, as when all the natural teeth have been removed.

EEG abbreviation for *electroencephalogram*.

E.E.S. abbreviation for antibacterial *erythromycin*.

EFFACEMENT n. shortening of the *vagina* and thinning of its walls as it is stretched and dilated during *labor*.

EFFERENT adj. carrying outward, away from the center, as a nerve carrying impulses from the brain to a muscle, gland, or other effector organ or as a vessel (e.g., blood vessel or lymphatic vessel) carrying fluid (e.g., blood, lymph) away from an organ or part (compare *afferent*).

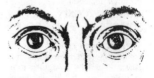

Ectropion

EFFLEURAGE n. rhythmic, firm or gentle, stroking, as in massage. Effleurage of the abdomen is commonly used in the *Lamaze method of natural childbirth*.

EFFUSION n. the escape of fluid (e.g., blood, lymph, serum) into a body cavity; often associated with circulatory or kidney disorders.

EGG n. ovum; the sex cell (*gamete*) of the female, which, when fertilized by the male *sperm*, becomes a *zygote*.

EGO n. a term used by Freud and now generally accepted to mean the self, esp. the conscious self (compare *id*, *superego*).

EGO- comb. form indicating a relationship to the self (e.g., **egocentric**, selfish, focusing especially or exclusively on oneself).

EGOMANIA n. abnormally excessive self-regard.

EJACULATE n. sperm-containing fluid (*semen*) emitted during *ejaculation*. The fluid volume of each ejaculate is usually between 2 and 5 milliters and it contains 50,000,000 to 150,000,000 *spermatozoa*.

EJACULATION n. a sudden discharge of something, esp. of *semen* during *coitus*, *masturbation*, or *nocturnal emission*. The sensation of ejaculation is called *orgasm*. (See also *premature ejaculation*.)   adj. **ejaculatory**

EJACULATORY DUCT n. duct, about 2 centimeters (1 inch) long, behind the bladder that transports sperm from the *ductus deferens* to the *urethra*.

EKG   abbreviation for *electrocardiogram* (the preferred abbreviation is ECG).

ELASTIC adj. having the ability to resume the original shape once the force that changed that shape is removed.

ELASTOSIS n. a condition in which elastic tissue breaks down.

ELAVIL n. trade name for a commonly used antidepressant drug (*amitriptyline* hydrochloride).

ELBOW n. 1. the joint at which the upper arm (*humerus*) and forearm (specifically the *ulna* of the forearm) meet; it is a common site of inflammation and injury (see also *tennis elbow*); 2. any L-shaped part or angle, as in an apparatus tube.

ELBOW

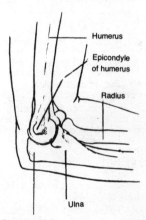

Humerus

Epicondyle of humerus

Radius

Ulna

Olecranon of ulna

ELECTIVE adj. decided on by the person and/or the physician, esp. with relation to procedures (e.g., surgery) that are not essential.

ELECTRIC adj. pertaining to, involving, or caused by electricity. Evidence shows that electric current may guide the development of embryos and the regeneration of tissue, including bone; the sources for this electric current are in dispute.

ELECTRIC BURN n. a burn caused by heat generated by an electric current (see also *burn*).

ELECTRIC(AL) HEALING n. use of electricity to increase the rate of natural repair of damaged tissues (e.g., fractures). Research suggests the electricity may keep the parathyroid hormone (which can destroy bone tissue) from acting on cells at the repair site.

ELECTRIC SHOCK n. a traumatic state caused by the passage of an electric current through the body. It usually results from accidental contact with exposed circuits in household appliances but may also result from contact with high-voltage wires or from being struck with lightning. The damage to the body depends on the type, intensity, and duration of the current; it commonly includes burns, heart rhythm abnormalities, and unconsciousness.

ELECTRO- comb. form indicating an association with electricity (e.g., **electrocoagulation**, the clotting of blood by applying an electric instrument—electrocautery).

ELECTROANESTHESIA n. loss of sensation resulting from application of an electric current to the body or to a part.

ELECTROCARDIOGRAM n. a graphic recording, produced by an *electrocardiograph*, of the electrical activity of the heart. Commonly referred to as an ECG (or EKG), it allows the detection of abnormalities in the transmission of the cardiac impulse through the heart muscle and serves as an important aid in the diagnosis of heart ailments.

ELECTROCARDIOGRAPH n. a device used to record the electrical activity of the heart. The patient is asked to lie down and rest quietly on a table, and electrodes, called leads, are positioned, usually using an adhesive gel, on certain sites on the chest. The leads detect the electrical impulses of the heart and transmit them to the recording device. adj. **electrocardiographic**

ELECTROCAUTERY n. the application of a needle or snare heated by an electric current to destroy tissue (e.g., to remove warts).

ELECTROCONVULSIVE THERAPY (ECT) n. treatment of certain mental disorders, esp. severe depression, in which a brief convulsion is induced by passing an electric current through the brain. The patient is placed in a comfortable supine position with limbs lightly restrained and a special tongue depressor between the teeth. Electrodes are placed on both sides of the forehead and an electric current delivered for a very

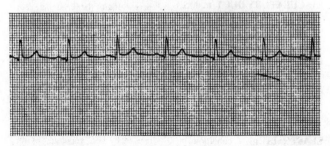

An electrocardiogram (ECG)

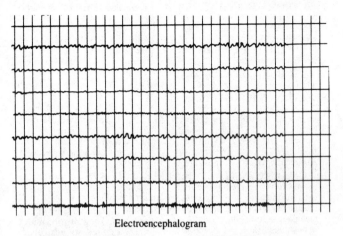

Electroencephalogram

brief time (less than one-half a second). The patient loses consciousness, experiences involuntary muscle contractions (convulsions) for a short period and then awakens with no memory of the shock. Electroconvulsive therapy is now less commonly used than it once was, largely replaced by psychoactive drugs; also called **electroshock therapy; shock therapy.**

ELECTROENCEPHALO-GRAM (EEG) n. a graphic recording, produced by an *electroencephalograph*, of the electrical activity of the brain. Electroencephalograms are helpful in detecting and locating brain tumors and in diagnosing *epilepsy*.

ELECTROENCEPHALO-GRAPH n. a device for receiving and recording the electrical activity of the brain. In most cases electrodes are attached to various areas of the head and the patient is asked to remain quiet while the brain-wave activity is recorded; during neurosurgery electrodes may be placed directly on the surface of or within the brain. adj. **electroencephalographic**

ELECTROLYSIS n. 1. an electrical action that causes a chemical (e.g., a salt) to break down into simpler forms; 2. the passing of an electric current into a hair root to remove superfluous or unwanted hair.   adj. **electrolytic**

ELECTROLYTE n. a chemical (element or compound) in the body that when dissolved produces ions, conducts an electric current, and is itself changed in the process. The proper amount and equilibrium of certain electrolytes (e.g., calcium, sodium, potassium) in the body is essential for normal health and functioning.

ELECTROLYTE BALANCE n. equilibrium between electrolytes in the body that is essential for normal functioning, with a deficiency or excess of a particular electrolyte usually producing characteristic symptoms. The normal electrolyte balance may be disturbed by many diseases, including prolonged diarrhea or vomiting, kidney malfunction, malnutrition, or disturbed activity of the adrenal cortex, pancreas, pituitary, or other gland.

ELECTROMYOGRAM (EMG) n. a recording of the electrical activity occurring when voluntary (skeletal) muscles work; it is helpful in diagnosing muscle and nerve abnormalities.

ELECTRONIC FETAL MONITOR n. see *fetal monitor*.

ELECTRON MICROSCOPE n. an instrument similar to a light microscope but which uses a beam of electrons, not light, to scan surfaces and create an image; magnification 1,000 times that of an optical microscope is possible.

ELECTROPHORESIS n. the movement of charged articles in a liquid medium in response to changes in an electric field. The technique allows the separation of component parts of a substance and is widely used to analyze certain substances (e.g., determining the proteins present in a sample of serum).

ELECTRORETINOGRAM n. a graphic recording of the electrical activity of the *retina*; it is made by flashing a light into the eye and recording the effects on the retina with special devices attached to the eye and the back of the head; it is used to help diagnose retinal disease.

ELECTROSHOCK THERAPY see *electroconvulsive therapy*.

ELECTROSLEEP n. sleep that is brought about by applying a controlled electric current to the head. The procedure has been used in treating mental and emotional disorders, e.g., anxiety, depression, and insomnia.

ELECTROSURGERY n. surgery performed using electrical devices (e.g., electrically wired needles).

ELEMENT n. the simplest chemical form, in which only one kind of atom is contained (e.g., oxygen) (compare *compound*).

ELEPHANTIASIS n. a condition characterized by enormous enlargement of certain body parts, esp. the legs and scrotum, often with a thickening and coarsening of the skin. It is the end stage of the disease *filariasis* and is due to blockage of the lymphatic vessels by infiltration of filarial worms.

ELIMINATION n. the process of getting rid of a material, as of waste products through the *urine*.

ELIXIR n. a sweetened, flavored liquid, usually containing a small amount of alcohol, used in compounding medicines to be taken by mouth.

ELIXOPHYLLIN n. trade name for a drug—*theophylline*—used as a *bronchodilator*.

ELSPAR n. trade name for an *antineoplastic* drug (asparaginase) sometimes used to treat acute lymphoblastic leukemia.

EMACIATION n. excessive thinness, due to disease or poor nutrition.

EMASCULATION n. 1. surgical removal of the penis and/or testes (see *castration*); 2. loss of a feeling of masculinity or of male characteristics.

EMBOLECTOMY n. surgical removal of an *embolus*, usually from an artery.

EMBOLISM n. blockage of a blood vessel, esp. an artery, by an *embolus*. Treatment depends on the nature of the embolus, the degree of obstruction and the blood vessel affected.

EMBOLUS n. a clot of blood (*thrombus*), foreign object, bit of tissue, or air or gas bubble that moves through the bloodstream until it becomes lodged in a vessel, causing an *embolism*.

EMBRYO n. the early developing organism, from the *zygote* to the *fetal* stage; in humans, from about week 3 to week 8 after conception, at which time the main organ systems have formed, at least in their early stages.   adj. **embryonic**

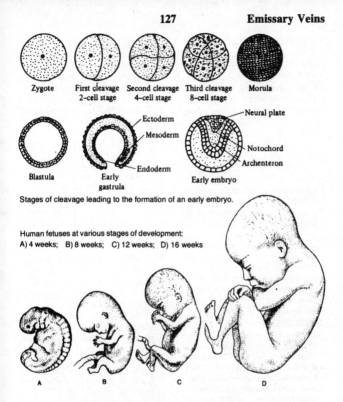

Stages of cleavage leading to the formation of an early embryo.

Human fetuses at various stages of development:
A) 4 weeks; B) 8 weeks; C) 12 weeks; D) 16 weeks

EMBRYO- comb. form indicating an association with an "embryo" (e.g., **embryotrophy**, nourishment of the embryo).

EMERGENCY n. an occasion of urgency; a situation that arises suddenly and requires immediate action to save the life or health of a person (e.g., as when someone has swallowed poison).

EMERGENCY MEDICINE n. medical subspecialty concerned with the diagnosis and prompt treatment of injuries, trauma, or sudden illnesses.

EMESIS n. vomiting.

EMETIC n. a substance that induces vomiting (e.g., ipecac), used in the treatment of some cases of drug overdose and in certain types of poisonings.

EMETROL n. trade name for a fixed-combination drug, containing fructose, glucose (sugars), and phosphoric acid, used to treat nausea and vomiting.

EMG n. abbreviation for *electromyogram*.

EMINENCE n. a raised bumplike projection on a part, esp. on a bone (e.g., the deltoid eminence, a rise on the shaft of the upper arm bone, where the deltoid muscle attaches).

EMISSARY VEINS n. small blood vessels in the skull that drain blood from sinuses in the *dura mater* to veins outside the skull.

EMISSION n. release of something, esp. the uncontrolled discharge of semen during sleep (*nocturnal emission*).

EMMENAGOGUE n. a drug used to bring on *menstruation*.

EMMETROPIA n. a state of normal vision, in which there is proper focus of light onto the retina. adj. **emmetropic**

EMOLLIENT n. an agent that soothes or softens the skin (e.g., lanolin).

EMOTION n. an intense feeling; a state of arousal, pleasant or unpleasant, often accompanied by physical changes such as release of epinephrine from the adrenal glands. Emotions include fear, anger, and love. adj. **emotional**

EMPATHY n. the ability to recognize and relate to, and to some extent share in, the emotions of another. adj. **empathetic**

EMPHYSEMA n. abnormal condition of the lungs in which there is overinflation of the air sacs (alveoli) of the lungs leading to a breakdown of their walls, a decrease in respiratory function, and, in severe cases, increasing breathlessness. Emphysema appears to be associated with chronic bronchitis, cigarette smoking, and advancing age; one form that occurs early in life is related to a hereditary lack of an enzyme. Early symptoms of emphysema include dyspnea, cough, rapid heart rate; advanced cases are marked by signs of oxygen lack (restlessness, weakness, confusion) and frequently by complications of pulmonary edema and congestive heart failure. Breathing exercises, drugs such as bronchodilators and the prevention of respiratory infections may be helpful; severe cases may require oxygen.

EMPIRIC adj. pert. to treatment of disease based on observation and experience, not on knowledge of the specific causes or mechanisms of the disease.

EMPIRIN n. trade name for a fixed combination drug containing *aspirin* and *phenacetin* (pain-relievers and fever-reducers) and *caffeine* (a central nervous system stimulant).

EMPYEMA n. pus in the lung cavity or other body cavity, usually due to bacterial infection; treatment is by antibiotics and surgical drainage of the pus.

EMULSION n. a combination of two liquids (e.g., oil and water) dispersed one in the other.

E-MYCIN n. trade name for the antibiotic *erythromycin*.

ENAMEL n. the hard white covering above the gum line of a tooth.

ENANTHEMA n. an eruption on a mucous membrane, e.g., the inside of the mouth.

ENARAX n. trade name for a fixed combination drug that inhibits gastric secretions and is used to treat peptic ulcer; it contains a minor tranquilizer (hydroxyzine hydrochloride) and an anticholinergic agent (oxyphencyclimine hydrochloride).

ENARTHROSIS see *ball-and-socket joint*.

EN BLOC adj. as a whole, in one piece.

ENCANTHIS n. a small growth at the inner angle of the eyelids.

ENCAPSULATION n. the process of enclosing something in a covering; the condition of being enclosed in a capsule, as the tendons or nerves are enclosed in membranous sheaths.

ENCEPHAL-, ENCEPHALO- comb. form indicating an association with the brain (e.g., **encephalospinal**, pert. to the brain and spinal cord).

ENCEPHALITIS n. an inflammation of the brain, usually due to viral infection but sometimes a complication of another infection (e.g., influenza, measles) or resulting from poisoning. Symptoms include headache, drowsiness, neck pain, nausea, and fever, followed sometimes by neurologic disturbances such as seizures, paralysis, and personality changes. The outcome depends on the cause, extent of brain inflammation, and general condition of the patient (see also *encephalomyelitis*).

ENCEPHALOCELE n. protrusion of the brain through a congenital defect of the skull.

ENCEPHALOGRAM n. radiograph of the brain made by withdrawing cerebrospinal fluid and replacing it with a gas (e.g., oxygen). It is a risky procedure, used when computed tomography is not definitive, and used in diagnosis of *hydrocephalus* and other abnormalities.

ENCEPHALOMALACIA n. brain softening.

ENCEPHALOMYELITIS n. acute inflammation of the brain and spinal cord, marked by fever, headache, neck and back pain, and vomiting; in severe cases and in weak or aged persons seizures, coma, and death may result (see also *encephalitis*).

ENCEPHALON n. the *brain*.

ENCEPHALOPATHY n. any brain disease or disorder.

ENCHONDROMA n. a benign, slow-growing tumor of cartilage cells at the ends of tubular bones, esp. those of the hands and feet.

ENCOPRESIS n. a condition, not caused by physical illness or defect, in which the passing of *feces* occurs without control.

ENCYSTED adj. surrounded by a capsule or membrane.

END-, ENDO- comb. form meaning "inward," "within" (e.g., **endocranial**, within the skull).

ENDARTERITIS n. inflamma-
tion of the inner lining of an artery or arteries, often associated with advanced *syphilis* and causing progressive thickening and blocking of the vessel.

ENDEMIC adj. indigenous to a given population or area; occurring frequently in a given group of community, esp. pert. to a disease.

ENDOCARDITIS n. inflammation of the membrane (endocardium) lining the inside of the heart and the heart valves, caused by bacterial infection or occurring as a complication of another disease (e.g., rheumatic fever). Symptoms include fever, and changes in heart rhythms; damage to heart valves may occur. Treatment consists of bedrest, antibiotics, and surgery, if necessary, to treat damaged valves.

ENDOCARDIUM n. the membrane that lines the chambers of the heart and the heart valves.

ENDOCERVICITIS n. inflammation of the epithelium and glands of the cervix of the uterus.

ENDOCRANIUM n. the membrane lining the inside of the skull.

ENDOCRINE GLAND n. any ductless gland (e.g., pituitary gland) that releases its secretion—a *hormone*—directly into the bloodstream through which it moves to specific "target organs" to produce an effect.

ENDOCRINE SYSTEM n. the network of endocrine glands that produce and secrete hormones directly into the bloodstream for transport to specific target organs where they exert their effect. Along with the *nervous system*, the endocrine system coordinates and regulates many of the activities of the body, including growth, metabolism, sexual development, and reproduction. The major endocrine glands, their location and main hormones and functions are listed in the chart.

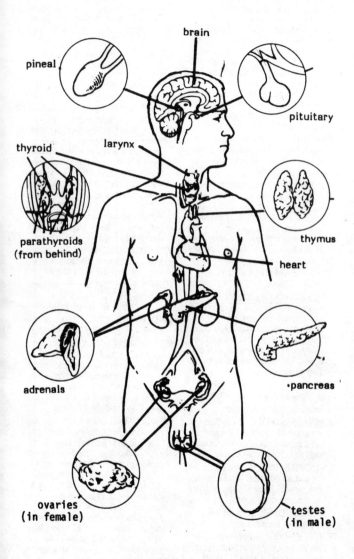

ENDOCRINE GLANDS

Endocrines and Their Hormones

Name of Gland	Location	Hormone	Normal Function	Excess Secretion	Diminished Secretion
Anterior pituitary	Base of brain forward portion	Growth hormone (STH)	Affect skeletal growth, protein synthesis, blood glucose concentration	Gigantism acromegaly	Dwarfism
		Trophic hormones TSH ACTH FSH LH	Stimulate target glands thyroid adrenal cortex ovarian follicles; testes gonads	Oversecretion of glands	Undersecretion of glands
Posterior pituitary	Hind portion	Vasopressin	Control of blood pressure; reabsorption of water by kidney tubules	Increased blood pressure; glycogen converted to sugar	Decreased blood pressure; excess sugar changed to fat; kidney tubules not reabsorbing water
		Oxytocin	Contractions of uterus		
Thyroid	2 lobes on either side of larynx	Thyroxin (65% iodine)	Controls rate of oxidation in cells	Increased oxidation; nervous exophthalmic goiter	Lowered oxidation; in a child-cretinism; in an adult myxedemic goiter due to lack of iodine in drinking water

Endocrines and Their Hormones (Continued)

Name of Gland	Location	Hormone	Normal Function	Excess Secretion	Diminished Secretion
Parathyroid	Four glands above thyroid	Parathyroxin	Regulates amount of calcium in blood	Trembling due to lack of muscular control	Contraction of muscles (tetany); death.
Stomach	Mucous lining (mucoos)	Gastrin	Stimulates secretion of gastric juice	Promotes ulceration of stomach wall	Inhibits gastric digestion
Small intestine	Mucous lining	Secretin	Activates the liver and pancreas to secrete and release their secretions	Excessive pancreatic and liver secretions	Diminished pancreatic and liver secretion
Adrenal medulla	Two glands above kidney	Adrenalin	Controls release of sugar from liver; contraction of arteries; clotting	Increases blood pressure; promotes clotting; releases glycogen; strengthens heart beat	
Adrenal Cortex		Glucocorticoids	Affects normal functioning of gonads; helps maintain normal blood sugar levels		Addison's disease: muscular weakness, darkening of skin, low blood pressure; death

Gland	Location	Hormone	Function		
		Mineralo-corticoids	Stimulates kidney tubules to reabsorb sodium		
Pancreas Isles of Langerhans	Embedded in pancreas	Insulin	Regulates storage of glycogen in liver; accelerates oxidation of sugar in cells		Diabetes; unused sugar remains in blood and is excreted with urine
Gonads	Abdominal region	Testosterone (Males) Estrogen Progesterone (Females)	Regulates normal growth and development of sex glands; regulates reproduction; controls sex characteristics	Premature development of gonads; effects on secondary sex characteristics	Interference with normal reproductive functions; diminished growth of sex characteristics
Thymus	Chest region	Thymosin	Stimulates immunological activity of lymphoid tissue		Breakdown of immune system
Pineal	Base of brain	Melatonin	Regulates gonadotropins by anterior pituitary		

ENDOCRINOLOGIST n. a physician who specializes in the diagnosis and treatment of diseases affecting the *endocrine system*.

ENDOCRINOLOGY n. the study of the structure, function, and diseases of the *endocrine system*. adj. **endocrinologic**

ENDODERM n. in the embryo, the inner layer of cells from which the epithelium of the trachea, bronchi, lungs, gastrointestinal tract, and many other organs arises and from which the lining of body cavities and the covering of internal organs arises. (The other cell layers are the outer *ectoderm* and the middle *mesoderm*.)

ENDOGENOUS adj. developed within an organism; arising within; for example, **endogenous obesity** is caused by an endocrine or metabolic disorder, not by overeating.

ENDOGENOUS DEPRESSION n. a serious and persistent form of *depression* believed due to a complex interrelationship of biochemical, genetic and psychological factors and frequently not traceable to a specific extrinsic event (e.g., death of a spouse).

ENDOMETRIAL adj. pert. to the *endometrium*, the mucous membrane lining of the *uterus* (e.g., endometrial carcinoma, cancer of the uterine lining).

ENDOMETRIOSIS n. a condition marked by the presence, growth, and function of endometrial tissue outside of its normal location as lining of the *uterus* in such sites as the uterine walls, the Fallopian tubes, the ovaries, and other sites within the pelvis, or rarely, outside the pelvis. Endometriosis is fairly common (est. 15% of women), esp. in childless women and women who have children late in life. Symptoms depend on the size and location of the displaced tissue but commonly include painful *menstrua-*tion, painful *coitus*, and sometimes painful urination and defecation and premenstrual staining. Endometriosis is a common cause of *infertility*. Treatment includes the use of *analgesics* to relieve pain and hormones to decrease the size and number of lesions, and in severe cases, surgery.

ENDOMETRITIS n. acute or chronic inflammation of the *endometrium*, usually caused by bacterial infection and most commonly occurring after *childbirth*, *abortion*, or the fitting of an *IUD*. Symptoms include fever, abdominal pain, enlargement of the uterus, and discharge (often foul-smelling). Treatment includes antibiotics and rest; untreated it may lead to blockage of the Fallopian tubes and resultant *sterility*.

ENDOMETRIUM n. the mucous membrane lining of the *uterus*, which, under hormonal control, changes in thickness and complexity during the *menstrual cycle* and if pregnancy does not occur is mostly shed during *menstruation*. adj. **endometrial**

ENDOMORPH n. a person whose body tends to be more heavily developed in the torso than in the limbs, with fat accumulations giving the body a generally round and soft appearance (compare *ectomorph*, *mesomorph*). adj. **endomorphic**

ENDOMYOCARDITIS n. acute or chronic inflammation of the heart muscle (myocardium) and the inner lining (endocardium) of the heart, due to disease or infection (see also *endocarditis*).

ENDONEURIUM n. the fragile tissue covering the separate fibers in a *nerve*.

ENDORPHIN n. any of several naturally occurring chemicals (proteins) in the brain, believed to be involved in reducing or eliminating pain and in enhancing pleasure. Studies show that *acupuncture* may induce activation of endorphins (compare *enkephalin*).

ENDOSCOPY n. viewing the inside of a body cavity by means of a special instrument (endoscope), inserted usually through a natural body opening (e.g., the mouth, vagina, urethra) but sometimes through an incision.   adj. **endoscopic**

ENDOSTEUM n. the membranous lining of a cavity inside a bone.

ENDOTHELIUM n. the layer of flat cells that lines the heart, blood and lymph vessels, and some body cavities.   adj. **endothelial**

ENDOTOXIN n. a toxin confined within a bacterium or other microorganism and released only when the microorganism is broken down or dies. Endotoxins may cause fever, chills, shock, and other symptoms in the infected person (compare *exotoxin*). adj. **endotoxic**

ENDOTRACHEAL TUBE n. a catheter inserted through the mouth or nose into the trachea to maintain an open airway (e.g., in severe inflammation and swelling of the pharynx), to deliver oxygen, to permit suctioning of mucous, or to prevent aspiration of stomach contents.

END-PLATE n. the end of the fiber of a motor nerve in a muscle that receives stimulus (*neurotransmitter*) from a motor nerve fiber.

ENDURON n. trade name for a *diuretic* and antihypertensive.

ENEMA n. the insertion of liquid into the rectum to remove feces, to help diagnose certain gastrointestinal disorders (barium enema), or to administer drugs.

ENERVATION n. 1. weakness, loss of strength or energy; 2. surgical removal of a nerve.

ENFLURANE n. a nonflammable gas (an ether) used as a general *anesthetic*.

ENGAGEMENT n. in obstetrics, fixation of the presenting part of the fetus, usually the head, in the maternal pelvis; it usually occurs in late pregnancy, after which fetal movements are curtailed.

ENGORGE v. to fill to the limit of expansion.

ENKEPHALIN n. any of a group of brain chemicals (proteins) that influence mental activity and behavior (sometimes grouped with the *endorphins* as "natural opiates"). Evidence shows that these chemicals influence the body's immune system and help fight disease (compare *endorphin*).

ENOPHTHALMOS n. a condition in which the eyeball is displaced back in the eye socket, because of injury or developmental defect.

ENOVID n. trade name for an *oral contraceptive* containing the *estrogen* mestranol and the *progestin* norethynodrel.

ENTER-, ENTERO- comb. forms indicating an association with the *intestine* (e.g., **enterogastric**, pert. to the intestine and stomach).

ENTERIC adj. pert. to the intestines.

ENTERITIS n. inflammation of the intestine, esp. the small intestine, due to viral or bacterial infection or other disorder, usually marked by diarrhea (compare *gastroenteritis*).

ENTEROBIASIS n. infection of the large intestine with the pinworm *Enterobius vermicularis*, occurring esp. in children. The females deposit eggs around the *anus*, which cause itching; if the patient scratches the area and then puts the fingers in or near the mouth, reinfection occurs. Treatment is by anthelmintics (agents that destroy worms).

ENTEROLITHIASIS n. the presence of stonelike formations in the intestines.

ENTEROPTOSIS n. unusually downward position of the intestine in the abdominal cavity.

ENTEROSPASM n. excessive, abnormal contraction of muscles in the intestine, usually causing pain.

ENTEROSTOMY n. surgical creation of a permanent opening in the intestine through the abdominal wall (compare *colostomy*).

ENTODERM see *endoderm*.

ENTOZYME n. trade name for a fixed combination drug containing bile salts and digestive enzymes (pepsin and pancreatin).

ENTROPION n. abnormal inward turning of an edge, esp. the eyelid toward the eyeball, resulting from spasm or from scar tissue on the *conjunctiva*.

Entropion

ENUCLEATION n. surgical removal of a whole tumor or whole organ (e.g., the eyeball).

ENURESIS n. the passing of urine without control, esp. during sleep (bedwetting). The condition can be caused by a urinary tract disorder but is usually a childhood phenomenon that is outgrown. Restriction of fluids, esp. near bedtime, and the use of a device that rings a bell to awaken the child when urination begins are sometimes helpful. See also *incontinence*. adj. **enuretic**

ENZYME n. a protein produced in cells that acts as a catalyst, speeding up the rate of biological reactions without itself being used up. Many enzymes are involved in digestion (e.g., lipase helps to break down fat) and respiration (e.g., cocarboxylase). The names of many enzymes end in -ase. adj. **enzymatic**

EOSIN n. a red dye commonly used to stain cells, bacteria, and other materials for examination under the microscope.

EOSINOPENIA n. a decrease in the number of *eosinophils* in the blood.

EOSINOPHIL n. a white blood cell readily stained with eosin. Eosinophils, normally about 1–3% of the total white blood cell count, are believed to function in allergic responses and in resisting some infections.

EOSINOPHILIA n. an increase in the number of *eosinophils* in the blood; it commonly occurs in allergic reactions and in some inflammatory conditions.

EP-, EPI- prefix meaning "on," or "above" (e.g., **epipial**, on the brain's inner covering (*pia mater*).

EPENDYMA n. the very thin membrane that lines the ventricles of the *brain* and helps to form *cerebrospinal fluid*.

EPHEDRINE n. a bronchodilator; a drug that widens the air passages of the lungs and is used to treat *asthma*, *bronchitis*, and other conditions; side effects include headache, nervousness, and insomnia.

EPICANTHUS n. a vertical fold of skin on the inner aspect of the eye. Normal in Oriental persons and sometimes occurring also in *Down's syndrome*; also: **epicanthic fold**. adj. **epicanthal, epicanthic**

EPICARDIA n. that part of the esophagus between the diaphragm and the stomach.

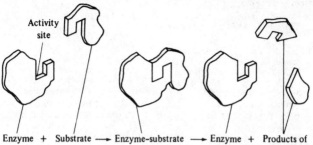

Enzyme + Substrate ⟶ Enzyme-substrate ⟶ Enzyme + Products of
complex   Reaction

EPICARDIUM n. the innermost of the two layers of the *pericardium*, the membranous covering of the heart.

EPICONDYLE n. a projection on a bone, above another part, the *condyle*.

EPICONDYLITIS n. painful inflammation of the muscles and soft tissue around the elbow, usually caused by excessive strain, as in tennis or golf, or by carrying a heavy load. Treatment includes rest and injection of pain-relieving drugs into the joint area (also called **tennis elbow**).

EPICRANIUM n. all layers of the scalp; the coverings of the skull.

EPIDEMIC n. an outbreak of infectious disease (e.g., influenza) in which many people in a given geographic area are readily affected with the disorder.   adj. affecting a large number of people at the same time (compare *endemic*, *pandemic*).

EPIDEMIOLOGY n. the study of the causes, occurrences, and control of disease.

EPIDERMIS n. the superficial, outer layers of the skin which contain numerous nerve endings but no blood vessels. Made up of *squamous epithelium* tissue, the epidermis is divided into an outer stratum corneum containing dead cells that are sloughed off as new cells from the inner stratum germinativum push upward; other layers are also sometimes found, esp. in thick skin (e.g., the palms and soles).   adj. **epidermal**, **epidermoid**

EPIDIDYMIS n. a long, coiled tube along the back side of the testis that connects the *seminiferous tubules* of the testis to the *vas deferens*. Sperm mature as they pass through the epididymis and are then stored before ejaculation.   adj. **epididymal**

EPIDIDYMITIS n. acute or chronic inflammation of the epididymis, producing tenderness, pain in the groin, chills and fever; it may result from *venereal disease*, inflammation of the *prostate*, or urinary tract infection. Treatment includes rest, support of the area, and antibiotics, if appropriate.

EPIDURAL adj. outside the *dura mater*, the outermost membranous covering of the brain and spinal cord; also: **extradural**.

EPIDURAL ANESTHESIA n. injection of a local anesthesia into the epidural space of the spinal column to achieve regional anesthesia of the abdominal, genital, or pelvic area; widely used in vaginal childbirth, Cesarean delivery, and gynecologic surgery.

EPIGASTRIC adj. above the stomach; in the epigastrium, the region of the abdomen just below the *sternum*.

EPIGLOTTIS n. a flap of mucous membrane-covered cartilage at the back of the mouth cavity that covers the opening to the windpipe during swallowing, thereby preventing choking.

EPIGLOTTITIS n. inflammation of the *epiglottis*.

EPIKERATOPHAKIA n. the shaping of a piece of donated *cornea* to the eye of a patient who has had a *cataract* removed. Called a "living contact lens," the added tissue bends the light to focus on the retina. The technique has been used on babies born with cataracts and also for correction of *keratoconus* and *myopia*.

EPILATION n. removal of hair by the roots.

EPILEPSY n. a neurological disorder characterized by recurrent episodes (ranging from several times a day to once in several years) of convulsive seizures, impaired consciousness, abnormal behavior, and other disturbances produced by uncontrolled electrical discharges from nerve cells in the brain. Trauma to the head, brain tumor, chemical imbalances, and other factors may be associated with epilepsy, but in most cases the cause is unknown. Treatment depends on the severity and frequency of episodes. Common types of epilepsy are *grand mal epilepsy* and *petit mal epilepsy*. adj. **epileptic**

EPIMYSIUM n. fibrous tissue surrounding a muscle.

EPINEPHRINE n. 1. a hormone of the adrenal medulla that acts as a powerful stimulant in times of fear or arousal and has many physiological effects, including increasing breathing, heart, and metabolic rates to provide quick energy, constricting blood vessels, and strengthening muscle contraction; 2. a synthetic drug used in the treatment of bronchial asthma to reduce bronchial spasm and dilate air passageways and during surgery to reduce blood loss by constricting blood vessels. Also called **adrenaline**.

EPINEURIUM n. connective tissue sheath surrounding a nerve fiber.

EPIPHYSIS n. the end portion of a long bone, separated by cartilage from the shaft (the *diaphysis*) until the bone stops growing, at which time the shaft and head unite. pl. **epiphyses** adj. **epiphyseal**

EPISCLERITIS n. inflammation of the *sclera* (the white of the eye) and overlying tissues.

EPISIOTOMY n. an incision made to enlarge the opening of the *vagina* during a difficult birth or forceps delivery. The purpose is to make the delivery easier or to hasten it and to avoid stretching and tearing adjacent muscle and tissue.

EPISPADIAS n. a congenital abnormality in males in which the opening for passing urine (the *urethra*) is on the upper surface of the penis.

EPISTAXIS n. bleeding from the nose; causes include a blow or other injury, violent sneezing, high blood pressure, and fragile mucous membranes. The bleeding may be controlled by applying pressure to the sides of the nose, by inserting cotton or gauze, or by holding an ice compress over the nose; also called **nosebleed**.

EPITHELIUM n. the cell layers covering the outside body surfaces as well as forming the lining of hollow organs (e.g., the *bladder*) and the passages of the respiratory, digestive, and urinary tracts. adj. **epithelial**

EPONYM n. name for a structure, condition, or process that includes or is formed from the name of a person (e.g., *Meniere's disease*, *parkinsonism*).

EPSOM SALT n. a bitter-tasting chemical (magnesium sulfate) commonly dissolved in water and swallowed to treat heartburn and constipation. It may also be prescribed to prevent seizures (esp. in pre-*eclampsia*) and is used as a soaking solution for treatment of *inflammations*.

EPSTEIN-BARR VIRUS (EBV) n. virus that causes *infectious mononucleosis* and in parts of Africa is associated with *Burkitt's lymphoma*.

EPSTEIN'S PEARLS n. small white pearl-like cysts occurring on the hard palate of a newborn that disappear within a few weeks.

EQUAGESIC n. trade name for a fixed combination drug containing *analgesics* (including aspirin) and the sedative *meprobamate*; it is used to treat anxiety and muscle spasm.

EQUANIL n. trade name for the sedative *meprobamate* used to treat anxiety.

EQUANITRATE n. trade name for a fixed combination drug, containing a *vasodilator* (pentaerythritol tetranitrate) and the sedative *meprobamate*, used to treat cardiovascular disorders.

EQUILIBRIUM n. a state of balance, in which opposing forces (e.g., body chemicals like calcium and phosphorus) exactly counteract each other.

EQUINE ENCEPHALITIS n. an infection characterized by inflammation of the brain and spinal cord, fever, headache, nausea, vomiting and neurological symptoms (e.g., tremor, visual disturbances). It is caused by a virus transmitted by a mosquito from an infected horse.

ERB'S PALSY n. paralysis of the arm due to injury to the brachial plexus, most often during childbirth; also called **Erb-Duchenne paralysis**.

ERECTILE TISSUE n. a type of spongy tissue (e.g., that found in the *penis* or *clitoris*) having large spaces within it that can fill with blood to stiffen the structure in which it is contained.

ERECTION n. a state of rigidity, esp. of the *penis*, which becomes enlarged and elevated when its tissues fill with blood, usually as a result of sexual arousal but also occurring normally during sleep and as a result of physical stimulation. Erection of the penis enables the penis to enter the vagina during *coitus*.

ERETHISM n. state of abnormal irritation, sensitivity, or excitement.

ERGO- comb. form indicating an association with work or exertion (e.g., **ergocardiogram**, a record of heart action during exertion).

ERGONOMICS n. the study and analysis of work as it relates to human physical and physiological processes.

Cilia   Goblet cell

Squamous cells   Cuboidal cells   Columnar cells   Columnar cells with cilia

Types of epithelial tissue

ERGONOVINE n. an ergot preparation used to contract the uterus to prevent or treat hemorrhage following childbirth or abortion.

ERGOT n. a fungus (*Claviceps purpurea*) that infects wheat, rye, and other cereal grains. It produces several alkaloids (ergonovine, ergotamine) used in medicine. Ingestion of food contaminated with ergot causes *ergotism*.

ERGOTAMINE n. an ergot alkaloid that causes constriction of blood vessels and contraction of uterine muscles and is used to treat migraine and postpartum (after childbirth) lack of muscle tone in the uterus.

ERGOTISM n. *ergot* poisoning, resulting from prolonged or excessive use of ergot-containing drugs or from accidental ingestion of ergot-contaminated food. Symptoms include excessive thirst, diarrhea, nausea, vomiting, cramping, abnormal cardiac rhythms, and, if severe, seizures and gangrene of the extremities.

ERGOTRATE MALEATE n. trade name for *ergonovine*.

EROGENOUS adj. pert. to stimulation of the sexual instinct, esp. to the areas of the body (erogenous zones) where such stimulation leads to sexual arousal.

EROSION n. wearing away of a surface, esp. a mucous membrane or epidermal surface, due to inflammation, injury, friction, or other factor.

EROTICISM n. 1. sexual instinct or desire; 2. unusually strong or persistent sexual drive. adj. **erotic**

ERUCTATION n. the act of bringing up air from the stomach with a characteristic noise; belching.

ERUPTION n. 1. the act of breaking out and becoming visible, esp. a rash or other skin lesion; 2. the emergence of a tooth as it breaks through the gum. adj. **eruptive**

ERYSIPELAS n. an acute skin disease, caused by infection with *Streptococci* bacteria (esp. *Streptococcus pyogenes*) and characterized by redness, swelling, fever, pain, and skin lesions. Treatment is by antibiotics.

ERYSIPELOID n. an infection of the hands characterized by reddish nodules and sometimes *erythema*. It is usually acquired by handling meat or fish infected with *Erysipelothrix rhusiopathiae*. Treatment is by antibiotics.

ERYTHEMA n. abnormal redness of the skin resulting from dilatation of the capillaries, as occurs in sunburn. adj. **erythematous**

ERYTHEMA MULTIFORME n. a red, slightly raised rash occurring on the body as a *hypersensitivity reaction* to a disease, drug, or other *allergen*. Treatment depends on the cause.

ERYTHEMA NODOSUM n. tender, reddened nodules on the shins, legs, and occasionally other body areas, often accompanied by fever, muscle and joint pain, and malaise; it occurs in certain diseases, as a drug reaction, and in certain allergic reactions.

ERYTHRO- comb. form meaning "red" (e.g., **erythroclasis**, the splitting of red blood cells).

ERYTHROBLAST n. a nucleated cell passing through maturation stages to become a mature *erythrocyte*. Erythroblasts are normally found in *bone marrow*, but they may appear in the blood circulation in certain diseases.

ERYTHROBLASTOSIS FETALIS n. a severe anemia in newborn babies resulting from an incompatibility between fetal and maternal blood, specifically involving the *Rh factor*. It typically occurs with the Rh-positive infant (the Rh factor being inherited from the father) of an Rh-negative mother, the mother transmitting to the fetal bloodstream antibodies against the Rh antigen that cause destruction of the fetal blood. The disorder rarely occurs in a first-born (unless the mother has already been sensitized to Rh antigen by a transfusion with Rh-positive blood), but the risk increases with each succeeding pregnancy. The condition can be diagnosed before birth through *amniocentesis* and treated by intrauterine transfusion. In some cases the development of Rh antibodies by the mother may be prevented by administration of anti-RH gamma globulin (RhoGAM) following birth or abortion of an Rh-positive fetus.

ERYTHROCIN n. trade name for antibacterial *erythromycin*.

ERYTHROCYTE n. a mature red blood cell, which contains the pigment *hemoglobin*, the main function of which is to transport oxygen to the tissues of the body. A red blood cell is a biconcave disc with no nucleus. It is the main cellular element in the blood; in one cubic milliliter of blood there are usually 4,500,000–5,000,000 erythrocytes in males, 4,000,000–4,500,000 in females.

ERYTHROCYTE SEDIMENTATION RATE (ESR) n. the rate at which red blood cells settle out in a tube (usually a 10-centimeter or 200 milliliter tube) of unclotted blood under standardized conditions. An ESR higher than normal usually indicates the presence of inflammation, and the test can be used as a diagnostic aid and to monitor the course of an inflammatory process (e.g., in chronic infections, rheumatic disorders). Colloquially called **sed rate**.

ERYTHRODERMA n. any skin disorder associated with abnormal redness (compare *erythema*).

ERYTHROMYCIN n. an antibiotic, known under several trade names (e.g., E-Mycin, Ilosone) used to treat infections caused by a wide variety of bacteria and other microorganisms. Adverse side effects are uncommon but may include nausea and diarrhea, or rarely, hypersensitivity reactions and liver inflammation.

ERYTHROPOIESIS n. the process of *erythrocyte* production; it normally occurs in the bone marrow.

ESCHAR n. a scab or crust that forms on the skin after a burn.

ESIDRIX n. trade name for a *diuretic* (hydrochlorothiazide) used to treat hypertension.

-ESIS suffix indicating an action or condition (e.g., *enuresis*)

ESKALITH n. trade name for the antipsychotic *lithium* carbonate.

ESOPHAG-, **ESOPHAGO-** comb. form indicating an association with the esophagus (e.g., **esophagectomy,** surgical removal of the esophagus).

ESOPHAGITIS n. inflammation of the esophagus, most often caused by backflow of acid stomach contents (gastroesophageal reflux) often associated with *hiatal hernia* but sometimes caused by infection or irritation.

ESOPHAGOSCOPE n. a special optical instrument used to examine the esophagus, to dilate the canal, or to remove a foreign object or material for biopsy.   n. **esophagoscopy**

ESOPHAGUS n. the gullet; the muscular canal, about 24 centimeters (10 inches) long, that connects the pharynx and stomach; food passes through it by waves of **peristalsis**.   adj. **esophageal**

ESOTROPIA n. a condition in which one or both eyes appear to turn inward; cross-eye (see *strabismus*).

ESP abbreviation for *extrasensory perception*.

ESR abbreviation for *erythrocyte sedimentation rate*.

ESSENTIAL AMINO ACID n. see *amino acid*.

ESSENTIAL HYPERTENSION n. high blood pressure (*hypertension*) for which no specific cause can be found.

EST n. see *electroconvulsive therapy*.

ESTAR n. trade name for a coal tar preparation used to treat *eczema*, *psoriasis* and other skin conditions.

ESTINYL n. trade name for an estrogen preparation (ethinyl *estradiol*) used to treat menstrual irregularities, menopause symptoms, and for contraceptive purposes.

ESTRADIOL n. the most powerful naturally occurring female hormone (see also *estrogen*).

ESTRATAB n. trade name for an *estrogen* preparation.

ESTRAVAL n. trade name for an *estrogen* preparation.

ESTRIOL n. a naturally occurring, rather weak *estrogen*.

ESTROGEN n. a general term for the female hormones (including estradiol, estrone, estriol) produced in the ovaries (and in small amounts in the testes and adrenals). In women estrogen functions in the *menstrual cycle* and in the development of secondary sex characteristics (e.g., breast development in adolescence). As a synthetic preparation, sold under many trade names, estrogen drugs are used to treat menstrual irregularities, to relieve symptoms of *menopause*, to treat cancer of the prostate, and in oral contraceptives. Long-term use of estrogen has been associated with some blood-clotting disorders and some forms of cancer and is controversial.

ESTRONE n. a form of estrogen.

ESTRONOL n. trade name for an *estrone* preparation.

ESTRUS n. the periodic occurrence of sexual activity in female mammals, marked by acceptance of the male (commonly known as being "in heat"). The term is not used in reference to human sexuality.

ETHACRYNIC ACID n. a diuretic, known under trade name Edecrin, used to treat *edema*. Adverse effects include muscle weakness, electrolyte imbalance, and hearing disorders.

ETHANOL n. ethyl alcohol; the alcohol found in alcoholic beverages and the alcohol used in solution as an antiseptic.

ETHER n. a liquid used as a solvent and general anesthetic. It is generally safe and provides excellent pain relief and muscle relaxation without greatly depressing the respiratory and circulatory systems. However, it is explosive and highly flammable and has an irritating odor and frequently causes postoperative nausea and vomiting, and its use as an anesthetic has been largely replaced by safer drugs.

ETHICAL DRUG n. a prescription drug; a drug available only by prescription.

ETHMOID n. one of the eight bones of the *cranium*; a small bone filled with air spaces that is between the eye sockets. adj. **ethmoidal**

ETHMOID SINUS n. a cavity in the ethmoid bone behind the bridge of the nose.

ETHOCAINE n. trade name for a local *anesthetic* (*procaine*).

ETHOSUXIMIDE n. an anticonvulsant, known under trade names Zarontin and Emeside, used to treat *petit mal epilepsy*. Adverse side effects include blood abnormalities and gastrointestinal disturbances.

ETHOTOIN n. an anticonvulsant, known under the trade name Peganone, used to treat *grand mal epilepsy*. Adverse reactions include nausea, fatigue, and chest pain.

ETHRANE n. trade name for the inhalation general anesthesia *enflurane*.

ETHRIL n. trade name for the antibiotic *erythromycin*.

ETHYL ALCOHOL n. *ethanol*.

ETHYL CHLORIDE n. a highly flammable topical anesthetic used to treat skin irritations and in minor skin surgery. Adverse side effects include pain and muscle spasm.

ETHYLENE n. a gas sometimes used as a general *anesthetic*. Nausea and vomiting commonly occur after its use.

ETIOLOGY n. the study of the causes of disease. adj. **etiologic**

ETRAFON n. trade name for a fixed-combination drug containing a *tranquilizer* (perphenazine) and an antidepressant (*amitriptyline*).

EU- prefix meaning "good," "well" (e.g., **eucapnia**, an optimal level of carbon dioxide in the arteries).

EUGENICS n. study concerned with controlling the characteristics of future generations through selective breeding techniques.

EUKARYOTE n. an organism containing cells that have a true nucleus. adj. **eukaryotic**

EUNUCH n. a male whose testes have been removed; a eunuch shows signs of a lack of male hormone (testosterone) such as feminine voice and lack of facial hair.

EUPHORIA n. 1. a feeling or state of well-being and optimism; 2. an exaggeration and unreal sense of well-being, commonly seen in some mental disorders. adj. **euphoric**

EUSTACHIAN TUBE n. the mucous membrane-lined tube that connects the nasopharynx and the middle ear; it allows pressure in the inner ear to be equalized with that of the atmosphere. Increased pressure in the tube, occurring, e.g., in a plane that is ascending, can usually be relieved by swallowing; also called **auditory tube**.

EUTHANASIA n. deliberately causing the death of a person who is suffering from an incurable disease either actively by the use of artificial means (e.g., drugs) or passively by withholding treatment necessary for the prolongation of life; also called **mercy killing**.

EVENTRATION n. 1. protrusion of the *intestine* through the abdominal wall; 2. surgical removal of the organs in the abdomen.

EVERSION n. the act of turning something inside out or turning it (e.g., a foot) outward.

EVEX n. trade name for an *estrogen* preparation.

EVISCERATION n. the act of removing an organ or the contents of the eyeball (see also **eventration; exenteration**).

EVOKED POTENTIAL n. an electrical response produced in the central nervous system by an external stimulus (e.g., a flash of light). The response can be monitored on recording equipment (see *electroencephalogram*) and used to verify the integrity of nerve connections.

EWING'S SARCOMA n. a malignant tumor developing in bone marrow, usually in long bones or the pelvis; it occurs most often in adolescent boys and produces pain, swelling, and an increase in white blood cells. Treatment is by radiotherapy and surgical removal (sometimes amputation); also called **Ewing's tumor**.

EX- prefix meaning "away from," "from," "out of," "outside" (e.g., **exsufflation**, the process of withdrawing the air from a cavity or organ, esp. the lungs).

EXACERBATION n. an increase in the seriousness of a disease or disorder, usually marked by a worsening of the symptoms.

EXAMINATION n. the act of viewing and studying the body, using various procedures, techniques, and equipment to ascertain the general health of the person and the presence or absence of any disease or disorder. The examination may include *palpation* (e.g., of the abdomen); percussion (tapping fingers or special instrument on a body surface to detect the presence of fluid or determine borders of an internal organ); auscultation (e.g., use of a stethoscope on the chest); the taking of tissue samples or body fluids (e.g., blood) for laboratory analysis; the analysis of X rays or other diagnostic procedures involving the internal organs; and the evaluation of subjective complaints (*symptoms*) of the patient.

EXANTHEM n. 1. any disease that includes fever and skin eruptions, such as measles; 2. a skin rash, like that seen in *rubella*, *measles*, or *chicken pox*.

EXCHANGE TRANSFUSION n. the removal of a person's blood in small amounts and its replacement with equal amounts of donor blood, esp. exchange transfusion of the newborn (neonate) or fetus (intrauterine exchange transfusion) to treat *erythroblastosis fetalis* (neonatorum) by removing the Rh and ABO antibodies and lysed erythrocytes (red blood cells) and substituting blood with normal oxygen-carrying capacity.

EXCISION n. surgical removal of a part or organ.

EXCORIATION n. injury to the surface of the skin caused by scratching, scraping, chemicals, or other means.

EXCREMENT n. feces.

EXCRESCENCE n. an abnormal projection or outgrowth, e.g., a wart.

EXCRETION n. 1. the discharge of waste from an organ or from the body; 2. waste matter, such as feces or urine (compare *secretion*). adj. **excretory** v. **excrete**

EXENTERATION n. 1. surgical removal of the organs within a body cavity, as those of the pelvis (see also *evisceration*); 2. removal of the entire contents of the eye socket.

EXERCISE n. activity to condition the body, maintain fitness, or correct a deformity (see also *aerobic exercise*; *isometric exercise*; *isotonic exercise*).

EXFOLIATION n. scaling off of dead skin; this occurs naturally but may be increased in some skin diseases and severe sunburn.

EXHALATION n. the process of breathing out, expelling air from the lungs. v. **exhale**

EXHAUSTION n. extreme fatigue; complete lack of energy (see also *heat exhaustion*).

EXHIBITIONISM n. a psychosexual disorder marked by exposure of the genitals to another person, usually of the opposite sex, for self-gratification in a socially unacceptable situation.

EXO- prefix meaning "outer," "outside," "outward" (e.g., **exoenzyme**, an enzyme whose action is outside the originating cell).

EXOCRINE GLAND n. a gland that discharges its secretion, usually through a duct, to an adjacent epithelial surface, as in the sweat glands discharging onto the skin surface. Included among the exocrine glands are the *sweat glands*, *sebaceous glands*, certain glands involved in digestion (e.g., ducts secreting pancreatic juice in the pancreas), *lacrimal* (tear) *glands*, *salivary glands*, wax-producing glands of the ear, and *mammary glands*. Also sometimes called **duct gland** (compare *endocrine gland*).

EXOGENOUS adj. originating or developing from outside the body (e.g., **exogenous obesity**, which is caused by overeating, not by bodily malfunction) (compare *endogenous*).

EXOMPHALOS n. umbilical hernia, in which some organs in the abdomen push into the umbilical cord at birth.

EXOPHTHALMIC GOITER n. *exophthalmos* occurring in association with *goiter*.

EXOPHTHALMOS n. abnormal protrusion of one or both eyeballs, due to *goiter*, injury, or disease of the eyeball or socket. Treatment depends on the cause.

EXOPHYTIC adj. growing outward, as a tumor that grows on the surface of an organ.

EXOSTOSIS n. benign outgrowth from a bone, usually covered with cartilage.

EXOTOXIN n. a poison produced by a living microorganism and secreted into the surrounding medium (compare *endotoxin*).

EXOTROPIA n. outward turning of one eye relative to the other (see also *strabismus*).

EXPECTORANT n. an agent that promotes *expectoration*.

EXPECTORATION n. the process of raising material (e.g., mucus or phlegm) from the respiratory tract by coughing and then spitting it out of the mouth. v. **expectorate**

EXPIRATION n. 1. that act of breathing out air from the lungs; 2. death. v. **expire**

EXPLORATION n. thorough examination of an area of the body, esp. in **exploratory surgery**.

EXPRESSION n. the act of forcing something out by pressing or squeezing (e.g., expressing milk from a breast).

EXSANGUINATION n. severe blood loss.

EXTENDED CARE FACILITY n. an institution that provides nursing, medical, and custodial care for a prolonged period, as in a chronic illness or rehabilitation from an acute illness.

EXTENDER n. a substance that increases the amount of another (e.g., plasma extender, used to add to the blood volume in emergencies).

EXTENSION n. stretching; the action of moving two joined parts away from one another.

EXTENSOR n. a muscle that, when flexed, causes *extension* of a joint, or straightening of an arm or leg.

EXTERIORIZE v. to place an internal organ or part of it (e.g., part of the colon in a *colostomy*) on the outside of the body.

EXTERNAL EAR n. the outer structure of the ear, consisting of the fleshy auricle and the canal (external acoustic meatus) leading to the *tympanic membrane* (eardrum).

EXTERNALIZE v. in psychology, to turn inner problems outward and express them in social relationships.

EXTINCTION n. in psychology, the loss of a learned response because of nonreward or nonreinforcement.

EXTIRPATION n. surgical removal of an entire part, organ, or growth.

EXTRA- comb. form meaning "additional," "beyond," "outside" (e.g., **extracorporeal**, outside the body).

EXTRACELLULAR adj. located on or outside a cell.

EXTRACELLULAR FLUID (ECF) n. protein and electrolyte (e.g., potassium, chloride) - containing fluid in blood plasma and interstitial fluid that helps control water and electrolyte movement in the body. Normally, the body has about 14 liters (15 quarts) of ECF.

EXTRACTION n. the act of pulling out, as a tooth.

EXTRASENSORY PERCEPTION (ESP) n. awareness or knowledge obtained by means other than the five senses; also: *clairvoyance, telepathy.*

EXTRAUTERINE adj. outside of the *uterus,* as in an extrauterine pregnancy (see *ectopic pregnancy*).

EXTRAVASATION n. leakage of fluid (e.g., blood) to the tissues outside of the vessel normally containing it; this may occur in injuries, burns, and allergic reactions.

EXTRAVERSION n. the directing of feelings and interests toward external things and the outside world rather than toward oneself; the person so inclined is an extrovert; also: **extroversion** (compare *introversion*).

EXTREMITY n. any of the limbs; an arm or a leg.

EXTRUSION n. the act of pushing something out by force.

EXUDATION n. the slow escape (oozing) of fluids and cellular matter from blood vessels or cells through small pores or breaks in the cell membranes, sometimes the result of inflammation.

EYE n. either of two organs of sight located in a bony socket at the front of the skull. The outer coat of the eye is made of the anterior transparent *cornea* and the posterior opaque *sclera* ("white of the eye"). Light enters through the cornea, passes through a fluid-filled anterior chamber, passes through the opening (*pupil*) in the *iris* (colored portion of the eye) and then through the *lens* and *vitreous body* to strike nerve cells (rods and cones) in the *retina* of the eye. The impulse is then transmitted from the retina through the *optic nerve* to the brain.

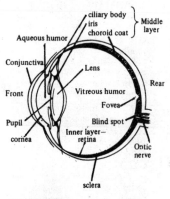

EYEBROW n. arch above the eye in the frontal bone, separating the eye socket from the forehead.

EYELASH n. one of many cilia growing along the margin of the *eyelid* that through their movement help to keep the eye free of debris.

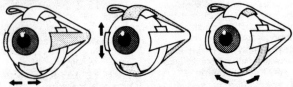

Six muscles attached to the outside of the eye control eyeball movement.

EYELID n. a movable fold of skin over the eye.

EYE STRAIN n. tiredness of the eyes brought about by prolonged close work or occurring in a person with an uncorrected eye problem; symptoms are aching and burning of the eyes, often accompanied by headache; also: **asthenopia**.

EYE TOOTH n. the sharp *canine* teeth in the upper jaw.

f

F symbol for the Fahrenheit temperature scale; symbol for the element fluorine.

FACE n. the front of the head, from the hairline to the chin, and including the forehead, eyes, nose, cheeks, and jaw.   adj. **facial**

FACE LIFT n. colloquial term for the repair of sagging tissues of the cheeks and eyelids by *cosmetic surgery* (see also *plastic surgery*; *ptosis*).

FACIAL NERVE n. the seventh (VII) cranial nerve, a mixed sensory and motor nerve that innervates much of the face, with sensory fibers extending from taste buds in the tongue and motor fibers extending to the scalp, muscles of facial expression, and some of the lacrimal (tear) and salivary glands.

FACILITATION n. in neurology, a phenomenon that occurs when two or more impulses, individually not powerful enough to produce a response in a neuron, combine to bring about a response (*action potential*) (compare *inhibition*).

FACTOR n. something that produces or influences a result (e.g., factor S, a sleep-promoting substance isolated from human urine).

FACTOR I - FACTOR XIII n. factors, most of which are present in blood plasma, involved in the process of *blood coagulation* (see also *fibrinogen*, *prothrombin*, *thromboplastin*).

FACULTATIVE adj. able to adjust to different environments or conditions (e.g., **facultative anaerobe**, an organism that normally lives without air [oxygen] but can survive in air).

FACULTY n. the ability to do something specific (e.g., the faculty of hearing).

FAHRENHEIT adj. a scale used to show temperature levels. Water freezes at 32° Fahrenheit and boils at 212° Fahrenheit; commonly abbreviated F (compare *Celsius*).

FAILURE n. loss of ability to function normally (see also *heart failure*; *renal failure*).

FAINT v. to become unconscious, usually as a result of insufficient blood flow to the brain, as a reaction to emotional or physical shock or to pain, hunger, or fear. Fainting is often preceded by a feeling of lightheadedness and can be prevented by placing the head between the knees, thus increasing the blood flow to the head; also: *syncope*.

FALCIFORM adj. sickle-shaped.

FALCIFORM LIGAMENT n. ligament attaching part of the liver to the *diaphragm* and abdominal wall.

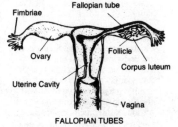

FALLOPIAN TUBES

FALLOPIAN TUBE n. either of two tubes or ducts, each of which extends from the *uterus* to the region of an *ovary*. The tube serves as passage for the movement of an ovum from the ovary (after *ovulation*) to the uterus and for the movement of sperm from the uterus upward toward the ovary. Fertilization normally occurs in the Fallopian tube (also called *oviduct*).

FALLOT'S SYNDROME (TETRALOGY) see *tetralogy of Fallot*.

FAMILIAL adj. pert. to some factor (e.g., a disease or characteristic), usually but not always inherited, that is present in some families but not in others; occurring in family members more frequently than would be expected by chance (compare *acquired*, *congenital*, *hereditary*).

FAMILIAL HYPERCHOLESTEROLEMIA n. inherited disorder characterized by a high level of serum *cholesterol* and early development of *atherosclerosis* that places affected individuals at a high risk for certain types of heart disease.

FAMILY HISTORY n. part of a patient's medical history in which questions are asked about the incidence and prevalence of specific diseases and disorders in his/her family in an attempt to ascertain if the patient has a hereditary or familial tendency toward a particular disease.

FAMILY PLANNING n. deliberate limiting or spacing of the number of children born to a couple (see *contraception*).

FAMILY THERAPY n. in psychiatry, treatment that focuses on the individual as a family member; in the same session two or more family members or the whole family may meet together with the therapist to discover how the various family members interact.

FANTASY n. 1. free play of the imagination; 2. conversion of disliked reality into invented, imagined experiences in order to fulfill hidden desires or to express unconscious conflicts.

FARMER'S LUNG n. a respiratory disorder caused by an allergic response to inhaled fungi from moldy hay and characterized by coughing, difficult breathing, nausea, chills, fever, and rapid heart beat.

FARSIGHTEDNESS see *hyperopia*.

FASCIA n. fibrous connective tissue that supports soft organs and sheaths structures such as muscles. pl. fasciae

FASCICLE n. a small bundle of nerve, muscle, or tendon fibers; also: **fasciculus**. adj. **fascicular**

FASCIOLIASIS n. infection with the liver fluke *Fasciola hepatica* obtained by eating aquatic plants (e.g., watercress) with encysted forms of the flukes and common in many parts of the world, including the southern United States. Symptoms include fever, abdominal pain, loss of appetite, jaundice, vomiting, and diarrhea; liver damage sometimes occurs. Treatment is by bithionol (TBP).

FASCIOLOPSIASIS n. an intestinal infection common in the Far East and caused by eating aquatic plants (e.g., water chestnuts) contaminated with *Fasciolopsis buski* flukes. Symptoms include abdominal pain, diarrhea, and, in severe cases, *edema*. Treatment is by *anthelmintics*.

FAST v. to go without all or certain food (compare *anorexia*; *diet*).

FAT n. 1. a water-soluble substance derived from fatty acids and found in animal tissues, where it serves as a source of energy; 2. a type of body tissue (*adipose*) containing stored fat that serves as a source of energy, as insulation, and as a protective cushion for vital organs.

FATALITY RATE n. the number of deaths during a given period for a stipulated population, as, e.g., the percentage of people who die of a particular disease.

FAT EMBOLISM n. a serious circulatory disease in which a fat *embolus* blocks an artery; the embolus enters the circulation after fracture of a long bone or traumatic injury to adipose (fatty) tissue or a fatty liver.

FATIGABILITY n. a tendency to become easily tired or to lose strength.

FATIGUE n. 1. exhaustion, weariness, loss of strength resulting from hard or prolonged mental or physical work; 2. temporary inability of tissues (e.g., muscle) to respond to stimuli that normally produce a response.

FATIGUE FRACTURE n. see under *fracture*.

FAT METABOLISM n. the biochemical processes in the body by which fats ingested in the diet are broken down (first into *fatty acids* and *glycerol* and then into simpler compounds) into substances that can be used by the cells of the body. Fats are a major energy source, providing approximately 9 kilocalories per gram, compared with about 4 kilocalories per gram in *carbohydrates*.

FATTY ACID n. an organic (carbon-containing) acid; fatty acids are the building blocks of many *lipids*. Some fatty acids are manufactured by the body; others, the essential fatty acids, must be supplied by the diet.

FATTY LIVER n. accumulation of certain fats (triglycerides) in the liver, due to alcoholic cirrhosis, exposure to certain drugs or toxic substances, or as complication of certain conditions (e.g., *kwashiorkor*, pregnancy); symptoms include enlarged liver, loss of appetite, and abdominal discomfort. Treatment depends on the cause.

FAUCES n. the opening at the back of the mouth into the *pharynx*.

FAVISM n. an anemia resulting from eating fava beans or breathing in the plant's pollen. It occurs in the Mediterranean area (e.g., Italy); victims have an inherited blood abnormality and enzyme deficiency. Symptoms include dizziness, headache, fever, vomiting, and diarrhea; blood transfusions may be required.

FAVUS n. a contagious fungal infection of the scalp, producing honeycomblike crusts, a musty odor, and itching. The condition occurs chiefly in the Middle East and Africa.

FDA n. see *Food and Drug Administration*.

FEBRILE adj. pert. to or characterized by an elevated body temperature (*fever*).

FECAL adj. pert. to *feces*.

FECAL IMPACTION n. an accumulation of hardened *feces* in the rectum or lower part of the colon which the person is unable to move. Treatment is by enemas and manual breaking of the stool with a gloved finger. Prevention includes a diet containing bulk foods, adequate water intake, exercise, and sometimes use of fecal softeners.

FECALITH n. a hard mass of *feces* in the colon evacuated manually or by means of an oil enema.

FECES n. the material discharged from the bowel in *defecation*. Formed in the colon, feces consist of water, undigested food residue, bacteria, and mucus; also: **stool**.   adj. **fecal**

FECUNDITY n. the ability to produce offspring, esp. in large numbers in a short period.   adj. **fecund**

FEEBLEMINDEDNESS n. see *mental retardation*.

FEEDBACK n. the coupling of the output of a gland or process to the input; the return of some portion of the energy or effect of a process to the originating source to regulate its further output. For example, a feedback mechanism controls the release of thyroxine from the thyroid gland; the level of thyroxine in the circulating blood is detected by the pituitary gland, which then responds to maintain the level at normal range, releasing a factor (thyroid-stimulating hormone) to stimulate the thyroid to release more thyroxine if needed.

FEEDING n. the taking in of food or the offering of food (see *breast feeding*; *demand feeding*; *forced feeding*).

FEHLING'S SOLUTION n. a solution of copper sulfate, potassium tartrate, and sodium hydroxide used to test for sugar (esp. glucose) in the urine, which, when present, turns the solution reddish.

FELLATIO n. sucking the penis or otherwise stimulating it with the mouth.

FEMALE adj. pert. to the sex that bears young (compare *male*); n. a woman or girl. adj. **feminine**

FEMINIZATION n. the development of womanlike changes (e.g., breast enlargement, loss of facial hair) in a male because of endocrine (hormonal) disorder or the administration of certain drugs.

FEMOGEN n. trade name for an *estrogen* preparation.

FEMORAL adj. pert. to the *femur* or to the thigh.

FEMORAL ARTERY n. the main artery of the thigh, arising from the external *iliac artery* in the region of the inguinal ligament and running down two thirds of the thigh, after which it divides into several branches.

FEMORAL NERVE n. the main nerve of the anterior (front) part of the thigh, receiving sensory impulses from the front and inner thigh and supplying the muscles of the anterior thigh; also sometimes called **anterior crural nerve**.

FEMORAL PULSE n. pulse of the *femoral artery*, felt in the groin.

FEMUR n. the thighbone, the longest and strongest bone in the body, extending from the hip to the knee. Largely cylindrical, the femur has a large rounded head that fits into the *acetabulum* of the hipbone; a neck and shaft with projections and ridges for the attachment of muscles; and an expanded distal end that articulates with the *tibia* of the lower leg. adj. **femoral**

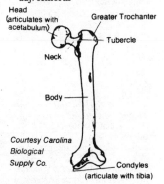

Head (articulates with acetabulum)

Greater Trochanter

Tubercle

Neck

Body

Condyles (articulate with tibia)

Courtesy Carolina Biological Supply Co.

FENESTRA n. a windowlike opening, sometimes closed by a membrane. The fenestra ovalis (fenestra vestibuli), or *oval window*, and the fenestra cochleae (fenestra rotunda), or *round window* are two openings in the ear.

FENESTRATION n. 1. surgical procedure in which a windowlike opening is created in the inner ear to restore hearing lost because of *osteosclerosis*; 2. any surgical procedure in which an opening is created to gain access to a cavity within an organ or bone.

FENOPROFEN n. an antiinflammatory agent used in the treatment of arthritis and other painful inflammatory disorders. Adverse side effects include gastrointestinal upsets, dizziness, and drowsiness.

FEOSOL n. trade name for an iron-containing drug used to treat some types of *anemia*.

FERGON n. trade name for an iron-containing compound used to treat some types of *anemia*.

FERMENTATION n. breakdown of complex substances, esp. sugar and other carbohydrates, by enzymes or microorganisms.

-FEROUS comb. form meaning "bearing," "yielding" (e.g., **lipoferous**, carrying fat).

FERR-, FERRI-, FERRO- comb. form indicating an association with iron (e.g., **ferrokinetics**, the rate of change in iron levels in the body).

FERRITIN n. an *iron* compound found in the intestines, liver, and spleen; it contains more than 20% iron and is one of the chief forms in which iron is stored in the body.

FERTILE adj. capable of reproducing, of bearing young. n. **fertility**

FERTILE PERIOD n. that time in the menstrual cycle in which *fertilization* is most likely to occur. Attempts to determine a woman's fertile period are based on knowledge of when ovulation (the release of an ovum, or egg, from the ovary) occurs (usually 14 days before onset of a period), of how long the ovum will survive (usually 24 hours), and of how long sperm will survive in the female genital tract (usually 48 to 72 hours). Thus the fertile period begins 2 or 3 days before ovulation and lasts 2 or 3 days afterward, but to allow for possible longer survival times of sperm and egg is usually considered to last 7 or 8 days around ovulation. Knowledge of the fertile period is used by some to help prevent conception and by others to try to increase the chances of conception. See also *basal body temperature method of family planning, calendar method of family planning, contraception*.

FERTILIZATION n. the union (fusion) of the male and female sex cells (*gametes, the sperm and ovum*) to form a single cell (*zygote*) that then divides to eventually form the *fetus* (see also *test-tube baby*). Fertilization takes place in the *Fallopian tube* of the female.

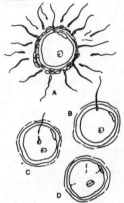

The fertilization process. (A) It is believed that at least several hundred sperm typically reach the ovum, and begin pushing their way through the cells remaining around it. The sperm release an enzyme that dissolves the substance holding these cells together. Eventually a single spermatozoon penetrates the zona pellucida which surrounds the ovum. B) As the ovum is penetrated, its outer surface seems to expand outward to help engulf the spermatozoon; it also becomes impenetrable to other sperm. (C) The sperm disintegrates after it has entered the ovum. (D) The head of the spermatozoon which contains the spermatozoon's genetic material expands into a cell nucleus which fuses with the nucleus of the ovum, combining with it to form a full complement of 46 chromosomes. The fertilized ovum is now called zygote.

FERTILIZATION MEMBRANE n. a membrane that develops around a fertilized ovum and prevents the penetration of additional sperm.

FESTER v. to become inflamed and form *pus*.

FESTINATION n. an involuntary quickening and shortening of steps in walking, as occurs in some diseases (e.g., *parkinsonism*).

FETAL adj. pert. to a *fetus*.

FETAL ALCOHOL SYN-DROME n. a condition in which mental ability, body formation, and facial development may be defective in a *fetus* as the result of the mother's consumption of alcohol (ethanol) while pregnant. The fetus may also be stillborn as a result (see also *teratogenicity*).

FETAL AGE n. the age of the *conceptus* counted from the time of *fertilization*. Since in most cases pregnancy is counted from the first day of the last menstrual period but fertilization occurs about two weeks after that, the fetal age is often about two weeks less than the calculated length of the pregnancy; also called **fertilization age**. (Compare *gestational age*.)

FETAL CIRCULATION n. the system of blood vessels and special structures through which blood moves in the *fetus*. The fetus is attached to the mother's *placenta* through the *umbilical cord*. Maternal oxygenated blood from the placenta travels through the umbilical vein to the liver of the fetus and from there through the inferior vena cava to the right atrium of the heart. It then passes through the *foramen ovale* into the left atrium and from there to the left ventricle and circulation through the head and upper body parts. The returning blood flows through the superior vena cava into the right atrium from which at low pressure it flows into the right ventricle and then through the pulmonary artery into the descending aorta and circulation through the lower body parts. The wastes of the fetus are carried by the blood through the umbilical arteries back to the placenta, where they diffuse into the mother's bloodstream for eventual excretion. This system, which differs in many ways from the circulatory path in an adult, allows oxy-

FETAL CIRCULATION

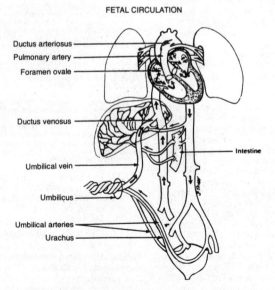

Ductus arteriosus
Pulmonary artery
Foramen ovale

Ductus venosus

Intestine

Umbilical vein

Umbilicus

Umbilical arteries
Urachus

gen and nutrients to be supplied to the fetus and wastes to be carried away. At birth several changes occur, including closure (at least partial) of the foramen ovale so that blood no longer flows from the right atrium to the left atrium. Circulation through the baby's lungs begins with the first breath.

FETAL DISTRESS n. a compromised or abnormal condition of the *fetus* usually characterized by abnormal heart rhythm and discovered during pregnancy or labor, sometimes through the use of a *fetal monitor*. If possible the cause of the problem is determined and corrected; if this is not possible immediate *Cesarean delivery* may be indicated.

FETAL HEART RATE n. the number of heartbeats in the fetus during a given time, normally between 100 and 160 beats per minute but varying with cycles of rest and activity and maternal condition. The fetal heart rate is detected through use of a *fetoscope* or *fetal monitor*.

FETAL MONITOR n. a device used during pregnancy, labor, and childbirth to observe the fetal heart rate and maternal uterine contractions. The device may be applied externally on the abdomen of the mother or less commonly inserted into the uterus through the vagina.

FETAL MEMBRANES n. collectively, the *amnion*, *chorion* (sac around the amnion) and umbilical cord (which includes the yolk stalk, *allantois*, and blood vessels), all of which function for the protection, nourishment, respiration, and excretion of the developing fetus. The *placenta*, made of both fetal and maternal tissue, also serves these functions.

FETAL MOVEMENT n. motion of the fetus itself within the uterus. The motion is usually first detected by a woman pregnant for the first time at about the 13th week of pregnancy, somewhat earlier in those who have had previous pregnancies.

FETISHISM n. the transfer of sexual or love interest to an object (fetish), either an inanimate object (e.g., underwear) or a part of the body not usually associated with sex (e.g., the foot). ''Partial fetishism'' or ''auxiliary fetishism'' refers to use of an object to heighten interest in heterosexual intercourse (e.g., the wearing of particular articles of clothing).

FETISHIST n. one who engages in fetishism.

FETO- comb. form indicating an association with a *fetus* (e.g., **fetoplacental**, pert. to the fetus and the *placenta*).

FETOLOGY n. that branch of medicine concerned with the *fetus* in the *uterus*, including the diagnosis and treatment of abnormalities.

FETOMETRY n. the measurement of a fetus, esp. the diameter of the head.

FETOPROTEIN n. an antigen that occurs naturally in the *fetus* and sometimes in adults with certain cancers. A greater-than-normal amount of *alpha fetoprotein* (AFP) in the fetus often indicates an abnormality of the neural tube (e.g., *hydrocephaly* or *spina bifida*).

FETOSCOPE n. a stethoscope placed on the mother's abdomen to detect the fetal heartbeat.

FETOSCOPY n. procedure that allows the direct observation of the *fetus* in the *uterus* through a fetoscope introduced through a small incision in the pregnant woman's abdomen.

FETOR n. a bad smell.   adj. **fetid**

FETUS n. the live offspring while it is inside the mother (*in utero*), in humans, from the beginning of the third month of pregnancy until birth.   adj. **fetal**

FEVER n. a rise in the temperature of the body (see *pyrexia*). Normal body temperature is 98.6° Fahrenheit (37.0° Celsius) taken orally, somewhat higher rectally. A rise in temperature can sometimes be caused by severe stress, strenuous exercise, or dehydration, but fever is most often a sign of infection (bacterial, viral, or other) or other disease. Fever is often accompanied by headache, chills, and feeling of malaise; high fevers can cause delirium and convulsions (esp. in young children). The onset, course, and duration of a fever vary with the cause; certain diseases are associated with characteristic rising and falling curves that may aid in diagnosis; also: **hyperpyrexia**. adj. **febrile**

FEVER BLISTER n. a cold sore caused by a herpesvirus (see *herpes simplex*).

FIBER n. 1. a long, threadlike structure (e.g., a nerve fiber); 2. food content (cellulose) that adds roughage to the diet.

FIBEROPTICS n. the technique in which thin, flexible, glass or plastic fibers in special instruments called *fiberscopes* are used to view inner parts of the body; the fibers transmit light and relay a magnified image of the body part.

FIBERSCOPE n. a flexible instrument containing light-carrying glass or plastic fibers used to view internal body structures. Fiberscopes are especially designed for examination of particular body parts. For example, the bronchoscope is designed for viewing the tracheal and bronchial region; the gastroscope is designed for viewing the interior of the stomach; the duodenoscope is designed for viewing the deodenum.

FIBRIL n. a very small fiber or a thread of a fiber (e.g., *myofibrils* of muscle fiber).

FIBRILLATION n. recurrent, involuntary, and abnormal muscular contraction in which a single or small number of fibers act separately rather than as a coordinated unit, esp. in the heart, as in atrial or *ventricular fibrillation*.

FIBRIN n. an insoluble protein in the blood that combines with similar molecules, red and white blood cells, and platelets to form a blood clot. Fibrin is formed by the action of *thrombin* on its precursor, *fibrinogen* (see *blood coagulation*).

FIBRINOGEN n. a protein present in the blood plasma and essential to the process of blood coagulation; the factor (Factor I) converted into fibrin by thrombin in the presence of calcium ions during the process of *blood coagulation*.

FIBRINOLYSIS n. process in which the protein *fibrin* dissolves and small clots are removed.

FIBROADENOMA n. a benign, nontender, hard, movable and firm tumor of the breast, most common in young women and caused by high estrogen levels.

FIBROBLAST n. an undifferentiated cell in connective tissue that gives rise to cells that are the precursors of bone, collagen, and other connective tissue cells.

FIBROCYSTIC DISEASE OF THE BREAST n. a common condition among women characterized by the presence of one or more cysts in the breast. The cysts are benign but should be watched carefully for any changes in size or consistency; women with fibrocystic breast disease have a higher-than-normal chance of developing breast cancer later in life. In many cases no treatment is necessary; in other cases aspiration of the cyst with/without *biopsy* is performed. Some investigators believe that consumption of caffeine (e.g., in coffee, soft drinks) in large amounts is associated with cystic breast disease;

also called **cystic breast disease**, **cystic mastitis**.

FIBROID TUMOR n. a benign tumor (fibroma) containing fibrous tissue, esp. that of the uterus. Fibroid tumors of the uterus are common and in many cases do not require treatment; if, however, they cause discomfort or hemorrhage, surgical removal is necessary.

FIBROMA n. a nonmalignant tumor of connective tissue.

FIBROMYOSITIS n. any of a large number of disorders marked by local inflammation of muscle and connective tissue, stiffness, and joint or muscle pain. It may result from infection, trauma, or other cause. Treatment includes rest, pain-relieving drugs, and sometimes massage.

FIBROSIS n. an increase in the formation of fibrous connective tissue, either normally as in scar formation, or abnormally to replace normal tissues, esp. in the lungs, uterus, or heart (see also *cystic fibrosis*).

FIBROUS adj. consisting of fibers.

FIBROUS JOINT n. an immovable joint, such as those in the skull (compare *cartilaginous joint*, *synovial joint*).

FIBULA n. the long, thin outer bone of the lower leg. It articulates with the *tibia* (the other lower leg bone) just below the knee and extends to the outer side of the ankle; also called **calf bone**.

FIELD n. 1. an area, as that seen through a microscope (microscopic field); 2. the area seen (visual field); 3. an open area during surgery (operative field); 4. an area of expertise (e.g., field of psychiatry).

FILARIASIS n. a disease, largely of the tropics, caused by filariae (long, threadlike worms) that enter the body through mosquito bites and infest primarily lymph glands and vessels. Symptoms include blockage of the lymph vessels and resultant swelling and pain in the limb distal to the blockage, which, over many years, may lead to *elephantiasis*. Treatment is by *anthelmintics*.

FILIFORM adj. thread-shaped.

FIMBRIA n. a fringe or fringelike structure, such as the fingerlike projections around the ovarian end of the *Fallopian tube*. pl. **fimbriae**

FIORINAL n. trade name for a fixed-combination drug containing the pain-relieving, fever-reducing, and anti-inflammatory agent *aspirin*; the pain-reliever *phenacetin*; the sedative-hypnotic butalbital, and the stimulant *caffeine*.

FIRST AID n. immediate care given an injured or ill person before treatment by medically trained personnel. The most critical concerns are dealt with first: maintenance of adequate heart function and an open airway and control of bleeding; after that, care depends on the nature of the injury or illness.

FISSION n. a splitting, as in the asexual formation of new bacterial or protozoan cells or in the splitting of an atomic nucleus, with the release of energy.

FISSURE n. 1. any of the deep grooves of the outer covering of the brain; 2. a cleft or groove in a part, whether normal or abnormal (e.g., an anal fissure, a long ulcerlike groove at the anus).

FISTULA n. an abnormal opening or channel connecting two internal organs or leading from an internal organ to the outside (e.g., urinary fistula, an abnormal channel of the urinary tract). Fistulas are due to ulceration, failure of a wound to heal, injury, tumors, or congenital defects. Surgical repair is not always possible. pl. **fistulae** adj. **fistular, fistulous**

FIT n. colloquial, a sudden attack (e.g., a fit of coughing) or a seizure (e.g., in epilepsy).

FIXATION n. 1. the process of securing a part, as by sewing with catgut or wire (suturing); 2. a halt in personality growth at a particular stage of phychological development; 3. hardening and preservation of tissues for examination under a microscope.

FIXED-COMBINATION DRUG n. a preparation containing multiple ingredients in specific amounts; it allows concomitant administration of two or more drugs.

FLACCID adj. limp, soft, weak, or flabby (e.g., a muscle).

FLACCID BLADDER n. a type of malfunctioning bladder caused by interruption of the normal reflex arc associated with voiding; symptoms include absence of bladder sensation, overfilling of the bladder and inability to urinate voluntarily.

FLACCID PARALYSIS n. abnormality characterized by weakness or loss of muscle tone due to disease or injury to the nerves affecting the involved muscles (compare *spastic paralysis*).

FLAGELLATION n. the action of whipping someone else (see *sadism*) or of being whipped (see *masochism*) for stimulation or sexual arousal.

FLAGELLUM n. a threadlike tail or other extension from an organism, as in *sperm*, to provide locomotion.   pl. **flagella**

FLAGYL n. trade name for an antiprotozoal (metronidazole) used to treat *trichomoniasis* (a vaginal infection) and certain other infections.

FLAP n. a section of tissue used to cover a burn or other injury, as the pedicle flap, a tubular gathering of skin, one end of which is left attached in the original site while the other end is freed for attachment in another part of the body. When the flap has healed at the new site, the other end is also detached and the remaining skin is sewn in place.

FLARE n. 1. a reddening of the skin around a lesion produced by an allergic reaction; 2. a reddening of the skin spreading outward from a focus of irritation or infection.

FLATFOOT n. a condition in which the instep is not arched and the bottom of the foot (plantar surface) is flat, sometimes causing footache and fatigue. Treatment, when needed, is by special shoes or other devices.

FLATULENCE n. an abnormal amount of abdominal gas, causing distension of the stomach or intestine and sometimes discomfort.

FLATUS n. gas in the stomach and/or intestines.   adj. **flatulent**

FLAVIN n. see *riboflavin* in the Table of Vitamins

FLAXEDIL n. trade name for a neuromuscular blocking agent *gallamine* often used with anesthesia in surgery.

FLEET THEOPHYLLINE n. trade name for smooth muscle relaxant administered rectally as a *bronchodilator*.

FLEXION n. a bending of a joint (e.g., the elbow) that causes two adjoining bones (e.g., those in the upper and lower arm) to come closer together (compare *extension*).

FLEXOR n. a muscle that bends a joint (e.g., flexor hallucis brevis, which bends the great toe upward).

FLEXURE n. an angle or fold, such as the hepatic flexure of the colon.

FLOATER n. a spot that appears in the visual field when one stares at a blank wall. Floaters are due to bits of protein and other debris that move in front of the retina. Usually they are harmless but a sudden increase in the number of floaters may indicate a disease (e.g., *detached retina*).

FLOCCULATION n. reaction in which material that is normally invisible in a solution forms a suspension or precipitate as a result of changes in the physical or chemical conditions. This reaction is the basis of flocculation tests used to diagnose certain diseases (e.g., *syphilis*).

FLOXURIDINE n. an antineoplastic drug used to treat certain cancers. Adverse effects include *alopecia*, dermatitis, gastrointestinal disturbances, and depression of bone marrow function.

FLU n. see *influenza*.

FLUORESCEIN n. a dye used in ophthalmology to detect certain defects of the cornea and other abnormalities and to determine whether the fit of a contact lens is correct.

FLUORESCENCE n. the emission of light by a material when it is exposed to certain types of radiation (e.g., X-ray or ultraviolet). This property is used in *fluoroscopy*.   adj. **fluorscent**

FLUORIDATION n. the addition of fluoride to drinking water to prevent or reduce tooth decay. The fluorine compounds enhance the ability of the tooth to withstand acid breakdown, and their use (although controversial) has led to a decline in the prevalence of dental caries in the United States and other countries. Too much fluoride in the water can lead to *fluorosis*.

FLUORINE n. an element (see Table of Elements).

FLUOROCARBON n. any of several chemical compounds of *fluorine* and *carbon*, which, because of their ability to carry large amounts of oxygen, may become useful in *artificial blood* for humans who cannot have, or refuse, transfusions of human blood.

FLUOROSCOPY n. a technique in which a special device (fluoroscope) allows the immediate projection of X-ray images of the body onto a special fluorescent screen. It eliminates the need for taking and developing X-ray photographs.

FLUOROSIS n. condition resulting from excessive intake of fluorine, usually from too-high concentrations in drinking water; it causes discoloration and pitting of tooth enamel in children and bone and joint changes in adults.

FLUOROURACIL n. an antineoplastic drug used to treat certain cancers. Adverse effects include alopecia, bone marrow depression, and gastrointestinal disturbances.

FLUPHENAZINE n. a *tranquilizer* used to treat psychotic disorders. Adverse effects include hypotension, liver toxicity, and blood abnormalities.

FLURAZEPAM n. a minor tranquilizer used to treat *insomnia*. Adverse side effects include drug hangover (next-day sleepiness), dizziness, and possibly the development of dependence.

FLUSH n. 1. a sudden reddening of the face; 2. a sudden sensation of heat.

FLUTTER n. rapid movement back and forth of a part, esp. of the heart chambers (*atria* and *ventricles*).

FLUX n. an excessive flow from an organ or cavity (e.g., diarrhea).

FOCAL DISTANCE n. in ophthalmology, the distance between the lens and the point behind the lens at which light from a distant point is focused. In a normal sighted person the point of focus is on the retina, but distortions in the shape of the eyeball may cause *myopia* (nearsightedness) or *hyperopia* (farsightedness).

FOCAL SEIZURE n. a transitory disturbance, caused by abnormal electrical activity of nerve cells in a particular localized area of the brain (produced by temporary lack of oxygen, a small lesion, or trauma) and manifested by disturbance in motor or sensory function, as, e.g., profuse salivation, lip smacking, or tingling feeling in a certain body part.

FOCUS n. 1. a point at which light, sound, or other rays meet, as determined by positions of lenses and other devices; the point of convergence of light after passing through a convex lens is the place at which there is the clearest image; 2. the main site of an infection or other diseased state. pl. **foci** adj. **focal**

FOLD n. a doubling back or infolding (e.g., the neural fold, which leads to the development of the neural tube in the embryo).

FOLIC ACID n. one of the B-complex vitamins, essential for cell growth and reproduction; it functions as a coenzyme with vitamins C and B_{12} in the metabolism of proteins and the formation of iron-carrying *hemoglobin* in red blood cells. Rich sources include green leafy vegetables, liver, kidney, and whole grain cereals. Also called **folacin; pteroylglutamic acid**.

FOLIE n. any of several abnormal reactions; a mental disorder.

FOLIE A DEUX n. *psychosis* in two persons closely involved with each other, that of one leading to the condition in the other.

FOLIE DU DOUTE n. a condition in which the person cannot make even the simplest decisions.

FOLLICLE n. 1. pouchlike cavity, as that in the skin enclosing a hair; 2. a saclike gland, as a sebaceous follicle that secretes sebum; 3. *Graafian follicle* of the ovary, from which an *ovum* erupts. adj. **follicular**

FOLLICLE - STIMULATING HORMONE (FSH) n. a substance given off by the anterior portion of the pituitary gland (one of the three *gonadotropic hormones*) that stimulates the growth and maturation of the *Graafian follicle* in the ovary and spermatogenesis (formation of sperm) in the testes. FSH is sometimes administered to stimulate *ovulation* and sperm production.

FOLLICULITIS n. inflammation of a *hair follicle*.

FOMENTATION n. application of warm, wet coverings to relieve pain or inflammation.

FOMES n. any object (as a utensil, towel, money) that can support and transmit disease-causing organisms. pl. **fomites**

FONTANEL n. one of two membrane-covered soft spots in the skull of a newborn infant, which close as the cranial bones develop; also: **fontanelle**.

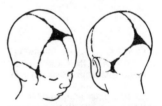

Diagrammatic representation of fontanels.

FOOD ALLERGY n. a *hypersensitivity reaction* to a substance—an antigen, most often a protein—ingested in food. Symptoms may include *rhinitis*, diarrhea, nausea, vomiting, itchy skin eruptions, bronchial asthma, colitis, and other signs. Food commonly associated with allergic reactions in sensitized people include eggs, wheat, milk, fish and seafoods, citrus fruits and tomatoes, and chocolate.

FOOD AND DRUG ADMINIS-TRATION (FDA) n. federal agency concerned with the enforcement of laws regulating the manufacture and distribution of food, drugs, and cosmetics.

FOOD POISONING n. acute illness caused by eating food containing toxic substances (e.g., insecticide) or organisms (bacteria and fungi, esp. certain mushrooms) and the toxins produced by them. The bacteria most commonly responsible for food poisoning are *Clostridium botulinum*, *Salmonella*, and *Staphylococcus*; the mushrooms are *Amanita* species. Symptoms vary with the type of poison and may range from mild abdominal discomfort, nausea, and diarrhea to severe symptoms including paralysis, coma, and death (see also *botulism*; *gastroenteritis*; *mushroom poisoning*; *ptomaine*; *salmonellosis*.

FOOT n. the part of the leg below the ankle.

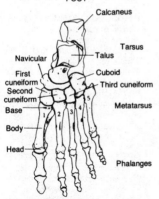

FOOT

Calcaneus

Tarsus

Navicular — Talus

First cuneiform — Cuboid

Second cuneiform — Third cuneiform

Base — Metatarsus

Body

Head

Phalanges

Courtesy Carolina Biological Supply Co.

FOOT-AND-MOUTH DISEASE n. a common viral disease of farm animals in Europe, Asia, and Africa that is sometimes transmitted to humans who come in contact with the animals and their products; symptoms include headache, fever, malaise, and small blisters on the oral membranes, tongue, hands, and feet.

FOOTDROP n. abnormal condition in which the foot is not in its normal flexed position, but rather drags; it is usually due to damage to the nerves and muscles of the foot.

FORAMEN n. a hole or opening, esp. in a bone or membrane (e.g., the **foramen ovale**, an opening between the two atria of the fetal heart that closes after birth).

FORCED FEEDING n. the forcible administration of food (e.g., through a nasal tube) to someone who will not or cannot otherwise eat.

FORCEPS n. any of a large variety of surgical instruments used to grasp, handle, pull or otherwise manipulate a body part or a fetus.

FORCEPS DELIVERY n. an obstetrical procedure in which forceps are inserted through the vagina to grasp the head of the fetus and draw it through the birth canal; performed to shorten labor or quickly deliver a baby in distress. The forceps usually leaves marks on the baby's skull and sometimes causes injury; use of forceps delivery has declined in recent years as the rate of Cesarean deliveries has increased.

FOREARM n. that part of the upper extremity between the elbow and the wrist.

FOREBRAIN n. the part of the brain controlling sensation, perception, emotion, learning, thinking, and other intellectual functions and including the olfactory bulb and tracts, cerebral hemispheres, and nasal ganglia as well as the thalamus, optic tracts, and hypothalamus.

FORENSIC MEDICINE n. a branch of medicine concerned with the legal aspects of medical care, such as the cause of unexplained death; forensic pathology provides evidence used in the resolution of crimes involving the death of a person.

FOREPLAY n. stimulation of sexual arousal between partners before actual intercourse.

FORESKIN n. the loose skin around the base of the head of the penis (glans) or clitoris; its removal constitutes *circumcision*; also: *prepuce*.

FORMALDEHYDE n. a poisonous gas that, when dissolved in water, has many uses as a disinfecting and preserving agent.

FORMICATION n. the sensation that worms or insects are crawling on the skin; it is sometimes a symptom of drug intoxication.

FORMULA n. 1. a simplified statement, using, as a rule, symbols and numerals that show the relationship among certain factors; for example, Fahrenheit (F) temperature can be converted to Celsius (C) by this formula: $C = \frac{5}{9}(F - 32)$, and water can be expressed as H_2O, signifying its makeup of 2 hydrogen (H) atoms and one oxygen (O) atom; 2. a preparation, containing proteins, carbohydrates, fats, minerals, and vitamins, usually in proportions similar to those of breast milk, used to feed infants. Most infant formulas are based on cow's milk, but some based on soybean or other substances are available for those infants who cannot tolerate milk products.

FORNIX n. a part shaped like an arch, as the fornix cerebri in the hippocampus of the brain or the vaginal fornix.

FOSSA n. a channel or shallow depression (e.g., the axillary fossa, the armpit). pl. **fossae**

FOVEA n. a surface pit or small depression, esp. the pit in the center of the *macula* of the *retina*; when light rays from an object converge on the fovea, there is the sharpest visual image.

FRACTURE n. a break, esp. of a bone. There are many kinds of fractures, including:

CLOSED FRACTURE n. a bone break in which the skin is not broken.

COMMINUTED FRACTURE n. a fracture in which there are several breaks in a bone, resulting in two or more fragments.

COMPLETE FRACTURE n. a break involving the entire width of the involved bone.

COMPLICATED FRACTURE n. a bone break that results in injury to another organ, as, for example, when a broken rib pierces a lung.

COMPOUND FRACTURE n. a fracture in which the broken end(s) of the bone break through the skin; also called **open fracture**.

COMPRESSION FRACTURE n. a bone break that collapses the bone, esp. in short bones (e.g., vertebrae).

DEPRESSED FRACTURE n. a break in the skull with the bone pushed inward.

DISPLACED FRACTURE n. a fracture in which the two ends of the broken bone are separated from each other.

FATIGUE FRACTURE n. a break that results from excessive physical activity, not from a specific injury; it sometimes occurs in the metatarsal bones of runners.

GREENSTICK FRACTURE n. an incomplete fracture in which the bone is bent and only the outer arc of the bend is broken; it occurs primarily in children and often heals quickly.

INCOMPLETE FRACTURE n. a break that does not involve the entire width of the involved bone.

IMPACTED FRACTURE n. a break in which one fragmented

end is wedged into the other fragmented end.

SIMPLE FRACTURE n. an uncomplicated closed fracture in which the skin is not broken.

FRANK BREECH n. position of the fetus within the mother's uterus in which the buttocks present at the maternal pelvic outlet, not the head as is normal for delivery.

FRATERNAL TWINS n. twins who developed from two separate fertilized eggs. Fraternal twins may be of the same or opposite sex; they do not contain the same genetic makeup and differ from each other in the same way as other siblings with the same parents do; also called **dizygotic twins** (compare *identical twins*; *siamese twins*).

FRECKLE n. a small, flat brown or tan discoloration on the skin, usually resulting from exposure to the sun; the tendency to freckle is hereditary and occurs primarily in redheaded persons and others with fair skin. Since these people tend to develop more serious skin changes, they should avoid overexposure to the sun.

FREE ASSOCIATION n. in psychoanalysis, a technique intended to reveal what is carried in the unconscious, whereby a person says spontaneously whatever comes to mind, esp. in giving the first word or thought that occurs when a word cue is given.

FREMITUS n. a flutter that can be felt by the hand of the examiner or by listening, as the chest vibrations that occur with speech or on coughing.

FRENULUM n. a band or fold of membrane that connects two organs and usually limits the movement of one, esp. the band of tissue (frenulum linguae) that extends from the floor of the mouth to the under surface of the tongue, limiting the movement of the tongue. (If the frenulum is too short, tongue movement is impaired; this condition, known as

tongue-tied, can usually be corrected surgically.) Also: **frenum**.

FREQUENCY n. 1. the need to have an action occur often (e.g., urinary frequency); 2. the number of times a phenomenon occurs in a certain time period (e.g., the number of heartbeats per minute); 3. in statistics, the number of events or instances of something for each unit (compare *incidence*).

FREUDIAN adj. pert. to Sigmund Freud or his theories, esp. those relating to sexual symbolism.

FRIEDMAN TEST n. a reliable means for determining whether or not a woman is pregnant, involving injecting some of her urine into an unmated female rabbit, and then, 2 days later, examining the ovaries of the rabbit. The finding of yellow bodies (corpora lutea) indicates that the woman is pregnant; also called **rabbit test** (see also *corpus luteum*).

FRIEDREICH'S ATAXIA n. an abnormal condition marked by muscular weakness, loss of muscular control, and an abnormal gait, usually beginning between the ages of 5 and 20 and progressing to affect the upper extremities and leading to severe disability and often death.

FRIGIDITY n. sexual passivity or unresponsiveness, esp. in a woman; coldness; inability to reach the climax of sexual intercourse (orgasm). adj. **frigid**

FRONTAL adj. pert. to the forehead.

FRONTAL LOBE n. that part of the cerebral cortex in either hemisphere of the brain, found directly behind the forehead; it helps to control voluntary movement and is associated with the higher mental activities (e.g., planning, judgment) as well as with personality.

FRONTAL SINUS n. one of a pair of hollow spaces (sinuses) in the frontal bone above the eye socket.

FROSTBITE n. tissue damage, esp. of the fingers, toes, ears, or nose, caused by freezing, generally due to prolonged exposure to very cold weather. The affected parts turn white and become numb. Gentle warming in tepid water, without rubbing, is the appropriate first aid measure. Severe freezing results in the death of the tissues, necessitating amputation of the affected part.

FROTTAGE n. sexual gratification obtained by rubbing against a person of the opposite sex, as in a crowded train.

FRUCTOSE n. a simple sugar found in honey and some fruits; also: **fruit sugar**, **levulose**.

FRUCTOSURIA n. presence of fructose (levulose) in the urine, a harmless condition.

FSH n. see *follicle-stimulating hormone*.

FUGUE n. a state in which a person appears to be conscious of his/her actions but later has no recollection of them. If the condition lasts for a long time, the person may leave the community and start a new life elsewhere. The condition is believed to be due to inability to handle a conflict or severe stress.

FULMINANT adj. occurring with suddenness and severity (e.g., disease, pain, fever). v. **fulminate**

FULVICIN n. trade name for the antifungal agent *griseofulvin*.

FUNCTIONAL DISORDER n. a condition in which a body part (e.g., an organ) functions (acts or works) abnormally, although it is physically normal; in other words, a disorder marked by symptoms and signs for which no anatomical or physiological cause can be identified (compare *organic disorder*).

FUNDUS n. the base of a hollow organ; the part of a structure farthest from its opening, as the inside of the eye farthest from the pupil, or the wide end of the *uterus* opposite the cervix. pl. **fundi**

FUNGAL INFECTION n. an inflammatory condition caused by a fungus. Common fungal infections are *candidiasis*, *tinea* (ringworm), and *coccidioidomycosis*.

FUNGUS n. one of a group of simple plantlike organisms, including mushrooms and yeasts, some of which cause disease (*fungal infection*). pl. **fungi** adj. **fungal**

FUNICULITIS n. inflammation of the *spermatic cord* or *spinal cord*.

FUNNY BONE n. a colloquial term for the back of the elbow, where the ulnar nerve is near the surface. A sharp blow to the site causes a most unpleasant shock or tingle.

FUROSEMIDE n. a commonly used diuretic, known under the trade name Lasix, used to treat hypertension and edema. Adverse effects include fluid and electrolyte imbalances.

FURUNCLE n. a small, painful lump in the skin that has a core of dead tissue and surrounding inflammation. Caused by bacterial (staphylococcal) infection through a sweat gland or hair follicle, it produces pain, redness, and swelling. Treatment is by antibiotics, applications of moist heat, and surgical incision and drainage if necessary; also: **boil**.

FURUNCULOSIS n. acute skin disease marked by presence of many furuncles.

FUSIFORM adj. spindle-shaped, tapering at both ends.

FUSION n. 1. normal or abnormal joining; 2. the combining of images from both eyes to form one image (optical fusion); 3. the surgical joining of two or more vertebrae (*spinal fusion*). v. **fuse**

g

GABA see *gamma-aminobutyric acid*.

GAG v. to feel like vomiting; to retch. n. an object used to hold the mouth open during surgery or to prevent swallowing of the tongue during a *seizure* (e.g., in *epilepsy*).

GAG REFLEX n. a normal retching reaction, which may be produced by touching the soft palate at the back of the mouth.

GAIT n. the way in which a person walks.

GALACTAGOGUE n. an agent that promotes the flow of milk.

GALACTOCELE n. 1. breast cyst containing milk and caused by closure of a milk duct; 2. an accumulation of milky fluid in the sac surrounding the testis.

GALACTORRHEA n. 1. excessive flow of milk; 2. secretion of milk not associated with breast-feeding, sometimes a sign of a pituitary gland disorder.

GALACTOSE n. a simple sugar derived from milk sugar (*lactose*) and found in other substances; it is readily absorbed in the digestive tract and converted into *glycogen* in the liver.

GALACTOSEMIA n. an inherited (autosomal recessive) disease in which a deficiency in or absence of the enzyme (galactose-1-phosphate uridyl transferase) necessary for the metabolism of galactose to glucose results in galactose accumulation, leading to mental retardation, spleen and liver enlargement, cataract formation, and other abnormalities. Symptoms of vomiting, diarrhea, and poor weight gain typically develop shortly after birth. The disease can be diagnosed through blood and urine tests; treatment is a galactose-free diet.

GALL see *bile*.

GALLAMINE n. a muscle relaxant, known under the trade name Flaxedil, used as an adjunct to *anesthesia*.

GALLBLADDER n. a pear-shaped organ, about 8 centimeters (3 inches) long and located on the lower surface of the liver, that is a reservoir for bile. Bile produced in the liver passes (through the hepatic duct) to the gallbladder, where it is stored; the presence of food, esp. fats, in the *duodenum* and hormonal influences cause the gallbladder to contract, releasing the bile to the common bile duct for transport to the duodenum. The gallbladder is a common site of stone formation (*cholelithiasis*) and inflammation (*cholecystitis*).

GALLBLADDER

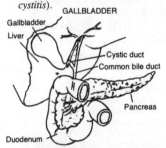

GALLOP RHYTHM n. a heart rhythm characterized by the presence of an extra sound on stethoscopic examination; it may indicate a heart abnormality.

GALLSTONE n. a stonelike mass (*calculus*) in the gallbladder or in its duct (see *cholelithiasis*).

GALVANIC SKIN RESPONSE n. a change in the electrical resistance of the skin, measurements of which are used in some studies involving reactions to stress and other psychological variables.

GAMETE n. a mature sex cell, with the *haploid* number of chromosomes; either the *sperm*, in the male, or the *egg* (or *ovum*) in the female. Union of male and female gametes in *fertilization* results in the formation of a *zygote* with the *diploid chromosome* number.

GAMETO- comb. form indicating an association with sex (reproductive) cells (e.g., **gametocyte**, a cell capable of developing into a *gamete*).

GAMETOCIDE n. an agent able to kill sex cells.

GAMETOGENESIS n. the development and maturation of sex cells; it occurs through the process of *meiosis*; in males it is called *spermatogenesis*, in females, *oogenesis*.

GAMMA-AMINOBUTYRIC ACID (GABA) n. an amino acid found in the central nervous system, esp. the brain, that functions in nerve impulse transmission processes.

GAMMA GLOBULIN see *immunoglobulin*.

GAMMA RAY n. electromagnetic wave of very short wavelength emitted by radioactive substances. Controlled radiation with gamma rays and rays of other wavelengths is used in medical diagnosis and in the treatment of some skin cancers and other cancers deep within the body.

GAMMOPATHY n. an abnormal condition in which proteins having antibody activity (*immunoglobulins*) increase greatly in the blood.

GANGLI-, GANGLIO- comb. form indicating an association with a *ganglion* (e.g., **gangliocyte**, a ganglion cell).

GANGLION n. 1. a collection of nerve cells forming a knotlike shape; they usually lie outside the brain and spinal cord; in the autonomic nervous system, chains of ganglia lie on either side of the spinal cord; 2. a cyst that forms on a tendon, esp. in the wrist. pl. **ganglia**

GANGLIOSIDOSIS see *Tay-Sachs disease*.

GANGRENE n. tissue death resulting from lack of nutrition when the blood supply to the affected part is decreased or lost because of disease (e.g., diabetes), injury, blood clot, tourniquet, frostbite, severe burn, or bacterial infection. The arms and legs are most commonly affected (compare *necrosis*).   adj. **gangrenous**

GANTANOL n. trade name for sulfamethoxazole, a *sulfonamide* antibacterial used to treat certain infections, esp. those of the urinary tract.

GANTRISIN n. trade name for sulfisoxazole, a *sulfonamide* antibacterial, used to treat urinary infections.

GARAMYCIN n. trade name for the antibacterial *gentamicin*.

GARGOYLISM see *Hurler's syndrome*.

GAS n. a basic form of matter; a gas lacks definite shape and its volume depends on temperature and pressure.

GAS EMBOLISM see *bends*.

GASTR-, GASTRO- comb. form indicating an association with the *stomach* (e.g., **gastroesophageal**, pert. to the stomach and esophagus).

GASTRECTOMY n. surgical removal of all or part of the stomach; it is usually done to stop hemorrhaging from an ulcer or to remove a chronic ulcer or cancer.

GASTRIC adj. pert. to the stomach.

GASTRIC DIGESTION n. the process of breaking down food (esp. protein) in the stomach through the action of chemicals in the *gastric juice*.

GASTRIC JUICE n. secretions given off by the gastric glands of the stomach and consisting chiefly of hydrochloric acid, the lubricant mucin, and the enzymes *pepsin*, *rennin*, and *lipase*.

GASTRIC LAVAGE n. washing out the stomach with sterile water or a salt-water solution to cleanse it before surgery or certain diagnostic procedures (e.g., *gastros-copy*) or to remove harmful contents (e.g., poisons).

GASTRIC ULCER n. an erosion or open sore of the lining of the stomach that may penetrate the muscle layers and wall of the stomach. Symptoms include burning pain, belching, and nausea; they tend to occur when the stomach is empty, after eating certain foods, or when the patient is under stress. Treatment includes avoidance of irritating foods and drugs to decrease the acidity of the stomach. If the ulcer perforates the stomach wall and hemorrhage occurs, surgery is usually needed; also called *peptic ulcer*.

GASTRIN n. a hormone secreted by the pylorus (the upper part of the stomach) that stimulates the release of *gastric juice* from stomach glands and helps stim- .ulate the secretion of *bile* and *pancreatic juice*.

GASTRITIS n. inflammation of the lining of the stomach characterized by loss of appetite, nausea, vomiting, and discomfort after eating. **Acute gastritis** is caused by the ingestion of an irritating substance (e.g., aspirin, too much alcohol) or by bacterial or viral infection; **chronic gastritis** is often a symptom of gastric (peptic) ulcer, stomach cancer, pernicious anemia, or other disorder.

GASTROCNEMIUS n. the superficial muscle in the back of the leg that forms the greater part of the calf.

GASTROENTERITIS n. inflammation of the stomach and intestines. Symptoms include abdominal discomfort, loss of appetite, nausea, vomiting, and sometimes diarrhea. Causes include bacterial or viral infection, the ingestion of toxic or irritating substances, allergic reactions to specific foods (e.g., milk intolerance), and other disorders.

GASTROENTEROLOGIST n. a physician who specializes in the diagnosis and treatment of diseases affecting the *gastrointestinal tract*.

GASTROENTEROLOGY n. medical specialty concerned with the study of the *gastrointestinal tract* (the stomach, intestines, and related structures) and the diseases that affect them.

GASTROENTEROSTOMY n. surgical creation of an artificial opening between the stomach and the small intestines, performed when the normal opening has been removed through removal of all or part of the stomach or of part of the small intestine.

GASTROESOPHAGEAL RE-FLUX n. the backflow of the contents of the stomach into the *esophagus*, usually caused by malfunction of the sphincter muscle between the two organs; symptoms include burning pain in the esophagus, commonly known as heartburn; (see also *hiatal hernia*).

GASTROGAVAGE n. artificial feeding of a nutrient solution through a tube inserted into a surgically created opening into the stomach; it is done in cases of prolonged unconsciousness or cancer of the esophagus; also called **gastrostomy feeding**.

GASTROINTESTINAL adj. pert. to the stomach and intestines; frequently abbreviated **GI**.

GASTROINTESTINAL TRACT n. the stomach and intestines; sometimes used more broadly to include the entire digestive tube from the mouth to the anus.

GASTROSCOPY n. visual examination of the stomach (esp. the upper part of the stomach) by means of a flexible, fiberoptic instrument (gastroscope) inserted through the esophagus; photographs may be taken and specimens removed for analysis.

GASTROSTOMY n. surgical creation of an artificial opening into the stomach through the abdominal wall, done to allow artificial feeding (*gastrogavage*) in cases of prolonged unconsciousness or esophageal cancer.

GASTRULA n. an early stage in embryo development, occurring after the *blastula* stage; the gastrula is a hollow cup-shaped stage consisting of an outer *ectoderm* layer and an inner layer that later differentiates into two layers (*endoderm* and *mesoderm*).

GAUCHER'S DISEASE n. a rare, familial disorder of fat metabolism that leads to spleen and liver enlargement and abnormal bone growth. Mortality is high in early childhood; those who survive through adolescence may live for many years.

GAVAGE n. artificial feeding of liquid or semiliquid food through a tube, most commonly one extending from the nose to the stomach (nasogastric tube) (see also *gastrogavage*).

GELATIN n. a jellylike protein derived from connective tissues such as bones and ligaments and used as food, in medicinal preparations (e.g., suppositories, capsules), and as a medium for growing microorganisms; also: **gel.** adj. **gelatinous**

GENDER n. the sex (male or female) of an animal.

GENDER IDENTITY n. the awareness of knowing to which sex (male or female) one belongs that normally begins in infancy, continues through childhood, and is reinforced during adolescence.

GENDER ROLE n. the sexual identity that a person assumes and presents to others.

GENE n. the basic unit of inheritance; the basic unit of genetic material, that part of a chromosome considered to be a single unit of heredity and which codes for the production of a specific polypeptide chain of a protein. In humans and many other animals genes occur as paired *alleles* (see also *chromatin*; *mutation*).

GENERAL ANESTHESIA n. an agent, usually given by inhalation or intravenous injection, that produces unconsciousness and complete loss of sensation throughout the body; it is used for major surgery (e.g., removal of a lung or of the stomach) (compare *regional anesthesia*; *local anesthesia*).

GENERIC adj. pert. to the descriptive or nonproprietary (nontrade) name of a drug or other product; for example, *diazepam* is the generic name for Valium.

GENESIS n. the origin, evolution or generation of something. adj. **genetic**

-GENESIS suffix meaning "the production of something" (e.g., **psychogenesis**, the development of the mind) (compare *-genic*).

GENE SPLICING n. a technique for recombining the chemical structures of a *gene* (see *recombinant DNA*).

GENETIC adj. 1. pert. to a *gene* or heredity; 2. pert. to origin, birth, development.

GENETIC COUNSELING n. the process of determining the risk of a particular genetic disorder occurring within a family and providing information and advice based on that determination; used to help couples in family planning and in the care of children affected or thought to be affected with a particular genetic disorder. An accurate diagnosis is essential and may require special biochemical and cell studies; a careful and complete family medical history is also needed. The subjects of prenatal diagnosis (see *amniocentesis*), artifical insemination, sterilization and termination of a pregnancy may be included in the counseling, depending on the particular disease and circumstances involved.

GENETIC DISEASE n. any disorder or abnormality that results from inherited factors (*genes*) (e.g., *Tay-Sachs disease*, *sickle-cell anemia*).

GENETIC ENGINEERING n. the process of altering and controlling the genetic makeup of an organism through manipulation and recombination of the genetic material, DNA (see *recombinant DNA*).

GENETIC MARKER n. a specific gene that produces a recognizable trait and can be used in family or population studies, e.g., to determine susceptibility to a certain disease.

GENETICS n. the science that studies inherited characteristics; the study of genes, their composition and function.   adj. **genetic**

GENETIC SCREENING n. the process of analyzing a specific group of people to detect the presence of or susceptibility to a particular disease or diseases. Examples include the screening of all infants for phenylketonuria and the screening of certain racial or ethnic groups who have a high incidence of a particular disease, such as sickle-cell anemia among blacks and Tay-Sachs disease among Ashkenazic Jews (see also *genetic counseling*).

-GENIC suffix meaning ''producing,'' ''causing,'' ''forming'' (e.g., **cytogenic**, producing cells).

GENICULUM n. a kneelike bend in a small structure, such as a vein.   pl. **genicula**

GENITALIA n. the male or female reproductive organs, esp. the external ones; also: **genitals**.   adj. **genital**

GENITAL HERPES   see *herpes*.

GENITAL STAGE n. the third stage (after the oral and anal phases) in the Freudian theory of psychosexual development, said to occur between the ages of two and seven, and involving increased sexual interest and pleasure, often focusing on the *penis* for boys and the *clitoris* for girls; also: **phallic phase**.

GENITOURINARY (GU) adj. pert. to the genital and urinary systems of the body; also: **urogenital**.

GENOME n. the complete set of hereditary factors (*genes*) contained in the chromosomes of each cell of an individual.

GENOTYPE n. the complete genetic makeup or constitution of an individual organism or a related group (compare *phenotype*).   adj. **genotypic**

GENTAMICIN n. an antibiotic, known under the trade name Garamycin, used to treat some severe infections. Adverse effects include kidney and hearing disturbances and hypersensitivity reactions.

GENTIAN VIOLET n. an agent with antibacterial, antifungal, and anthelmintic properties used to treat pinworms and infections of the skin and vagina.

GEOGRAPHIC MEDICINE n. a medical specialty concerned with the geographic distribution of diseases and their causes as related to climate, elevation, topography, and culture; also: **geomedicine**.

GERIATRICS n. a medical specialty that deals with the problems of aging and the diagnosis and treatment of diseases affecting the aged.   adj. **geriatric**

GERM n. 1. a microorganism, esp. one that causes disease; 2. a unit from which a structure or part originates (e.g., **germ layer**, the layer from which new tissue develops).   adj. **germinal**

GERMAN MEASLES see *rubella*.

GERM CELL n. a sexual reproductive cell (*spermatozoon* or *ovum*) in any stage of its development (compare *somatic cell*).

GERONTOLOGY n. the scientific study of aging or of old age.

GESTALTISM n. a school of psychology that maintains that the mind perceives integrated wholes, not discrete parts; for example, that a triangle is perceived as a triangle, not as three lines. In Gestaltism, behavior is seen as an integrated response to a situation, not as a series of sensations and reflexes; also: **Gestalt psychology**

GESTATION n. the period of time in humans and other viviparous animals from fertilization of the ovum to birth; the length of pregnancy. In humans, gestation averages 266 days, or about 280 days from the first day of the last menstrual period (see also *pregnancy*).

GESTATIONAL AGE n. the age of a fetus or newborn, usually expressed in weeks since the onset of the mother's last menstrual period (compare *fetal age*).

GH see *growth hormone*.

GIARDIASIS n. infection of the intestines with *Giardia protozoa* found in contaminated food and water throughout the world; symptoms include diarrhea (the stools are typically pale and fatty), nausea, abdominal discomfort, and flatulence; also called **traveler's diarrhea**.

GIBBUS n. a lump or protrusion on the body surface, esp. of the spine, resulting from fracture or collapse of a vertebra.   adj. **gibbous**

GIGANTISM n. an abnormal condition characterized by excessive size, caused most frequently by oversecretion of *growth hormone* from the pituitary gland. Treatment is by irradiation or removal of the pituitary gland (see also *acromegaly*).

GILLES DE LA TOURETTE SYNDROME n. an abnormal, sometimes intermittent, condition characterized by facial grimaces, tics, involuntary grunts, shouts, movements of the upper body, and compulsive use of obscene and offensive language (coprolalia). Treatment with agents that block the effects of the neurohumor *dopamine* has been found effective.

GINGIVA n. the mucous membrane and fibrous tissue that encircles the neck of each tooth; also: **gum**.   pl. **gingivae**   adj. **gingival**

GINGIVITIS n. condition in which the gums are red, swollen, and bleeding. It most commonly results from poor oral hygiene and the development of bacterial plaque on the teeth, but is also common in pregnancy and may be a sign of another disorder (e.g., *diabetes mellitus*, *vitamin deficiency*).

GIRDLE n. a ringlike arrangement or part (e.g., pelvic girdle, the bony structure to which the lower limbs are attached) (see *pelvic girdle*; *shoulder girdle*).

GI SERIES n. a sequence of diagnostic tests involving the alimentary canal, esp. the stomach and intestines. It is usually done by inserting (e.g., by enema) a contrast medium (e.g., barium sulfate) into the parts to be studied, X-raying or otherwise obtaining images of those parts, and having films or other images reviewed by a radiologist to detect the presence of any abnormality (e.g., tumor, ulcer).

GLABELLA n. the smooth bump between the eyebrows, most noticeable in men.

GLAND n. any of numerous organs in the body (e.g., thyroid gland), each of which is made up of specialized cells that secrete or excrete materials not related to their own metabolism but which are needed by the body. There are two main types of glands: endocrine, or ductless, glands that secrete *hormones* directly into the bloodstream; and exocrine, or duct, glands that release materials into ducts or onto adjacent epithelial surfaces; included among the exocrine glands are sweat glands, sebaceous glands and tear glands.

GLANDERS n. a bacterial (*Pseudomonas mallei*) infection, endemic in Africa, Asia, and South America, where it is transmitted to humans from infected horses and other domesticated animals. Symptoms include purulent (pus-filled) inflammation of the mucous membranes and ulcerating skin lesions that, if untreated by antibiotics, may spread to internal tissues and lead to death.

GLANDULAR FEVER see *infectious mononucleosis*.

GLANS n. a glandlike part, esp. that at the end of the *clitoris* or *penis*.

GLAUCOMA n. a disease in which elevated pressure in the eye, due to obstruction of the outflow of *aqueous humor*, damages the optic nerve and causes visual defects. Acute (angle-closure) glaucoma is an hereditary disorder with the iris blocking the flow of aqueous humor; symptoms, which may occur suddenly, include dilated pupil, red eye, blurred vision, and severe eye pain, sometimes accompanied by nausea and vomiting; if untreated—by special eye drops or surgery—angle-closure glaucoma may result in permanent blindness within a few days. The much more common open-angle, or chronic, glaucoma, also hereditary, is one of the leading causes of blindness in the United States. Caused by blockage of the canal of Schlemm, it produces symptoms very slowly with gradual loss of peripheral vision over a period of years, sometimes with headache, dull pain, and blurred vision. Treatment involves the use of special eye drops. Glaucoma can also occur as a congenital defect or as a result of another eye disorder.

GLEET n. mucus or pus discharged from the *penis* or *vagina*, esp. after *gonorrhea*.

GLENOID CAVITY n. the socket of the shoulder joint into which the head of the humerus fits.

GLIA see *neuroglia*.

GLIDING JOINT n. a type of *synovial joint* in which the articulations of the bones allows only gliding motion; examples of gliding joints are the ankle and the wrist.

GLIOMA n. a tumor of *neuroglia* cells.

GLOBIN n. the protein in *hemoglobin*, the oxygen-carrying compound of red blood cells.

GLOBULIN n. any of a group of simple proteins found in the blood (see also *immunoglobulins*).

GLOBUS HYSTERICUS n. transitory feeling of a lump in the throat that cannot be swallowed or coughed up, often accompanying anxiety or emotional experience; it is thought to be due to a functional disturbance of nerves and muscles affecting the lower throat region.

GLOMERULAR CAPSULE see *Bowman's capsule*.

GLOMERULONEPHRITIS n. disease of the glomerulus of the *kidney* characterized by decreased production of urine, the presence of protein and blood in the urine, and edema; the cause is unknown, but it sometimes follows an acute upper respiratory infection, perhaps as an allergic reaction to the infective organism (e.g., streptococcal).

GLOMERULUS n. a cluster, esp. the network of blood capillaries contained in Bowman's capsule of a kidney nephron that is the main site where waste products from the blood are filtered into the kidney tubules. pl. **glomeruli** adj. **glomerular**

GLOMUS n. a group of small arterial blood vessels, richly supplied with nerves, and connecting to veins.

GLOSSA see *tongue*.

GLOSSALGIA n. painful tongue.

GLOSSITIS n. inflammation of the tongue. **Acute glossitis**, characterized by swelling and pain, usually results from infection or injury. **Chronic glossitis** with atrophy of tongue tissue sometimes occurs in pernicious anemia, and one superficial form of glossitis (Moeller's glossitis, or glossodynia exfoliativa) marked by irregular red patches on the tongue and sensitivity to hot and spicy foods occurs in some middle-aged women.

GLOSSODYNIA n. pain in the tongue.

GLOSSOLALIA n. 1. repetitive nonsense speech, not related to the subject or situation involved; 2. speaking in an unknown language—"speaking in tongues"—during a religious experience.

GLOSSOPTOSIS n. abnormal downward or backward placement of the tongue.

GLOSSOPYROSIS n. burning sensation in the tongue.

GLOSSOPHARYNGEAL adj. pert. to the tongue and pharynx.

GLOSSOPHARYNGEAL NERVE n. either of a pair of *cranial nerves* (IX) with mixed sensory and motor fibers essential to taste, sensation in the *palate*, and secretion of the *parotid glands*.

GLOTTIS n. the voice-producing part of the larynx consisting of the vocal cords and the opening (covered by the *epiglottis*) they form. adj. **glottic**

GLUCAGON n. a hormone produced in the *pancreas* that stimulates the conversion of *glycogen* in the liver to *glucose*; preparations of glucagon are sometimes used to treat certain hypoglycemic (low blood sugar) conditions.

GLUCOCORTICOID n. any of several hormones, including cortisol, corticosterone, and cortisone, released by the cortex of the *adrenal gland* that exert an anti-inflammatory effect and affect protein, fat, and carbohydrate metabolism to help the body respond to stress and avoid fatigue.

GLUCOSE n. a simple sugar that is the major energy source in the body. Ingested in certain foods, esp. fruits, and the product of the breakdown of other carbohydrates, glucose is absorbed into the blood from the intestines; excess amounts are stored in the form of *glycogen*, chiefly in the liver. Determination of glucose levels in the blood is important in the diagnosis of many disorders, including *diabetes mellitus*. Pharmaceutical preparations of glucose (e.g., dextrose) are widely used in medicine.

GLUCOSE TOLERANCE TEST n. a test of the body's ability to metabolize carbohydrates used in the diagnosis of diabetes mellitus, *hypoglycemia*, and other disorders. After an overnight fast, the level of glucose in the blood is measured; then the patient is given a 100-gram dose of glucose to drink, and glucose levels in the blood and urine are tested periodically during several hours.

GLUCOSURIA n. abnormal presence of glucose in the urine, resulting from ingestion of large amounts of carbohydrates, kidney disease, *diabetes mellitus*, or other metabolic disorder (compare *glycosuria*).

GLUTAMIC ACID n. a nonessential *amino acid*, preparations of which are used in digestive aids.

GLUTEAL adj. pert. to the *buttocks*.

GLUTEN n. insoluble protein found in wheat, rye, and other grains; an inability to handle gluten is the cause of *celiac disease*.

GLUTEN-FREE DIET n. diet used in the treatment of *celiac disease* and related disorders that eliminates products such as wheat, rye, oats, beans, cabbage, turnips, and cucumbers, which are rich in gluten.

GLUTETHIMIDE n. a sedative, known under the trade name Doriden, used to treat some sleep disorders. Adverse effects include skin rashes and the possibility of dependence.

GLUTEUS n. any of three paired muscles in the buttocks, involved in movements of the thigh.

-GLYCEMIA suffix meaning "sugar in the blood" (see *hypoglycemia*; *hyperglycemia*).

GLYCERINE n. sweet, colorless preparation of glycerol used as a moisturizing agent for chapped skin; in suppositories; and as a sweetening agent in drugs; also: **glycerin**.

GLYCEROL n. an alcohol found in fats (see *glycerine*).

GLYCINE n. a nonessential amino acid widely found in proteins and preparations of which are used in antacids and to treat some muscle disorders.

GLYCOGEN n. a polysaccharide that is the principal form in which carbohydrates are stored in the body. Stored primarily in the liver and in muscle, glycogen is readily broken down to *glucose* when needed by the body.

GLYCOGENESIS n. the formation of *glycogen* from *glucose*.

GLYCOLYSIS n. the breakdown of *glucose* and other sugars through a series of enzyme-catalyzed reactions to either pyruvic acid (aerobic glycolysis—in the presence of oxygen) or lactic acid (anaerobic glycolysis—without oxygen), releasing energy for the body in the form of ATP (adenosine triphosphate).

GLYCOSURIA n. the presence of abnormally high levels of sugar, esp. glucose, in the urine, due to ingestion of large amounts of carbohydrates, kidney disease, *diabetes mellitus*, or other metabolic disorder.

GOITER n. an enlargement of the thyroid gland at the front of the neck; it may be caused by deficiency of iodine in the diet, by tumor, or by overactivity (Graves' disease) or underactivity of the thyroid gland. Treatment depends on the cause; it often involves surgical removal of all or part of the thyroid gland. (See also *exophthalmic goiter*.)

GOLD n. a metallic element; gold salts are sometimes used in the treatment of *rheumatoid arthritis*, and radioactive gold isotopes are used to treat some forms of cancer (see Table of Elements).

GOLGI APPARATUS n. a small, membranous structure found in most cells that functions to store and transport proteins manufactured in other parts of the cell. The structure is usually well-developed and abundant in cells that produce secretions (e.g., those in endocrine and exocrine glands); also called: **Golgi body**; **Golgi complex**.

GOLGI CELLS n. a type of nerve cell (neuron) found in the brain and spinal cord.

GONAD n. a gland that produces sex cells (gametes); in males the gonads are the testes; in females, the ovaries. adj. **gonadal**

GONADOTROPIN n. a hormone that stimulates the function of the *gonads*. The anterior pituitary gland secretes two gonadotropins: *follicle stimulating hormone (FSH)* and *luteinizing hormone*; during pregnancy the placenta secretes chorionic gonadotropin, which helps to maintain the pregnancy; also: **gonadotrophin**.   adj. **gonadotropic**, **gonadotrophic**

GONOCOCCUS n. a bacteria (*Neisseria gonorrhoeae*) that causes *gonorrhea*.

GONORRHEA n. a common venereal disease caused by the bacteria *Neisseria gonorrhoeae* and transmitted through contact with an infected person or with secretions containing the bacteria. Symptoms include painful urination and burning, itching and pain around the urethra and in women the vagina, accompanied by a greenish-yellow and pus-containing discharge. If untreated the infection spreads, esp. in women, infecting the reproductive organs, causing inflammation of the liver, and, if widespread, leading to septicemia and polyarthritis, with painful lesions in joints and tendons and infection of the conjunctiva of the eye that can lead to blindness. Treatment is by antibiotics.   adj. **gonorrheal**

GOOSE BUMP n. collquial term for a skin reaction occurring in cold, fright, or stress; the arrector pili contract causing the hairs of the skin to stand up; also: **gooseflesh**.

GOUT n. a disease in which a defect in uric acid metabolism causes the acid and its salts to accumulate in the blood and joints, causing pain and swelling of the joints (esp. the big toe area), accompanied by fever and chills. The disease is more common among men than women and usually has a genetic basis. If untreated, the disease causes destructive tissue changes in the joints and kidneys. Treatment includes a purine-free diet and use of drugs to reduce inflammation and to increase the excretion of uric acid salts or decrease their formation; also called: **gouty arthritis.**

GRAAFIAN FOLLICLE n. a fully, developed, egg-containing sac in the ovary that ruptures during ovulation to release an egg, or ovum. Many primary follicles, each containing an immature ovum, are embedded in the wall of the ovary. Under the influence of follicle-stimulating hormone (FSH) released by the pituitary, one follicle ripens into a mature Graafian follicle containing a mature ovum in the early phase of each menstrual cycle. At ovulation the follicle ruptures and the ovum is released. The collapsed follicle—now the *corpus luteum*—produces the hormone progesterone and prepares the uterus to receive a fertilized egg; if fertilization does not occur, the corpus luteum is shed in *menstruation*.

follicle   ruptured follicle   corpus luteum   breakdown in corpus luteum

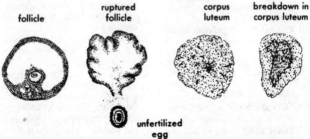

unfertilized egg

In the normal menstrual cycle, once each month a Graafian follicle in the ovary ruptures, releasing an ovum (egg). The ruptured follicle then is the corpus luteum.

GRACILIS n. the slender, superficial muscle that runs along the inside of the thigh and functions in movement of the thigh and leg.

GRAFT n. a tissue or organ that is taken from one site and transplanted to another site on the same person (autograft), as in transplanting thigh skin to the arm to replace badly burned skin, or that is taken from one person and inserted in another, as in a kidney transplant. (See also *transplant*.)

-GRAM suffix indicating something written, drawn, or otherwise recorded, as in *electrocardiogram*.

GRAM'S STAIN n. a method of staining bacteria that is used as a means of identifying and classifying them. A series of stains and solutions is applied to a bacteria; those that appear violet or blue are termed Gram-positive; those that appear pink or red are termed Gram-negative. Also called **Gram's method**.

GRAND MAL n. 1. an attack, suffered in epilepsy, during which the patient becomes unconscious, develops bluish discoloration (cyanosis) of the skin and lips due to oxygen lack, and experiences convulsions; 2. a type of epilepsy characterized by recurrent grand mal attacks (compare *petit mal*).

GRANULATION n. the growth of small projections of tiny blood vessels and connective tissue that form on the surfaces of a wound during the healing process.

GRANULE n. a small particle or grain.   adj. **granular**

GRANULOCYTE n. a type of white blood cell characterized by granules in the cytoplasm; it includes the *basophil*, *eosinophil*, and *neutrophil*.

GRANULOCYTOPENIA n. an abnormal condition characterized by a decrease in the number of granulocytes in the blood (see *neutroperia*); also: **granulopenia**.

GRANULOMA n. a mass of nodular granulation tissue resulting from injury, infection or inflammation. Treatment depends on the cause and probable course of the granuloma.

GRANULOMA INGUINALE n. a venereal disease caused by the bacterium *Calymmatobacterium granulomatis* and characterized by a pimply rash that develops into ulcers of the skin and subcutaneous tissue of the genital and groin region. Treatment is by antibiotics.

GRANULOMATOSIS n. condition characterized by the development of widespread granulomas.

GRAPHOSPASM n. pain in the hand and arm due to prolonged writing; also called **writer's cramp**.

GRAVE'S DISEASE   see *exophthalmic goiter*.

GRAVID adj. pregnant.

GRAVIDA n. 1. a pregnant woman; 2. a designation of the numbered pregnancy a woman is in, gravida I indicating her first pregnancy, gravida III her third.

GRAVID-, -GRAVIDA comb. forms meaning "pregnant" or a "pregnant woman" (e.g., **secundigravida**, a woman pregnant for the second time) (compare *para-*).

GRAY MATTER n. the gray tissue of the central nervous system made up primarily of nerve cell bodies and *neuroglia* cells. It is found in the cerebral cortex and other parts of the brain and forms an H-shaped center of the spinal cord surrounded by lighter, so-called white matter; gray matter in the spinal column functions as the center for spinal reflex activity (compare *white matter*).

GREENSTICK   FRACTURE see under *fracture*.

GRIEF n. the pattern of responses, physical (faster heart and breathing rates, sweating, increased energy reserves, slowed or disturbed digestive processes) and emotional (typically proceeding from disbelief and denial to anger and guilt to final acceptance) to the loss of a loved one or separation from him or her.

GRIPPE see *influenza*.

GROIN n. the area where the abdomen and thighs join; also called **inguen**.

GROOVE n. a narrow channel or depression in a structure (e.g., the costal groove lodges the blood vessels and nerves between two ribs) (see also *sulcus*).

GROSS adj. visible to the unaided eye, as a gross (vs. microscopic) examination.

GROSS ANATOMY n. study of the structure of the body and its parts without the aid of a microscope.

GROUP THERAPY n. psychotherapy involving several (usually six to eight) persons and a therapist with the interactions of the group members considered an important part of the therapy.

GROWTH n. an increase in size of an organism or any of its parts, as occurs normally in a child or abnormally in a tumor.

GROWTH HORMONE (GH) n. a hormone synthesized and released by the *anterior pituitary gland* that stimulates the growth of long bones in the limbs and increases protein synthesis and the use of fats for energy. Excessive production results in *gigantism* or *acromegaly;* a deficiency, in *dwarfism.* Also called **somatotropin**.

GROWTH HORMONE RELEASING FACTOR (GHRF) n. substance released by the *hypothalamus* that stimulates the release of growth hormone by the *anterior pituitary gland*.

GSF see *galvanic skin response*.

GUANINE n. an organic compound, one of the bases found in DNA (deoxyribonucleic acid) and RNA (ribonuclecic acid).

GUBERNACULUM n. a structure that guides (e.g., **gubernaculum testis**, the cord that is involved in the descent of the testes). pl. **gubernacula**

GUILLAIN-BARRE SYNDROME n. a form of peripheral *polyneuritis* marked by pain, weakness, and sometimes paralysis of the limbs that may spread to the trunk of the body. The cause is unknown; it usually develops one to three weeks after a viral infection or immunization. There is no treatment; in most cases symptoms resolve within a few weeks or months.

GULLET see *esophagus*.

GUM see *gingiva*.

GUMBOIL n. an abscess of the gingiva (gum) and tooth root resulting from injury, infection, or dental decay. The gums are usually red, swollen, and painful. Treatment includes antibiotics, special mouthwashes, and sometimes incision and drainage of the abscess.

GUMMA n. a soft tumor—a *granuloma*—characteristic of the tertiary stage of syphilis found in the liver, brain, or other tissues.

GUSTATION n. the sense of *taste* or the process of tasting.

GUT n. intestine.

GYN-, GYNE-, GYNECO-, GYNO- prefixes indicating a relationship to women or the female sex (e.g., **gynopathy**, a disease of women).

GYNECOLOGY n. the medical specialty concerned with the health care of women, including function and diseases of the reproductive organs. It combines both medical and surgical concerns and is usually practiced in combination with *obstetrics*.

GYNECOLOGIST n. one who practices *gynecology*.

GYNECOMASTIA n. abnormal development of one or more breasts in males, usually the result of hormonal imbalance, liver malfunction, or treatment with steroid compounds.

GYRUS n. a curved portion (*convolution*) of the surface of the *brain*, caused by infolding of the cortex.   pl. **gyri**

h

H symbol for hydrogen (see Table of Elements).

HABIT n. a customary practice or behavior; an automatic response or pattern of behavior learned by frequent repetition (compare *addiction*).

HABITUAL ABORTION   see under *abortion*.

HABITUATION n. 1. the process of becoming accustomed to something; 2. in pharmacology, the dependence on a drug (including alcohol or tobacco) resulting from repeated use but without severe physiological signs of addiction or need to increase dosage; 3. in psychology, the decrease or loss of response to a particular stimulus after repeated exposure to that stimulus.

HABITUS n. 1. the general physical build of a person (e.g., an athletic habitus); 2. a person's tendency to require or be affected by something, as a disease.

HAIR n. a threadlike, keratin-containing appendage of the outer layer of the skin present over most of the body surface except the palms, soles, lips, and a few other small areas. A hair develops inside a tubular *hair follicle* beneath the skin with the root of the hair expanded into a bulb. The part above the skin consists of an outer *cuticle* that covers the cortex, which contains pigment and gives the hair its color, and an inner medulla. A hair may be raised by small arrector pili muscles attached to the follicle.

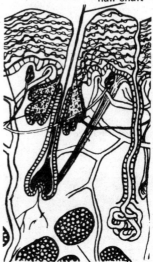

hair shaft

A hair shaft arises from a follicle in the dermis layer of the skin.

HAIR FOLLICLE n. tubular sheath of cells in the epidermis layer of the skin that surrounds the root of a hair. *Sebaceous glands* and small arrector pili muscles are associated with hair follicles.

HAIRY TONGUE n. dark overgrowth of the papilla (tiny projections) of the tongue that is a side effect of some antibiotics; it is benign and gradually subsides; also called **furry tongue**; **black tongue**.

HALDOL n. trade name for *haloperidol*.

HALF-LIFE n. the amount of time needed for a radioactive substance to lose one half of its radioactivity or to decay by one half.

HALITOSIS n. offensive breath; it may result from poor mouth hygiene, diseased teeth or gums, some systemic diseases, or the ingestion of certain foods or drugs.

HALITUS n. an exhaled breath.

HALLUCINATION n. the perception of something that is not actually present; it may be visual (seeing objects that are not present), auditory (hearing noises that are not present), olfactory, gustatory, or tactile. Hallucinations are a common symptom of severe mental illness (e.g., schizophrenia); they also occur following injury to the head, in delirium accompanying severe illness, in toxic states, and from the use of *hallucinogenic drugs*. adj. **hallucinative**, **hallucinatory**

HALLUCINOGEN n. a substance (e.g., LSD [lysergic acid diethylamide], mescaline, peyote, phencyclidine) that excites the central nervous system, producing hallucinations (false perceptions); mood changes; increases in pulse, blood pressure, and body temperature; dilation of the pupils of the eyes; and other physiological and psychological changes. adj. **hallucinogenic**

HALLUCINOSIS n. an abnormal mental state in which the patient has almost continual hallucinations.

HALLUX n. the great toe; pl. **halluces** adj. **hallucal**

HALOGEN n. any of a family of chemicals, including chlorine, bromine, fluorine, and iodine, used in drugs and disinfectants.

HALOPHIL n. a microorganism favoring a high-salt environment for growth; also: **halophile**. adj. **halophilic**

HALOPERIDOL n. a tranquilizer, commonly known under the trade name Haldol, used in the treatment of psychotic disorders and Gilles de la Tourette syndrome; also sometimes used to treat sleep disorders. Adverse effects include hypotension and muscular incoordination.

HALOTHANE n. an inhalation anesthetic widely used to produce general anesthesia for many types of surgical procedures; it is most often used in combination with analgesics and muscle relaxants. Among its advantages are its properties of being nonexplosive, nonflammable, and nonirritating to the respiratory passages. Serious adverse reactions include hypotension, heart arrhythmia, and liver damage.

HAMARTIA n. a defect in development due to abnormal tissue combination. adj. **hamartial**

HAMARTOMA n. a benign tumor made up of an overgrowth of mature cells that normally occur in the affected part, but often with one element predominating.

HAMATE BONE n. the wrist (carpal) bone that projects a hook-shaped (hamate) part on its palmar surface, in line with the fourth and fifth fingers. adj. **hamate**, **hamular**, hooked

HAMMERTOE n. condition in which one or more toes (most commonly the second toe) is permanently flexed, giving a claw-like appearance.

HAMSTRING MUSCLE n. any of three powerful muscles at the back of the thigh.

HAMSTRING TENDON n. any of the tendons at the back of the knee; they connect the *hamstring muscles* with the bones of the knee area.

HAND n. that part of the upper limb distal to the forearm and extending from the wrist to include the fingers. It contains 27 bones, including 8 in the wrist, 5 in the metacarpal region, and 14 in the fingers.

HANDEDNESS n. the preference to use either the left or right hand for writing and other delicate manipulations. Handedness is thought to be hereditary and is related to cerebral dominance with left-handedness being associated with dominance of the right hemisphere of the brain and vice versa. Of 100 persons, usually about 67 are right-handed.

HANSEN'S DISEASE   see *leprosy.*

HANGNAIL n. a narrow loose strip of skin near the base of a fingernail in the region of the nailfold and cuticle. Tearing the fragment usually produces a painful, easily infected sore.

HAPLOID adj. pert. to a cell, specifically a gamete, or sex cell, that has half the chromosome number characteristic of the species. Thus, in humans, the sex cells—the ovum (egg) and sperm—each has the haploid chromosome number 23; at fertilization when the gametes fuse to form a zygote, the zygote has the chromosome number 46, charac-

teristic for humans (compare *diploid*).

HAPTOGLOBIN n. a protein found in *plasma* that binds *hemoglobin* and clears it from wounds; the amount of haptoglobin is increased in certain inflammatory diseases, decreased in hemolytic anemia.

HARDENING OF THE ARTERIES   see *arteriosclerosis.*

HARD PALATE n. the bony portin of the roof of the mouth, bounded on the front and sides by the gums and in the back continuous with the *soft palate*.

HARELIP n. a congenital deformity in which there is one or more clefts in the upper lip; it results from failure of the upper jaw and nasal processes to close during embryonic development. It is often associated with cleft palate. It can be repaired surgically during infancy.

HARTNUP DISEASE n. an hereditary defect of the metabolism of certain amino acids, characterized by dry, scaly skin lesions; gastrointestinal problems; extreme photosensitivity; and often psychological and mental abnormalities.

HASHIMOTO'S DISEASE n. an autoimmune disorder of the thyroid gland in which antibodies are produced against thyroid tissue. It is most common in middle-aged women. Symptoms include an enlarged, lumpy thyroid and an enlarged thymus. Treatment is by administration of thyroid hormones.

HASHISH n. a drug prepared from the Indian hemp plant *Cannabis sativa* that produces euphoria, distorted perceptions, and sometimes hallucinations (see also *cannabis; marihuana*).

HAUSTRUM n. a pouch, esp. in the colon.   pl. **haustra** adj. **haustral**

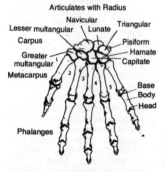

HAND
Articulates with Radius
Navicular
Lesser multangular Lunate Triangular
Carpus   Pisiform
Greater   Hamate
multangular   Capitate
Metacarpus
                                  Base
                                  Body
                                  Head
Phalanges

Courtesy Carolina Biological Supply Co.

HAY FEVER n. a type of allergic *rhinitis*, with symptoms of sneezing, runny nose, and watery eyes, that occurs seasonally on exposure to pollen. Antihistamines are frequently used to alleviate the symptoms; if the specific allergen can be identified desensitization may be possible.

HAVERSIAN CANAL n. one of many tiny (about 0.05 millimeter) canals, containing blood vessels, nerve filaments, and connective tissue, found as the central tube in the Haversian systems of *compact bone*.

HAVERSIAN SYSTEM n. a basic unit of compact bone, consisting of a central *Haversian canal* around which bone matrix and bone cells occur.

HB abbreviation for *hemoglobin*.

HCG abbreviation for human chorionic *gonadotropin*.

HEAD n. 1. the upper part of the body, esp. that which contains the brain and organs of sight, hearing, taste, and smell; 2. the rounded portion of a bone, which fits into a groove in another to form a joint (e.g., the head of the humerus [upper arm bone] fits into the shoulder joint); 3. that part of a muscle that is away from the bone that it moves.

HEADACHE n. pain, ranging from mild to severe, that occurs in the head. There are many causes of headache and treatment depends on the cause. See *histamine headache*, *migraine*, *sinus headache*, *tension headache*; also: **cephalgia**.

HEALING n. the process of restoring health or normal function or of natural repair of damaged or cut tissue.

HEARING n. the sense of receiving and interpreting sounds. Sound waves enter the outer ear, cause vibrations of the eardrum and bones of the middle ear and are transmitted to the inner ear from which they are transmitted along the *auditory nerve* to the brain for interpretation.

HEARING AID n. a device, usually worn in or near the ear, that intensifies sound; it is used to help some people with hearing impairment.

HEARING IMPAIRMENT n. a decrease or limitation in sensitivity to sound.

HEART n. the muscular, roughly cone-shaped organ that pumps blood throughout the body. Lying behind the sternum between the lungs, it is about the size of a closed fist, about 12 centimeters (5 inches) long, 8 centimeters (3 inches) wide at its broadest upper part, and about 6 centimeters (2¼ inches) thick and weighs about 275–345 grams (10–12 ounces) in males, 225 to 275 grams (8–10 ounces) in females. Under outer *epicardium* membranes, the heart wall—*myocardium*—consists of cardiac muscle; the innermost layer—the endocardium—is continuous with lining of the blood vessels. The heart is divided into left and right sides by a septum; each side has an upper atrium (auricle) and lower ventricle. Through coordinated nerve impulses and muscular contractions, initiated in the *sinoatrial node* of the right atrium, the heart pumps blood throughout the body. Deoxygenated blood, carried to the heart by the vena cava, flows into the right atrium and passes into the right ventricle, from which it flows through pulmonary arteries to the lungs, where it gives up its wastes and becomes freshly oxygenated. The oxygenated blood then passes through the pulmonary veins into the left atrium and from there into the left venticle. From the left ventricle it is pumped throughout the body. The heart normally beats about 70 times per minute. It is nourished by coronary blood vessels.

HEART, CUT VIEW

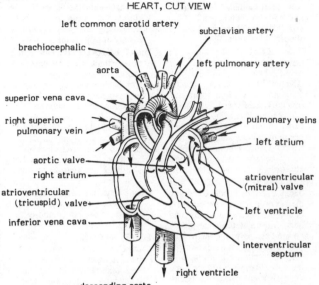

left common carotid artery

subclavian artery

brachiocephalic

aorta

left pulmonary artery

superior vena cava

right superior
pulmonary vein

pulmonary veins

left atrium

aortic valve

right atrium

atrioventricular
(mitral) valve

atrioventricular
(tricuspid) valve

left ventricle

inferior vena cava

interventricular
septum

right ventricle

descending aorta

HEART ATTACK n. popular term
for a disruption of the normal
function of the heart; see *myocardial infarction*.

HEART BLOCK n. a condition in
which the conduction of the electrical impulses generated by the
heart (the sinoatrial node, or natural pacemaker) is impaired,
slowing down the pumping action of the heart. The block may
be partial (often causing no
symptoms) or complete (in which
cases the ventricles beat at their
own slow rate); it may be congenital or the result of any heart disorder; it is most often seen in the
elderly.

HEARTBURN a painful, burning
sensation in the chest, below the
sternum, resulting from irritation
in the esophagus most often due
to backflow of acidic stomach
contents into the esophagus. It is
often a symptom of *hiatal hernia*,
peptic ulcer, or other disorder;
also: **pyrosis**.

HEART FAILURE n. inability of
the heart to pump enough blood
to maintain normal body requirements. It may be caused by congential defects or by any condition (e.g., *atherosclerosis* of
coronary arteries, *aortic stenosis*,
myocardial infarction) that damages or overloads the heart muscle. Symptoms include edema,
shortness of breath, and feelings
of faintness. Treatment depends
on the specific cause of the heart
malfunction and on the age and
general condition of the patient.

HEART-LUNG MACHINE n. an
apparatus that takes over the
functions of the heart and lungs
temporarily, used during heart
surgery. It includes a pump and a
means of oxygenating blood.

HEART MASSAGE   see *cardiac massage*.

HEART MURMUR n. an abnormal heart sound. Some heart murmurs are benign and of no significance; others are signs of abnormal heart function.

HEART RATE n. the number of heart contractions (beats) per minute. Normal adult heart rate is about 70-72 beats per minute; an abnormally rapid heart rate (over 100 beats per minute in an adult) is *tachycardia*; an abnormally slow rate (below 60 beats per minute in an adult) is *bradycardia*. Children normally have a heart rate faster than an adult (see also **pulse**).

HEART SOUND n. any of four distinct sounds produced within the heart during its normal cycle of contraction and relaxation and heard with a stethoscope placed on the chest over the heart. The first sound (a dull, prolonged "lub") is caused by closure of the valves between the atria and ventricles and marks the beginning of ventricular contraction; the second (a short, sharp "dub") occurs with closing of the semilunar valves as the ventricle begins to relax; the third (a weak, dull sound) occurs as the ventricles fill with blood during their relaxed phase; the fourth (usually not heard, except in abnormal conditions) occurs as the atria contract. Changes in the characteristic sounds usually indicate abnormalities in heart structure or function and are important diagnostic aids.

HEART SURGERY n. any surgical procedure involving the heart. In closed heart surgery, a small incision is made into the heart; the heart-lung machine is not used. In open-heart surgery, the heart is opened, the chambers of the heart made visible, and blood detoured from the operating field through the heart-lung machine.

HEART VALVE n. any of four structures (two semilunar valves, the mitral valve, and the tricuspid valve) within the heart that by closing and opening control blood flow in the heart and permit flow in only one direction.

HEAT EXHAUSTION n. condition characterized by dizziness, nausea, weakness, muscle cramps, and pale, cool skin caused by overexposure to intense heat and depletion of body fluids and electrolytes. It is most common in infants and the elderly. Recovery usually occurs with rest, replacement of water and electrolytes, and removal from the intense heat; also **heat prostration** (compare *heat stroke*).

HEAT RASH n. a fine papular inflammation of the skin resulting from heat or high humidity (see also *prickly heat*).

HEAT STROKE n. a severe, sometimes fatal, condition caused by prolonged exposure to intense heat and failure of the body's temperature regulating capacity; symptoms include high body temperature, rapid heart beat, hot dry skin, confusion, and possibly convulsions and loss of consciousness. Treatment includes cooling of the body, fluid and electrolyte replacement, and sedation; also: **sunstroke**, **heat hyperpyrexia** (compare *heat exhaustion*).

HEBEPHRENIA n. a form of *schizophrenia* marked by a severe disintegration of personality. It typically becomes evident during puberty with symptoms of extreme silliness; inappropriate laughter; facial grimaces; talking and gesturing to oneself; withdrawal from contact with others; and delusions and hallucinations; also called **disorganized schizophrenia**.   adj. **hebephrenic**

HEBERDEN NODE n. an enlargement of a terminal joint of a finger sometimes occurring in *osteoarthritis* or other degenerative joint disease.

HEEL n. the posterior part of the foot, formed by the *calcaneus* bone.

HEGAR'S SIGN n. a softening of the uterine cervix that occurs in early *pregnancy*.

HEIMLICH MANEUVER n. an emergency procedure to help someone who is choking because food or other material is lodged in the trachea. The rescuer should grab the choking person from behind and place one fist, thumb side in, just below the sternum (breastbone) and the other hand placed over the fist. Then he/she should sharply and abruptly push upward to force the obstruction up the trachea.

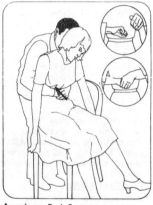

American Red Cross

HELIATION n. the use of sunlight for treatment.

HELIX n. a coil-shaped part; the hereditary material DNA (deoxyribonucleic acid) has a double helix configuration.

HELMINTH n. any of various parasitic worms, including flatworms, tapeworms, and roundworms, some of which infest humans, causing disease. adj. **helminthic**

HELMINTHIASIS n. infestation of the body with worms that may affect the skin, the intestines, or other internal organs.

HELOMA n. a hard-tissue formation; a corn or callosity. pl. **helomata**

HELPER T CELL see *T cell.*

HEM-, HEMA-, HEMATO-, HEMO- prefix indicating an association with blood (e.g., **hemodilution**, adding fluid to blood thus reducing the number of red blood cells per unit of volume).

HEMAGGLUTINATION n. the clumping together of red blood cells. adj. **hemagglutinative**

HEMANGIOMA n. a benign tumor consisting of blood vessels. Some occur as birthmarks (*strawberry hemangioma*), often spontaneously disappearing; others develop later in life, often in the elderly. pl. **hemangioma**, **hemangiomata**

HEMARTHROSIS n. the flow of blood out of its vessels and into a joint or joint cavity, causing pain and swelling of the joint area; it may result from injury or certain diseases (e.g., *hemophilia*).

HEMATEMESIS n. the vomiting of blood, most often caused by bleeding in the esophagus (e.g., from varicose veins), stomach, or upper intestine (e.g., from an ulcer).

HEMATIN see *heme.*

HEMATINIC n. a drug (e.g., ferrous sulfate or other iron-containing compound) that increases the *hemoglobin* content of the blood; it is used to treat or prevent iron-deficiency anemia.

HEMATOCOELE n. a tumor or swelling caused by leakage of blood from blood vessels, esp. a swelling of the membrane covering the testis.

HEMATOCHEZIA n. the passage of stools containing blood.

HEMATOCOLPOMETRA n. accumulation of menstrual blood in the vagina because of an unopened *hymen*.

HEMATOCRIT n. a measure of the volume of red blood cells as a percentage of the total blood volume. The normal range is 43-49% in males, 37-43% in females (see also *blood count*; *differential blood count*).

HEMATOCYTOPENIA n. an abnormally low number of cells in the blood.

HEMATOCYTURIA n. the presence of red blood cells (erythrocytes) in the urine.

HEMATOGEN n. any blood-producing material; also: **hematinogen.**

HEMATOHIDROSIS n. the secretion of sweat containing blood; also: **hematidrosis.**

HEMATOLOGIST n. a specialist in *hematology*.

HEMATOLOGY n. the science of blood and blood-forming tissues, including its functions, diseases, and use in treatment. adj. **hematologic, hematological**

HEMATOMA n. a localized collection of blood, usually clotted, in an organ, space, or tissue due to escape of blood from a blood vessel, often the result of trauma; when the hematoma occurs near the skin surface, it causes discoloration (e.g., a black eye).

HEMATOPOIESIS n. the process by which blood cells are produced, esp. as occurring in the bone marrow; also: **hemopoiesis.** adj. **hematopoietic**

HEMATURIA n. the presence of blood in the urine, often a symptom of disease in the urinary tract.

HEME n. the red pigment, nonprotein, iron-containing part of the *hemoglobin* molecule of red blood cells.

HEMERALOPIA n. abnormal condition in which bright light causes a blurring of vision; a side effect of some anticonvulsant drugs; also: **day blindness.**

HEMI- comb. form meaning "half" (e.g., **hemifacial**, affecting only one side of the face).

HEMIANOPIA n. blindness to one half of the visual field in one or both eyes; also: **hemianopsia.** adj. **hemianopic**

HEMIC adj. pert. to blood.

HEMIPLEGIA n. paralysis affecting only one side of the body; also called **unilateral paralysis.** adj. **hemiplegic**

HEMISPHERE n. half of a ball-like part; in medicine, half the lateral half of the *cerebrum* or *cerebellum* of the brain.

HEMOCHROMATOSIS n. a disorder of iron metabolism in which iron accumulates in tissues; it is characterized by bronze pigmentation of the skin, an enlarged and impaired liver, diabetes mellitus, and abnormalities of the pancreas and joints. It may be hereditary (idiopathic, or classic, hemochromatosis) or acquired through iron-overload from repeated transfusions or intake of iron-containing compounds. Also called **bronzed diabetes**; **iron-storage disease** (compare *hemosiderosis*).

HEMODIALYSIS n. a procedure, used in toxic conditions and renal (kidney) failure, in which wastes and impurities are removed from the blood by a special machine. The blood is shunted to and from a dialyzer where, through diffusion and ultrafiltration, wastes are removed; popularly known as **artificial kidney.**

HEMOFIL n. trade name for human antihemophilic factor used in the treatment of *hemophilia*.

HEMOGLOBIN n. the complex compound, containing the nonprotein, iron-containing pigment *heme* and the protein *globin*, found in red blood cells (erythrocytes) that transports oxygen to cells throughout the body and carries carbon dioxide away from body cells. In the high oxygen concentration of the lungs, hemoglobin binds with oxygen to form *oxyhemoglobin*. In the tissues of the body, the oxygen is given off and the hemoglobin combines with carbon dioxide to form *carboxyhemoglobin*, which is carried back to the lungs. There the carbon dioxide is given off and more oxygen picked up for transport to the body cells. Normal hemoglobin concentration in blood is 13.5 to 18 grams per deciliter for males, 12 to 16 for females.

HEMOGLOBINEMIA n. the presence of excessive *hemoglobin* in blood plasma.

HEMOGLOBINOPATHY n. any of a group of inherited disorders characterized by an alteration in the normal structure of *hemoglobin*. Types of hemoglobinopathies include *sickle-cell disease* and *thalassemia*. adj. **hemoglobinopathic**

HEMOGLOBINURIA n. the abnormal presence of free *hemoglobin* in the urine. adj. **hemoglobinuric**

HEMOLYSIN n. a substance that breaks down or dissolves red blood cells. Hemolysins are found in some bacteria, some venom, and some foods.

HEMOLYSIS n. the breakdown of red blood cells and the release of hemoglobin. It occurs normally at the end of the life span of a red blood cell, abnormally in certain antigen-antibody reactions, on exposure to certain bacteria and venoms; in hemodialysis and in certain other conditions. See also *hemolytic anemia*.

HEMOLYTIC ANEMIA n. a disorder in which there is premature destruction of red blood cells. Anemia—abnormally low *hemoglobin* levels— may or may not be present, depending on the ability of bone marrow to increase red blood cell production. It can result from certain infections or inherited disorders of red blood cells but most often is a response to drugs or toxic substances (e.g., snake venom) (compare *aplastic anemia*).

HEMOPHILIA n. an inherited disorder characterized by excessive bleeding and occurring only in males. Several forms of the disease—including hemophilia A and hemophilia B (also called Christmas disease)—occur; in all forms one of the factors necessary for normal *blood coagulation* is missing or present in abnormally low amounts. Greater than usual blood loss in dental extractions and simple injuries and bleeding into joint areas commonly occur; severe internal hemorrhage is less common. Treatment involves administration of missing blood coagulation factors in some cases and transfusions to replace lost blood.

HEMOPTYSIS n. coughing up blood from the respiratory tract; it may occur in small amounts in mild upper respiratory infection and bronchitis; profuse bleeding usually indicates severe infection or disease of the bronchi or lungs. adj. **hemoptysic**

HEMORRHAGE n. the loss of a large amount of blood during a short time, either externally or internally. The bleeding may be from an artery (the blood flows in spurts and is bright red), from a vein (the blood flows slowly and is dark), or from a tiny vessel or capillary (the blood oozes). External bleeding may be controlled by pressure and ice on the wound or by a tourniquet applied proximally to the wound; internal bleeding requires prompt medical attention. Loss of large amounts of blood can lead to shock and death. adj. **hemorrhagic**

HEMORRHAGIC FEVER n. any of several kinds of arbovirus infection, usually occurring in a specific geographic area; symptoms include fever, malaise, respiratory or gastrointestinal symptoms, followed by capillary hemorrhage.

HEMORRHOID n. swelling of a vein or veins (varicosity) in the lower rectum or anus, either internal, above the anal sphincter, or external, outside the anal sphincter. Often associated with constipation, straining to defecate, pregnancy, or prolonged sitting, hemorrhoids are often painful and sometimes bleed with defecation. Treatment includes topical agents to shrink and anesthetize the hemorrhoids, compresses, and, if severe, ligation or surgical excision. adj. **hemorrhoidal**

HEMORRHOIDECTOMY n. surgical procedure for tying and excising hemorrhoids.

HEMOSIDEROSIS n. abnormal deposition of an iron-containing compound (hemosiderin) in tissues, often associated with diseases in which there is extensive destruction of red blood cells (e.g., *thalassemia*) (compare *hemochromatosis*).

HEMOSTASIS n. cessation of bleeding either naturally through the blood coagulation process or mechanically (e.g., with surgical clamps) or chemically (e.g., with drugs). adj. **hemostatic**

HEMOSTAT n. a plierslike instrument used to compress a blood vessel to check bleeding.

HEMOTHORAX n. accumulation of blood in the pleural cavity (the space between the lungs and chest wall); it is usually the result of injury, sometimes of blood vessel rupture associated with lung disease. The blood must be drained or impaired lung function and infection may occur.

HEPARIN n. 1. a chemical produced in certain white blood cells (basophils) and connective tissue cells (mast cells), esp. in the lungs and liver, that inhibits the activity of the *thrombin factor* in blood coagulation and thus prevents clotting within the blood vessels; 2. a drug (heparin sodium) used as an anticoagulant in the treatment of thromboembolic disorders.

HEPAT-, HEPATO- comb. form indicating an association with the liver (e.g., **hepatalgia**, pain in the liver).

HEPATIC adj. pert. to the liver.

HEPATIC DUCT n. tube that carries bile from the liver toward the intestine; it joins with the cystic duct from the gall bladder to form the common bile duct.

HEPATITIS n. an inflammation of the liver, characterized by *jaundice*, loss of appetite, abdominal discomfort, an enlarged and abnormally functioning liver, and dark urine. It may be caused by bacterial or viral infection, infestation with parasites, alcohol, drugs, toxins, transfusions of incompatible blood, or as a complication of another disease (e.g., infectious mononucleosis) and may be mild and brief or prolonged and severe, even life-threatening. See also *serum hepatitis*; *viral hepatitis*.

HEPATOMA n. a primary malignant tumor of the liver, most common in tropical parts of the world, esp. where fungus-produced aflatoxins may contaminate food; also sometimes associated with hepatitis or cirrhosis of the liver. Symptoms include an enlarged liver, pain, loss of appetite, weight loss, and the presence of alphafetoprotein in the plasma.

HEPATOMEGALY n. abnormal enlargement of the liver, usually a sign of liver disease.

HEPATOTOXIC. adj. damaging to the liver, e.g., certain drugs or alcohol. n. **hepatotoxicity**

HEREDITARY adj. pert. to transmission from parents to offspring; inherited (e.g., an hereditary disorder, a disorder that is passed from parents to offspring).

HEREDITY n. 1. the process by which specific traits or characteristics are transmitted, through genes, from parents to offspring; 2. the total genetic makeup of an individual. adj. **hereditary**

HERMAPHRODITE n. a person who has the tissues of both testes and of ovaries; true hermaphroditism is rare among humans.

HERNIA n. protrusion of an organ through an abnormal opening in the muscular wall surrounding the organ area. It may be congenital or acquired as a result of injury, muscular weakness, or disease. Common types of hernia include *hiatal hernia*, *inguinal hernia*, and *umbilical hernia*. adj. **hernial**

HERNIATED DISC n. rupture of the fibrocartilage of the disc between vertebrae of the spinal column, occurring most often in the lumbar region. With the ruptured disc there is a lack of cushioning between the vertebrae above and below and resultant pressure on spinal nerves, causing pain; also called **slipped disc**; **ruptured intervertebral disc**.

HEROIN n. a strongly addictive drug made from *morphine*; it has no medical uses in the United States but is widely abused.

HERPANGIA n. a viral infection, occurring most often in children, characterized by sore throat; papules on the tongue, pharynx, and palate; fever; headache; and pain in the abdomen and extremities. It usually subsides within a short time.

HERPES n. any of a group of viruses that cause painful blister-like eruptions on the skin. See *herpes genitalis*, *herpes simplex*, *herpes zoster*.

HERPES GENITALIS n. an infection, caused by type 2 herpes simplex virus, usually transmitted by sexual contact, characterized by recurrent attacks of painful eruptions on the skin and mucous membranes of the genital area. Symptoms include fever, malaise, urinary problems, painful coitus, swelling of lymph glands in the inguinal area, and lesions on the glans or foreskin of the penis in males and lesions on the vagina and cervix, sometimes with a discharge from the cervix, in females. Treatment is aimed at relieving symptoms; there is no cure. Also called **genital herpes**.

HERPES SIMPLEX n. an infection, caused by herpes simplex virus, that usually affects the skin and nervous system, producing small, transient, sometimes painful blisters on the skin and mucous membranes. Herpes simplex 1 (HS1) most commonly affects the facial region, esp. the area near the mouth and nose. Symptoms include tingling and burning, followed by blisterlike eruptions that dry and crust before healing. Treatment involves keeping the area clean to prevent secondary infection and topical use of drying medications. Also called **cold sore**. Herpes simplex 2 (HS2) commonly affects the genital region (see *herpes genitalis*).

HERPES ZOSTER n. an infection with herpes zoster virus, usually occurring in adults, and characterized by blisterlike eruptions along the course of an inflamed nerve. Symptoms include pain—chronic or intermittent, mild or severe—along the course of the lesions, sometimes with fever, malaise, and headache. Treatment is symptomatic and includes cold compresses and calamine applications on the lesions. Complications, occurring most often in the elderly, include postherpetic neuralgia, which may last for months. Also called **shingles**.

HERPES ZOSTER VIRUS see *chickenpox*.

HETEROGENEOUS adj. made up of unlike, dissimilar parts or materials; not of the same consistency throughout (compare *homogeneous*).

HETEROGENOUS adj. not from the same source (compare *homogenous*).

HETEROGRAFT n. tissue from an individual of one species used as a temporary graft, as in cases of severe burn, on an individual of another species. A heterograft is usually rapidly rejected but provides temporary cover for an injured area, reducing fluid loss; also called **xenograft** (compare *homograft*).

HETEROPHIL TEST n. a blood test that when positive usually indicates *infectious mononucleosis*.

HETEROPLOIDY n. the condition of having an abnormal number of chromosomes, either more or less than the number normal for body cells of the species.

HETEROSEXUAL n. a person whose sexual preference is for persons of the opposite sex (compare *homosexual*).

HETEROZYGOUS adj. having two different alleles of a *gene* at corresponding loci (sites) on homologous chromosomes. A person heterozygous for a given trait inherits one allele from each parent and the dominant allele usually manifests itself (compare *homozygous*).

HEXACHLOROPHENE n. a topical antiinfective agent used as a disinfectant and antiseptic scrub.

HEXADROL n. trade name for *dexamethasone*, an antiinflammatory agent.

HEXESTROL n. an *estrogen* compound used to treat menstrual irregularities and menopausal symptoms and to prevent pregnancy.

HEXOBARBITAL n. a short-acting sedative and hypnotic.

HIATUS n. a normal opening in a membrane or other tissue. adj. **hiatal**

HIATUS HERNIA n. protrusion of part of the stomach through the *diaphragm*. It is a common disorder and in many cases produces no symptoms. Symptoms, when present, include gastroesophageal reflux (heartburn), the flow of acid stomach contents into the esophagus; also **hiatal hernia**.

HICCUP n. a characteristic sound produced by involuntary spasm of the diaphragm and rapid closure of the glottis as air is breathed in. Hiccups sometimes indicate indigestion, or too-rapid eating, but in most cases have no identifiable cause; also: **hiccough, singultus**.

HIDROSIS n. the production and secretion of sweat.

HIDROTIC adj. pert. to sweat.

HIGH BLOOD PRESSURE see *hypertension*.

HIGH DENSITY LIPOPROTEIN (HDL) n. a protein of plasma that contains relatively more protein and less fats; it serves to transport cholesterol and other lipids from plasma to tissues. According to some studies high HDL levels are associated with lowered risks of cardiovascular disorders.

HILUS n. a depression or small pit in an organ, esp. the entry site for blood vessels and nerves; also: **hilum**. pl. **hila, hili** adj. **hilar**

HINGE JOINT n. a freely movable (synovial) joint in which bones are articulated in such a way as to permit extensive motion in one plane. The elbow, knee, and interphalangeal joints are hinge joints (compare *ball and socket joint*, *gliding joint*, *pivot joint*).

HIP n. area of the body formed by the lower part of the torso (pelvis) and the upper part of the thigh.

HIP JOINT n. a ball-and-socket joint in which the head of the *femur* (thigh bone) fits into the acetabulum of the innominate bone of the pelvis. The joint involves several ligaments and permits extensive motion; also **coxa joint**.

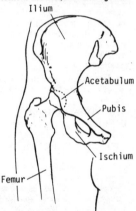

Front view of the hip joint. The innominate, or hip, bone is formed by the ilium, ischium, and pubis.

HIPPOCAMPUS n. a structure of the brain, part of the *limbic system*.   adj. **hippocampal**

HIPPOCRATIC OATH n. a statement, attributed to the ancient Greek physician Hippocrates, that serves as an ethical guide for physicians and is incorporated into the graduation ceremonies at many medical schools.

HIRSCHSPRUNG'S DISEASE n. congenital condition in which the colon does not have a normal nerve network; there is little urge to defecate, feces accumulate, and

the colon becomes dilated (megacolon). Symptoms include intermittent diarrhea and constipation, loss of appetite, and distended abdomen. Surgical repair involves joining the normal colon section to the rectum; also called **megacolon**.

HIRSUTISM n. excessive hairiness, sometimes the result of heredity, endocrine (hormonal) imbalance, disease, or drug intake.

HIST-, HISTIO-, HISTO- comb. form indicating an association with tissue (e.g., **histogenesis**, tissue development).

HISTAMINE n. a compound found in all cells and released in allergic responses and inflammatory conditions; it causes small blood vessels to widen, decreases blood pressure, increases gastric secretions, and constricts smooth muscles of the bronchi and uterus.

HISTAMINE HEADACHE n. headache associated with the release of *histamine* from cells. Symptoms include sharp pain on one side of the head, runny nose, and watery eyes. Treatment is by antihistamines and agents to constrict dilated arteries. Also called **cluster headache**. (Compare *migraine*, *sinus headache*, *tension headache*).

HISTOCOMPATIBILITY n. the ability of the cells of one tissue to survive in the presence of cells of another tissue, as in the ability of cells of a transplanted organ to survive in the presence of cells of another organism. A high degree of histocompatibility is necessary for a successful *graft* or *transplant*.

HISTOLOGY n. the science of tissues, including their cellular composition and organization.

HISTOPLASMOSIS n. infection caused by inhaling spores of the fungus *Histoplasma capsulatum*, most common in the Ohio and

Mississippi River valleys; symptoms include fever, malaise, cough, and enlarged lymph nodes. In most cases the disease subsides spontaneously; in a few cases it progresses to a severe infiltration of the lungs and death.

HIVES see *urticaria*.

HODGKIN'S DISEASE n. a malignant disorder in which there is painless, progressive enlargement of lymph tissue. Symptoms include generalized itching, weight loss and loss of appetite, low-grade fever, and night sweats. It occurs more often among males and usually manifests itself between the ages of 15 and 35. Treatment with radiotherapy and/or chemotherapy effects long-term remissions in more than one half of cases and cures in a large percentage of those with localized disease.

HOLISTIC MEDICINE n. a system of medical care based on the concept that a person is an integrated entity, more than the sum of his/her physiological, mental, psychological and social parts.

HOMEOPATHY n. medical system, based on the idea that "like cures like," which uses drugs or other substances that would produce in healthy persons the symptoms shown by the sick person, e.g., treating a fever by giving small doses of a drug that raises body temperature.

HOMEOSTASIS n. a steady state in the internal environment of the body (e.g., temperature, electrolyte balance, respiration, heart rate) maintained by various feedback and control mechanisms, involving primarily the nervous and endocrine systems. adj. **homeostatic**

HOMOGENEOUS adj. consisting of like parts; having a uniform quality; also: **homogenous** (compare *heterogeneous*).

HOMOGENOUS adj. derived from the same source (compare *heterogenous*).

HOMOGRAFT n. tissue from one person transplanted to another person of the same species but of different genetic makeup. The recipient's immune system must be repressed to prevent rejection of the graft or transplanted organ.

HOMOSEXUAL n. a person whose sexual preference is for persons of the same sex (compare *heterosexual*).

HOMOZYGOUS adj. having two identical alleles of a *gene* at corresponding loci (sites) on homologous chromosomes, having inherited the same allele from each parent. The recessive trait usually manifests itself when homozygous (compare *heterozygous*).

HOMUNCULUS n. a dwarf with no deformity or abnormality and all parts of the body proportionate.

HOOKWORM DISEASE n. condition resulting from intestinal infestation by hookworms, which most often enter the body by penetratng the skin, esp. that of the feet when walking barefoot in hookworm-infested soil areas. Symptoms include abdominal discomfort, diarrhea, and blood loss sometimes leading to anemia.

HORDEOLUM n. a localized, pus-containing bacterial infection—a boil—of the eyelid. Treatment includes antibiotics and hot compresses. Also called **stye.**

HORMONE n. a complex chemical produced and secreted by endocrine (ductless) glands that travels through the bloodstream and controls or regulates the activity of another organ or group of cells—its target organ. (For example, growth hormone released by the pituitary gland controls the growth of long bones of the body.) Secretions of hormones is regulated by feedback mechanisms and neurotransmitters. See *endocrine gland*; *endocrine system*.   adj. **hormonal**

HORNER'S SYNDROME n. a group of symptoms—drooping upper eyelid, constricted pupil, absence of facial sweating—occurring as a result of damage to nerves in the cervical (neck) region of the spine.

HORRIPILATION n. gooseflesh; the standing up of the hairs on the body in cold or fear.

HOST n. 1. an organism in which another, usually parasitic, organism lives; 2. the recipient of a transplanted organ or tissue (compare *donor*).

HOT FLASH n. a transient feeling of warmth experienced by some women during *menopause*; the frequency and severity of the flashes vary widely.

HUMAN CHORIONIC GONADOTROPIN (HCG) n. hormone produced by the placenta in early *pregnancy* that functions to maintain the pregnancy. It can be detected in the urine of pregnant women.

HUMERUS n. the upper arm bone, extending from the shoulder to the elbow. Its head articulates with the *scapula* (shoulderbone); its body is cylindrical; and its condyle end has depressions for articulations with the *ulna* and *radius* of the lower arm at the elbow. adj. **humeral**

HUMOR n. a fluid in the body, esp. the *aqueous humor* of the eye.   adj. **humoral**

HUMPBACK   see *kyphosis*.

HUNTINGTON'S CHOREA n. an abnormal hereditary condition (*autosomal dominant disease*) characterized by progressive chorea (involuntary rapid, jerky motions) and mental deterioration, leading to dementia. Symptoms usually first appear in the third or fourth decade of life and progress to death, often within 15 years.

HURLER'S SYNDROME n. a hereditary disease (*autosomal recessive disease*) in which mucopolysaccharides and lipids accumulate in the tissues causing mental retardation, enlarged liver and spleen, enlarged head (sometimes *hydrocephalus*), low forehead; it usually leads to death in childhood from cardiac or pulmonary complications.

HYALIN n. a clear glassy material that results from the breakdown of certain tissues.

HYALINE CARTILAGE n. the most common type of cartilage; the bluish-white elastic cartilage covering the ends of bones, connecting the ribs to the breastbone, and supporting facial structures and the trachea.

HYALINE MEMBRANE DISEASE n. see *respiratory distress syndrome of the newborn*.

HYALOID MEMBRANE n. transparent membrane that surrounds the vitreous humor of the eye and separates it from the *retina*.

HUMERUS

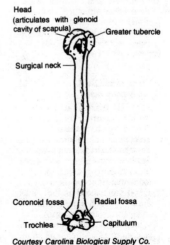

Head
(articulates with glenoid
cavity of scapula)

Greater tubercle

Surgical neck

Coronoid fossa

Radial fossa

Trochlea

Capitulum

Courtesy Carolina Biological Supply Co.

HYALURONIC ACID n. a chemical present in the vitreous humor of the eye, in movable joints, and certain other tissues; it is a cementing and protective substance, forming a gel in intercellular spaces.

HYALURONIDASE n. an *enzyme*, found in testes, semen, and other tissues, that increases the permeability of connective tissue and the absorption of fluids; injected to increase the absorption of other drugs.

HYAZYME n. trade name for *hyaluronidase*.

HYBRID n. offspring of a cross between two individuals of different species (e.g., a mule is a hybrid, the result of the mating of a male donkey and a female horse); most hybrids are *sterile*.

HYDANTOIN n. any of a group of anticonvulsant drugs, similar to barbiturates, used in the management of epilepsy. The most widely used hydantoin is phenytoin (diphenylhydantoin), commonly known under the trade name Dilantin.

HYDATID n. a cystlike, usually fluid-filled structure, esp. that which forms around the dog tapeworm *Echinococcus granulosus* (see *echinococcosis*).

HYDATID DISEASE see *echinococcosis*.

HYDATIDIFORM MOLE see *hydatid mole*.

HYDATID MOLE n. an abnormality occurring in pregnancy during which chorionic villi degenerate forming grapelike masses throughout the placenta, causing death of the embryo and sometimes leading to a malignancy in the uterus. It occurs in about 1 in 1,500 pregnancies in the United States; is much more common in some Far Eastern countries. Early symptoms include extreme nausea, uterine bleeding, and an unusually large uterus. It is important that all molar tissue be removed from the uterus to minimize the risk of developing choriocarcinoma.

HYDATIDOSIS see *echinococcosis*.

HYDERGINE n. trade name for fixed-combination drug containing *ergot* alkaloids.

HYDRALAZINE n. a drug, commonly known under the trade name Apresoline, that dilates blood vessels and is used, often in combination with a diuretic, in the treatment of hypertension. Adverse effects include headache, rapid heart rate, and gastrointestinal disturbances.

HYDRAMNIOS n. an abnormality of pregnancy in which there is an excess of amniotic fluid surrounding the fetus; sometimes associated with toxemia or diabetes mellitus in the mother, multiple pregnancy, or fetal disorder.

HYDRARTHROSIS n. swelling of a joint because of excess synovial fluid; it most often affects the knee (colloquially called "water on the knee") and usually indicates *inflammation*.

HYDREMIA n. excess fluid volume compared with cell volume of the blood.   adj. **hydremic**

HYDROA n. eruption of small, usually very itchy, blisters on skin exposed to sunlight, occurring most often in children.

HYDROCELE n. a condition in which watery fluid accumulates in a sac, esp. the scrotum (the sac surrounding the testes). The condition may subside spontaneously or the fluid may be drained.

HYDROCEPHALUS n. an abnormal condition in which *cerebrospinal fluid* accumulates in the ventricles (central spaces) of the brain due to blockage of normal fluid outflow from the brain or failure of fluid to be absorbed into the bloodstream quickly enough.

The result is enlargement of the head (esp. in infants and young children) and increased pressure that damages the brain. The condition may be congenital—it is estimated to occur in 1 out of every 500 births—and manifest itself immediately after birth or more slowly during early childhood with abnormally rapid head growth, bulging fontanelles, and small face; if untreated it progresses to cause lethargy, defective reflex actions, seizures, and eventually death. When acquired later in life, e.g., as a result of trauma, brain tumor, or infection, the symptoms are primarily neurological, resulting from pressure on the brain, and include headache, loss of muscular coordination, and visual abnormalities. Treatment usually involves surgical procedures to remove or shunt the excess fluid. The outcome depends on the cause and severity of the condition. Also: **hydrocephaly**. adj. **hydrocephalic**

HYDROCHLORIC ACID n. a chemical secreted in the stomach and a major constituent of *gastric juice*.

HYDROCHLOROTHIAZIDE n. a diuretic, commonly known under the trade names Esidrix and HydroDIURIL, used in the treatment of hypertension. Adverse effects include *electrolyte imbalance*.

HYDROCORTISONE   see *cortisol*.

HYDROCORTONE n. trade name for *cortisol*.

HYDRODIURIL n. trade name for the diuretic *hydrochlorothiazide*.

HYDROFLUMETHIAZIDE n. a *diuretic* used to treat hypertension and edema. Adverse effects include electrolyte imbalances.

HYDROGEN n. an element, a constituent of water and many biological compounds (see Table of Elements).

HYDROGEN PEROXIDE n. a clear liquid compound (H_2O_2) applied in water solution to cleanse wounds and as a mouthwash.

HYDROMORPHONE n. a narcotic analgesic used to treat moderate to severe pain. Adverse effects include drowsiness, dizziness, constipation, and the potential for addiction.

HYDRONEPHROSIS n. distension of the kidney caused by accumulation of urine that cannot flow out because of an obstruction (e.g., tumor, calculus [stone], edema) of the *ureter*. Symptoms include pain, high fever, and the presence of blood and pus in the urine. Treatment involves removal of the obstruction in the ureter.   adj. **hydronephrotic**

HYDROPHOBIA n. 1. rabies; 2. an irrational fear of water.

HYDROPRES n. trade name for a fixed combination drug containing the diuretic *hydrochlorothiazide* and the antihypertensive *reserpine*; used to treat *hypertension*.

HYDROPS n. abnormal accumulation of watery fluid in the tissues or cavities of the body; formerly called **dropsy**; also: **edema**.

HYDROTHERAPY n. the use of water to treat disorders; mostly limited to exercises in special pools for rehabilitation of paralyzed patients.

HYDROXYINE n. a minor tranquilizer used to treat anxiety and motion sickness.

HYDROTHORAX n. accumulation of fluid in the pleural cavity (the cavity surrounding the lungs).

HYMEN n. a fold of tissue at the opening of the vagina that may be absent, thin and pliant, or, rarely, tough and dense, completely occluding the opening. If the vaginal opening is completely closed, coitus and the escape of menstrual fluid are impossible.

HYOID BONE n. small, isolated υ-shaped bone that supports the tongue.

HYOSCINE see *scopolamine*.

HYOSCYAMINE n. a drug used to treat excess motility of the gastrointestinal tract.

HYPER- prefix meaning "above," "beyond," "excessive" (e.g., **hyperacidity**, excess acid, as in the stomach).

HYPERACTIVITY n. a condition characterized by excessive movement and restlessness, seen esp. in children (see *attention deficit syndrome*).

HYPERADRENALISM see *Cushing's disease*.

HYPERADRENOCORTICISM see *Cushing's syndrome*.

HYPERALDOSTERONISM see *aldosteronism*.

HYPERBARIC CHAMBER n. a roomlike chamber in which the oxygen pressure is higher than in the atmosphere; used to treat carbon monoxide poisoning and certain breathing disorders.

HYPERBETALIPOPROTEIN-EMIA n. a genetic disorder of lipid metabolism in which there are abnormally high levels of serum *cholesterol* and a tendency to develop *atherosclerosis* and heart disease at an early age. Treatment involves a low-cholesterol diet and sometimes the use of drugs to lower blood lipid levels.

HYPERBILIRUBINEMIA n. abnormally high amounts of the bile pigment *bilirubin* in the blood, usually characterized by jaundice, loss of appetite, and malaise. It may occur in liver or biliary tract disease, and in diseases in which there is excessive red blood cell destruction (hemolytic anemia), and is common in newborns (see *hyperbilirubinemia of the newborn*).

HYPERBILIRUBINEMIA OF THE NEWBORN n. an excess of the bile pigment *bilirubin* in the blood of a newborn, characterized by jaundice. A common disorder, it is usually due to immaturity of the liver, deficiency of enzymes, and normal destruction of fetal red blood cells; in many cases it subsides spontaneously, in other cases is treated by *phototherapy*. Severe cases, more often due to an abnormal condition (e.g., *erythroblastosis fetalis*), produce signs of spleen and liver enlargement, anemia, *kernicterus* (sometimes leading to mental retardation), and other complications, sometimes leading to death. The mild physiologic condition is also called **neonatal hyperbilirubinemia**.

HYPERCALCEMIA n. abnormally high levels of calcium in the blood, usually the result of excessive bone resorption in *osteoporosis*, *hyperparathyroidism*, *Paget's disease*, or other disorders of bone and calcium function. Symptoms include muscle pain and weakness, loss of appetite, and if severe, kidney failure and death. adj. **hypercalcemic**

HYPERCALCIURIA n. the presence of abnormally large amounts of calcium in the urine, usually resulting from excess bone resorption (e.g., in *osteoporosis*, *hyperparathyroidism*). Also: **hypercalcinuria**. adj. **hypercalciuric**

HYPERCAPNIA n. the presence of excess carbon dioxide in the blood.

HYPERCHOLESTEROLEMIA n. the presence of higher-than-normal amounts of cholesterol in the blood; the condition is associated with an increased risk of atherosclerosis and cardiovascular disease. A low-cholesterol diet is usually recommended. Some forms of the condition are familial (see *familial hypercholesterolemia*).

HYPEREMESIS n. severe vomiting, esp. **hyperemesis gravidarum**, an abnormal condition of pregnancy characterized by severe vomiting, weight loss, fluid and electrolyte imbalance, and, if severe, resultant brain, liver, and kidney damage. Treatment is by drugs to arrest vomiting and maintenance of adequate food intake and fluid and *electolyte balance*.

HYPEREMIA n. increased blood in part of the body, caused by inflammatory response or blockage of blood outflow; the skin typically becomes reddened and warm in the affected area.   adj. **hyperemic**

HYPERGLYCEMIA n. higher-than-normal amount of glucose in the blood, most often associated with *diabetes mellitus* but sometimes occurring in other conditions (compare *hypoglycemia*).

HYPERHIDROSIS n. excessive perspiration, sometimes caused by strong emotion, heat, hyperthyroidism, or menopausal changes.

HYPERKALEMIA n. higher-than- normal potassium levels in the blood, with symptoms of nausea, diarrhea, muscle weakness, and, if severe, heart abnormalities; occurs in kidney failure and sometimes as an adverse effect following *diuretic* use.

HYPERKINETIC SYNDROME see *attention deficit syndrome*.

HYPERLIPOPROTEINEMIA n. any of a large group of disorders of lipoprotein and cholesterol metabolism resulting in higher-than-normal cholesterol and lipoprotein levels in the blood. Some of the disorders are hereditary (e.g., *familial hypercholesterolemia*), others acquired.

HYPERMOTILITY n. excessive movement, esp. in the intestines.

HYPERNATREMIA n. higher-than-normal levels of sodium in the blood, resulting from too-frequent urination, *diabetes insipidus*, profuse sweating, diarrhea, or other disorder.

HYPEROPIA n. farsightedness; a condition in which light rays are brought to a focus behind the *retina* (compare *myopia*).

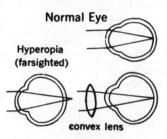

Normal Eye

Hyperopia (farsighted)

convex lens

In a normal eye, the image comes to a focus on the retina. In hyperopia, the image comes to a focus behind the retina. The defect can be corrected by convex lenses.

HYPERPARATHYROIDISM n. condition characterized by excessive secretion of parathyroid hormone from the parathyroid glands due to disease of the parathyroid glands or resulting from another disorder (e.g., too-low blood calcium levels). Higher-than-normal levels of calcium in the blood result, with effects on many systems of the body, including kidney damage, *osteoporosis*, gastrointestinal disturbances, muscle weakness, and central nervous system changes leading to personality disturbances, and, if severe, coma. Treatment may involve surgical removal of all or part of the parathyroid glands or correction of any underlying causes.

HYPERPITUITARISM n. overactivity of the *pituitary gland*, causing excess secretion of all or some of the pituitary hormones, esp. overactivity of the anterior lobe leading to excess secretion of growth hormone and the disorders *acromegaly* and *gigantism*.

HYPERPLASIA n. excessive formation of cells. adj. **hyperplastic**

HYPERPIGMENTATION n. an unusual darkening of the skin; it may be caused by exposure to the sun, by certain drugs, or by adrenal gland disorder (compare *hypopigmentation*).

HYPERPNEA n. deep, rapid breathing that occurs normally after excercise or abnormally with fever, pain, hysteria or respiratory or cardiac disorder (compare *dyspnea*).

HYPERPYREXIA n. an extremely elevated body temperature, sometimes occurring with acute infections in children or in others during general anesthesia. Treatment is by sponging the body with tepid water and administering antipyretic drugs.

HYPERSENSITIVITY REACTION n. an inappropriate and excessive response to an antigen—an allergen. Common allergens are pollen, dust, animal hairs, and certain foods. The degree of the response depends on the nature and amount of the allergen, how it enters the body, and other factors. Reactions range from mild allergic symptoms such as runny nose and watery eyes to severe systemic reactions leading to *anaphylactic shock*.

HYPERSPLENISM n. a condition marked by an enlarged spleen and a decrease in number of one or more blood cells; it is associated with many disorders, treatment depending on the underlying cause.

HYPERSTAT n. trade name for a vasodilator (diazoxide) used to treat severe *hypertension*.

HYPERTENSIN n. trade name for a vasoconstrictor (angiotensin) used to raise blood pressure.

HYPERTENSION n. a common disorder, often with no symptoms, in which the blood pressure is persistently above 140/90 mg Hg. Causes of hypertension include adrenal and kidney disorders, toxemia of pregnancy, and thyroid disorders, but in most cases—*essential hypertension*—the cause is unknown, though obesity, *hypercholesterolemia*, and high sodium levels are predisposing factors. Symptoms, when present, include headache, palpitations, and easy fatiguability. Severe hypertension damages the cardiovascular system and frequently results in heart disorders. Treatment is by diuretics, vasodilators, central nervous system depressants and inhibitors, and ganglionic blocking agents (beta blockers, e.g., propranolol). Adequate rest and a low-sodium, low-fat diet are also usually advised. adj. **hypertensive**

HYPERTHERMIA n. extremely high body temperature, sometimes induced as a treatment, as in some forms of cancer (see also *malignant hyperthermia*).

HYPERTHYROIDISM n. overactivity of the *thyroid gland* due to tumor, overgrowth of the gland, or Graves disease.

HYPERTROPHY n. increase in the size of an organ or other part, resulting from enlargement of the individual cells. (compare *atrophy*; *hyperplasia*). adj. **hypertrophic**

HYPERVENTILATION n. a ventilation rate in the lungs that is greater than demanded by body needs, the result of too frequent and/or too deep breathing; often associated with emphysema; asthma; hyperthyroidism; central nervous system disorders; increased metabolic needs from fever, infection, or excercise; or acute anxiety or pain. The carbon dioxide level in the blood decreases and the oxygen level increases. Symptoms include faintness, tingling of the fingers and toes, and, if continued, chest pain and respiratory alkalosis.

HYPERVITAMINOSIS n. an abnormal condition resulting from excessive intake of vitamins. Serious effects may occur with excessive intake of vitamins A, D, and K (compare *avitaminosis*). (See Table of Vitamins).

HYPERVOLEMIA n. an increase in the volume of circulating blood. adj. **hypervolemic**

HYPESTHESIA n. lessened sensitivity to touch.

HYPHEMA n. bleeding into the anterior chamber of the eye, usually the result of injury.

HYPNAGOGUE n. an agent that tends to induce sleep.

HYPNOSIS n. a passive, sleeplike state in which perception and memory are altered, and the person is more responsive to suggestion and has more recall than usual; used in psychotherapy and in medicine to induce relaxation and relieve pain. Susceptibility to hypnosis varies widely.

HYPNOTHERAPY n. the use of *hypnosis* in psychotherapy.

HYPO- prefix meaning "under" "beneath," "deficient" (e.g., **hypoacidity,** lower than normal acidity, as in the stomach).

HYPOADRENALISM see *Addison's disease.*

HYPOBETALIPOPROTEINE- MIA n. hereditary disorder in which the levels of beta lipoproteins, lipids, and cholesterol are lower than normal. There are no symptoms and there is no treatment.

HYPOCALCEMIA n. an abnormally low level of calcium in the blood, due to *hypoparathyroidism*, vitamin D deficiency, kidney malfunction, or other disorder. Mild hypocalcemia produces few signs; severe cases lead to cardiac arrhythmias and *tetany*. adj. **hypocalcemic**

HYPOCHONDRIASIS n. a condition in which a person has excessive concern about his/her health, unrealistic interpretations of real or imagined symptoms, often accompanied by anxiety and depression. Also: **hypochondria**. adj. **hypochondriachal**

HYPOGAMMAGLOBULINE- MIA n. a lower-than-normal concentration of gamma globulins (*immunoglobulins*) in the blood, associated with an increased risk of infection. It may be congenital and transient (as in some infants), congenital and permanent (as in some sex-linked immune disorders), or acquired, due to kidney disease, exposure to certain drugs, or other factors (compare *agammaglobulinemia*).

HYPOGLOSSAL NERVE n. either of a pair of cranial nerves (XII) involved in swallowing and movements of the tongue (see also *cranial nerve*).

HYPOGLYCEMIA n. a lower-than-normal level of *glucose* in the blood, usually resulting from administration of too much *insulin* (in *diabetes mellitus*), excessive insulin secretion from the *pancreas*, or poor diet. Symptoms include headache, weakness, anxiety, personality changes, and, if severe and untreated, coma and death. Treatment is by administration of glucose. adj. **hypoglycemic**

HYPOGLYCEMIC AGENT n. any of a large group of drugs, including insulin and tolbutamide, that decrease the level of *glucose* in the blood and are used in the treatment of *diabetes mellitus*.

HYPOKALEMIA n. abnormally low level of potassium in the blood, leading to weakness and heart abnormalities; it may result from *diuretic* intake, adrenal tumor, starvation, or other disorder. adj. **hypokalemic**

HYPOLIPOPROTEINEMIA
see *abetalipoproteinemia*; *hypobetalipoproteinemia*.

HYPONATREMIA n. a lower-than-normal concentration of sodium in the blood, caused by dehydration (as from prolonged vomiting, diarrhea) or excessive water in the bloodstream or from diuretic intake. adj. **hyponatremic**

HYPOPARATHYROIDISM n. underactivity of the *parathyroid glands*, causing a lowering of calcium levels in the blood; symptoms include muscle spasms and nervous system changes, and, if untreated, *tetany*.

HYPOPHYSIS n. the pituitary gland (see *anterior pituitary gland*; *posterior pituitary gland*).

HYPOPIGMENTATION n. unusual lack of skin color, as in *albinism* and *vitiligo* (compare *hyperpigmentation*).

HYPOPLASIA n. underdevelopment of an organ due to decrease in the number of cells (compare *aplasia*; *hyperplasia*).

HYPOPNEA n. shallow or slow respiration; it is a normal sign in athletes but in others a sign of brain disorder.

HYPOPROTEINEMIA n. an abnormally low level of protein in the blood, usually with signs of abdominal pain, nausea, diarrhea, and edema. It may be caused by inadequate dietary intake of protein or intestinal or renal disease.

HYPOSMIA n. lessened sensitivity to smell. adj. **hyposomic**

HYPOSPADIAS n. the opening of the *urethra* in an abnormal location on the underside of the *penis*.

HYPOTENSION n. blood pressure that is abnormally low; it may result from hemorrhage, excessive fluid loss, heart malfunction, Addison's disease, or other disorder. In some people blood pressure drops when they rise from a horizontal position (**orthostatic hypotension**). Mild, transient hypotension may cause light-headedness and syncope. Severe hypotension leads to inadequate blood circulation and shock (compare *hypertension*).

HYPOTHALAMUS n. part of the brain that controls the endocrine system, the autonomic nervous system, and many other body functions (e.g., body temperature, thirst, hunger). adj. **hypothalmic**

HYPOTHERMIA n. 1. a condition in which the body temperature is below 35° Celsius (95° Fahrenheit), most often occurring in the elderly or very young who are exposed to excessive cold; symptoms include pallor, slow, shallow respiration, and slow, faint heartbeat; 2. deliberate reduction of body temperature to slow metabolic rate and lower oxygen demands for therapeutic reasons or certain surgical procedures.

HYPOTHROMBINEMIA n. lower-than-normal levels of prothrombin (Factor II) in the circulating blood, leading to poor clot formation, long clotting time, and sometimes excessive bleeding. It often results from vitamin K deficiency or anticoagulant therapy.

HYPOTHYROIDISM n. decreased activity of the thyroid gland (see *cretinism*; *myxedema*).

HYPOVITAMINOSIS see *avitaminosis*; Table of Vitamins.

HYPOVOLEMIC SHOCK n. physical collapse caused by severe blood loss and circulatory malfunction; symptoms include feeble pulse, rapid heart beat, clammy skin, low blood pressure.

HYPOXIA n. inadequate amounts of available oxygen in the blood. Symptoms include bluish discoloration of the skin, high blood pressure, rapid heart rate, mental confusion, and, if severe, irregular breathing and finally respiratory and cardiac failure.

HYSTERECTOMY n. surgical removal of the *uterus*, done to remove tumors or to treat hemorrhage, severe pelvic inflammatory disease, or a cancerous or precancerous condition. In a total hysterectomy, the uterus and cervix are removed; in a radical hysterectomy, the ovaries, oviducts, uterus, cervix, and associated lymph nodes are removed.

HYSTERIA n. a disorder marked by abnormal emotional response, as shown in unusual sensory, circulatory, intestinal, or other responses. In severe cases, paralysis of a limb may be a chief symptom.

HYSTERO- comb. form indicating a relationship with the *uterus* (e.g., *hysterocele*, protrusion (hernia) of the uterus).

HYSTEROSALPINOGRAM n. an X ray of the *uterus* and *Fallopian tubes*, usually done to determine if there is a blockage; useful in diagnosing causes of *infertility*.

HYSTEROSCOPY n. visual inspection of the *uterus*, using an endoscope introduced through the vagina, done to examine the uterine lining, to remove a specimen for analysis, or to excise small polyps.

HYSTEROTOMY n. surgical incision of the *uterus*, sometimes done as a means of abortion.

i

I symbol for the element *iodine* (see Table of Elements).

-IASIS suffix indicating "disease produced," "disease producing characteristics" (e.g., *elephantiasis*).

IATROGENIC adj. pert. to a condition caused by medical diagnostic procedures, or exposure to medical treatment, facilities and personnel.   n. **iatrogenesis**

IBUPROFEN n. a nonsteroid, antiinflammatory agent, known under the trade name Motrin, used in the treatment of arthritis. Adverse effects include gastrointestinal disturbances and skin irritation.

ICHTHAMMOL n. a thick, black liquid used topically as an antiinfective to treat certain skin diseases.

ICHTHYOSIS n. any of several *congenital* diseases in which the skin is dry and scaly—fishlike.

ICSH abbreviation for interstitial cell-stimulating hormone, also known as *luteinizing hormone*.

ICTERO- comb. form indicating an association with *jaundice* (e.g., **icterogenic**, producing jaundice).

ICTERUS n. *jaundice* (see also *hyperbilirubinemia; kernicterus*). adj. **icteric**

ICTERUS NEONATORUM see *hyperbilirubinemia of the newborn.*

ICTUS n. a seizure (e.g., in *epilepsy*) or sudden attack (e.g., *cerebrovascular accident*).   pl. **ictuses**   adj. **ictal, ictic**

ICU abbreviation for *intensive care unit.*

ID n. in psychoanalysis, the unconscious; the unconscious part of one's psyche, the source of instincts and drives, based largely on the tendency to avoid pain and to pursue pleasure (compare *ego*; *superego*).

IDEATION n. the process of forming ideas, images, impressions, or concepts.   adj. **ideational**

IDENTICAL TWINS see *monozygotic twins.*

IDENTIFICATION n. in psychology, the adoption of the traits and characteristics of another person; it is a normal part of personality development, as in a child identifying with the parent of the same sex.

IDENTITY CRISIS n. a period of confusion about one's identity and role in society, occurring most often during a transition from one stage of life to another, esp. at adolescence.

IDIOPATHIC adj. of unknown cause. An **idopathic disease** is a disease for which no identifiable cause can be determined.   n. **idiopathy**

IDIOSYNCRASY n. 1. a characteristic or manner unique to an individual or group; 2. a peculiar or unusual variation, as in an unusual reaction to a drug or particular food.   adj. **idiosyncratic**

IDIOT n. obs. for a person who is severely mentally retarded (I.Q. under 20) (compare *imbecile*; *moron*) (see also *mental retardation*).   n. **idiocy**

IDIOT SAVANT n. a person who is severely mentally retarded but able to carry out specific limited intellectual functions (e.g., calculate square roots or calendar dates).

Ig abbreviation for *immunoglobulin*.

IgA abbreviation for *immunoglobulin A*.

IgD abbreviation for *immunoglobulin D*.

IgE abbreviation for *immunoglobulin E*.

IgG abbreviation for *immunoglobulin G*.

IgM abbreviation for *immunoglobulin M*.

ILEITIS n. inflammation of the *ileum* (see also *Crohn's disease*).

ILEO- comb. form indicating an association with the *ileum* (e.g., **ileocecal**, pert. to the *ileum* and *cecum*).

ILEOCECAL VALVE n. valve between the *ileum* of the small intestine and the *cecum* of the large intestine that prevents the backflow of material from the large to the small intestine.

ILEOSTOMY n. surgical formation of an opening of the ileum onto the abdominal wall through which feces pass; performed in cases of cancer of the colon, severe or recurrent Crohn's disease, or ulcerative colitis (compare *colostomy*).

ILEUM n. the distal portion of the *small intestine*, starting at its attachment with the *jejunum* and ending at the *cecum*, the beginning of the large intestine.   adj. **ileac, ileal**

ILEUS n. an intestinal obstruction.

ILIAC ARTERIES n. the arteries that supply most of the blood for the pelvis and lower extremities. The right and left common iliac arteries are the terminal branches of the abdominal *aorta*.

ILIAC VEINS n. the veins that drain blood from the pelvis and lower limbs; the right and left common iliac veins join to form the inferior vena cava.

ILIO- comb. form indicating an association with the *ilium* (e.g., **iliococcygeal**, pert. to the ilium and *coccyx*).

ILIUM n. one of the three bones (the other two being the *ischium* and *pubis*) that unite before birth to form the *innominate*, or hip, bone.   pl. **ilia**   adj. **iliac**

ILLUSION n. a false impression; a wrongful interpretation of what has been perceived by the senses (compare *hallucination*) (see also *optical illusion*).   adj. **illusional**

ILOSONE n. trade name for the antibacterial *erythromycin*.

IMAGERY n. in psychiatry, the formation of images, concepts, and ideas.

IMAVATE n. trade name for the antidepressant *imipramine*.

IMBECILE n. obs. for a person who is moderately mentally retarded (I.Q. 20 to 49) (compare *idiot*; *moron*) (see also *mental retardation*). adj. **imbecilic**

IMBRICATION n. the overlapping arrangement of parts, like tiles on a roof.

IMIPRAMINE n. an antidepressant, known under the trade name Imavate, used to treat *depression*. Adverse effects include sedation, gastrointestinal upset, and cardiovascular disturbances.

IMMINENT ABORTION see under *abortion*.

IMMUNE adj. protected from, not susceptible to a disease, esp. an infectious disease.

IMMUNE GAMMA GLOBULIN n. immunizing agent, made from pooled human plasma, used for immunization against certain infectious diseases (e.g., measles, poliomyelitis) and to treat immunodeficiencies (e.g., *hypogammaglobulinemia*). Adverse reactions include pain and inflammation at the injection site; also: **immune globulin**.

IMMUNE GLOBULIN see *immune gamma globulin*.

IMMUNE RESPONSE n. a defense reaction of the body whereby an invading substance—an antigen, such as grafted tissue, a transplanted organ, bacteria, virus, or fungus—is recognized as foreign and antibodies specific against that antigen are produced to neutralize and/or destroy it. There are two basic kinds of immune response: the humoral, mediated by B lymphocytes, or B cells, (chiefly against bacterial invasion) and the cell-mediated, involving T cells (chiefly against viral and fungal invasion and transplanted tissue).

IMMUNE SYSTEM n. the complex interactions that protect the body from pathogenic organisms and other foreign invaders (e.g., transplanted tissue), including the humoral response, chiefly involving B cells and the production of antibodies, and the cell-mediated response, chiefly involving T cells and the activation of specific leukocytes. The organs involved include the bone marrow, the thymus, and lymphoid tissue.

IMMUNITY n. the state of being not susceptible to a particular disease. Immunity may be natural, or innate, or it may be acquired during life (e.g., as a result of infection or vaccination) (see also *acquired immunity*; *active immunity*; *natural immunity*; *passive immunity*).

IMMUNIZATION n. the process by which resistance to an infectious disease is induced or increased.

IMMUNODEFICIENCY n. an abnormal condition in which some part of the body's immune system is inadequate and consequently resistance to infectious disease is decreased. Immunodeficiency may be congenital or acquired (see also *acquired immune deficiency syndrome*; *acquired immunodeficiency*; *agammaglobulinemia*; *hypogammaglobulinemia*).

IMMUNOGEN n. an organism or substance that provokes an *immune response*; an antigen. adj. **immunogenic**

IMMUNOGLOBULIN n. any of five classes of structurally distinct antibodies, produced in lymph tissue in response to the invasion of a foreign substance. The five major kinds are immunoglobulin A, D, E, G, and M; also called **immune serum globulin**. (See also *antibody*; *antigen*).

IMMUNOGLOBULIN A n. one of the five classes of immunoglobulins; one of the most common immunoglobulins, it is present in body secretions and is the chief antibody in the mucous membranes of the gastrointestinal tract, saliva, tears, and respiratory tract.

IMMUNOGLOBULIN D n. one of the five classes of immunoglobulins; it is present in small amounts in serum and is thought to function in certain allergic responses.

IMMUNOGLOBULIN E n. one of the five classes of immunoglobulins; it is present primarily in the skin and mucous membranes and is believed to function in response to environmental antigens and to play a role in allergic reactions characterized by skin eruptions.

IMMUNOGLOBULIN G n. one of the five major classes of immunoglobulins; widespread in the body, it is the main antibody defense against most bacterial invasions and other antigens.

IMMUNOGLOBULIN M n. one of the five classes of immunoglobulins; a large molecule, it is found in blood and is involved in combatting blood infections and in triggering **immunoglobulin G** production.

IMMUNOLOGIST n. a specialist in *immunology*.

IMMUNOLOGY n. the study of the body's response to foreign invasion (e.g., bacteria, virus, fungus, transplanted tissue). adj. **immunologic; immunological**

IMMUNOSUPPRESSION n. 1. the lowering of the body's normal immune response to the invasion of foreign material. It may be deliberate, as in the administration of drugs to decrease the immune response to prevent rejection in cases of transplanted organs; or it may be accidental, resulting from chemotherapy or radiotherapy in cancer treatment; 2. an abnormal condition in which the body's normal immune responses are in-

adequate (see *immunodeficiency*). See also *acquired immunodeficiency*; *acquired immune deficiency syndrome*. adj. **immunosuppressed**

IMMUNOSUPPRESSIVE adj. pert. to a substance that causes a lowering of the body's normal *immune response*.

IMPACTED TOOTH n. a tooth, usually a wisdom tooth, so firmly wedged in the socket that it cannot break through the gum.

IMPACTION n. the cramping or tight wedging of materials or parts in a limited space, esp. feces lodged in the lower colon.

IMPAIRMENT n. an injury, disability, functional loss, or weakened state (e.g., hearing impairment).

IMPERFORATE adj. lacking an opening, as an imperforate hymen completely closing the vagina and preventing the outflow of menstrual blood (see also *imperforate anus*).

IMPERFORATE ANUS n. any of several congenital defects in which there is partial or complete obstruction of the anal opening due to a developmental defect. Treatment is by surgery.

IMPERMEABLE adj. not allowing fluid to pass through, as with a membrane.

IMPETIGO n. a bacterial (usually streptococcal and/or staphylococcal) infection of the skin, common in children and very contagious, in which localized skin redness develops into fluid-containing small blisters that gradually crust and erode. Treatment is by topical and sometimes oral antibiotics, careful washing, and steps to prevent the spread of the infection.

IMPLANT v. to attach a part or tissue to a host (e.g., to insert a tooth); n. the part of tissue inserted into a host for repair of a damaged part (e.g., a blood vessel graft) or for therapeutic reasons (e.g., pacemaker inserted in the chest).

IMPLANTATION n. the putting and attaching of an organ part or cell into a new place, esp. the attachment and penetration of the fertilized egg (blastocyst) into the wall of the *uterus* during early prenatal development.

IMPOTENCE n. 1. weakness; 2. the inability of the male to achieve erection of the penis or, less commonly, to ejaculate. Impotence may be organic, due to disease (e.g., *diabetes mellitus*) or ingestion of certain drugs, or psychogenic; (compare *sterility*). Also: **impotency** adj. **impotent**

IMPREGNATE v. 1. to inseminate and make pregnant; 2. to saturate with another substance. n. **impregnation**

IMPRESSION n. a mold of a part of the body from which a replacement can be made, esp. in dentistry, the mold of the mouth from which dentures are made.

IMPULSE n. 1. a sudden urge to do something; 2. the electrochemical changes in the membrane of a nerve through which a signal is transmitted (see *nerve impulse*).

IMURAN n. trade name for immunosuppressive drug *azathioprine*.

INANITION n. condition of exhaustion and weakness caused by inadequate nutrition, resulting from starvation, malnutrition, or disease.

INACTIVE COLON n. a lack of normal tone in the large intestine, resulting in decreased contractions and propulsive movements, a delay in the normal passage of material through the intestine to the anus, often an enlargement of the colon, and constipation. It may be congenital (e.g., *Hirschsprung's disease*) or acquired (e.g., through inadequate food and fluid intake, faulty elimination habits, intake of certain drugs, certain diseases). Treatment includes efforts to establish regular elimination habits, use of stool softeners and agents to increase fecal bulk, and a diet containing adequate bulk and fluids (see also *megacolon*).

INBORN n. present at birth, either as a result of heredity or acquired during intrauterine life (e.g., certain developmental abnormalities) (see also *congenital*; *hereditary*; *inborn error of metabolism*).

INBORN ERROR OF METABOLISM n. any of a number of diseases, including *galactosemia*, *phenylketonuria*, and *Tay-Sachs disease* in which an inherited defect—usually missing or inadequate levels of a specific enzyme—produces an abnormality in metabolism.

INBORN REFLEX see under *reflex*.

INBREEDING n. the production of offspring by the mating of closely related persons (or other animals or plants).

INCEST n. sexual intercourse between persons closely related. adj. **incestuous**

INCIDENCE n. the number of times an event occurs in a given period of time, as the number of times a given disease occurs during a year (compare *prevalence*).

INCISION n. a slit or opening made by cutting, as with a scalpel.

INCISOR n. any of eight front teeth, four in each jaw, used for cutting and tearing food (compare *canine tooth*, *molar tooth*, *premolar tooth*).

INCISURE n. in anatomy, a notch or small hollow.

INCLUSION n. a small body found within another, as inclusions in the cytoplasm of a cell.

INCOHERENT adj. disordered; lacking logical connection or orderly continuity; unable to express oneself in an intelligible manner. n. **incoherence**

INCOMPATIBLE adj. unable to exist together.

INCOMPATIBILITY n. 1. condition in which two substances (organisms, tissues, drugs) cannot exist together, as, for example, one drug cancelling out or altering the therapeutic effect of another drug given at the same time; 2. in immunology, the degree to which the body's immune system will reject or otherwise react to foreign material, such as transfused blood or transplanted tissue. (When a person's tissues cannot be transplanted to another, the term is **histoincompatibility**.)

IMCOMPETENCE n. inability of an organ or part to function normally (e.g., **valvular incompetence**, inability of a valve to close an opening completely). adj. **incompetent**

INCOMPETENT CERVIX n. in obstetrics, a condition in which the opening of the cervix of the *uterus* becomes dilated (without labor) before term, often causing miscarriage or premature birth. Treatment is by surgical suturing.

INCOMPLETE ABORTION see under *abortion*.

INCOMPLETE FRACTURE see under *fracture*.

INCONTINENCE n. the inability to control urination and/or defecation (see also *enuresis*). adj. **incontinent**

INCOORDINATION n. inability to produce controlled, harmonious muscular movement.

INCUBATION PERIOD n. the time between exposure to a disease-causing organism and the appearance of the symptoms of the disease (e.g., the 2-to-3-week interval between exposure to the chickenpox organism and the appearance of symptoms).

INCUBATOR n. 1. a special transparent device that provides a controlled environment (e.g., a particular temperature) for a premature or low-birth-weight infant; 2. a laboratory device for the cultivation of eggs or microorganisms.

INCUS n. one of three small bones in the *middle ear* (the others are the *malleus* and *stapes*); also called **anvil**.

INDERAL n. trade name for *propranolol*.

INDEX CASE n. the first, or model, case of a disease, as contrasted with subsequent cases.

INDEX FINGER n. the forefinger; the finger between the thumb and middle finger.

INDICATION n. in medicine, a reason to prescribe a drug or perform a procedure, as the presence of a bacterial infection is an indication for the use of a specific antibiotic. v. **indicate**

INDICATOR n. a substance (e.g., paper, tablet, tape) used to test for a particular reaction because of a predictable easy-to-detect change.

INDIGENOUS adj. occurring naturally or native to a particular environment (e.g., the gastrointestinal tract) or geographic region.

INDIGESTION see *dyspepsia*.

INDOCIN n. trade name for the antiinflammatory agent *indomethacin*.

INDOLENT adj. 1. slow in growth or development (e.g., a tumor); 2. inactive, sluggish, slow to heal (e.g., indolent ulcer).

INDOMETHACIN n. a nonsteroid antiinflammatory agent, known under the trade name Indocin, used to treat arthritis and certain other inflammatory conditons. Averse effects include peptic ulcer and gastrointestinal disturbances; dizziness; and tinnitus.

INDUCE v. to start, cause, or stimulate the beginning of an activity, e.g., to induce anesthesia or to induce labor.

INDUCTION OF LABOR n. in obstetrics, the artificial starting of the childbirth process by puncturing the *amniotic sac* surrounding the fetus or by administration of drugs (oxytocin) to stimulate contractions of the muscles of the *uterus*. Labor may be induced to speed childbirth in cases of maternal or fetal distress or electively (e.g., to avert the possibility of a woman delivering outside of a hospital).

INDURATION n. the hardening of a tissue or part, esp. the skin due to edema, inflammation, or other abnormality.   adj. **indurated**

INDUSTRIAL DISEASE   see *occupational disease*.

INERT adj. 1. not moving; 2. in pharmacology, not active, acting e.g., as a binder or flavoring agent in a drug; 3. in chemistry, not taking part in a chemical reaction or acting as a catalyst.

INERTIA n. a state of inactivity or sluggishness, e.g., uterine inertia in which the contraction of the muscular wall of the uterus is inadequate.

INEVITABLE ABORTION see under *abortion*.

INFANT n. a child from birth to one year (some extend it to 2 years).   adj. **infantile**

INFANT DEATH   see *sudden infant death syndrome*.

INFANT FEEDING   see *demand feeding*; *breast-feeding*.

INFANTICIDE n. the killing of an infant.

INFANTILE PARALYSIS   see *poliomyelitis*.

INFANTILISM n. a condition in which childhood characteristics (mental and/or physical) continue into adulthood.

INFANT MORTALITY RATE n. number of deaths of infants under one year per 1,000 live births in a given geographic region or institution in a given period (usually 1 year).

INFARCT n. small localized area of dead tissue resulting from diminished or stopped blood flow to the tissue area.

INFARCTION n. the formation of dead tissue as a result of diminished or stopped blood flow to the tissue area (see also *myocardial infarction*).

INFECT v. to transmit a disease-causing organism.

INFECTION n. 1. the invasion of disease-producing microorganisms into a body where they may multiply, causing a disease; 2. a disease caused by disease-producing microorganisms (e.g., certain bacteria) (compare *infestation*; *contagion*).

INFECTIOUS adj. 1. caused by an infection; 2. capable of producing an infection.

INFECTIOUS HEPATITIS see *viral hepatitis*.

INFECTIOUS MONONUCLEOSIS n. an acute infection, caused by the Epstein-Barr herpes virus and most common among young people; it is not highly contagious. Symptoms include fever, swollen lymph glands, sore throat, enlarged spleen and liver, abnormal liver function, fatigue, and malaise. Treatment is symptomatic, including bed rest to prevent spleen rupture or other spleen or liver complications. One attack usually confers immunity; sometimes called **glandular fever**.

INFECTIOUS POLYNEURITIS see *Guillain-Barré syndrome*.

INFERIOR adj. in anatomy, below or lower than a given reference.

INFERIOR VENA CAVA n. the large vein that returns deoxygenated blood to the heart from the body below the *diaphragm*. It is formed by junction of the common iliac veins in the lower back region and travels upward along the vertebral column, pierces the diaphragm and empties into the right atrium of the heart.

INFERTILITY n. the condition of being unable to bear young—in a woman an inability to conceive, in a male, an inability to impregnate. Female infertility may be due to a defective ovum, an ovulation disorder, a blockage of the Fallopian tubes, a uterine disorder, or a hormonal imbalance; in a male, infertility may be due to a lower-than-normal number of sperm produced or to sperm with abnormal shape or motility. Many cases of infertility can be corrected through surgery, drugs, or other medical procedures (compare *sterility*).

INFEST v. to attack and live on the skin or internal organs of a host, as ringworm infestation of the skin.

INFESTATION n. the presence, and usually the growth and increase, of parasites on the skin or within the body, usually producing signs of disease (compare *infection*).

INFLAMMATION n. response of the tissues of the body to irritation or injury, characterized by pain, swelling, redness, and heat. The severity, specific characteristics, and duration of the inflammation depends on the cause, the particular area of the body affected, and the health of the person. adj. **inflamed; inflammatory**

INFLAMMATORY BOWEL DISEASE see *ulcerative colitis*.

INFLUENZA n. an acute, contagious, virus-caused infection of the respiratory tract; symptoms usually begin suddenly and include fever, sore throat, cough, muscle aches, headache, fatigue, and malaise, and often signs of the common cold (watery eyes, runny nose). Treatment is symptomatic and includes rest, pain relievers and fever reducers, and increased fluid intake. The disease usually subsides within a week; complications (e.g., bacterial pneumonia) usually affect only the very young, the old, or those weakened by another condition. Several strains of the virus have been identified and new strains emerge at intervals, often named for the geographic region in which they are first discovered (e.g., Asian flu). Also called **flu; grippe**.

INFORMED CONSENT n. permission obtained from a patient for the performance of a particular procedure or test, after being told fully the risks, options, and expected results. Informed consent, usually in a signed statement, is generally required before any invasive procedure (e.g., surgery or diagnostic procedures in which instruments are inserted into the body), before admission to any experimental or research study, and in certain other situations.

INFRA- comb. form meaning situated or occurring below (e.g., **infraclavicular**, below the clavicle).

INFRARED THERAPY n. the use of infrared radiation, in, e.g., hot water bottles, heating pads, incandescent lights, to relieve pain and increase blood circulation to a particular area of the body.

INFUNDIBULUM n. a funnel-shaped part, esp. the part of the brain (the hypophyseal stalk) that connects to the *hypothalamus* and *pituitary gland*. pl. **infundibula** adj. **infundibular**

INFUSION n. 1. the introduction of a substance (e.g., fluid, drug, electrolyte) directly into a vein or between tissues, often by gravitational force (compare *injection*); 2. the substance introduced into the body by infusion.

INGEST v. to take in; to eat or drink.

INGESTA n. the solid and liquid materials taken into the mouth.

INGESTION n. the act of putting food and other material into the mouth. adj. **ingestive**

INGROWN HAIR n. a hair that does not emerge from the follicle but remains embedded in the skin, usually causing inflammation.

INGROWN TOENAIL n. a toenail whose free ends grow into or become pressed into the skin, causing inflammation and sometimes secondary infection.

INGUEN see *groin*. adj. **inguinal** (e.g., *inguinal hernia*).

INGUINAL adj. pert. to the groin.

INGUINAL HERNIA n. hernia in which a loop of the intestine enters the inguinal canal, and, in males, sometimes fills the scrotum; the most common type of hernia, it is usually treated surgically.

INH abbreviation for *isoniazid*.

INHALATION n. the act of breathing in, whereby air or other gas or vapor (e.g., anesthetic gas) is taken into the lungs.

INHALATION ANESTHESIA n. general anesthesia achieved by inhalation of an anesthetic gas or volatile liquid; widely-used inhalation anesthetics include cyclopropane, halothane, enflurane, and isoflurane.

INHALATION THERAPY n. treatment in which oxygen, water, or a drug is introduced into the respiratory tract with inhaled air. It may be used to provide oxygen or to administer drugs to liquefy mucus or dilate the bronchial passageways.

INHALE v. to breath in; to inspire.

INHERENT adj. inborn, innate (compare *acquired*; *indigenous*).

INHERITANCE n. the acquisition of characteristics and conditions by transmission (by genetic material) from parents to offspring; the total genetic makeup of an individual.

INHERITED DISORDER see *genetic disease*.

INHIBITION n. the slowing or stopping of an otherwise normal response, as, e.g., the restriction of a specific impulse, drive, or activity; in psychology, evidence shown by a person's actions that he/she is restraining a display of an instinctual drive (e.g., averting any encounter with sexual activity).

INION n. the bump that protrudes at the back of the head.

INJECTION n. 1. the act of putting a liquid into the body forcefully by means of a syringe; the fluid may be injected into a vein (intravenous), muscle (intramuscular), under the skin (subcutaneous), or into the skin (intradermal); 2. the substance inserted into the body by force.

INNATE adj. inborn, hereditary or congenital; an essential characteristic of someone or something.

INNATE IMMUNITY see *natural immunity*.

INNERVATION n. the distribution and action of nerve fibers to an organ or body region.

INNOCUOUS adj. harmless.

INNOMINATE ARTERY n. the artery arising from the arch of the aorta that divides into the right subclavian artery and the right common carotid artery, supplying the right side of the head and neck and the right shoulder and arm.

INNOMINATE BONE n. the hip bone, formed by the fusion of the ilium, ischium, and pubis. The innominate bone together with the *sacrum* and *coccyx* forms the pelvis.

INOCULUM n. the substance introduced into the body to produce or increase immunity to a specific disease. The substance may be a live, weakened, or killed virus; a toxin; or immune serum; also called **inoculant**.

INOCULATION n. the process of deliberately injecting a substance into the body to produce or increase immunity to the disease associated with the substance; it may be done by placing a drop of the substance on the skin and scratching the skin in that area, by puncturing the skin, or by intradermal, subcutaneous or intramuscular injection. v. **inoculate**

INSANITY n. 1. a legal term meaning an inability to distinguish right from wrong, an inability to control one's life, or to act in a socially acceptable manner; 2. colloquial, severe mental illness.

INSEMINATION n. the introduction of semen into the vagina, either during *coitus* or through other techniques (see *artificial insemination*).

INSIDIOUS adj. pert. to gradual, subtle or hard-to-discern development, as in a disease (e.g., glaucoma) that develops without early symptoms (compare *acute*).

IN SITU n. in its natural place or place of origin, as in a cancer that has not spread (carcinoma in situ).

INSOMNIA n. a condition characterized by difficulty falling asleep or staying asleep or by seriously disturbed sleep (e.g., frequent short awakenings). It may result from a variety of psychological and physical causes; treatment depends on the cause and condition of the person (compare *narcolepsy*).

INSPIRATION n. the act of drawing air into the lungs. Contraction of the diaphragm causes the lungs to expand and air to flow in.

INSTINCT n. a complex, unlearned pattern of response and behavior that is specific to the species and released by certain environmental stimuli (e.g., sucking in a newborn infant). adj. **instinctive**

INSUFFLATION n. the blowing of a material (e.g., gas or powder) into a tube, cavity, or organ of the body to allow visual examination, to determine if an obstruction is present, or to introduce a drug (e.g, introduction of gas into the Fallopian tubes to determine whether or not they are open—*Rubin's test*).

INSULIN n. 1. a hormone secreted by the beta cells of the *islands of Langerhans* of the *pancreas*; it regulates the metabolism of glucose and secondarily intermediary processes in the metabolism of carbohydrates and fats. Inadequate insulin levels lead to too-high glucose levels and other disturbances of metabolism, often associated with *diabetes mellitus*; 2. a drug made from the natural hormones used to treat *diabetes mellitus*.

INSULIN SHOCK n. an abnormal physiological state in which the blood glucose level is too low; it may be caused by an overdose of insulin, decreased food intake, or excess exercise. Symptoms include sweating, trembling, nervousness, irritability, and pallor; if not corrected, it can lead to convulsions and death. Treatment requires the administration of glucose (compare *diabetic coma*; *ketoacidosis*).

INTEGRATION n. the organization, unification, and use of experiences, insights, and reactions into a functional whole with coordinated thinking, feeling and acting. v. **integrate**

INTEGUMENTARY SYSTEM

n. the skin and its appendages: nails, hair, *sebaceous glands*.

INTEGUMENT n. the skin, a covering. adj. **integumentary**

INTELLECT n. the capacity to know, perceive, and understand, in contrast to the capacity for emotion.

INTELLECTUALIZATION n. in psychiatry, a defense mechanism in which reasoning is used to block emotional conflict and stress.

INTELLIGENCE n. the ability to learn, to understand, to apply experience, and to make judgments (see also *intelligence quotient*).

INTELLIGENCE QUOTIENT (IQ) n. a numerical expression of a person's intellectual level measured against the statistical average of his/her age or as mental age (measured by standardized tests) as a ratio of chronological age. Virtually all intelligence tests are designed so that the average IQ in the population is about 100.

INTENSIVE CARE UNIT (ICU) n. a hospital unit in which patients with life-threatening conditions are provided with constant care and close monitoring, and often involving the use of sophisticated machines for caring for and maintaining the patient.

INTER- prefix meaning ''between'' (e.g., **intercellular**, between cells).

INTERCOURSE see *coitus*.

INTERN n. a physician (a graduate of a medical school) in the first postgraduate year, learning under the supervision of more experienced physicians in a hospital; sometimes called a first-year resident.

INTERNAL adj. within, inside (e.g., internal organs, organs inside the body).

INTERNAL MEDICINE n. that branch of medicine concerned with the function of internal organs and the diagnosis and treatment of disorders affecting these organs.

INTERNALIZATION n. the unconscious process of adopting and absorbing the beliefs, values, and attitudes of another or of the society to which the person belongs.

INTERNIST n. a specialist in *internal medicine*.

INTEROCEPTOR n. a sensory nerve ending inside the body that responds to stimuli within the body (e.g., digestion, blood pressure).

INTERSEX n. a person who has the characteristics of both sexes or who has external genitalia that is ambiguous or not appropriate to the normal male or female (see also *hermaphrodite*; *pseudohermaphrodite*). n. **intersexuality**

INTERSTICE n. a space in a tissue or between parts of the body. adj. **interstitial**

INTERSTITIAL adj. pert. to the space between tissues.

INTERSTITIAL FLUID n. part of the *extracellular fluid*; the fluid found between cells of the body that helps to provide a large part of the fluid environment of the body.

INTERSTITIAL PNEUMONIA n. chronic inflammation of the lungs, characterized by progressive dyspnea, fever, and bluish discoloration of the skin. It may be caused by a hypersensitivity reaction to a particular drug or by an autoimmune disorder. Treatment is symptomatic, but the disease often progresses to pulmonary or heart failure (compare *bronchopneumonia*).

INTERTRIGO n. an irritation of two skin surfaces that are in contact, as in the armpits, under the breasts, or between the thighs. Prevention is by weight reduction, keeping the surfaces clean and dry, and the application of antifungal preparations if needed.

INTERVERTEBRAL adj. pert. to the space between two *vertebrae*, as the intervertebral discs.

INTERVERTEBRAL DISC n. a fibrocartilaginous disc found between all of the vertebrae of the spinal column, except the first two (the axis and the atlas).

INTERVAL n. the space between parts or time between events (e.g., the Q-T interval in the activity of the ventricles of the heart).

INTESTINAL adj. pert. to the intestine.

INTESTINAL BYPASS n. surgical procedure, used in the treatment of obesity, in which a large part of the small intestine is bypassed so food is not absorbed there and weight is lost.

INTESTINAL FLORA n. the microorganisms (e.g., *Escherichia coli*) normally present in the intestinal tract and essential to its normal function.

INTESTINAL FLU n. inflammation of the stomach and intestine caused by a virus; symptoms include abdominal discomfort, nausea, vomiting, and diarrhea (see also *gastroenteritis*).

INTESTINAL JUICE n. the secretions of glands lining the intestine.

INTESTINAL OBSTRUCTION n. a blockage in the intestine that results in a failure of the contents of the intestine to pass through to the lower bowel. It may be caused by tumor, adhesions, hernia, narrowing from inflammatory bowel disease, or other cause. Symptoms include pain, abdominal distension, constipation, and vomiting of fecal matter. Treatment involves evacuation of the contents of the intestines and removal of the obstruction.

INTESTINE n. that part of the alimentary canal extending from the pyloric opening of the stomach to the *anus*. It is divided into two major parts: the small intestine (made up of the *duodenum*, *jejunum* and *ileum*), where most digestion and absorption of food occurs; and the large intestine (consisting of the *cecum*; *appendix*; ascending, transverse and decending *colon*; and the *rectum*), where water is absorbed from material passing from the small intestine. Waves of muscular contractions—*peristalsis*—propels material through the intestine. adj. **intestinal**

INTIMA n. the innermost lining of a part, esp. of a blood vessel. adj. **intimal**

INTOXICATION n. the state of being poisoned or inebriated due to ingestion of excessive alcohol, another drug, or a toxic substance. adj. **intoxicated**

INTRA- prefix meaning "within" (e.g., **intraabdominal**, within the abdomen).

INTRACELLULAR adj. within a cell.

INTRACELLULAR FLUID n. fluid, usually containing dissolved solutes, contained within cell membranes (compare *extracellular fluid*; *interstitial fluid*).

INTRACEREBRAL adj. within the *brain*.

INTRACRANIAL adj. within the *cranium*.

INTRACRANIAL ANEURYSM n. an aneurysm of a cranial artery. Symptoms include headache, stiff neck, nausea, and sometimes loss of consciousness; rupture of the aneurysm is a serious, often fatal, condition.

INTRACTABLE adj. not readily responsive to treatment; not easily cured or treated.

INTRACUTANEOUS adj. within the skin.

INTRADERMAL adj. within the skin, e.g., an intradermal injection.

INTRADERMAL TEST n. a procedure used in allergy testing in which a small amount of the suspected allergen is injected within the skin. Wheal formation and reddening of the skin within 30 minutes of the injection indicates a positive result; also called **subcutaneous test** (compare *patch test*; *scratch test*).

INTRAMUSCULAR adj. within a muscle, as an intramuscular injection.

INTRAOCULAR PRESSURE n. the internal pressure of the eye regulated by resistance to the outward flow of *aqueous humor* (see also *glaucoma*).

INTRAUTERINE DEVICE (IUD) n. a contraceptive device, made up of a bent plastic or metal (a coil, loop, or other shape) inserted through the vagina into the *uterus* where it functions to prevent pregnancy. Complications of IUD use include infection, undetected expulsion, perforation of the uterus, bleeding, and pain (see also *contraception*).

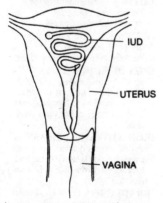

An IUD after insertion into the uterus.

INTRAVASATION n. the entry of a foreign substance into a blood vessel.

INTRAVENOUS adj. into or within a vein.

INTRAVENOUS FEEDING

(I.V.) n. the administration of nutrients through a vein.

INTRAVENOUS INJECTION n. hypodermic injection into a vein to instill a fluid, withdraw blood, or begin a blood transfusion or intravenous feeding.

INTRAVENOUS PYELOGRAPHY (IVP) n. a radiological technique for examining the structures of the urinary system to detect tumors, cysts, stones, or structural or functional abnormalities. A contrast medium is injected intravenously and a series of X rays traces the clearance of the medium by the urinary system.

INTRINSIC FACTOR n. a substance secreted by the mucous membranes of the stomach that is essential for absorption of vitamin B_{12}; lack of intrinsic factor leads to deficiency of vitamin B_{12} and resultant *pernicious anemia*.

INTROITUS n. the entrance or opening to a hollow organ or hollow tube (e.g., the introitus of the vagina).

INTROPIN n. trade name for *dopamine*.

INTROVERSION n. the tendency to turn one's interests inward toward the self (compare *extroversion*).

INTROVERT n. one whose interests are turned inward toward the self.

INTUBATION n. the placement of a tube into an opening, esp. the passage of a breathing tube into the trachea to allow passage of oxygen or anesthetic gas.

INTUMESCENCE n. a swelling or increase in volume. adj. **intumescent**

INTUSSUSCEPTION n. prolapse or infolding of one part of the intestine into the lumen of another part, causing an obstruction. Symptoms include abdominal pain and bloody stool. Treatment is by surgery.

IN UTERO adj./adv. within the uterus.

INVAGINATION n. condition in which one part of an organ folds into or becomes telescoped into another part of the organ, as in the intestine, sometimes causing an obstruction.

INVERSION n. an abnormal condition in which an organ is turned inward or turned inside out (e.g., uterus after childbirth when its upper part is pulled into the cervical canal.

IN VITRO adj./adv. pert. to an artificial condition, as within a test tube or other laboratory apparatus (compare *in vivo*).

IN VIVO adj./adv. in the living organism (compare *in vitro*).

INVOLUNTARY adj. done without conscious thought or control of the will.

INVOLUNTARY MUSCLE see *smooth muscle*.

INVOLUTION n. decrease in the size of an organ, as in the return of the *uterus* to its normal size after childbirth.

IODINE n. a nonmetallic element that is an essential nutrient (in small amounts) and is used in antiseptics, in radioisotope scanning procedures, and in certain treatments of thyroid cancer (see Table of Elements).

IODOCHLORHYDROXYQUIN n. drug, known under the trade name Clioquinol, used to treat certain fungal infections (e.g., athlete's foot eczema). Adverse effects include skin irritation.

IODOPSIN n. a photosensitive chemical in the cones of the retina that plays a part in color vision.

ION n. an electrically charged particle.

IPECAC n. a drug used to induce vomiting in some types of poisoning and drug overdose. Adverse effects include gastrointestinal irritation, or, if vomiting does not occur and the ipecac is retained, cardiac abnormalities.

IQ abbreviation for *intelligence quotient*.

IRIDECTOMY n. surgical removal of part of the *iris* of the eye, usually performed to remove a foreign body or tumor or to enhance drainage of aqueous humor in cases of *glaucoma*.

IRIDOCYCLITIS n. inflammation of the iris and ciliary body of the eye.

IRIDONCUS n. swelling of the iris of the eye.

IRIDOKERATITIS n. inflammation of the iris and cornea of the eye.

IRIDOTOMY n. a surgical procedure in which an incision is made in the iris to enlarge the pupil or to treat *glaucoma*.

IRIS n. the circular, colored part of the eye suspended in the aqueous humor and perforated by the *pupil*. adj. **iritic**

IRITIS n. inflammation of the iris, causing tearing, pain, and decreased visual sharpness.

IRON n. a metallic element essential for *hemoglobin* synthesis in the body and used in various drugs.

IRON-DEFICIENCY ANEMIA n. a type of *anemia* caused by lack of adequate iron to synthesize hemoglobin. Symptoms include fatigue, pallor, and weakness.

IRON STORAGE DISEASE n. any of several disorders in which excessive iron is stored in the body (see *hemochromatosis*; *hemosiderosis*).

IRRADIATION n. exposure to heat, light, X-ray, or other form of radiant energy for diagnostic or therapeutic purposes.

IRREDUCIBLE adj. not able to be returned to normal, as an irreducible hernia.

IRRIGATION n. washing out of a body part by water or other fluid.

IRRITABLE BOWEL SYNDROME n. a condition characterized by recurrent abdominal pain and diarrhea. Occurring most often in young adults, it has no known organic cause and is often associated with emotional stress (compare *Crohn's disease*; *ulcerative colitis*); also called **spastic colon**; **mucous colitis**.

ISCHEMIA n. decreased blood supply to a given body part sometimes resulting from vasoconstriction, thrombosis, or embolism (see also *infarct*).

ISCHIUM n. one of the three parts of the hip (*innominate bone*), the other two being the *ilium* and *pubis*. pl. **ischia** adj. **ischiatic**

ISLANDS OF LANGERHANS n. cell clusters within the *pancreas* that form the *endocrine* part of the organ, secreting hormones important in controlling sugar metabolism. Beta cells secrete *insulin*; alpha cells *glucagon*; and other cells pancreatic peptide. Also called **islets of Langerhans**.

ISLETS OF LANGERHANS see *islands of Langerhans*

-ISM suffix indicating a condition of or theory of (e.g., *hyperthyroidism*).

ISMELIN n. trade name for antihypertensive drug *guanethidine*.

ISO- comb. form indicating equality or sameness (e.g., **isomorphous**, of the same form).

ISOAGGLUTINATION n. process in which antibodies (isoagglutinins) occurring naturally in blood cause clumping of red blood cells of a different group, carrying a corresponding antigen (isoagglutinogen) but of the same species.

ISOANTIBODY n. an antibody that occurs naturally against foreign tissues of a person of the same species.

ISOCARBOXAZID n. a *monoamine oxidase inhibitor*, known under the trade name Marplan, used to treat *depression*.

ISOLATION n. 1. the process of separating one thing from all others like it; 2. the separation of a patient from others, as, e.g., to prevent the spread of an infectious disease; 3. in surgery, the separation of a structure from surrounding structures.

ISOMETRIC EXERCISES n. exercises that increase muscle tension by applying pressure against stable resistance, as in pressing hands together (compare *isotonic exercises*); also **isometrics**.

ISONIAZID n. a drug used to treat *tuberculosis*. Adverse effects include disturbances of peripheral nerve function; liver toxicity, rashes, and fever.

ISOPROTERENOL n. drug, known under the trade name Isuprel, used to treat bronchial asthma and to stimulate the heart. Adverse effects include hypotension and abnormalites of cardiac rhythm.

ISORDIL n. trade name for *isosorbide* used to treat angina.

ISOSORBIDE n. drug, known under the tradename Isordil, used to treat angina pectoris and congestive heart failure. Adverse effects include hypotension, dizziness, and headache.

ISOTONIC adj. of equal pressure or concentration, esp. in a solution.

ISOTONIC EXERCISES n. a form of exercise in which the muscle contracts and there is movement; joint mobility and muscle strength are improved (compare *isometric*).

ISOTOPE n. one of two or more forms of an element having the same atomic number and the same or nearly the same properties but differing in atomic weight (due to difference in number of neutrons in the nucleus); see also *radioisotope*.

ISTHMUS n. a narrow connecting part, as the band of tissue connecting the lobes of the *thyroid gland*.

ISUPREL n. trade name for *isoproterenol*.

ITCH n. an annoying sensation on the skin that impels the person to scratch the site (compare *pruritus; scabies, tinea*).

-ITIS suffix meaning inflammation (e.g., **neuritis**, nerve inflammation).

IUD abbreviation for *intrauterine device*.

I.V. abbreviation for *intravenous*, esp. *intravenous feeding*.

j

JACKET n. a covering, as of plaster of Paris, leather, or other material, placed over the torso to provide support or help correct a deformity.

JACKSONIAN EPILEPSY n. a type of *epilepsy* characterized by recurrent motor seizure episodes that typically start as a twitching or convulsive movement of a small group of muscles and then spread (''marche'') to other muscles on the same side of the body, as, for example, twitching of the fingers of one hand spreading to muscles of the hand, forearm, and arm. The affected person usually remains conscious during the attack.

JACQUEMIER'S SIGN n. bluish or purplish coloration of the mucous membrane lining of the *vagina* that occurs in early pregnancy.

JACTITATION n. tossing, twitching, and jerking movements of a person with a severe illness.

JAKOB-CREUTZFELDT DISEASE see *Creutzfeldt-Jakob disease*.

JÁMAIS VU n. the sensation of being strange or unfamiliar with a person or surroundings that are familiar; it can occur in normal persons but is most often associated with certain types of *epilepsy* (compare *déjà vu*).

JARGONAPHASIA n. a stream of words that are inappropriate or meaningless (compare *logorrhea*).

JAUNDICE n. a yellowing of the skin and whites (sclerae) of the eyes caused by an accumulation of the bile pigment *bilirubin* in the blood. Jaundice is a symptom of many disorders, most commonly obstruction of the ducts (biliary tract) that carry bile to the intestine, as by a gallstone; disease of the liver, due to infection, alcoholism, poisons, or other factor; and anemia in which there is excessive destruction of red blood cells. Also called **icterus**. (See also *kernicterus hyperbilirubinemia*.) adj. **jaundiced**

JAUNDICE OF THE NEWBORN n. physiological jaundice occurring in some infants in the first few weeks of life caused by destruction of excess hemoglobin in red blood cells; it usually disappears spontaneously; also called **physiological jaundice of the newborn**; **icterus neonatorum**.

JAW n. the bones that form the framework of the mouth and serve for the attachment of teeth. The upper jaw bone is the *maxilla*; the lower jaw bone is the *mandible*.

JEJUNE adj. lacking in nutritive value.

JEJUNITIS n. inflammation of the *jejunum*.

JEJUNO- comb. form indicating an association with the *jejunum* (e.g., **jejunostomy**, surgical creation of an opening between the jejunum and the anterior abdominal wall, sometimes made to allow artificial feeding).

JEJUNOILEITIS n. inflammation of both the *jejunum* and *ileum* parts of the small intestine.

JEJUNUM n. that part of the *small intestine* between the *duodenum* and the *ileum*; in humans, it is about 2.4 meters (8 feet) long. adj. **jejunal**

JERK n. a sudden movement; a muscle reflex. Efforts to elicit certain jerks (e.g., the knee jerk) are used to help diagnose specific nerve transmission disorders.

JET LAG n. a condition marked by fatigue, sleep disturbances, and sluggish body functions, caused by a disruption of the body's normal circadian (daily) rhythm resulting from travel through several time zones.

JOINT n. the point where two or more bones meet. A joint may be immovable (fibrous), as those of the skull; slightly movable (cartilaginous), as those connecting the vertebrae; or freely movable (synovial), as those of the elbow and knee; also: **articulation**. (See also *cartilaginous joint; fibrous joint; synovial joint*.)

JUGULAR adj. pert. to the throat or neck.

JUGULAR VEINS n. any of several veins in the neck that drain blood from the head and empty into larger veins leading to the heart.

JUICE n. any of several liquids of the body (e.g., **cancer juice**, a milklike substance found in certain cancerous growths); also: **succus** (see also *gastric juice, pancreatic juice*).

JUMENTOUS adj. smelling strongly like an animal.

JUNCTION n. the point where two parts come together (e.g., neuromuscular junction, the point where a nerve and muscle come together).

JUVANTIA n. drugs or devices that ease pain or discomfort.

JUVENILE DIABETES see *diabetes mellitus*.

JUXTA- comb. form indicating proximity, nearness (e.g., **juxtaspinal**, near the spine).

JUXTAPOSITION n. a side-by-side position.

k

K symbol for the element *potassium*; abbreviaton for the *Kelvin* temperature scale.

K: VITAMIN n. any of a group of fat-soluble vitamins essential for blood coagulation and important in certain energy-transfer reactions. Rich sources include green leafy vegetables, egg yolk, yogurt, and fish-liver oils (see *vitamin*; Table of Vitamins).

KAFOCIN n. trade name for a *cephalosporin* antibiotic (cephaloglycin) no longer commonly used.

KAKKE DISEASE see *beriberi*.

KALA-AZAR n. a visceral form of *leishmaniasis*. Occurring mainly in warm regions of Asia, Africa, Central and South America, and parts of the Mediterranean area, it is caused by the protozoan *Leishmania donovani*, transmitted by the bite of a sand fly. Symptoms include anemia, enlarged spleen and liver, fever, and loss of weight. Treatment includes antimony preparations, blood transfusions, and rest. Also: **Assam fever, dumdum fever**.

KALEMIA n. the presence of *potassium* in the blood.

KALIURESIS n. the presence of *potassium* in the urine; also: **kaliuresis**. adj. **kaliuretic, kaliuretic**

KANAMYCIN n. an antibiotic, commonly known under the trade name Kantrex, used to treat certain severe infections. Adverse effects include hypersensitivity reactions and kidney and hearing disturbances.

KANTREX n. trade name for the antibiotic *kanamycin*.

KAOCHLOR n. trade name for *potassium* chloride solution used to treat *electrolyte imbalance*.

KAOLIN n. an aluminum-and-silicon-containing product used internally, often with pectin in the trade-name product Kaopectate, as an adsorbent to treat diarrhea and externally as a dusting powder, or, in an ointment base, as a *poultice*.

KAOPECTATE n. trade name for a fixed-combination antidiarrheal drug containing the adsorbent *kaolin* and the emollient *pectin*.

KAPOSI'S SARCOMA n. a malignant neoplasm that starts as soft purplish or brownish spots on the feet and then spreads from the skin to the lymph nodes and internal organs. Until the early 1980's it occurred almost exclusively among older Jewish, Italian, and Negro men, but after that time it increased in incidence and is one of the common manifestations of *acquired immune deficiency syndrome* (AIDS).

KARYO- comb. form indicating an association with a nucleus (e.g., **karyogamy**, the fusion of cell nuclei, as in fertilization).

KARYOKINESIS n. division of the cell nucleus during *mitosis* and *meiosis*.

KARYOLYMPH n. clear fluid of the cell nucleus in which the nucleolus, chromatin, and other structures are dispersed.

KARYOLYSIS n. the breakdown of the cell *nucleus*. adj. **karyolytic**

KARYON n. the cell *nucleus*.

KARYOPLASM see *nucleoplasm*.

KARYOTYPE n. 1. the appearance of the chromosomal makeup of a cell, including the number, arrangement, size, and structure of the *chromosomes* as determined by a photomicrograph taken during mitosis; 2. diagrammatic representation of the chromosomal makeup of a cell arranged according to a given classification system. adj. **karyotypic**

KARYOTYPING n. the process of analyzing and classifying the chromosomes of a cell and preparing a *karyotype* diagram; used in the diagnosis of certain chromosomal abnormalities (e.g., *Down's syndrome*).

KATABOLISM see *catabolism*.

KAVRIN n. trade name for a smooth muscle relaxant (*papaverine*) used to treat visceral and cardiovascular spasm.

KAWASAKI DISEASE n. an acute illness, primarily in children, characterized by a rash, swollen lymph glands, fever, inflammation of the mucous membranes of the mouth, and a "strawberry tongue"; joint pain, pneumonia, meningitis, cardiac abnormalities, and aneurysms develop in some cases. The cause is unknown, and diagnosis is difficult, based on the exclusion of all known diseases. Treatment is largely symptomatic. Also called **mucocutaneous lymph node syndrome**.

KAYSER-FLEISCHER RING n. a pigmented ring at the outer edge of the cornea of the eye that is a sign of *Wilson's disease*.

KEFLEX n. trade name for the *cephalosporin*-family antibiotic cephalexin.

KEFLIN n. trade name for the *cephalosporin*-family antibiotic cephalothin.

KEGEL EXERCISES n. a regimen of exercises for women designed to improve the ability to retain urine and to increase the muscular contractility of the *vagina*; sometimes advised to help overcome weakness of the pubococcygeus muscles that may occur after childbirth. The exercises involve the squeezing, pulling-up action required to stop the stream of urine when voiding; also called **pubococcygeus exercises**.

KELOID n. overgrowth of collagenous scar tissue at the site of a wound on the skin. The lesion is generally rounded and raised, often with clawlike margins; it may flatten and become less noticeable with time, or it may be treated by cryosurgery, corticosteroid injections, surgery, or other means.

KELVIN n. a temperature scale used in science in which 0° Kelvin (absolute zero) is equivalent to $-273.16°$ Celsius.

KEMADRIN n. trade name for a skeletal muscle relaxant (*procyclidine*) used to treat *parkinsonism*.

KENALOG n. trade name for a glucocorticoid (*triamcinolone*) used to treat inflammatory conditions.

KERAT-, KERATO- comb. form indicating a relationship to the *cornea* of the eye (e.g., **keratectomy**, removal of part of the cornea); or to horny cells or horny tissue, esp. of the skin (e.g., **keratolysis**, a loosening of the horny layer of the outer skin).

KERATALGIA n. pain in the *cornea*.

KERATECTASIA n. a bulging or protrusion of the *cornea* of the eye.

KERATIN n. a protein that forms horny tissues such as the nails, and is also found in the outer skin and hair.   adj. **keratic**

KERATINIZATION n. the process by which cells become horny due to the deposit of *keratin* in them; it occurs in outer layers of the skin and associated structures (e.g., nails and hair).

KERATITIS n. inflammation of the *cornea* that produces watery, painful eyes and blurred vision; it may be caused by irritation, as

from exposure to dust or certain vapors, or by infection.

KERATOACANTHOMA n. a *keratin*-containing skin nodule, most often occurring on the face, hands, or arms; it usually disappears spontaneously, often leaving a scar.

KERATOCOELE n. hernia of the cornea.

KERATOCONJUNCTIVITIS n. inflammation of the *cornea* and *conjunctiva*, tissues lining the eyelids and covering the front of the *eyeball*.

KERATOCONUS n. cone-shaped protrusion of the *cornea*; it may be treated by special contact lenses or by *epikeratophakia*.

KERATODERMA n. any surface growth or covering that appears horny.

KERATOIRITIS n. inflammation of the *cornea* and the *iris*.

KERATOMALACIA n. a softening, drying, and ulceration of the *cornea*, usually resulting from severe vitamin A deficiency in the diet or from a disease that impairs vitamin A absorption or storage in the body (e.g., *cystic fibrosis*, *sprue*).

KERATOMYCOSIS n. fungus infection of the *cornea*.

KERATONOSIS n. general term for any abnormal condition of the outer skin.

KERATONOSUS n. general term for a disease of the cornea.

KERATOPATHY n. any disease of the *cornea* without inflammation.

KERATOPLASTY n. a surgical procedure in which diseased tissue of all or part of the *cornea* of the eye is replaced by healthy corneal tissue from a donor; corneal graft.

KERATORHEXIS n. a tear or break in the *cornea*.

KERATOSCLERITIS n. inflammation of the *cornea* and *sclera*.

KERATOSCOPY n. examination of the *cornea* to detect abnormal curvature; a special instrument, called a keratoscope, is used to study light reflected from the front surface of the cornea.

KERATOSIS n. a skin condition characterized by an overgrowth of horny skin layers. pl. **keratoses** adj. **keratotic**

ACTINIC KERATOSIS n. an overgrowth of outer skin layers caused by long-term overexposure to the sun.

SEBORRHEIC KERATOSIS n. a condition marked by well-circumscribed wartlike lesions that are often itchy and covered with a greasy crust and occurring most often on the face, neck, upper chest, and upper back. Treatment is by curretage, cryotherapy, or electrodesiccation.

KERATOSIS FOLLICULARIS n. an uncommon hereditary disorder characterized by dark, sometimes purulent (containing pus) crusted patches. Treatment includes vitamin A orally and topically and sometimes *corticosteroids*.

KERION n. pustule-covered swelling that oozes fluid; occurring in some with a fungus infection of the scalp (*Tinea capitas*).

KERNICTERUS n. an abnormal accumulation of the bile pigment bilirubin (*hyperbilirubinemia*) in the brain and other nerve tissue, causing yellow staining and damage to the involved tissues. In newborns it may cause mental retardation and sensory and motor disturbances (see also *hyperbilirubinemia of the newborn*).

KERNIG'S SIGN n. a symptom of *meningitis* in which the patient is unable to extend the leg at the knee when the thighs are held at right angles to the body due to stiffness of the hamstring muscles.

KEROID adj. hornlike or cornealike.

KETALAR n. trade name for a general anesthetic (*ketamine hydrochloride*).

KETAMINE HYDROCHLORIDE n. a nonbarbiturate general anesthetic, known under the trade name Ketalar, that does not cause complete muscle relaxation and is used mainly for brief, minor surgical procedures and for pediatric and geriatric patients. On emergence from anesthesia, hallucinations, delirium, and other psychological signs may occur; increased blood pressure and intracranial pressure are also sometimes found.

KETOACIDOSIS n. *acidosis* with an accumulation of *ketone* bodies, occurring primarily as a complication of uncontrolled *diabetes mellitus*. It is characterized by a fruity breath odor, nausea and vomiting, shortness of breath, mental confusion, and, if untreated, coma (*diabetic coma*). Treatment includes the administration of *insulin* and fluids and the correction of electrolyte imbalance (compare *insulin shock*). adj. **ketoacidotic**

KETOACIDURIA see *ketonuria*.

KETONE n. any of a group of organic chemicals derived by oxidation of alcohol and containing a carbon-oxygen group. Among the ketones are acetone and acetoacetic acid.

KETONE BODY n. products (acetone, B-hydroxylbutyric acid, and acetoacetic acid) of the breakdown of fats in the body. Excessive fat metabolism and production of ketone bodies leads to their excretion in urine, as in uncontrolled *diabetes mellitus*.

KETONEMIA n. presence of abnormally high levels of ketone bodies in the blood, as in uncontrolled *diabetes mellitus*.

KETONURIA n. the presence of excessive amounts of *ketone bod-*

ies in the *urine*; it is usually the result of uncontrolled *diabetes mellitus*, starvation, or metabolic disorder affecting fat metabolism; also: **ketoaciduria**.

KETOSIS n. an abnormal accumulation of ketones in the body resulting from inadequate intake or metabolism of carbohydrates and increased fatty acid metabolism, leading to the formation of ketone bodies. Ketosis occurs most often in starvation and uncontrolled *diabetes mellitus*. It is characterized by a fruity breath odor and the presence of ketone bodies in the urine; if untreated, it can lead to *ketoacidosis*, coma, and death.

KIDNEY n. either of two bean-shaped excretory organs that filter wastes (esp. *urea*) from the blood and excrete them and water in *urine* and help to regulate the water, electrolyte, and pH balance of the body. The kidneys are located in the dorsal part of the abdominal cavity, one on each side of the vertebral column. Each kidney, about 11 centimeters (4.5 inches) long, 6 centimeters (2.5 inches) wide, and 2.5 centimeters (1 inch) thick, consists of an outer cortex and inner medulla and contains one million or more fil-

tering units, called *nephrons*. Blood passes through tufts of capillaries (glomeruli) in the nephrons, where it is filtered; the filtrate then passes through renal tubules, where some substances (e.g., sugar, some salts) are selectively reabsorbed, into collecting ducts. The final product—known as urine—passes out of the kidney through tubes known as *ureters* and is carried to the *bladder*. The function of the kidney is controlled by hormones, esp. the *antidiuretic hormone* (ADH) produced by the *pituitary gland*. The kidney is subject to inflammation, infection, the formation of stones (*renal calculi*), and other disorders (see also *excretory system*).

KIDNEY FAILURE   see *renal failure*.

KIDNEY STONE   see *renal calculus*.

KILO- prefix meaning ''one thousand'' of a given unit (e.g., **kilogram**, one thousand grams).

KILOCALORIE   see *calorie*.

KILOGRAM CALORIE   see *calorie*.

KINANESTHESIA n. inability to sense movement.

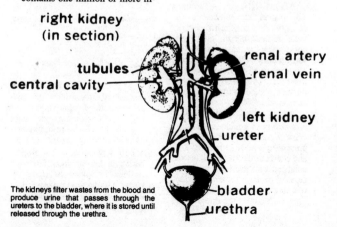

**right kidney
(in section)**

tubules

central cavity

renal artery
renal vein

left kidney
ureter

bladder
urethra

The kidneys filter wastes from the blood and produce urine that passes through the ureters to the bladder, where it is stored until released through the urethra.

KINE-, KINESIO- comb. form indicating an association with movement, esp. body movement and muscle action (e.g., **kinesalgia**, pain from muscle action).

KINEMATICS n. the study of motion, including flexion, abduction, adduction, and rotation; it is important in orthopedics and rehabilitation medicine.

KINESIOLOGY n. the study of muscular activity and the anatomy, physiology, and mechanics of the movement of the body and its parts.

KINESTHESIA n. the perception of body position and movement. adj. **kinesthetic**

KINETICS n. the study of motion, including the study of the forces producing and modifying motion (compare *kinematics*).

KINETOSIS n. illness or abnormality caused by movement (e.g., airsickness, carsickness).

KISSING DISEASE see *infectious mononucleosis*.

KLEBSIELLA n. a genus of gram-negative bacteria, some of which cause respiratory infections (e.g., bronchitis, pneumonia) and infections affecting other parts of the body.

KLEPTOMANIA n. a compulsion to steal. The objects are usually not taken for their monetary value or need but for their symbolic meaning associated with some emotional conflict; they are often returned or hidden. Treatment usually involves psychotherapy to uncover the underlying emotional problems.

KLINEFELTER'S SYNDROME n. a defect in which at least one extra X chromosome (XXY) is present in a male (normally XY) and characterized by small testes, enlarged breasts, long legs, decreased or absent sperm production, and mental retardation. Persons with more than one extra X

(e.g., XXXY) usually show marked physical and mental abnormalities.

K-LOR n. trade name for a *potassium* chloride solution used to treat *electrolyte imbalances*.

KLORVESS n. trade name for a *potassium* chloride solution used to treat *electrolyte imbalance*.

K-LYTE/Cl n. trade name for a *potassium* chloride solution used to treat *electrolyte imbalances*.

KNEE n. the joint complex, fronted by the kneecap (*patella*), at which the thighbone (*femur*) and lower leg connect. It includes joints at which the femur and tibia (a lower leg bone) meet, a joint where the femur and patella meet, and numerous *ligaments* and *bursae*.

KNEE JOINT

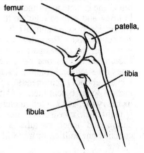

The patella, or kneecap, is in front of the articulation of the femur with the lower leg bones—the tibia and fibula.

KNEECAP see *patella*.

KNEE JERK n. see *patellar reflex*.

KNEE JOINT n. a hinged joint made up of three articulations: two at which the *femur* (thighbone) and *tibia* (a lower leg bone) meet and one at which the femur and *patella* (kneecap) meet.

KNOCK-KNEE n. a condition in which the legs are curved inward so that the knees are close together and the ankles far apart as the person stands or walks; also **genu valgum**.

KNUCKLE n. the joints of the fingers, esp. the joints where the fingers attach to the main part of the hand.

KOILONYCHIA n. a condition in which the nails are thin and concave (spoon-shaped), sometimes associated with iron-deficiency anemia.

KOPLIK'S SPOTS n. small red spots with bluish-white centers found on the mucous membrane of the mouth and tongue and characteristic of *measles*, usually appearing one or two days before the measles rash.

KORSAKOFF'S PSYCHOSIS (syndrome) n. a condition, occurring most often in chronic alcoholics, marked by disorientation, impaired memory, and other mental abnormalities. It is thought to be due to degenerative changes in the thalamus of the brain caused by vitamin B deficiency associated with excessive alcohol intake. Treatment includes adequate nutrition and the administration of vitamins, esp. B complex vitamins (compare *Wernicke's encephalopathy*).

KRAUROSIS n. a drying, thickening, and shrivelling of the skin, esp. that of the external genitalia of a woman (*kraurosis vulvae*).

KREB'S CYCLE n. the complex sequence of enzyme-catalyzed reactions occurring in cells through which sugars, fatty acids, and amino acids are broken down to produce carbon dioxide, water, and energy (in the form of *ATP*). The final step in the metabolism of carbohydrates, fats, and proteins, it is the body's chief source of energy; also: **Krebs citric acid cycle; tricarboxylic acid cycle**.

KUPFFER'S CELLS n. specialized cells found in the *liver* that destroy bacteria, foreign proteins, and worn-out blood cells.

KURU n. a progressive disease of the central nervous system characterized by tremors and increasing lack of coordination leading to paralysis and death, usually within a year after the onset of symptoms. The disease, known only among the Fore people of New Guinea, is thought to be caused by a slow virus (the incubation period may be 30 years or more) and thought to have been transmitted through cannibalistic practices in which the diseased brain tissue of the dead was eaten or wiped on the body; with the abandonment of cannibalism the disease has now virtually disappeared.

KWASHIORKOR n. a disease, primarily of children, caused by a severe protein deficiency; it is characterized by retarded growth, changes in skin and hair coloring, loss of appetite, diarrhea, anemia, degenerative changes in the liver edema, and signs of multiple vitamin deficiencies.

KWELL n. trade name for a drug, available in cream and shampoo form, used to kill lice and itch mites.

KYPHOSIS n. an abnormality of the *vertebral column* in which there is increased convex curvature in the upper spine, giving a hunchback or humped back appearance. Mild cases are often

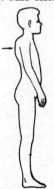

In kyphosis, there is increased convexity in the curvature of the thoracic spine.

self-limiting and asymptomatic; severe or progressive cases may cause back pain and are sometimes treated with special back braces (compare *lordosis*; *scoliosis*). adj. **kyphotic**

l

LABIAL adj. pert. to the *labium* or the lips.

LABIA MAJORA n. two long folds of skin that form the outer and larger lips of the external female genitalia, one on each side of the vaginal opening outside the *labia minora*; in some women the outer surface of the labia majora is covered with pubic hair. sing. **labium majus**

LABIA MINORA n. two folds of skin that form the inner, smaller lips of the female genitalia extending from the *clitoris* backwards on each side of the vaginal opening, inside the *labia majora*. sing. **labium minus**

LABILE adj. unstable; tending to change. n. **lability**

LABIO- comb. form indicating an association with the lips or liplike structures (e.g., **labiodental**, pert. to the lips and teeth).

LABIUM n. a liplike edge or liplike structure, esp. the structures (*labia majora* and *labia minora*) enclosing the vulva. pl. **labia** adj. **labial**

LABOR n. the process by which a baby is born and the *placenta* is expelled from the *uterus*. Labor has three stages: the first, or stage of dilatation, characterized by contractions of the uterine wall and dilatation of the opening of the *cervix*; the second, or stage of expulsion, during which the baby is born; and the third, or afterbirth stage, in which the *placenta* is expelled. The average duration of labor is about 13 hours in first pregnancies (12 hours in first stage, 1 hour in second, few minutes in third); about eight hours in subsequent pregnancies. (See also *Braxton-Hicks contractions*).

LABOR COACH n. a person (often the father) who assists a woman in labor by providing emotional support and encouragement to use breathing, concentration, and exercise techniques learned in childbirth-preparation classes (see also *Bradley method of childbirth*; *Lamaze method of childbirth*).

LABOR PAIN n. the discomfort and pain caused by contractions of the *uterus* during *labor*.

LABRUM n. a lip-edge or liplike structure, e.g., **labrum glenoidule**, the cartilage of the glenoid cavity in the shoulder). pl. **labra**.

LABYRINTH n. the intricate communicating channels of the inner ear. adj. **labyrinthine**

LABYRINTHITIS n. inflammation of the inner ear; it usually produces vertigo, loss of balance, and vomiting; also: **otitis interna**.

LACERATION n. a wound with a jagged edge, resulting from a tearing or scraping action. v. **lacerate**

LACRIMAL adj. pert. to tears.

LACRIMAL APPARATUS n. the structures that secrete and drain tears from the eye. Tears produced in the lacrimal gland drain through small openings at the corner of the eye into special ducts that pass into the nasal cavity.

LACRIMAL APPARATUS

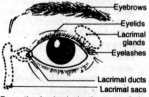

From the lacrimal glands, tears drain through the lacrimal ducts and lacrimal sacs into the nasal passageways.

LACRIMAL BONE n. a small, fragile facial bone located at the inner part of the orbital cavity.

LACRIMAL GLAND n. either of two oval-shaped structures (exocrine glands) located to the upper outer side of the eye that secrete tears that moisten the *conjunctiva* of the eye.

LACRIMAL SAC n. either of two oval-shaped dilated ends of the nasolacrimal duct that fill with tears secreted by the lacrimal glands.

LACRIMATION n. 1. the normal continuous secretion of tears by the lacrimal glands; 2. copious tear production, as in weeping.

LACTALBUMIN n. a protein found in milk.

LACTASE n. an enzyme secreted by glands in the small intestine that converts lactose (milk sugar) into simpler sugars.

LACTASE DEFICIENCY n. an abnormality in which a deficiency in the amount of the enzyme lactase results in an inability to digest *lactose* (milk sugar). It is usually congenital, more common in people of Asian and African heritage, but may also result from gastrectomy, disease of the small intestine or certain other disorders; see also *lactose intolerance*.

LACTATION n. 1. the synthesis and secretion of milk by the mammary glands of the breast; 2. the time during which an infant or child is nourished with breast milk. adj. **lactational**

LACTEAL n. a lymph channel in the *villi* of the *small intestine* that absorbs digested fat (chyle).

LACTIC adj. pert. to milk.

LACTIC ACID n. 1. a chemical formed by the process of *glycolysis*; during strenuous exercise it may accumulate in muscle cells; 2. the acid formed by the action of certain bacteria on milk and milk products.

LACTIFEROUS adj. pert. to a structure that produces and/or conveys milk, as the lactiferous tubules of the *breast*.

LACTIFEROUS DUCT n. any of several ducts that transport milk from the lobes of the breast to the nipple.

LACTIFUGE n. an agent that reduces milk secretion, as, e.g., a drug given to suppress milk production in a woman not breast feeding.

LACTOGEN n. a drug or other substance that enhances milk production. adj. **lactogenic**

LACTOGENIC HORMONE see *prolactin*.

LACTOSE n. a sugar (made up of glucose and galactose) found only in milk; it is split into its constituent sugars by the enzyme lactase.

LACTOSE INTOLERANCE n. a disorder, due to a defect or deficiency of the enzyme lactase, resulting in an inability to digest lactose and symptoms of bloating, flatulence, abdominal discomfort, nausea, and diarrhea on ingestion of milk and milk products (see also *lactase deficiency*).

LACTOSURIA n. the presence of milk in the urine, occurring during pregnancy or lactation.

LACUNA n. a small hollow or cavity in or between body parts, esp. a cartilage-filled depression in bone. pl. **lacunae** adj. **lacunar**

LAETRILE n. a chemical (amygdalin), derived from the seeds of apricots, plums, and some other fruits, that, when taken into the body, causes cyanide production; it has been publicized as a treatment for cancer, but there is no evidence that it is therapeutic.

LAGOPHTHALMOS n. an abnormal condition in which an eye cannot be closed completely, due to disorder of the *cornea* or neurological or muscular disorder.

LALLATION n. 1. unintelligible speechlike utterances, as the babbling of an infant; 2. a speech disorder in which the sound "l" is used in place of other sounds, esp. "r" sounds, or the sound "l" is mispronounced.

LAL-, LALIO-, LALO- comb. form indicating a relationship with speech (e.g., **lalopathy**, a speech disorder).

LAMARCKISM n. a theory of evolution, postulated by Jean Baptiste Lamarck in the 19th century, that holds that adaptations to environmental conditions lead to structural changes in organisms, through the increased use or the disuse of certain parts, and that these acquired characteristics are then transmitted to the offspring. adj. **Lamarckian**

LAMAZE METHOD OF CHILDBIRTH n. a method of psychophysical preparation for childbirth, developed by the French obstetrician Fernand Lamaze in the 1950's, that is now the most widely used method of *natural childbirth*. In classes during pregnancy and in practice sessions at home, the pregnant woman, usually with the help of a coach (called a "monitrice"), learns the physiology of pregnancy and childbirth, techniques of relaxation, concentration, and breathing, and exercises certain muscles to promote control during labor and childbirth (compare *Bradley method of childbirth*; *Read method of childbirth*).

LAMBDACISM n. a speech disorder marked by incorrect or excessive pronunciation of the sound "l" or substitution of the sound "r" for "l" (compare *lallation*).

LAMELLA n. any platelike part, as a bone. pl. **lamellae** adj. **lamellar**

LAMINA n. a thin membrane or platelike structure, as the two parts of a vertebra that join to hold the spinous process of the vertebra over the spinal cord. pl. **laminae** adj. **laminar**

LAMINECTOMY n. a surgical procedure in which the bony arches of one or more vertebrae are chipped or removed to relieve pressure on the spinal cord, to remove tumors, or to treat disorders involving the vertebral column (e.g., *ruptured intervertebral disk*).

LANCE v. to pierce, open, or cut into, as a boil for drainage.

LANCINATING adj. cutting, sharp, knifelike, as in lancinating pain.

LANOXIN n. trade name for the cardiotonic *digoxin*.

LANUGO n. fine, downy hair covering a fetus; it is normally shed during the ninth month of *gestation* but may be present on newborns, esp. premature newborns.

LAPARO- comb. form indicating an association with the abdomen, loin, or flank (e.g., **laparocele**, a hernia through the abdomen).

LAPAROSCOPY n. examination of the abdominal cavity, esp. the ovaries and Fallopian tubes, through a laparoscope (a type of endoscope) introduced through a

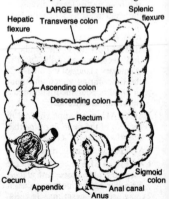

LARGE INTESTINE

Hepatic flexure
Transverse colon
Splenic flexure
Ascending colon
Descending colon
Rectum
Cecum
Appendix
Sigmoid colon
Anal canal
Anus

The large intestine includes the cecum, the ascending colon, the transverse colon, the descending colon, the sigmoid colon, and the anal canal.

small incision in the abdominal wall; also used in women as a sterilization procedure in which the Fallopian tubes are ligated.

LAPAROTOMY n. any surgical procedure in which an incision is made into the abdominal wall; often done for exploration, as, e.g., to examine abdominal organs.

LARGE INTESTINE n. that portion of the digestive tract containing the *cecum*; *appendix*; ascending, transverse and descending colons; and the *rectum*.

LARODOPA n. trade name for *levodopa*, a drug used to treat *parkinsonism*.

LAROTID n. a trade name for the antibacterial *amoxicillin*.

LARYNGECTOMY n. surgical removal of all or part of the *larynx*, usually performed to treat carcinoma of the larynx. After a laryngectomy a person must learn esophageal speech or use artificial means for speaking.

LARYNGISMUS n. spasm of the *larynx* caused by sudden contraction of the muscles of the larynx, often marked by sudden and noisy indrawing of breath; sometimes associated with croup, or irritation of the larynx (e.g., from inhaled anesthetic or a foreign body).

LARYNGITIS n. inflammation of the mucous membrane of the *larynx* and swelling of the *vocal cords*, characterized by loss or hoarseness of voice, cough, and sometimes difficult breathing. It may be acute, caused by bacterial or viral infection or irritation (e.g., from irritating fumes); or chronic, from excessive use of the voice or excessive smoking or long-term exposure to irritants. Treatment depends on the cause, but usually includes rest of the voice, a moist atmosphere, and the avoidance of irritants. (In young children spasm of the larynx and difficulty in breathing may result.)

LARYNGO- comb. form indicating an association with the *larynx* (e.g., **laryngostenosis,** narrowing of the larynx).

LARYNGOPHARYNGEAL adj. pert. to the *larynx* and the *pharynx*.

LARYNGOPHARYNGITIS n. inflammation of the *larynx* and *pharynx*.

LARYNGOSCOPE n. an instrument for examining the *larynx*.

LARYNGOSPASM n. closure of the larynx that blocks the passage of air to the lungs; usually associated with severe allergic reaction or severe laryngeal inflammation, esp. in young children.

LARYNGOTRACHEOBRON-CHITIS n. inflammation of the larynx, trachea, and bronchial passageways; it may be caused by bacterial or viral infection and is characterized by hoarseness, difficulty in breathing, and cough. Treatment depends on the cause; it may include steam inhalation, cough suppressants, and antibiotics, if indicated.

LARYNX n. the organ which contains the vocal cords and is responsible for sound production; it is part of the air passageway connecting the *pharynx* and the *trachea*, and it produces a bump—the Adam's apple—in front of the neck. adj. **laryngeal**

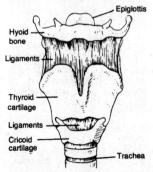

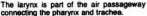

The larynx is part of the air passageway connecting the pharynx and trachea.

LASER n. acronym for Light Amplification by Stimulated Emission of Radiation; an instrument that produces a very thin beam of light—of one wavelength—with radiation intense enough to be used surgically to destroy tissue or to separate parts.

LASIX n. trade name for the diuretic furosemide used to treat *hypertension* and *edema*.

LASSA FEVER n. a highly contagious viral desease, largely confined to central West Africa; it is characterized by fever, inflammation of the pharynx, difficulty in swallowing, and bruises, frequently with complications of renal failure leading to cardiac failure and death.

LATENCY PHASE n. in psychology, a period in psychosexual development, generally between the ages of 5 and puberty, during which the sex drive is not active, but is sublimated into other activities (compare *anal phase*; *oedipal phase*; *oral phase*; *phallic phase*).

LATENT adj. dormant; existing as a potential (e.g., **latent diabetes**, a mild disorder of carbohydrate metabolism occurring only when stress loads of *glucose* are given).

LATENT SCHIZOPHRENIA n. a form of schizophrenia characterized by mild symptoms and/or a preexisting tendency to the disease in its usual form; also called **borderline schizophrenia**.

LATERAL adj. pert. to a side; away from the center plane, as the cheeks are lateral to the nose.

LATERO- comb. form indicating an association with the side of something (e.g., **lateroabdominal**, at or toward the side of the abdomen).

LAUGHING GAS see *nitrous oxide*.

LAVAGE n. the process of washing out an organ, esp. the stomach (gastric lavage), bladder, or paranasal sinuses (see also *irrigation*).

LAW n. in science, a reliable principle, standard, relationship, or observation; a fact, e.g., the Bell-Magendie law states that, in the spinal nerves, the forward (anterior) roots relate to motor function and the back (posterior) roots relate to sensory function. (See also *all-or-nothing law*).

LAXATION n. a bowel movement.

LAXATIVE n. an agent that promotes bowel evacuation by a mild action, by increasing the bulk of the stool or softening it, or by lubricating the intestinal tract (compare *cathartic*).

L-DOPA see *levodopa*.

LE abbreviation for lupus erythematosus (see *systemic lupus erythematosus*).

LEAD n. 1. a metallic element (see Table of Elements) (see also *lead poisoning*); 2. a connection attached to the body to record electrical activity, as in an *electrocardiograph* or *electroencephalograph*.

LEAD POISONING n. a toxic condition caused by inhaling or ingesting lead or lead compounds (e.g., in some paints). Acute poisoning causes gastrointestinal disturbances, mental disturbances, and paralysis of the extremities, sometimes followed by convulsions and collapse. Chronic poisoning causes irritability, anorexia, and anemia, and often progresses to produce acute symptoms.

LEARNING DISABILITY n. any of several abnormal conditions of children who, although having at least average intelligence, have difficulty in learning specific skills—e.g., reading (dyslexia) or writing (dysgraphia)—or have other problems associated with normal learning procedures. It may result from psychological or organic causes or from slow development of motor skills, but in many cases the cause is unknown (see also *attention deficit syndrome*).

LEBOYER METHOD OF CHILDBIRTH n. an approach to childbirth, formulated by the French obstretrician Charles Leboyer, that aims to minimize the trauma of birth and to provide as gentle and pleasant an introduction to life outside the uterus as possible for the newborn. Delivery typically occurs in a quiet, dimly lit room; the infant's head is not pulled and the infant is not overstimulated in any way; immediate maternal-infant bonding is encouraged (compare *Bradley method of childbirth*; *Lamaze method of childbirth*; *Read method of childbirth*) (see also *natural childbirth*).

LECITHIN n. any of a group of phospholipids essential for the metabolism of fats; a deficiency leads to liver and kidney disorders, high serum cholesterol levels, and *atherosclerosis*. Rich food sources include egg yolk, corn, and soybeans. Lecithins are also used in the processing of foods, drugs, and cosmetics.

LEDERCILLIN VK n. trade name for an antibacterial (penicillin V potassium) of the *penicillin* family.

LEECH n. a worm, some species of which are parasitic, sucking blood from humans and other animals. Leeches were once used in medicine for *blood-letting*.

LEFT-HANDEDNESS n. a tendency to prefer use of the left hand in performing tasks, such as writing, grasping, and throwing; also: **sinistrality**.

LEG n. a supporting limb; in humans, either of the lower extremities, including femur, patella, tibia, and fibula bones; specifi-

cally, the lower leg, from the ankle to the knee and including the tibia and fibula.

LEGIONNAIRE'S DISEASE n. an acute pneumonia caused by the bacterium *Legionella pneumophilia*; symptoms include muscle pain, fever, cough, chills, and chest pain. Treatment is by *erythromycin*.

LEIO- comb. form indicating an association with smoothness (e.g., **leiodermia**, smooth, glossy skin).

LEIOMYOMA n. a benign tumor of smooth muscle, most often occurring in the *uterus* (leiomyofibroma) or digestive tract.

LEIOMYOSARCOMA n. a malignant tumor of smooth muscle, occurring most often in the bladder, prostate, uterus, or digestive tract.

LEISHMANIASIS n. an infection, most common in warm climates, with protozoa of the genus *Leishmania*; it occurs in two forms: visceral (see *kala-azar*) and cutaneous, affecting skin tissues (see also *oriental sore*). Treatment often involves the use of antimony preparations.

LENS n. 1. in anatomy, the transparent crystalline structure of the eye, behind the pupil, that helps to focus light onto the *retina*. (In a *cataract*, the lens becomes cloudy); 2. a transparent material—glass or plastic—that is ground and shaped to refract light in a certain way; used in eyeglasses, contact lens, microscopes, and cameras. (see also *contact lens*; *lens implant*).

LENS IMPLANT n. an artificial clear plastic lens implanted in the eye, usually when the natural lens has been removed because of a *cataract* but sometimes to treat other eye abnormalities.

LENTE ILETIN n. trade name for an *insulin* preparation used in the treatment of *diabetes mellitus*.

LENTE INSULIN n. trade name for an *insulin* preparation used in the treatment of *diabetes mellitus*.

LENTIGO n. a brown, roundish, flat spot on the skin, often the result of exposure to the sun. pl. **lentigines**

LEONTIASIS n. a condition in which a person has a somewhat lionlike facial expression or head structure; occurs in some diseases (e.g., *leprosy*).

LEPER n. a person who has *leprosy*.

LEPROSY n. a chronic, communicable disease, caused by *Mycobacterium leprae*, that is widespread throughout the world, chiefly in tropical and subtropical regions. In **tuberculoid leprosy** tumorlike changes occur in the skin and cutaneous nerves; in the more serious and progressive **lepromatous leprosy**, lesions spread over much of the body with widespread nerve involvement affecting many systems of the body. Treatment usually involves the use of *sulfones* (esp. dapsone); a vaccine with promising results is also being used; also called **Hansen's disease**. adj. **leprous**

-LEPSIA, -LEPSIS, -LEPSY comb. form indicating an association with seizures (e.g., *epilepsy*).

LEPTO- comb. form indicating meaning "thin," "narrow," "fragile" (e.g., **leptocephaly**, an abnormally narrow head).

LEPTOMENINGES n. the *arachnoid* membrane and *pia mater*, the inner two of the three layers covering the brain and spinal cord (see also *meninges*).

LEPTOMENINGITIS n. inflammation of the *leptomeninges*—the *arachnoid* and *pia mater*.

LEPTOSPIROSIS n. an infection caused by the spirochete *Leptospira interrogans*, transmitted to humans from infected animals (esp. dogs and rats), often from their urine. Symptoms include chills, fever, muscle pain, and jaundice. Treatment is by antibiotics, and most cases are mild, but severe cases (*Weil's disease*) can cause liver and kidney damage.

LERESIS n. talkativeness, rambling speech, esp. in the aged.

LESBIAN n. a female homosexual; a female whose sexual preference is for other women. n. **lesbianism**

LESION n. general term for any visible, local abnormality of tissue, such as an injury, wound, boil, sore, rash.

LET-DOWN n. sensation in the breasts of nursing women as the milk flows into the ducts of the breast, as when the infant begins to suck or when the mother prepares to nurse; also: **milk-ejection reflex**.

LETHAL adj. pert. to or causing death.

LETHAL DOSE n. the amount of a drug that will cause death.

LETHAL GENE n. any gene that produces an effect that causes the death of the organism at any stage, from fertilized egg to advanced age. The gene that causes *Huntington's chorea* is an example of a lethal gene.

LETHARGY n. a state of sluggishness, apathy, unresponsiveness; found in certain diseases.

LEUCINE n. an amino acid, obtained by the digestion of proteins, that is essential for growth.

LEUKEMIA n. one of the major types of cancer; a malignant neoplasm of blood-forming tissues, characterized by abnormalities of the bone marrow, spleen, lymph nodes, and liver and by rapid and uncontrolled proliferation of abnormal numbers and forms of leukocytes (white blood cells).

Leukemia may be acute, rapidly progressing from signs of fatigue and weight loss to extreme weakness, repeated infections, and fever; or it may be chronic, progressing slowly over a period of years. Leukemia is usually classified according to the type of white blood cell that is proliferating abnormally. Treatment involves chemotherapy, blood transfusions, antibiotics to control infections, and sometimes, bone marrow transplants. Also called **cancer of the blood**. See also *acute myelocytic leukemia*; *acute lymphoid leukemia*; *chronic lymphocytic leukemia*; *chronic myelocytic leukemia*.   adj. **leukemic**

LEUKERAN n. trade name for the antineoplastic *chlorambucil* used to treat certain cancers.

LEUKOCYTE n. a white blood cell. There are five types of leukocytes: three granulocytes with granules in the cytoplasm—neutrophils, basophils, and eosiniphils—and two agranulocytes, lacking granules in the cytoplasm—lymphocytes and monocytes. An important part of the body's defense mechanism, leukocytes phagocytose bacteria and fungi and function in allergic reactions and the response to cellular injury.

LEUKO- comb. form indicating an association with white blood cells (e.g., **leukopoiesis**, the development of white blood cells).

LEUKOCYTOSIS n. an abnormal increase in the number of white cells in the blood; it frequently occurs as a result of infection, esp. bacterial infection; a very large increase occurs in *leukemia*.

LEUKODERMA n. loss of skin pigment in a localized area (compare *vitiligo*).

LEUKOENCEPHALITIS n. inflammation of the white matter of the brain.

LEUKOMA n. a white opacity in the cornea of the eye, most often the result of corneal inflammation or ulceration, sometimes congenital; also: **leucoma**.

LEUKONYCHIA n. white discoloration of the nails; it may result from trauma, certain systemic disorders, or from unknown causes.

LEUKOPENIA n. an abnormal decrease in the number of leukocytes (white blood cells) in the blood, to fewer than 5,000 per cubic millimeter; it may affect one type or all types of white blood cells. It may occur as an adverse drug reaction or as a result of radiation exposure, poisoning, or other abnormal condition (e.g., *aplastic anemia*) (compare *leukocytosis*).   adj. **leukopenic**

LEUKOPLAKIA n. thickened white patches on mucous membranes, esp. those of the mouth region and genitalia; they can become malignant (compare *lichen planus*).

LEUKORRHEA n. a whitish discharge from the *vagina*; it occurs normally, varying in amount during different phases of the *menstrual cycle* and during pregnancy, lactation, and after menopause. A large increase in amount or a change in color or odor usually indicates infection in the reproductive tract.

LEUKOTRICHIA n. the condition of having white hair.

LEVALLORPHAN n. a drug, sometimes known under the trade name Lorfan, that counteracts the respiratory depression produced by narcotics (such as *morphine*), without affecting their pain-reducing effects.

LEVATOR n. 1. a muscle that lifts or raises a structure (e.g., the levator scapulae lifts the shoulder blade); 2. a surgical instrument used to lift depressed bone fragments in a fracture.

LEVO- comb. form meaning "left" (e.g., **levorotation**, turning to the left).

LEVODOPA (L-DOPA) n. a drug, known under several trade names, including Bendopa, Brocadopa, and Larodopa, that is used to treat *parkinsonism*. Adverse side effects include anorexia, gastrointestinal disturbances, and movement disorders.

LEVORPHANOL n. a narcotic drug, known under the trade name Dromoran, used to treat severe pain. Adverse effects include gastrointestinal disturbances, hypotension, cardiac arrhythmias, and the potential for dependence.

LEYDIG CELLS n. cells in the *testes* that secrete the hormone *testosterone*.

LEVULOSE see *fructose*.

LH abbreviation for *luteinizing hormone*.

LIBIDO n. the sexual drive; in psychoanalytic theory, one of the major drives that is a source of energy.

LIBRAX n. trade name for fixed combination drug containing the sedative *chlordiazepoxide* (Librium) and the anticholinergic clidinium, used to treat gastrointestinal spasm and discomfort.

LIBRITABS n. trade name for the antianxiety agent *chlordiazepoxide*.

LIBRIUM n. trade name for the antianxiety agent *chlordiazepoxide*.

LICHEN n. any of several skin disorders characterized by thickened, hardened lesions grouped closely together.

LICHEN PLANUS n. a skin disorder characterized by small, flat purplish, usually itchy, papules, occurring most often on the wrists, forearms, and thighs (compare *leukoplakia*).

LICHENIFICATION n. a thickening and hardening of skin, often resulting from scratching or irritation.

LIDOCAINE n. a local anesthetic agent, known under the trade names Lidocaine and Xylocaine, used topically on the skin and mucuous membranes and parenterally to treat cardiac arrhythmia. Adverse effects from systemic use include cardiac arrest and central nervous system disturbances; from topical use, hypersensivity reactions.

LIDOSPORIN n. trade name for a fixed combination drug, containing the antibacterial *polymyxin* and the local anesthetic *lidocaine*, used to treat ear infections.

LIEN see *spleen*.

LIENO- comb. form indicating an association with the *spleen* (e.g., **lienocele**, rupture of the spleen).

LIGAMENT n. a shiny, usually whitish, band of fibrous connective tissue that binds joints together and connects bones and cartilage (compare *tendon*).

LIGATION n. tying with silk thread, wire, or other filament a blood vessel or duct; it is done to prevent bleeding (e.g., during surgery) or to prevent passage of material through a duct (e.g., to prevent fertilization from occurring in the *Fallopian tube*) (see also *tubal ligation*).

LIGATURE n. a filament (catgut), thread (silk), or wire (chromic) used to encircle a part to close it off (as a blood vessel) or to fasten or tie the part.

LIGHT ADAPTATION n. reflex changes in the eye to allow vision in increased light (e.g., in normal light after being in the dark or in very bright light after being in normal light); it involves a contraction of the *pupil* so that less light enters (compare *dark adaptation*).

LIGHT DIET n. a diet consisting of easily digested foods and avoiding highly seasoned and fried foods; suitable for convalescent and bedridden persons.

LIGHTENING n. descent of the *uterus* into the pelvic cavity occurring in late pregnancy; it leaves more room in the upper abdomen and changes the profile of the pregnant woman's abdomen. The baby is said "to have dropped."

LIGHT REFLEX see *pupillary reflex*.

LIMB n. an extremity of the body; an arm or leg.

LIMBIC SYSTEM n. a group of structures in the brain, including the *hippocampus*, cingulate gyrus, and amygdala, that is connected to and normally controlled by other parts of the brain (e.g., *hypothalamus*); the system is associated with emotions and feelings, such as anger, fear, and sexual arousal, but little is known about its function.

LIMBUS n. the outer edge or border of a part (e.g., **limbus corneae**, the edge where the cornea and sclera of the eye join). pl. **limbi** adj. **limbal, limbic**

LINCOCIN n. trade name for the antibacterial *lincomycin*.

LINCOMYCIN n. an antibiotic known under the trade names Lincocin and Mycivin, used to treat certain bacterial infections (e.g., *osteomyelitis*). Adverse effects include diarrhea and other, sometimes serious, gastrointestinal disturbances.

LINE n. 1. an elongated mark or stripe on the body; 2. the origin of an organisms or cell (as in cell line); also: **linea**. pl. **lineae**

LINGUA see *tongue*. pl. **linguae** adj. **lingual**

LINGUAL adj. pert. to the tongue (e.g., **lingual artery**, the artery that supplies the tongue and surrounding area).

LINGULA n. a tonguelike part, esp. lingula cerebelli, the thin forward projection of the *cerebellum* of the brain.

LINGUO- comb. form indicating an association with the *tongue* (e.g., **linguogingival**, pert. to the tongue and gingiva).

LINIMENT n. a preparation (usually containing an alcohol or oil) applied to the skin to relieve discomfort.

LINKED GENES n. genes located close together on the same chromosome that tend to be transmitted as a unit.

LIP n. 1. the soft external structures that form the top and bottom borders of the *mouth* cavity; 2. the liplike enclosures of the *vulva* (see *labia majora*; *labia minora*); 3. any liplike border of an organ or groove.

LIPASE n. any of several enzymes, secreted in the digestive tract, that catalyze the breakdown of fats.

LIPEMIA n. an abnormally high amount of fat in the blood.

LIPID n. any of a group of greasy organic compounds, including fatty acids, waxes, phospholipids, and steroids. Lipids are stored in the body and serve as energy reserves.

LIPIDOSIS n. any of several disorders of fat metabolism in which abnormal levels of certain lipids accumulate in the body. Among the disorders are *Gaucher's disease*, *Niemann-Pick disease*, and *Tay-Sachs disease*.

LIPO-HEPIN n. trade name for the anticoagulant *heparin*.

LIPO-LUTIN n. trade name for a *progesterone* compound.

LIPO- comb. form indicating an association with fats or lipids (e.g., **lipopexia**, the accumulation of fat in body tissues).

LIPOMA n. a benign tumor consisting of fat cells; also called **adipose tumor**. adj. **lipomatous**

LIPOMATOSIS n. a condition in which fat accumulates in tumorlike masses (*lipomas*) in the body.

LIPOPROTEIN n. a protein combined with a lipid; lipoproteins are found in blood plasma and lymph and transport lipids in the body.

LIPOSARCOMA n. a malignant tumor of fat cells.

LIQUAEMIN n. trade name for the anticoagulant *heparin*.

LIQUAMAR n. trade name for the anticoagulant *phenprocoumon*.

LIQUEFACTION n. the process of changing a solid or a gas into a liquid.

LIQUID DIET n. a diet consisting of foods that can be served in liquid or strained form, plus custards, puddings, and similar foods. It is prescribed after certain types of surgery and in some infectious and inflammatory conditions.

LISTERIOSIS n. an infectious disease, caused by the bacteria *Listeria monocytogenes*, common in many animals and occasionally transmitted to humans, esp. newborns or immunosuppressed persons. In humans, it causes a dark red rash, enlargement of the spleen and liver, *endocarditis*, fever, malaise, and other abnormalities, frequently progressing to *meningitis* and encephalitis. Treatment is by *antibiotics*.

LITHANE n. trade name for a *lithium* preparation used to treat some forms of depression and *bipolar disorder*.

LITHIUM n. a metallic element (see Table of Elements) (see also *lithium carbonate*).

LITHIUM CARBONATE n. a drug, known under the trade names Lithane and Lithonate, used to treat manic episodes of bipolar (manic-depressive) disorder. Adverse effects include kidney damage, salt and water retention, and sometimes disturbances in normal mental and muscular functioning.

LITHIASIS n. the formation of stones (calculi) in an internal organ (e.g., the gallbladder or kidney) (see also *cholelithiasis*; *renal calculus*).   adj. **lithiasic**

LITHONATE n. trade name for *lithium carbonate*.

LITHOTOMY n. surgical removal of a stone (calculus), esp. from the urinary tract.

LITHOTOMY POSITION n. position in which the person lies on his/her back with knees bent, thighs spread and rotated outward; used for a vaginal or rectal examination.

LITHURESIS n. passing of small stones or small pieces of a stone with the *urine*.

LIVE BIRTH n. the birth of an infant that exhibits any sign of life (e.g., respiration, movement of voluntary muscle, heartbeat), not dependent on the length of *gestation*. A live birth may not be *viable*.

LIVEDO n. a discolored area on the skin.

LIVER n. one of the largest and most complex organs of the body, located in the upper right part of the abdominal cavity. The liver weighs about 1 pound (1.6 kg) in males, a little less in females; is dark reddish-brown, soft, and solid; is divided into four lobes; and is supplied by two blood systems, the hepatic artery, bringing freshly oxygenated blood to the liver and the hepatic portal vein (part of the portal blood system) carrying nutrients from the stomach and intestines to the liver. The liver has numerous functions: it is a site of protein, carbohydrate, and fat metabolism; it helps regulate the level of blood sugar, converting excess *glucose* into *glycogen* and storing it; it secretes *bile*, which is stored in the gallbladder before its release into the intestinal tract; it synthesizes substances involved in blood clotting (e.g., fibrinogen); it produces plasma proteins; it synthesizes vitamin A; it detoxifies poisonous substances; and it breaks down worn out erythrocytes (red blood cells).   adj. **hepatic**

Front view of the liver.

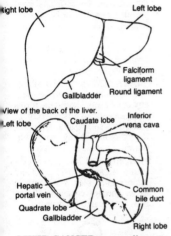
View of the back of the liver.

LIVER CANCER n. a malignant neoplastic disease of the liver occurring most often as a metastasis from another cancer. Primary liver cancer is common in parts of Africa and Asia, where it is often associated with aflatoxins, but it is rare in the United States, often associated with cirrhosis of the liver. Symptoms include loss of appetite, weakness, bloating, jaundice, and enlarged, tender liver and mild upper abdominal discomfort. The lesions often matastasize through the portal and lymphatic systems. Treatment depends on the nature and extent of the neoplasm; it may involve removal of a primary tumor and/or chemotherapy.

LOBAR PNEUMONIA n. a severe, bacterial (often streptococcal) infection of one or more lobes of the lung; it is characterized by fever, cough, rapid swallow breathing, cyanosis, inflammation of the membrane lining of the lung, nausea, and vomiting, and, if untreated, consolidation of lung tissue. Treatment is by antibiotics (compare *bronchopneumonia*).

LOBE n. a rounded part of an organ, separated from other parts of the organ by connective tissue or fissures; the brain, liver, and lungs are divided into lobes.

LOBECTOMY n. surgical procedure in which a lobe of the lung is removed; performed to treat intractable tuberculosis or bronchiectasis or to remove a malignant tumor.

LOBOTOMY n. a surgical procedure in which certain nerve fibers in the frontal lobe of the brain are severed (usually by a wire inserted through the eye socket) to prevent transmission of various impulses; it was once commonly used to treat certain mental illness, but is now rarely performed because it has many undesirable effects; also: **leukotomy**

LOBULE n. a small lobe or part of a lobe.   adj. **lobular**

LOCAL adj. pert. to a small circumscribed area.

LOCAL ANESTHESIA n. the administration of a local anesthetic agent to induce loss of sensation in a small area of the body. It may be applied topically, as in spraying on the skin before removing a small lesion; or it may be injected subcutaneously. Brief dental and surgical operations are the most common indications for use (compare *general anesthesia*; *regional anesthesia*; *topical anesthesia*).

LOCAL ANESTHETIC n. an agent that reduces or eliminates sensation, esp. pain, in a limited area of the body by blocking the transmission of nerve impulses in the area.

LOCALIZATION n. limiting a condition, effect, or finding to a given area or part.   v. **localize** adj. **localized**

LOCHIA n. the discharge from the *vagina* after childbirth. The discharge gradually decreases in amount and changes in color (from red to yellowish to gray-white) during the six weeks following childbirth.

LOCKJAW n. a common term for *tetanus*, during the late stages of which the jaw muscles sometimes spasm.

LOCULUS n. a small cavity or space. pl. **loculi** adj. **locular, loculate**

LOCUS n. a specific site, esp. the location of a *gene* on its chromosome. pl. **loci**

LOCUS OF INFECTION n. the specific site in the body where an infection originates.

LOESTRIN n. trade name for an *oral contraceptive*, containing *estradiol* and *norethindrone*.

LOGO- comb. form indicating an association with words (e.g., **logomania**, talking excessively).

LOGORRHEA n. rapid flow of words, often incoherent; associated with some mental disorders.

LOIN n. region of the back and side of the body between the lowest rib and the pelvis; the lumbus.

LOMOTIL n. trade name for a fixed-combination antidiarrheal drug.

LOMUSTINE n. an antineoplastic drug, known as CeeNU, used in the treatment of several types of cancer. Adverse effects include nausea, vomiting and bone marrow depression.

LONG-ACTING DRUG n. a drug that has prolonged effect due to the slow release of its active principle or to the continued absorption of the drug over an extended period (compare *short-acting drug*).

LONG-TERM MEMORY n. the ability to recall ideas, sensations, events for a long period.

LONITEN n. trade name for the vasodilator *minoxidil*, used in the treatment of severe and hard-to-control *hypertension*.

LOOP n. 1. a band that forms a circle or U-shaped curve (e.g., the loop of Henle, a U-shaped part of the inner *kidney*); 2. colloquial, a type of *intrauterine device*.

LO/OVRAL n. trade name for an *oral contraceptive* containing *estradiol* and *norgestrel*.

LORAZEPAM n. a benzodiazepine *tranquilizer* used to treat anxiety, tension, and some forms of insomnia. Adverse effects include drowsiness, and, after prolonged or high-dosage use, withdrawal symptoms.

LORDOSIS n. 1. the normal curvature of the cervical (neck) and lumbar spine seen from the side as an anterior concavity; 2. an increased degree of curvature.

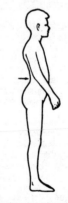

In lordosis, there is increased curvature in part of the back.

LOTION n. a liquid applied externally to treat a skin disorder or to protect the skin.

LOU GEHRIG'S DISEASE see *amyotrophic lateral sclerosis*.

LOW-BIRTH-WEIGHT INFANT (LBW) n. an infant born

weighing less than 2,500 grams regardless of gestational age. These babies are at risk for developing lack of oxygen during labor, and low blood sugar and slow growth and development after birth.

LOWER RESPIRATORY TRACT n. that part of the respiratory tract that includes the left and right bronchi and the lungs (compare *upper respiratory tract*).

LOW-FAT DIET n. a diet containing limited amounts of fat; omitting cream, fried foods, and foods prepared in oil, gravy, and butter; and stressing high carbohydrate foods. It is used in some gallbladder conditions and other disorders.

LOW-SALT DIET   see *low sodium diet*.

LOW-SODIUM DIET n. a diet that limits the intake of sodium chloride (salt); it is often used in treatment of *hypertension*, *edema*, kidney or liver disease, and certain other disorders. Foods such as bacon, frankfurters, salted butter, ham, sausage, cheese and many canned or frozen foods are prohibited.

LOXAPINE n. a *tranquilizer*, known under the trade name Loxitane, used to treat *schizophrenia*. Adverse effects include low blood pressure, liver toxicity, and hypersensitivity reactions.

LOXITANE n. trade name for the tranquilizer *loxapine*.

LSD abbreviation of *lysergic acid diethylamide*.

LUCID adj. clear, understandable, as in lucid statements.   n. **lucidity**

LUMBAGO n. pain in the lumbar region of the back, usually caused by muscle strain, arthritis, vascular insufficiency, or ruptured intervertebral disk.

LUMBAR adj. pert. to that part of the back between the ribs and the pelvis.

LUMBAR NERVES n. the five pairs of spinal nerves arising from the lumbar portion of the *spinal cord*.

LUMBAR PLEXUS n. a network of nerves formed by the ventral divisions of some of the lumbar nerves; it is located inside the posterior abdominal wall and supplies the caudal part of the abdominal wall, the front of the thigh, and part of the middle leg.

LUMBAR PUNCTURE n. the insertion of a hollow needle into the subarachnoid space of the lumbar region of the *spinal cord* for diagnostic (e.g., to obtain a sample of *cerebrospinal fluid* for analysis) or therapeutic (e.g., to remove blood or pus or inject a drug) purposes. Side effects of the procedure include headache, nausea, and infection. Also called **spinal tap**.

LUMBO- comb. form indicating an association with the lumbar region of the spinal column, the small of the back (e.g., **lumbocostal**, pert. to the loins and ribs).

LUMBOSACRAL adj. pert. to the loins (small-of-the-back area) and sacrum (the back part of the pelvis between the hips).

LUMBOSACRAL PLEXUS n. a network of nerves formed by the ventral divisions of the lumbar, sacral, and coccygeal nerves; it supplies the lower limbs, perineum, and coccygeal area.

LUMBUS   see *loin*.

LUMEN n. a cavity, canal, or channel within an organ or tube; the space inside a structure. pl. **lumina**   adj. **lumenal**

LUMINAL n. trade name for the anticonvulsant and sedative *phenobarbital*.

LUMPECTOMY n. surgical removal of a tumor without removal of much surrounding tissue or nearby lymph nodes; performed in some cases of breast tumor and other tumors.

LUMPY JAW see *actinomycosis*.

LUNATE BONE n. one of the *carpal* (wrist) bones.

LUNG n. either of a pair of highly elastic, spongy organs in the chest that are the main organs of respiration, inhaling air from which oxygen is taken and exhaling carbon dioxide. The lungs are composed of lobes, the right with three, the left with two. The lobes are divided into lobules, each of which contains blood vessels, lymphatics, nerves, and ducts connecting the *alveoli*, or air spaces, where the actual oxygen-carbon dioxide exchange takes place.

LUNG CANCER n. one of the most common types of cancer. Predisposing factors include cigarette smoking and exposure to asbestos, vinyl chloride, coal products, and other industrial and chemical products. Symptoms include cough, difficulty in breathing, blood-tinged sputum, and repeated infections. Treatment depends on the type, site, and extent of the cancer and may include surgery, chemotherapy, and radiation.

LUPUS see *systemic lupus erythematosus (SLE)*; *lupus vulgaris*;

LUPUS ERYTHEMATOSUS see *systemic lupus erythematosus*.

LUPUS VULGARIS n. a rare form of *tuberculosis* characterized by skin ulcers that heal slowly and leave deep scars.

LUTEAL adj. pert. to the *corpus luteum*.

LUTEAL PHASE n. the second half of the menstrual cycle during which the *corpus luteum* secretes the hormone *progesterone*, which, in turn, causes the *endometrium*

TRACHEA AND LUNGS

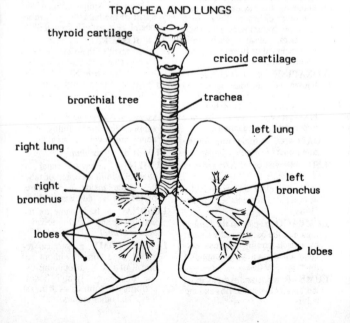

thyroid cartilage

cricoid cartilage

bronchial tree

trachea

left lung

right lung

right bronchus

left bronchus

lobes

lobes

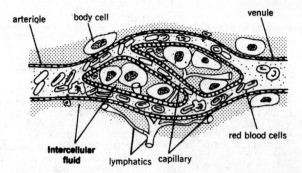

Lymph circulation

(uterine lining) to become rich and developed for implantation of a fertilized egg. If fertilization does not occur, progesterone secretion decreases and about 14 days after *ovulation*, the endometrium is shed in *menstruation*.

LUTEINIZING HORMONE (LH) n. a hormone produced by the *anterior pituitary gland* that stimulates the secretion of sex hormones by the *testes* and *ovaries* and is involved in the production of mature *sperm* and *ova*; also called **interstitial cell stimulating hormone (ICSH)**.

LUTEOTROPIN see *prolactin*.

LUXATION n. misalignment, displacement, or dislocation of an organ or joint (see also *subluxation*).

LYME ARTHRITIS n. an acute inflammatory disease, thought to be caused by a tick-borne virus, that affects one or more joints (esp. the knees and other large joints), causing heat, swelling, and skin redness, often accompanied by chills, fever, and malaise. Cardiac abnormalities and neurological complications sometimes occur. Treatment is by pain relievers (e.g., aspirin) and corticosteroids.

LYMPH n. a thin fluid that bathes the tissues of the body, circulates through lymph vessels, is filtered in lymph nodes, and enters the blood system through the thoracic duct at the junction of the subclavian vein and jugular vein. It contains chyle and leukocytes (mostly lymphocytes), but otherwise is similar to *plasma*.   adj. **lymphatic, lymphoid, lymphous**

LYMPH-, LYMPHO- comb. form indicating an association with lymph (e.g., **lymphadenopathy**, any disease of the lymph system).

LYMPHADENITIS n. inflammation of the lymph nodes; it usually occurs as a result of systemic neoplastic disease, bacterial infection, or inflammatory condition.

LYMPHANGIECTASIS n. dilatation of lymph vessels; also: **lymphangiectasia**.

LYMPHANGIOMA n. a benign tumor made up of dilated lymph vessels.

LYMPHANGITIS n. inflammation of a lymphatic vessel that usually results from a streptococcal infection, causing red streaks extending from the infected area, accompanied by fever, headache, and muscle pain. Treatment is by *antibiotics*.

LYMPHATIC adj. pert. to the *lymphatic system*.

LYMPHATIC SYSTEM n. a network of capillaries, vessels, ducts, nodes, and organs that help maintain the fluid environment of the body and help to protect the body by producing lymph and conveying it around the body. Lymphatic capillaries unite to form lymph vessels, which have numerous valves to control lymph flow and nodes to filter the lymph. The lymphatic vessels lead to two large vessels: the thoracic duct and right lymphatic duct, both in the neck, from which the lymph drains into the bloodstream. Specialized lymph organs include the *spleen*, *thymus*, and *tonsils*.

LYMPHEDEMA n. an accumulation of lymph in tissues, leading to swelling; it occurs most often in the legs. It can be congenital or result from lymph vessel obstruction from tumor or imflammation.

LYMPH NODE n. any of the many small structures that filter lymph and produce *lymphocytes*. Lymph nodes are concentrated in several areas of the body, such as the armpit, groin, and neck. Also called **lymph gland**.

LYMPHOCYTE n. an agranulocytic leukocyte (white blood cell) that normally makes up about 25% of the total white blood cell count but increases in the presence of infection. They occur in two forms: B cells, the chief agents of the humoral immune system, that

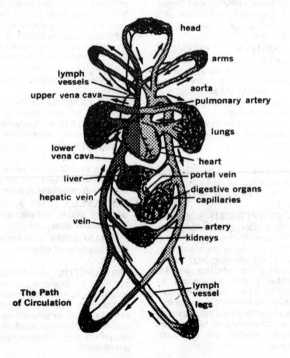

The Path of Circulation

head
arms
lymph vessels
upper vena cava
aorta
pulmonary artery
lower vena cava
lungs
liver
heart
hepatic vein
portal vein
digestive organs
capillaries
vein
artery
kidneys
lymph vessel
legs

recognize the specific antigens and produce antibodies against them; and T cells, the agents of the cell-mediated immune system, that secrete immunologically active compounds and assist B cells in their function.

LUMPHOCYTOPENIA n. a lower-than-normal number of *lymphocytes* in the blood circulation, due to malignancy, nutritional deficiency, blood disorder, or certain other diseases.

LYMPHOGRANULOMA VENEREUM (LGV) n. an infectious disease, caused by the bacterium *Chlamydia trachomatis* and transmitted by sexual contact. It is characterized by genital lesions and swelling of lymph nodes in the groin area, headache, fever, and malaise. Treatment is by *antibiotics*, usually *tetracyclines*. Also called **lymphopathia venereum**.

LYMPHOMA n. a neoplasm of lymph tissue, usually malignant; one of four major types of cancer. Lymphomas differ widely in the types of cells affected and the prognosis; general characteristics include enlarged lymph nodes, weakness, fever, weight loss, and malaise followed by enlargement of the spleen and liver. Types of lymphomas include *Burkitt's lymphoma* and *Hodgkin's disease*. Treatment is usually by chemotherapy and radiotherapy. adj. **lymphomatoid**

LYMPHOPENIA see *lymphocytopenia*.

LYMPHOPOIESIS n. the production of lymphocytes, occurring mainly in the bone marrow, lymph nodes, spleen, and thymus.

LYMPHURIA n. the presence of lymph in the *urine*.

LYPRESSIN n. an antidiuretic and vasoconstrictor used to treat *diabetes insipidus*. Adverse effects include angina and nausea.

LYSERGIC ACID DIETHYLAMIDE (LSD) n. a hallucinogen; a drug that produces illusions, hallucinations, distorted perceptions, feelings of panic, depression, or paranoia, and widespread physical symptoms (e.g., increased body temperature and blood pressure, dilation of the pupils, muscle weakness). Psychological dependence may occur. The drug is not used therapeutically but is a drug of abuse. Treatment of LSD intoxication involves attempts to calm the person and the use of tranquilizers and barbiturates. Slang: **acid**.

LYSINE n. an essential amino acid, needed for growth in children.

LYSINE INTOLERANCE n. a disorder in which a lack of or defect in certain enzymes produces an inability to utilize the amino acid lysine, resulting in symptoms of weakness, vomiting, and coma. Treatment is by limiting lysine content in the diet.

LYSINEMIA n. an inborn error of metabolism in which a defect in or lack of enzymes leads to an inability to metabolize the amino acid lysine; it is characterized by muscle weakness and mental retardation. Treatment is by limiting the intake of lysine in the diet. (compare *lysine intolerance*).

LYSIS n. destruction or breakdown of one substance (e.g., a cell or microorganism) by a specific agent.

LYSOGENIC adj. producing *lysis*.

LYSOSOME n. an *organelle* found in the *cytoplasm* of most cells, esp. *leukocytes* and kidney and liver cells, which contains enzymes that function in digestive processes within cells.

LYSOZYME n. an enzyme, found in tears, saliva, and sweat and certain other substances, that functions in the destruction of the cell walls of certain bacteria; also: **muramidase**

m

MACERATE v. to soften something, as an organ or part. n. **maceration** adj. **macerative**

MACR-, MACRO- comb. form indicating abnormally large size (e.g., **macroblepharia**, oversized eyelids).

MACRENCEPHALY n. an abnormally large brain. adj. **macroencephalic**

MACROCEPHALY n. a congenital disorder characterized by an abnormally large head and brain, usually resulting in mental and growth retardation. It differs from *hydrocephalus*, in that the overgrowth is symmetrical, and there is no increased intracranial pressure.

MACROCYTE n. an abnormally large *erythrocyte* (red blood cell) occurring in *megaloblastic anemia*. adj. **macrocytic**

MACROCYTIC ANEMIA n. a blood disorder, often caused by deficiency of folic acid and vitamin B_{12}, in which red blood cell production is impaired and abnormally large and fragile red blood cells are present.

MACRODANTIN n. trade name for the antibacterial *nitrofurantoin*, used to treat urinary tract infections.

MACROGLOSSIA n. a congenital disorder characterized by an abnormally large tongue, seen in Down's syndrome and certain other disorders.

MACROPHAGE n. a *phagocyte*, a cell that engulfs and digests invading microorganisms and cell debris. Some are fixed (e.g., in the liver and spleen); others circulate in the blood.

MACULA n. 1. a small pigmented spot, such as a freckle, that is different from surrounding tissue; 2. macula lutea, a small yellow spot on the *retina* where vision is most acute. pl.

maculae adj. **macular, maculated**

MACULE n. a small blemish or discoloration that is not raised above the skin surface (e.g., freckle) (compare *papule*). adj. **macular**

MAGNESIUM n. a metallic element essential to normal body functioning (see Table of Elements).

MAGNESIUM SULFATE n. a salt of magnesium used orally to treat constipation and heartburn and parenterally to prevent seizures, esp. in *pre-eclampsia*.

MAJOR AFFECTIVE DISORDER n. any of a group of psychotic disorders not caused by organic abnormality of the brain and characterized by persistent disturbances of mood and thought processes and inappropriate emotional responses, as occurs in some forms of *bipolar disorder*.

MAJOR SURGERY n. any surgical procedure that requires general anesthesia or assistance in respiration (compare *minor surgery*).

MALA n. the cheek or cheek bone.

MALACIA n. a state of abnormal softening or sponginess (e.g., *osteomalacia*). adj. **malacic**

MALABSORPTION n. abnormal absorption of nutrients from the digestive tract, occurring in malnutrition, *celiac disease*, *sprue*, and other disorders that impair normal absorption; see also *malabsorption syndrome*.

MALABSORPTION SYNDROME n. a complex of symptoms, including loss of appetite, bloating, weight loss, muscle pain, and stools with high fat content, that result from abnormal intestinal absorption and occur in celiac disease, sprue, cystic fibrosis, and certain other disorders.

MALAISE n. a vague feeling of weakness or illness, often an early sign of illness.

MALARIA n. a serious infectious illness characterized by reccurrent episodes of chills, fever, headache, anemia, muscle ache, and an enlarged spleen. It is caused by *Plasmodium* protozoa, transmitted from human to human through the bite of an infected *Anopheles* mosquito or through blood transfusions or infected hypodermic needles; it is largely confined to tropical and subtropical areas. Treatment is by *chloroquine*, or in hard to treat cases, a combination of *quinine*, *sulfonamides*, and other drugs. Prevention includes removal of swampy areas where *Anopheles* mosquitos breed, the use of insecticides and mosquito netting, and the use of antimalarial drugs when travelling in malaria areas.

MALATHION POISONING n. a toxic condition caused by ingestion or inhalation of the insecticide malathion; it is characterized by vomiting, nausea, abdominal cramps, weakness, breathing difficulties, and confusion. Treatment includes atropine, gastric lavage, respiratory assistance, cathartics, and oxygen.

MALE n. the organism that produces sperm to fertilize the female's eggs for the production of children; men and boys. adj. **masculine**

MALIGNANT adj. worsening or progressing toward death, esp. a cancer that is invasive and metastatic (spreading) (compare *benign*).

MALIGNANT HYPERTENSION n. the most lethal form of *hypertension* (either essential or secondary), characterized by very elevated blood pressure that produces damage in the inner linings of the blood vessels and in the heart, spleen, kidneys, and brain, often leading to death.

MALIGNANT HYPERTHERMIA (MH) n. a hereditary condition (*autosomal dominant disorder*) in which very high body temperatures and muscle rigidity occur when the person is exposed to certain anesthetics (e.g., halothane, methoxyflurane). Treatment includes cooling, the administration of oxygen, and the reestablishment of normal electrolyte balances.

MALIGNANT NEOPLASM n. a tumor that tends to grow and spread to other body parts, in most cases leading to death unless treated.

MALIGNANT TUMOR see *malignant neoplasm*.

MALINGERING n. the deliberate feigning of the symptoms of a disease to achieve some desired end; pretending illness. v. **malinger**

MALLEOLUS n. a bumplike projection on a bone, as on the inner and outer sides of the ankle. pl. **malleoli** adj. **malleolar**

MALLEUS n. one of the three small bones of the middle ear (the others are the incus and the stapes), connecting the *tympanic membrane* to the incus.

MALNUTRITION n. a state of poor nutrition, resulting from an insufficient, excessive, or unbalanced diet or from impaired ability to absorb and assimilate foods.

MALOCCLUSION n. a condition in which the teeth of the opposing jaws do not contact or mesh normally; it is often corrected by orthodontics (see also *occlusion*).

MALPHIGIAN CORPUSCLE n. any of a number of small bodies in the cortex of the *kidney* that contain a Bowman's capsule and *glomerulus*.

MALTA FEVER see *brucellosis*.

MAMA n. the breast; the milk-giving gland in the female. pl. **mammae** adj. **mammary**

MAMM-, MAMMO- comb. form indicating an association with the breast or milk-secreting glands (e.g., **mammogenesis**, the formation and development of the milk-giving glands).

MAMMOGRAM n. an X-ray film of the soft tissue of the *breast*.

MAMMOGRAPHY n. procedure in which the soft tissues of the breast are X rayed to detect benign or malignant tumors. Periodic mammography is generally recommended for women thought at high risk for breast cancer and in certain other situations.

MAMMOTHERMOGRAPHY n. a diagnostic procedure in which infrared detectors are used to detect warm and cold areas (thermography) of the breast as a means of detecting tumors (compare *mammography*).

MANDELAMINE n. trade name for the antibacterial *methenamine*, used to treat urinary tract infections.

MANDIBLE n. the large bone making up the lower jaw, consisting of a horizontal part, a horseshoe-shaped body, and two perpendicular branches that connect to the body. The mandible contains sockets for the 16 lower teeth and grooves and attachments for

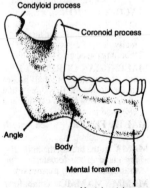

MANDIBLE

Condyloid process

Coronoid process

Angle

Body

Mental foramen

Mental protuberance

Lateral view of the mandible, or lower jaw.

the facial artery and various muscles (compare *maxilla*).

MANDOL n. trade name for a *cephalosporin* antibiotic (cefamandole nafate).

MANEUVER n. a manipulation; a movement of parts or a change of position, usually done by use of the hands (e.g., a manipulation of the fetus to aid delivery).

MANGANESE n. a metallic element important in trace amounts in metabolism (see Table of Elements).

MANIA n. a mood disorder, occurring in *bipolar disorder*, *delirium*, and certain other major affective disorders, in which the person tends to respond excessively, as with abnormal amounts of motion, overtalkativeness, elation, hyperactivity, and sometimes violent and destructive behavior. adj. **maniacal**

MANIC-DEPRESSIVE PSYCHOSIS see *bipolar disorder*.

MANIC-DEPRESSIVE n. a person whose mental state periodically swings from mania to depression (see *bipolar disorder*).

MANIPULATION n. the skillful use of hands to reduce a fracture; to diagnose, as in palpation; or to perform other diagnostic or therapuetic maneuvers (e.g., move a fetus before birth).

MANNITOL n. a diuretic, sometimes known under the trade name Osmitrol, used to promote the excretion of urine, to decrease abnormally high pressure in the eye or cranium, or to test kidney function. Adverse effects include heart abnormalities, edema of the lungs, headache, and vomiting.

MANTOUX TEST n. a skin test to determine past or present infection with *tuberculosis*. A protein derivative of the tubercle bacillus is injected intradermally; a hardened red area appearing 1 to

3 days after injection signifies a positive reaction and past or present exposure to the tubercle bacillus (see also *tuberculin test*).

MANUBRIUM n. the part of the *sternum* (breastbone) nearest the head. pl. **manubria**

MANUS see *hand*.

MAO abbreviation for *monoamine oxidase*.

MAO INHIBITOR see *monoamine oxidase inhibitor*.

MAPLE SYRUP URINE DISEASE n. an inherited disorder of metabolism in which the enzyme necessary for the breakdown of amino acids lysine, leucine, and isoleucine is lacking and the person has hyperreflexia and urine with a characteristic maple syrup odor. Treatment includes a diet low in these amino acids; untreated, the disorder leads to *mental retardation* and often death in early childhood.

MAPPING n. in genetics, the process of locating genes on a *chromosome*; also called **chromosome mapping**.

MAPROTILINE n. an antidepressant. Adverse effects include sedation; and gastrointestinal, cardiac, and neurological disturbances; the drug interacts with many others and must be used with caution in combination with other drugs.

MARASMUS n. extreme malnutrition, emaciation, and wasting, esp. in a young child; it usually results from inadequate protein and calorie intake but may also result from *malabsorption*, metabolic disorders, repeated vomiting and diarrhea, or certain infectious diseases. Symptoms include wasting of subcutaneous tissue and muscle and often a pallid appearance and subnormal body temperature. Treatment includes reestablishment of fluid and electrolyte balance and gradual introduction of foods.

MARAX n. trade name for a fixed-combination drug, containing the smooth muscle relaxant theophylline, the adrenergic ephedrine, and the tranquilizer hydroxyzine; used to treat asthma and bronchitis.

MARBLE BONE DISEASE see *osteopetrosis*.

MARBURG DISEASE n. a viral disease of vervet (green) monkeys transmitted to humans by contact with the infected animal, esp. blood or tissues used in laboratory studies. In humans it causes a serious and often fatal illness, characterized by fever, rash, headache, vomiting, diarrhea, and gastrointestinal hemorrhage. There is no treatment, but antiserum and measures to reduce blood loss are sometimes effective. Also called **green monkey disease**; **Marburg-Ebola disease**.

MARFAN'S SYNDROME n. an inherited abnormality (*autosomal dominant disorder*) characterized by elongation of bones, esp. the arms, legs, fingers, and toes; joint hypermobility; and abnormalities of the eyes (e.g., dislocation of the lens) and circulatory system (e.g., fiber fragmentation in the *aorta*, leading to *aneurysm*). There is no specific treatment.

MARIE-STRUMPELL DISEASE see *ankylosing spondylitis*.

MARIHUANA n. drug, made from the dried leaves of the *Cannabis sativa* plant, which, when smoked, provides a sense of euphoria often accompanied by changes in mood, perception, memory and fine motor skills. The drug has been used to help relieve the nausea associated with cancer chemotherapy. Street names include **pot, grass**, and **weed**.

MARPLAN n. trade name for the antidepressant isocarboxazid.

MARROW see *bone marrow*.

MARSEILLES FEVER n. a disease, common around the Mediterranean area and in India, caused by a rickettsia (*Rickettsia conorii*) transmitted by the brown dog tick (*Rhipicephalus sanguineus*); it is characterized by chills, fever, a black crusted ulcer at the site of the tick bite, and a rash. Also called **boutonneuse fever**; **Indian tick fever**; **Kenya fever**.

MARSUPIALIZE v. to form a pouch surgically, as in treatment of a cyst by opening it and draining it and suturing the edges to adjacent tissues.

MASCULINIZATION n. the acquisition of male secondary sexual characteristics (e.g., excess body and facial hair, deeper voice) by a female, usually as the result of hormonal treatment or malfunction of the adrenal glands; also: **virilism**.

MASK v. to conceal or obscure something, as the masking of one disease by the symptoms of another; n. 1. a masklike appearance, as sometimes occurs during pregnancy (see *chloasma*); 2. a cover worn over the nose and mouth to prevent inhalation of toxic or irritating substances or to deliver oxygen or anesthetic gas.

MASK OF PREGNANCY see *chloasma*.

MASOCHISM n. sexual pleasure derived from receiving mental, emotional, or physical abuse (compare *sadism*). adj. **masochistic**

MASSAGE n. manipulation of the soft tissues of the body through rubbing, stroking, kneading, or gripping to improve muscle tone, relax the person, or improve circulation (see also *cardiac massage*; *effleurage*).

MASTALGIA n. pain in the breast.

MAST CELL n. a large connective tissue cell that contains histamine, heparin, serotonin, and bradykinin, which are released in response to injury, inflammation, or allergic reaction.

MASTECTOMY n. the surgical removal of one or both breasts to remove a malignant tumor.
　modified radical mastectomy n. the removal of a breast with the underlying pectoralis minor muscle and some adjacent lymph nodes (the major chest muscle—pectoralis major—is not removed).
　radical mastectomy n. surgical removal of a breast, underlying chest muscles (both pectoralis major and pectoralis minor), lymph nodes in the armpit area, and fat and other tissues in the surrounding area.
　simple mastectomy n. the removal of a breast with the underlying chest muscles and adjacent lymph nodes and tissues left intact.

MASTICATION n. chewing and grinding food with the teeth.

MASTITIS n. inflammation of the breast, usually due to bacterial (streptococcal or staphylococcal) infection; it is most common in the first two months of lactation with pain, swelling, fever, malaise, and swelling of the lymph nodes in the armpit area occurring. Treatment includes antibiotics, analgesics, and rest; nursing can usually continue. A rare chronic form sometimes occurs in association with severe tuberculosis (see also *fibrocystic disease of the breast*).

MASTOID adj. breastlike in shape or appearance, esp. the bump (mastoid process of the temporal bone) behind the ear. adj. **mastoidal**

MASTOIDECTOMY n. surgical removal of part of the mastoid part of the temporal bone, done to treat chronic *otitis media* or *mastoiditis*, when antibiotics are not effective.

MASTOIDITIS n. infection of the mastoid bones, usually resulting from a middle ear infection; it is most common in children and is characterized by pain, fever, earache, and malaise. Treatment is by antibiotics; some residual hearing loss sometimes occurs.

MASTURBATION n. manipulation and stimulation of one's own genitals to achieve sexual pleasure, usually orgasm. It is practiced by most people at some point in their lives.

MATERIA MEDICA n. the study of the origins, preparation, uses, and effects of drugs and other substances used therapeutically in medicine.

MATERNAL adj. pert. to the mother.

MATERNAL-INFANT BONDING n. the process of a mother being attached to her newborn infant and vice versa. It is considered important to the emotional and physical development of the child and the interaction of mother and child. Skin-to-skin and eye-to-eye contact immediately after birth and frequently in the early postpartum period are considered helpful in establishing this bonding.

MATRIX n. the substance of an organ or tissue in which other specialized structures are embedded, as, e.g., the ground substance of connective tissue.

MATURATION n. the process of obtaining full development, as in the development of mature ova and sperm, or the development of physical, mental, and emotional abilities during childhood and adolescence.

MAXILLA n. one of a pair of large bones that form the upper jaw. It consists of a pyramidal body and four processes; contains sockets for the 16 upper teeth; and forms part of the structure of the orbits, nasal cavity, and roof of the mouth (compare mandible).   pl. **maxillae**   adj. **maxillary**

MAXILLARY ARTERY n. either of two branches of the external carotid arteries that arise near the parotid gland and divide into branches supplying the deep parts of the face.

MAXILLARY SINUS n. one of a pair of air cells forming a cavity in the *maxilla*; the mucous membrane lining is continuous with that of the nasal cavity (compare *frontal sinus*; *sphenoidal sinus*).

MAXILLO- comb. form indicating an association with the *maxilla*, or upper jaw (e.g., **maxillo-facial**, pert. to the lower jaw and face).

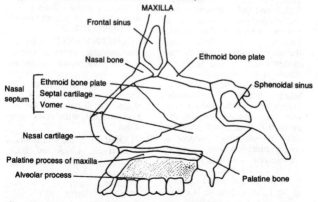

Lateral view of the maxilla, or upper jaw

McARDLE'S DISEASE n. an inherited disease in which larger than normal amounts of *glycogen* accumulate in skeletal muscle, causing muscle cramping and weakness after exercise.

McBURNEY'S POINT n. the point of maximum sensitivity in acute *appendicitis*; it lies one third of the way on a line drawn from the projection of the right hip to the umbilicus.

MEASLES n. an acute, contagious, viral disease, occurring primarily in children who have not been immunized and involving the respiratory tract and a spreading rash. Highly contagious, measles is spread by direct contact with droplets from the nose, mouth, or throat of infected persons, often in the prodromal stage. After an incubation period of about two weeks, fever, malaise, cough, loss of appetite, and photophobia develop, followed by characteristic blue-centered, small red spots on the membranes of the tongue and mouth (Koplik's spots). Two or three days later the characteristic rash appears, starting as pinkish spots in the head region and spreading to a red maculopapular rash over the trunk and extremities. Fever to 103° Fahrenheit (39.5° Celsius) or higher and inflammation of the pharynx and trachea occur. About five days later the lesions flatten, become brownish and fade, and the fever subsides. Treatment includes pain-relievers, fever reducers, rest, and lotions (e.g., calamine) to soothe the skin and relieve itching. Complications include *otitis media*, *pneumonia*, *laryngitis*, and occasionally *encephalitis*. One attack provides life-long immunity. Prevention is by immunization with live measles vaccine, usually done when the child is 1-1½ years old; or, in those unvaccinated and exposed to the disease, passive immunization with immune globulin.

MEATUS n. an opening or tunnel through any part of the body, as the acoustic meatus, leading from the external ear to the *tympanic membrane*.

MEBARAL n. trade name for the anticonvulsant and sedative *mephobarbital* used in the treatment of anxiety and some forms of epilepsy.

MEBENDAZOLE n. an anthelmintic used to treat pinworm, roundworm, and hookworm infestations. Adverse effects include gastrointestinal disturbances.

MECAMYLAMINE n. a drug, known under the trade name Inversine, used to lower blood pressure.

MECKEL'S DIVERTICULUM n. a congenital sac protruding from the *ileum* (last part of the small intestine), caused by incomplete closure of the yolk sac; it occurs in about 2% of the population. It usually produces no symptoms but may cause signs of appendicitis, intestinal obstruction, or bleeding in children. Treatment is by surgery, done if symptoms are present and/or to avoid obstruction or inflammation of the area.

MECLIZINE n. an antihistamine used to treat and prevent motion sickness. Adverse effects include drowsiness, skin rash, dry mouth, and rapid heart beat.

MECLOFENAMATE n. an antiinflammatory agent, known under the trade name Meclomen, used to treat rheumatoid arthritis and osteoarthritis. Adverse effects include dizziness and gastrointestinal disturbances; the drug also interacts with many other drugs.

MECONIUM n. the first stools of a newborn, which are thick, sticky, greenish-to-black, and composed of bile pigments, gland secretions, amniotic fluid, and other intrauterine debris. The presence of meconium in the amniotic fluid usually indicates *fetal distress*.

MEDI-, MEDIO- comb. form indicating a relationship to the middle, midline, or middle plane (e.g., **mediodorsal**, pert. to the middle and back).

MEDIAL adj. situated toward the midline of the body or the central part of an organ or tissue.

MEDIASTINUM n. the space in the chest cavity between the *pleural sacs* that contains the heart, aorta, esophagus, trachea and thymus.

MEDICATION n. 1. a drug or other substance used to remedy an illness; 2. the administration of a medicine.

MEDICINE n. 1. a drug or other substance used to remedy an illness; 2. the art and science of diagnosing and treating and preventing illness and maintaining good health; 3. that area of medical science concerned with the diagnosis and treatment of disease as distinct from *surgery*.

MEDICO- comb. form indicating a relationship to the art and science of medicine (e.g., **medicodental**, pert. to both medicine and dentistry).

MEDICOLEGAL adj. pert. to medicine and law, esp. to topics such as malpractice, patient consent for operations, and patient information.

MEDITERRANEAN ANEMIA see *thalassemia*.

MEDITERRANEAN FEVER see *brucellosis*.

MEDIUM n. 1. a substance through which something moves or acts. A contrast medium, for example, has a density different from body tissues and when used with X ray or similar technique allows visual comparison of structures; 2. a substance (e.g., agar) used as food for microorganisms; a culture medium.

MEDROXYPROGESTERONE n. a progestin compound, known under the trade name Provera, used to treat menstrual disorders. Adverse effects include thrombophlebitis, stroke, pulmonary embolism, and hepatitis.

MEDULLA n. the innermost part of an organ or structure, as in adrenal medulla (compare *cortex*). pl. **medullae** adj. **medullary**

MEDULLA OBLONGATA n. the lowest part of the brainstem, an extension in the skull of the upper end of the spinal cord; it is the most vital part of the brain, containing centers controlling respiration, heart and blood vessel function, and other activities as well as pathways for impulses entering and leaving the skull. Injury to the medulla is often fatal.

MEDULLARY adj. 1. pert. to the *medulla oblongata*; 2. pert. to *bone marrow*; 3. pert. to the central nervous system.

MEFENAMIC ACID n. a nonsteroid antiinflammatory agent and analgesic, known under the trade name Ponstan, used to treat mild or moderate pain. Adverse effects include gastrointestinal disturbances and drowsiness.

MEFOXIN n. a trade name for a *cephalosporin* antibacterial compound (cefoxitin).

MEGA-, MEGALO- comb. form meaning "great" "huge" "large" (e.g., **megacardia**, an abnormally large heart; **megalocyte**, an abnormally large red blood cell).

MEGACOLON n. abnormal enlargement of the colon, by an accumulation of impacted feces. It may be congenital (*Hirschsprung's disease*); acquired (as in chronic refusal to defecate, esp. in children); or toxic, a complication of ulcerative colitis. Treatment is by surgery, esp. for congenital and toxic forms, and by enemas and laxatives.

MEGALOBLASTIC ANEMIA n. a blood disorder in which large, immature and dysfunctional red blood cells circulate; associated with *pernicious anemia* and folic acid deficiency.

MEGALOMANIA n. an abnormal state of mind in which the person has delusions of grandeur and believes himself/herself to be of great power, importance, or achievement.

-MEGALY comb. form indicating an enlargement (e.g., **dactylomegaly**, an enlargement of the fingers or toes).

MEGESTROL n. a progestational compound used to treat endometrial cancer.

MEGAVITAMIN THERAPY n. theory that the intake of very large doses of vitamins—much above recommended daily doses—will prevent or cure many physical and psychological disorders.

MEIBOMIAN CYST see *chalazion.*

MEIOSIS a type of cell division that produces daughter cells with the haploid chromosome number. It occurs during the production of mature sperm and ova; the diploid chromosome number characteristic of the species is restored at fertilization. Meiosis consists of two consecutive divisions, each divided into four phases (*see accompanying illustration*); also called **reduction division** adj. **meiotic**

MELANCHOLIA n. extreme sadness; extreme depression (see *bipolar disorder; depression*)

MELANIN n. a dark brown to black pigment that occurs in skin, hair, and parts of the eye.

MELANOCYTE n. a melanin-producing cell found throughout the basal layer of the epidermis and controlled by melanocyte-stimulating hormone.

MELANOCYTE - STIMULATING HORMONE (MSH) n. a hormone, secreted by the *anterior pituitary gland*, that controls the intensity of pigmentation in melanocytes.

MELANODERMA n. abnormal darkening of the skin by increased *melanin* deposits.

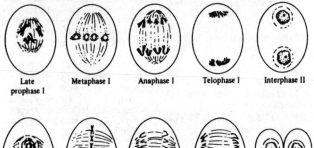

| Late prophase I | Metaphase I | Anaphase I | Telophase I | Interphase II |

| Prophase II | Metaphase II | Anaphase II | Telophase II | Four Haploid Cells |

Stages of meiosis

MELANOMA n. any of several malignant neoplasms, primarily of the skin, consisting of melanocytes. Most melanomas develop from a pigmented nevus (mole); any change in color or shape of such a mark suggests melanoma. Prognosis depends on the location, depth, and size of the lesion, and on the general health of the patient.

MELASMA　　see *chloasma*.

MELATONIN n. the only hormone secreted by the *pineal gland*; it is thought to inhibit endocrine function and decrease skin pigmentation. Decreased secretion leads to *diabetes mellitus*, hypogonadism, and, in boys precocious puberty.

MELENA n. abnormal dark, tarry stool, containing blood, usually from gastrointestinal bleeding.

MELIOIDOSIS n. an uncommon and serious, often fatal, infectious disease caused by the bacterium *Pseudomonas pseudomallei*, occurring mostly in China and Southeast Asia, characterized by pneumonia, lung abscesses, and septicemia. Treatment is by antibacterials (e.g., *chloramphenicol*, *tetracycline*).

MELLARIL n. trade name for the tranquilizer *thioridazine*.

MELPHALAN n. an antineoplastic drug, known under the trade name Alkeran, used to treat multiple myeloma and certain other malignancies. Adverse effects include bone marrow depression, nausea, and vomiting.

MEMBRANE n. a thin layer of tissue that covers an organ or lines a cavity or part (e.g., the *pleura* is a membrane enclosing the lung). Membranes may be mucous, serous, or synovial.　　adj. **membranous**

MEMBRANOUS LABYRINTH n. a network of membranous, semicircular ducts, containing the fluid endolymph, that are suspended within the bony semicircular canals of the inner ear and function in the maintenance of balance.

MEMORY n. the ability to retain and recall into consciousness previously experienced ideas and sensations and information learned. The retention and recall is associated with specific chemical changes in the brain and can be affected by organic brain disorders and various psychological disorders. In general memory is classified as recent or long-term.

MENARCHE n. the first *menstruation*, usually occurring between the ages of 9 and 16. adj. **menarchal**, **menarcheal**

MENDELISM n. the theory of inheritance based on Mendel's laws.

MENDEL'S LAWS n. basic principles of inheritance, developed in the 19th century by the Austrian monk Gregor Mendel on the basis of breeding experiments, which form the basis of the modern understanding of heredity. According to the laws each characteristic of a person is determined by a pair of units—now known as *genes*. One unit (*allele*) of each pair is contributed by each parent, carried in the gamete (egg or sperm). At fertilization the alleles combine to form a unit that determines the characteristic in the offspring. Some units are *dominant* over others, called *recessives*; some interact in other ways. These basic principles formed the foundation on which subsequent biochemical studies of genes and chromosomes were made, leading to the development of modern genetics.

MENIERE'S DISEASE n. a disease of the inner ear, characterized by recurrent episodes of dizziness, progressive hearing loss (usually unilateral), and tinnitus, often accompanied by nausea and vomiting. The cause is unknown, but the disease sometimes follows middle ear infection or injury to the head. Treatment is symptomatic, including the use of antihistamines.

MENINGES n. the three connective tissue membranes that protect and enclose the brain and spinal cord. The outer layer is the tough, thick *dura mater*; the middle layer the delicate spiderweb-like *arachnoid*; and the inner layer the highly vascularized *pia matter*. The inner two layers are called collectively the *leptomeninges*; the cerebrospinal fluid circulates between them.

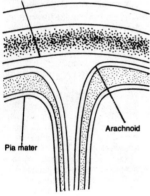

The meninges protect the brain. They include the outer dura mater, the arachnoid, and the inner pia mater.

MENINGIOMA n. a usually slow-growing tumor arising from the membranes enclosing the brain and spinal cord (meninges); symptoms arise from pressure on underlying nerve tissue. Some tumors are malignant. Treatment is by surgery, if the tumor is accessible.

MENINGISM n. symptoms (e.g., stiff neck) that mimic those of *meningitis* but in which there is no inflammation of the *meninges*; occurs most often in children.

MENINGITIS n. inflammation of the *meninges*, most commonly due to bacterial infection, but sometimes caused by viral or fungal infection, spreading tuberculosis, neoplasm, or chemical irritation. Symptoms include headache, stiff neck, fever, nausea, vomiting, and intolerance to light and sound, often followed by convulsions and delirium. Treatment depends on the cause; bacterial meningitis is treated by antibiotics; viral, fungal, or other forms of meningitis are more serious and difficult to treat.

MENINGO- comb. form indicating an association with the *meninges* (e.g., **meningoarteritis**, inflammation of the arteries of the meninges).

MENINGOCELE n. a congenital sacklike protrusion of either the cerebral (brain) meninges or the spinal meninges, containing *cerebrospinal fluid* but no nerve tissue. Treatment is by surgery.

MENISCECTOMY n. surgical removal of crescent-shaped cartilage (meniscus) of the knee, done when torn cartilage in the knee joint area causes chronic pain or difficulty in movement.

MENOPAUSE n. the stoppage of the *menstruation*, usually occurring naturally between the ages of 45 and 55. The term is also used to refer to that stage of a woman's life during which gradual hormonal changes, sometimes accompanied by vasomotor symptoms, such as hot flashes, and other signs (e.g., dryness of vaginal membranes and palpitations), lead to the cessation of menstrual periods. The production of gonadotropins from the pituitary and estrogens from the ovaries gradually decreases; ovulation ceases, and menstrual periods stop. The periods may become scanty and irregular in occurrence, or they may be episodes of heavy bleeding or abrupt cessation. Emotional disturbances may result from hormonal imbalances during the period, but many of the symptoms once believed due to menopause cannot be reliably attributed to it. Also called **climacteric, change of life**.   adj. **menopausal**

MENORRHAGIA n. abnormally heavy or prolonged menstrual periods; it occurs occasionally in many women, sometimes caused by benign uterine tumors, but if chronic, it may lead to *anemia*; also **hypermenorrhea** (compare *oligomenorrhea*).

MENOSTASIS n. condition in which menstrual products cannot leave the uterus or vagina, due to narrowing or closure of the normal openings.   adj. **menostatic**

MENOTABS n. trade name for an *estrogen* preparation.

MENRIUM n. trade name for a fixed-combination drug, containing an estrogen preparation and a tranquilizer (*chlordiazepoxide* [Librium]) used to treat symptoms of *menopause*.

MENSES n. the flow of blood and other material from the *uterus* during *menstruation*.

MENSTRUAL CYCLE n. the recurring cycle, beginning at *menarche* and ending at *menopause*, in which the endometrial lining of the *uterus* proliferates in preparation for *pregnancy* and when pregnancy does not occur is shed at *menstruation*. The average menstrual cycle is 28 days, with day 1 the first day of menstrual flow, but the length of the cycle varies greatly among women.

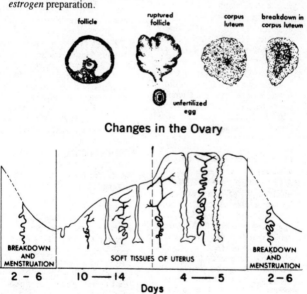

follicle   ruptured follicle   corpus luteum   breakdown in corpus luteum

unfertilized egg

Changes in the Ovary

BREAKDOWN AND MENSTRUATION   SOFT TISSUES OF UTERUS   BREAKDOWN AND MENSTRUATION

2 – 6   10 —— 14   4 —— 5   2 – 6

Days

Changes in the Uterus Wall

The Menstrual Cycle

MENSTRUAL FLOW n. the flow of blood and other material from the uterus at roughly monthly intervals during a woman's reproductive years. The average blood loss in the flow is about 30 milliliters, but this varies greatly among women.

MENSTRUAL PHASE n. that phase of the menstrual cycle during which the lining of the uterus is shed. The first day of the menstrual flow is considered day 1 of the menstrual cycle.

MENSTRUATION n. the discharge of blood and uterine material from the vagina at intervals of about a month during a woman's reproductive years; also: **catamenia** (see also *menses; menstrual cycle*).   adj. **menstrual**

MENTAL adj. 1. pert. to the mind; 2. pert. to the chin.

MENTAL AGE n. the age at which a person functions intellectually determined by standardized tests (compare *chronological age; developmental age*).

MENTAL DISORDER n. any disorder of the mind, such as disturbance of perceptions, memory, emotional equilibrium, thought or behavior; it may be genetic, congenital, or acquired as a result of physical, psychological, chemical, or social factors. Also called **mental illness; emotional disorder**.

MENTAL RETARDATION n. a disorder characterized by below average intellectual capability with defects in the ability to learn and adapt. More males than females are affected. It may be genetic, congenital, biological, or psychosocial. On standardized intelligence tests where the average intelligence quotient (IQ) is considered 90 to 110, mental retardation is generally classified as borderline with IQ 71 to 84; mild with IQ 50 to 70; moderate with IQ 35 to 49, severe with IQ 20 to 34; and profound with IQ below 20.

MENTATION n. any mental activity.

MENTO- comb. form indicating an association with the chin (e.g., **mentolabial**, pert. to the chin and lip).

MENTUM n. the chin.

MEPERIDINE n. a narcotic analgesic, known under the trade name Demerol, commonly used to treat moderate to severe pain. Adverse effects include drowsiness, gastrointestinal disturbances, circulatory and respiratory depression, and the potential for addiction.

MEPHENESIN n. a muscle relaxant, known under the trade name Myanesin, used to treat skeletal muscle spasm. Adverse effects include gastrointestinal disturbances, weakness, and disturbances of eye movement and function.

MEPHENYTOIN n. an anticonvulsant, known under the trade name Mesantoin, used to treat epilepsy. The drug is highly toxic and its use is limited to cases where other anticonvulsants are not effective. Adverse effects are common and include liver toxicity, blood abnormalities, fever, and rash.

MEPHOBARBITAL n. an anticonvulsant and sedative, known under the trade name Mebaral, used to treat epilepsy and anxiety. Adverse effects include gastrointestinal disturbances, paradoxical hyperexcitability, and the potential for dependence.

MEPROBAMATE n. a sedative and tranquilizer, known under many trade names, including Equanil, Miltown, and Meprin, used to treat anxiety and muscle tension. Adverse effects include drowsiness, ataxia, allergic reactions, and interaction with other drugs acting on the central nervous system.

MERALGIA n. pain in the thigh.

MERCAPTOPURINE n. an antineoplastic and immunosuppressive drug, known under the trade name Purinethol, used in the treatment of *acute lymphocytic leukemia* and certain other neoplasms. Adverse effects include nausea, vomiting, and bone marrow depression.

MERCURY n. a metallic element (see Table of Elements).

MERCURY POISONING n. a toxic condition caused by the ingestion or inhalation of mercury or mercury-containing products (e.g., fungicides and certain pigments); contamination of waters with industrial wastes containing mercury had led to contaminated fish and seafood in some areas. Acute poisoning causes a metallic taste in the mouth, gastrointestinal symptoms (e.g., vomiting, diarrhea), and kidney disturbances that may lead to death. Chronic poisoning, resulting from exposure to small amounts over a long period, causes irritability, slurred speech, staggering gait, and teeth and gum disorders. Treatment includes gastric lavage. (See also *Minamata disease*.)

MERCY KILLING see *euthanasia*.

MEROMELIA n. congenital absence of any part of a limb, including *phocomelia* and *adactyly* (compare *amelia*).

MEROZOITE n. stage in the life cycle of the malaria parasite and of certain other parasites.

MESANTOIN n. trade name for the anticonvulsant *mephenytoin*.

MESCALINE n. a psychoactive alkaloid derived from a cactus (*Lophophora williamsii*) that produces euphoria, hallucinations, anxiety, heart palpitations, and other signs of excitement. It is used by some Amerindian tribes to produce feelings of ecstasy during ceremonies and as a street drug; also called **peyote**.

MESENCEPHALON n. the midbrain.

MESENCHYME n. embryonic tissue that forms connective tissue, blood, and smooth muscles. adj. **mesenchymal**

MESENTERY n. a fold of *peritoneum* that holds abdominal organs (e.g., stomach, parts of the small intestine, spleen) to the posterior wall of the abdomen. adj. **mesenteric**

MESIAL see *medial*.

MESOCOLON n. fold of *peritoneum* that holds the lower parts of the colon to the inside of the abdominal wall. adj. **mesocolic**

MESODERM n. in the embryo, the middle germ cell layer from which muscle, bone, cartilage, blood, vascular and lymph tissue, and other tissues develop. (The other two cell layers are the inner *endoderm* and the outer *ectoderm*).

MESOMORPH n. a person with well developed skeletal and muscular structure, intermediate between the *ectomorph* and *endomorph*. adj. **mesomorphic**

MESOSALPINX n. the free end of the broad ligament, within which the Fallopian tubes lie.

MESOTHELIOMA n. a rare, malignant tumor of the mesothelial lining of the pleura or peritoneum, usually associated with exposure to asbestos.

MESSENGER RNA n. that form of *ribonucleic acid* (RNA) that transmits information from DNA in the *nucleus* to the *ribosome* sites of protein synthesis in the cell.

MESTRANOL n. an *estrogen* preparation that is used in combination with a progestin in *oral contraceptives*.

METABOLISM n. the combined chemical and physical processes that take place in the body involving the distribution of nutrients and resulting in growth, energy production, the elimination of wastes, and other body functions. There are two basic phases of metabolism: *anabolism*, the constructive phase, during which small molecules resulting from the digestive process are built up into complex compounds that form the tissues and organs of the body; and *catabolism*, the destructive phase, during which larger molecules are broken down into simpler substances with the release of energy. adj. **metabolic**

METABOLIC adj. pert. to *metabolism*.

METABOLIC RATE n. the amount of energy expended in a given period (see *basal metabolic rate*.

METABOLITE n. a substance taking part in metabolism, either a product of a metabolic process or a substance necessary for a metabolic process.

METACARPUS n. any of the five bones of the hand between the wrist (*carpus*) and the finger (*phalanges*); they are usually numbered I through V, starting on the thumb side. adj. **metacarpal**

METACARPAL adj. pert. to the bones of the hand between the wrist and fingers.

METAMORPHOPSIA n. a vision defect in which objects appear distorted; it is usually due to a defect in the *retina*.

METAMORPHOSIS n. a change in shape or structure, esp. a change from one distinct form to another (e.g., in insects, from larva to pupa to adult).

METAPHASE n. a stage in *mitosis* and meiosis during which chromosomes become aligned along the equatorial plane of the spindle in preparation for separation and distribution to the daughter cells.

METAPHYSIS n. the growing portion of a long bone, between the diaphysis (shaft) and epiphyses (ends). pl. **metaphyses** adj. **metaphyseal**

METASTASIS n. the spread of a tumor from its site of origin to distant sites, usually through the bloodstream, the lymphatic system, or across a cavity such as that contained in the peritoneum. v. **metastasize** adj. **metastatic**

METATARSAL adj. pert. to a *metatarsus*.

METATARSUS n. any of the five bones of the foot, between the ankle and toes (phalanges); they are usually numbered I to V, starting at the medial (great toe) side. adj. **metatarsal**

METATENSIN n. trade name for a fixed combination drug, containing the diuretic trichlormethiazide and the antihypertensive *reserpine*, used to treat cardiovascular abnormalities.

METENCEPHALON n. part of the brain, including the *pons* and the *cerebellum*.

METEORTROPISM n. the effects of climate on biological occurrences (e.g., angina, joint pains).

METHADONE n. a synthetic narcotic pain-reliever used in the treatment of opiate (esp. heroin)-addicted persons and sometimes to relieve severe pain. Adverse effects include drowsiness, gastrointestinal disturbances, respiratory and circulatory depression, and the potential for addiction.

METHAMPHETAMINE n. a central nervous system stimulant used to treat *narcolepsy* and certain other disorders. Adverse effects include central nervous system excitation, an increase in blood pressure, nausea, and the potential for drug dependence.

METHAPYRILENE n. an antihistamine used in the treatment of rhinitis, dermatitis, pruritus and other allergic responses. Adverse effects include drowsiness, dry mouth, skin rash, rapid heart beat, and hypersensitivity reactions.

METHAQUALONE n. a sedative-hypnotic, known under the name Quaalude; used as a street drug. Adverse effects include loss of inhibition, gastrointestinal disturbances, and drug dependence.

METHARBITAL n. an anticonvulsant, known under the trade name Gemonil, used to treat epilepsy. Adverse effects include ataxia, irritability, and gastric distress.

METHENAMINE n. an antibacterial contained in many products (e.g., Urotone) used to treat urinary tract infections. Adverse effects include rashes and gastrointestinal distress.

METHICILLIN n. an antibiotic of the *penicillin* family that is not rendered inactive by the penicillinase enzyme released by certain bacteria; it is used to treat certain staphylococcal infections. Adverse effects include allergic reactions, kidney disturbance, and occasionally inflammation or phlebitis at the site of injection.

METHOCARBAMOL n. a skeletal muscle relaxant, known under the trade names Methocarbamol and Robaxin, used to treat spasms of skeletal muscles. Adverse effects include low blood pressure, dizziness, drowsiness, and nausea.

METHOTREXATE n. an antineoplastic drug used to treat certain cancers. Adverse effects include mouth sores, digestive upsets, bone marrow depression, and rashes.

METHYCLOTHIAZIDE n. a diuretic and antihypertensive, known under the trade name Enduron, used to treat hypertension.

Adverse effects include electrolyte imbalance and hypersensitivity reactions.

METHYLDOPA n. an antihypertensive, known under the trade name Aldomet and combined with a diuretic in Aldoril; it is used to treat high blood pressure. Adverse effects include sedation, dry mouth, and liver and blood abnormalities.

METHYLENE BLUE n. a crystalline powder, used in kidney function tests, as a urinary antiseptic, and in the treatment of cyanide poisoning and certain other disorders.

METHYLPHENIDATE n. a central nervous system stimulant, known under the trade name Ritalin, used to treat hyperkinesis in children and *narcolepsy* in adults. Adverse effects include loss of appetite, insomnia, nervousness, and allergic reactions.

METHYL SALICYLATE n. oil of wintergreen; a liquid used as a counterirritant and pain-reliever, applied externally for minor muscle and joint pain. Adverse effects include skin reactions.

METHYLTESTOSTERONE n. an androgen preparation contained in Estratest and Metandren; it is used to treat testosterone deficiency and female breast cancer and to stimulate growth and weight gain. Adverse effects include edema, masculinization of females, and jaundice.

METHYPRYLON n. a sedative-hypnotic, known under the trade name Noludar, used to treat sleep disorders. Adverse effects include dizziness, gastrointestinal disturbances, headache, paradoxical excitement, and the possibility of dependence.

METHYSERGIDE n. a vasoconstrictor, known under the trade name Sansert, used to treat migraine. This drug is used only when other attempts to treat severe and frequent migraine are unsuccessful, because of serious potential adverse effects, including retroperitoneal fibrosis, pulmonary and cardiac abnormalities, blood disorders, and pains in various parts of the body.

METRALGIA n. pain in the *uterus*.

METRITIS n. inflammation of the *uterus* (see also *endometritis*).

METROPTOSIS n. prolapse of the uterus; a downward displacement of the uterus, with the neck (cervix) of the uterus sometimes protruding from the vagina. It most often occurs in women who have had children. Treatment is by surgery.

METRORRHAGIA n. bleeding from the *uterus* other than that of *menstruation*, usually indicative of uterine disease (e.g., cervical cancer).

MICR-, MICRO- comb. form indicating smallness (e.g., **microblepharon**, abnormally small eyelids).

MICROBE n. a small organism, visible only with the aid of a microscope (see *microorganism*). adj. **microbic, microbial**

MICROBIOLOGY n. that branch of biology concerned with the study of microorganisms, including bacteria, viruses, rickettsiae, fungi, and protozoa.

MICROBRACHIA n. a defect in development characterized by abnormally small arms.

MICROCEPHALY n. a congenital abnormality in which the head is abnormally small and the brain is underdeveloped, resulting in some degree of mental retardation (compare *macrocephaly*); also microcephalus. adj. **microcephalic**

MICROCYTOSIS n. a blood disorder characterized by abnormally small erythrocytes (red blood cells); often associated with iron-deficiency anemia.

MICRODACTYL n. an abnormality characterized by unusually small fingers and toes.

MICROGLIA n. small interstitial cells of the central nervous system that act as phagocytes, collecting waste products of nerve tissue.

MICRONOR n. trade name for an oral contraceptive, containing the progestin compound *norethindrone*.

MICRONUTRIENT n. a compound, such as a vitamin or mineral (e.g., riboflavin, zinc, copper, iodine) needed only in small amounts for normal body function.

MICROORGANISM n. a very small organism, usually visible only with the help of a microscope; included among microorganisms are bacteria, viruses, rickettsiae, fungi, and protozoa.

MICROPHAGE n. a *neutrophil* (type of white blood cell) that can ingest small things, like bacteria (compare *macrophage*).

MICROPHALLUS n. an abnormally small penis; also called **micropenis**.

MICROPHTHALMOS n. a developmental defect characterized by abnormal smallness of one or both eyes.

MICROSCOPE n. an instrument for producing a magnified image of an object that may be so small as to be invisible to the naked eye. There are several types of microscopes, including the light microscope, which uses light as source of radiation and a combination of lenses to magnify and focus the object; and an electron microscope in which a beam of electrons is used to scan and produce an image of the object.

MICROSCOPIC adj. 1. pert. to a microscope; 2. very small, visible only when magnified and illuminated by a microscope.

MICROSCOPIC ANATOMY n. the study of the microscopic structure of tissues and organs; included are *histology* and *cytology* (compare *gross anatomy*).

MICROSCOPY n. the use of a microscope to view objects. adj. **microscopic**

MICROSOMIA n. the condition of having an abnormally small and undeveloped, but structurally normal body.

MICROSURGERY n. that branch of surgery performed using special operating microscopes and miniaturized precision instruments to perform delicate and intricate procedures on very small structures and structures not previously accessible to surgery, such as parts of the eye, brain, and spinal cord and to reattach amputated digits and limbs, requiring suturing of very small nerves and blood vessels.

MICTURITION see *urination*

MICTURITION REFLEX n. normal response to increased pressure in the bladder, with relaxation of the urethral sphincter allowing passage of urine from the body.

MIDBRAIN n. a part of the brain stem, joining the hindbrain and forebrain, and serving as passageway for impulses to higher brain centers; also: **mesencephalon**

MIDDLE EAR n. that part of the ear consisting of air-filled space in the temporal bone and extending from the *tympanic membrane*, which separates it from the external ear, to the inner ear. It contains three ossicles (the *maleus*, *incus*, and *stapes*) that transmit sound vibrations from the *tympanic membrane* to the inner ear. The middle ear is connected to the pharynx through the *Eustachian tube*.

MIDWIFE n. a person who assists women in labor and childbirth.

MIGRAINE n. a recurring vascular headache, occurring more frequently in women. The cause is unknown but the pain is associated with dilation of extracranial blood vessels; attacks are often triggered by allergic reactions, menstruation, alcohol, or relaxation after a period of stress. A typical attack, which may last from several hours to several days, starts with a prodromal episode of visual disturbances (e.g., aura or flashing lights), numbness, tingling, vertigo, or other sensations, followed by the onset of severe, usually unilateral pain, sometimes accompanied by nausea, vomiting, photophobia, irritability, and fatigue. Ergotamine preparations that constrict cranial arteries are helpful if taken at the onset of an attack; aspirin does not usually provide relief. Also: **megrim, hemicrania** (see also *cluster headache*; *histamine headache*).

MILIA n. minute white cysts of epidermis caused by obstruction of hair follicles and sweat glands. **milia neonatorum** n. normal skin condition of newborns characterized by minute epidermal cysts on the face and sometimes trunk that disappear spontaneously within a few weeks.

MILIARIA n. minute vesicles and papules, often surrounded by a reddened area, caused by obstruction of sweat glands during times of high heat and humitity; itching and prickling may result; also called **prickly heat**.

MILIARY TUBERCULOSIS see under *tuberculosis*.

MILK n. the fluid secreted by the mammary glands (breasts), usually the first food of newborn mammals. After breast feeding, humans consume the milk of cows and certain other mammals (e.g., goats, yak). Milk contains carbohydrates (lactose), protein (casein), fat, the minerals calcium and phosphorus, and vitamins A, riboflavin, niacin, thiamine, and, when fortified, vitamin D.

MILK-EJECTION REFLEX see *let-down reflex*.

MILK INTOLERANCE n. a condition, caused by a lack of or defect in an enzyme that renders a person unable to digest milk sugar (lactose) (see *lactase deficiency*; *lactose intolerance*).

MILK OF MAGNESIA n. a laxative and antacid, containing magnesium hydroxide; it is used to treat constipation and acid indigestion.

MILK SUGAR see *lactose*.

MILK TEETH see *deciduous teeth*.

MILONTIN n. trade name for the anticonvulsant *phensuximide* used to treat some forms of *epilepsy*.

MILTOWN n. trade name for the sedative *meprobamate*.

MINAMATA DISEASE n. a form of mercury poisoning that occurred among people eating fish from mercury-contaminated waters of Minamata Bay, off Japan in the 1950's; it is characterized by severe neurological degeneration with symptoms of paresthesia of mouth and limbs, tunnel vision, difficulties with concentration and muscular coordination, weakness, and emotional instability, progressing with continued exposure to cause damage to the gastrointestinal tract and kidneys, coma, and in some cases death (see also *mercury poisoning*).

MINERAL n. in nutrition, an inorganic substance, such as copper, zinc, or magnesium, needed in small amounts by the body for normal growth and function.

MINERAL DEFICIENCY n. a lack of a mineral essential to normal nutrition and metabolism; it may be due to a lack of the mineral in the diet or to inability to absorb the mineral. The symptoms of a mineral deficiency vary, depending on the functions of the specific mineral in maintaining the health of the body. Treatment of a deficiency is by adding the element to the diet or correcting the cause of its malabsorption, if possible.

MINERALOCORTICOID n. any of several hormones secreted by the adrenal cortex, the most important of which is *aldosterone*, which functions to maintain normal blood volume and salt and fluid balance in the body.

MINERAL OIL n. a laxative and stool softener used to treat constipation. Adverse effects include possible laxative dependence, fat-soluble vitamin deficiency, and abdominal cramps.

MINIMAL BRAIN DYSFUNCTION (MBD) see *attention deficit syndrome*.

MINIPRESS n. trade name for the antihypertensive prazosin.

MINOCIN n. trade name for the antibacterial *minocycline*.

MINOCYCLINE n. a tetracycline antibiotic, known under the trade name Minocin, used to treat a wide variety of bacterial and rickettsial infections. Adverse effects include gastrointestinal disturbances, allergic reactions, the danger of superinfection, and in children, discoloration of the teeth.

MINOR SURGERY n. any surgical procedure that does not require general anesthesia or respiratory assistance.

MINOXIDIL n. a vasodilator used to treat severe and hard-to-control *hypertension*. Adverse effects include rapid heart beat, salt-and-water retention, cardiac abnormalities, and gastrointestinal upsets.

MIOSIS n. 1. contraction of the sphincter muscle of the *iris*, causing the pupil to become smaller; it may be caused by an increase

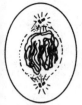 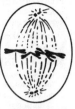

| Mid-prophase | Metaphase | Late anaphase | Late telophase |

Stages of mitosis

in light or by certain drugs; 2. abnormal constriction of the sphincter muscle of the iris, causing abnormally small pupils. adj. **miotic**

MIOTIC adj. pert. to or causing constriction of the *pupil* of the eye, as a miotic drug (e.g., pilocarpine).

MIRAGE n. an optical illusion caused by the refraction of light through layers of air of different temperatures.

MISCARRIAGE n. a spontaneous (non-induced) *abortion*.

MISSED ABORTION see under *abortion*.

MITE n. any of a group of small arachnids (relative of spiders and ticks), some of which cause local skin irritation and itching in humans.

MITHRACIN n. trade name for the antineoplastic *mithramycin*.

MITHRAMYCIN n. an antineoplastic, known under the trade name Mithracin, used to treat cancer of the testes. Adverse effects include blood clotting disorders, gastrointestinal upsets, and mouth inflammation.

MITOCHONDRION n. a self-replicating organelle found in the cytoplasm of cells, where it functions in cellular metabolism and respiration, providing the cell's major source of energy.

MITOGEN n. a substance that triggers *mitosis*.

MITOMYCIN n. an antineoplastic used to treat certain malignancies. Adverse effects include bone marrow depression and gastrointestinal disturbances.

MITOSIS n. type of cell division in which a cell divides into two genetically identical daughter cells; it is the way in which new body cells are produced for growth. Division of the cell nucleus takes place in four stages and the resulting daughter cells have the same number of chromosomes as the parent cell (compare *meiosis*). adj. **mitotic**

MITRAL STENOSIS see *mitral valve stenosis*.

MITRAL VALVE n. one of four valves of the heart; it is situated between the left atrium and left ventricle and allows blood to flow from the left atrium to the left ventricle but prevents backflow. It consists of two flaps or cusps; also called the **bicuspid valve** and **left atrioventricular valve** (compare *semilunar valve; tricuspid valve*).

MITRAL VALVE STENOSIS n. an obstruction or narrowing of the *mitral valve*, due to scarring from recurrent rheumatic fever; it causes reduced cardiac output, leading to breathlessness, fatigue, and cyanosis. Treatment is by surgery.

MITTELSCHMERZ n. pain in the area of the *ovary*, occurring at the time of *ovulation*, usually midway in the *menstrual cycle*.

MOBAN n. trade name for the antipsychotic *molindone*.

MODICON n. trade name for an oral contraceptive containing *estradiol* and *norethindrone*.

MODIFIED RADICAL MASTECTOMY see under *mastectomy*.

MOELLER'S GLOSSITIS n. chronic burning and pain of the tongue and sensivitity to spicy and hot foods.

MOLAR PREGNANCY see *hydatidosis*.

MOLECULAR GENETICS n. that branch of genetics concerned with the chemical structure, functions, and replication of molecules involved in the transmission of hereditary information, DNA and RNA.

MOLINDONE n. an antipsychotic drug, known under the trade name Moban, used in the treatment of *schizophrenia*. Adverse effects include low blood pressure, sedation, and disturbances of motor functions.

MOLLUSCUM n. a skin disease characterized by soft round masses.
Molluscum Contagiosum n. a virus disease of the skin characterized by white, rounded swellings that may resolve spontaneously or may be removed through surgery or other techniques. It is transmitted from person to person, occurring most often in children and adults with impaired immune function.

MONGOLIAN SPOT n. a benign, dark spot on the lower back and buttocks of some newborns, usually disappearing during early childhood.

MONGOLISM see *Down's syndrome*.

MONILIA see *Candida*. adj. **monilial**

MONILIASIS see *candidiasis*.

MONISTAT n. trade name for the antifungal *miconazole*.

MONITRICE n. a labor coach.

MONOAMINE OXIDASE (MAO) n. an enzyme, found in most tissues, esp. the liver and nervous system, that catalyzes the oxidation of many monoamines, including epinephrine, norepinephrine, and serotonin.

MONOAMINE OXIDASE (MAO) INHIBITOR n. any of a group of drugs used to treat depression. Adverse effects include dry mouth, drowsiness, and constipation. The drugs interact with many other drugs and with foods (such as cheeses, red wine, beer, and yogurt) containing tyramine, sometimes causing an acute hypertensive episode with headache and palpitations.

MONOBLAST n. a large immature *monocyte*, normally found in the bone marrow but present in the blood in certain diseases, esp. *monoblastic leukemia*.

MONOBLASTIC LEUKEMIA n. a malignancy of blood-forming tissues characterized by the proliferation of *monoblasts* and monocytes; also called **monocytic leukemia.**

MONOCLONAL adj. pert. to a group of identical cells or organisms derived from a single cell.

MONOCYTE n. a type of granular leukocyte (white blood cell) that functions in the ingestion of bacteria and other foreign particles.

MONOCYTIC LEUKEMIA n. a malignancy of the blood-forming tissues characterized by proliferation of monocytes and monoblasts. Symptoms include anorexia, fatigue, fever, weight loss, enlarged spleen, bleeding gums, and anemia. There are two forms: Schilling's leukemia and Naegeli's leukemia; also called **mon-**

oblastic leukemia; histiocytic leukemia.

MONOCYTOSIS n. an increase in the number of *monocytes* in the blood, occurring in some infections and in monocytic leukemia.

MONONEUROPATHY n. any disorder affecting a single nerve trunk, as in nerve compression from a fractured bone (see also *multiple mononeuropathy*) (compare *polyneuropathy*).

MONONUCLEOSIS see *infectious mononucleosis*

MONOPLEGIA n. paralysis of one limb.

MONORCHISM n. a condition in which only one testicle has descended into the scrotum; also: **monorchidism**. (See also *cryptorchidism*.)

MONOSOMY n. a chromosomal abnormality characterized by the absence of one chromosome from the normal diploid number for the species, as in humans 45, instead of the normal complement of 46 (compare *trisomy*) (see also *Turner's syndrome*).

MONOZYGOTIC TWINS n. twins developing from a single fertilized egg that splits in half at an early stage of cleavage and develops into two complete fetuses. Monozygotic twins are always of the same sex; have the same genetic makeup; and closely resemble each other in all characteristics. About one third of all twins are monozygous; such twinning is not hereditary and occurs in all races. Also called **identical twins** (compare *dizygotic twins*).

MONS n. a rounded eminence, esp. the **mons pubis**, the mound of fatty tissue overlying the pubic symphysis.

MONSTER n. a grossly malformed, usually nonviable, fetus.

MONTGOMERY'S TUBERCLE n. any of several sebaceous glands on the areolae of the breast that lubricate and protect the breast during breast-feeding.

MOON FACE n. a rounded, puffy face occurring in people treated with large doses of corticosteroids.

MORBID adj. diseased, abnormal.

MORBIDITY n. 1. the state of being diseased; 2. the ratio of persons who are diseased to those who are well in a given community.

MORBILLI see *measles*.

MORBILLIFORM adj. describing a rash that resembles that of measles.

MORIBUND adj. dying.

MORNING-AFTER PILL n. a large dose of an estrogen, given orally, within 24 to 72 hours after sexual intercourse to prevent conception; it is most commonly used after rape or incest. Effects include severe nausea and vomiting, blood clot formation, and harmful effects on the fetus, if pregnancy is not prevented.

MORNING SICKNESS n. nausea and vomiting that is a common occurrence in pregnancy, usually occurring in the morning but sometimes at other times during the day; it often disappears after the first three or four months of pregnancy. Symptomatic relief is often provided by not allowing the stomach to be empty and eating small, frequent meals (see also *hyperemesis gravidarum*).

MORON n. obsolete for a retarded person with an IQ between 50 and 70 (compare *idiot*; *imbecile*) (see also *mental retardation*).

MORO REFLEX n. normal reflex of a young infant, elicited by a sudden loud noise, in which the child flexes the legs and outstretches the arms, often with a cry; also called **startle reflex**.

MORPHEA n. a localized form of *scleroderma*, consisting of patches of rigid, dry, smooth skin.

MORPHINE n. a narcotic analgesic used to relieve pain. Adverse effects include respiratory depression, cardiovascular abnormalities, and the potential for dependence.

MORPHOGENESIS n. the development of the form and structure of an organism. adj. **morphogenetic**

MORTALITY RATE n. the death rate; the number of deaths per unit of population (e.g., per 100, 10,000, or 1,000,000) in a specific region, age group, or other group.

MORULA n. stage in human embryonic development between the *zygote* and *blastocyst*, consisting of a solid spherical mass of cells.

MOSAICISM n. a condition in which an organism contains two or more cell populations that differ in genetic makeup.

MOTION SICKNESS n. condition characterized by headache, nausea, and vomiting and caused by motion, as in a car or boat. Kinds of motion sickness are *air sickness*; *car sickness*; *sea sickness*. Prevention and treatment is by antihistamines.

MOTOR APHASIA n. an inability to utter remembered words, due to lesion in the Broca speech area of the cerebrum, most commonly the result of a stroke.

MOTOR AREA n. that part of the cerebral cortex associated with the function of voluntary muscles.

MOTOR END PLATE n. band of terminal fibers of a motor nerve that merges with the fibers of a voluntary muscle, allowing the impulse to be transmitted from the nerve to the muscle.

MOTOR NERVE n. a nerve that conducts impulses from the brain or spinal cord to muscles or organs of the body (compare *sensory nerve*).

MOTOR NEURON n. a nerve cell that makes up the pathway between the brain or spinal cord and an effector organ—a muscle or gland.

MOTOR NEURON DISEASE n. any of several diseases, often familial, characterized by loss of muscle mass, increasing paralysis, and other signs of impaired muscular function.

MOTOR SEIZURE n. a transitory disturbance in neuron function in a localized motor area of the cerebral cortex. The manifestations depend on the specific motor area affected. Also called **focal motor seizure**.

MOTOR SENSE n. perception allowing a person to undertake deliberate and purposeful movement.

MOTRIN n. trade name for the anti-inflammatory *ibuprofen*, used to treat rheumatoid arthritis, osteoarthritis, and certain other disorders.

MOUNTAIN FEVER see *Rocky Mountain spotted fever*.

MOUNTAIN SICKNESS see *altitude sickness*.

MOUTH

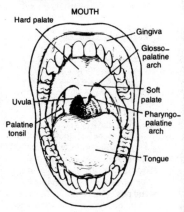

MOUTH n. 1. the oval cavity of the face, bounded by the lips and containing the gums, teeth and tongue, which is the anterior end of the digestive tube. In the mouth food is broken apart by the teeth and tongue and mixed with saliva, as the first step in the digestive process. 2. an opening into an organ or chamber, e.g. the mouth of the uterus; also: **orifice, os, ostium, stoma.**   adj. **oral**

MOUTH-TO-MOUTH RESUSCITATION see *cardiopulmonary resuscitation*.

MOXIBUSTION n. a method of pain relief or therapy, used mostly in the Far East, in which certain plant products are ignited and the burning substance held close to the body.

MSH abbreviation for *melanocyte-stimulating hormone*.

MUCIN n. the chief ingredient of *mucus*; the lubricant protecting body surfaces.

MUCOCUTANEOUS adj. pert. to the mucous membrane and the skin.

MUCOCUTANEOUS LYMPH NODE SYNDROME   see *Kawasaki disease*.

MUCOPOLYSACCHARIDE n. any of a group of complex carbohydrates that are structural parts of connective tissue.

MUCOPOLYSACCHARIDOSIS n. any of a group of genetic disorders, including *Hunter's syndrome* and *Hurler's syndrome*, in which greater than normal levels of mucopolysaccharides accumulate in the tissues; the diseases are characterized by skeletal deformity, mental retardation, and shortened life expectancy. The diseases can be detected through *amniocentesis*.

MUCOPURULENT adj. characteristic of a combination of mucus and pus.

MUCOSA   see *mucous membrane*.

MUCOUS adj. pert. to mucus.

MUCOUS COLITIS   see *irritable bowel syndrome*.

MUCOUS MEMBRANE n. a thin sheet of tissue that covers or lines parts of the body. It consists of a layer of epithelium overlying thicker connective tissue. It protects underlying organs, secretes mucus, and absorbs water and solutes.

MUCOUS PLUG n. in obstetrics, a collection of thick mucus, often streaked with blood that is expelled from the cervix of the uterus just before *labor* begins or during the early stages of labor.

MUCUS n. viscous secretions of mucous membranes and glands, containing mucin, water, white blood cells, and salts.   adj. **mucous**

MULTIFACTORIAL adj. pert. to a disease or condition resulting from the interaction of many factors, esp. many genes.

MULTIPLE FRACTURE   see under *fracture*.

MULTIPLE MONONEUROPATHY n. a condition in which there is impaired function of several individual nerve trunks; it may result from uremia, diabetes mellitus, or other disorders.

MULTIPLE MYELOMA n. a malignant neoplasm of bone marrow, causing bone pain and fractures, skeletal deformities, anemia, weight loss, and pulmonary and kidney complications.

MULTIPLE PERIPHERAL NEURITIS   see *peripheral polyneuritis*.

MULTIPLE PERSONALITY n. a disorder characterized by the presence of two or more distinct personalities in the same person, any of which may dominate at a given time ranging from a few minutes to years with transitions from one to the other personality usually occurring quickly and at a time of stress. Each personality is complex with developed behavioral patterns and mental and emotional processes and may or may not be known to the other. Clearcut examples are rare, but various symptoms appear in some schizophrenics, esp. among young women. Treatment is by psychoactive drugs and long-term psychotherapy.

MULTIPLE SCLEROSIS n. a progressive disease in which nerve fibers of the brain and spinal cord lose their *myelin* cover. It begins usually in early adulthood and progresses slowly with periods of remission and exacerbation. Early symptoms of abnormal sensations in the face or extremities, weakness, and visual disturbances (e.g., double vision) progress to ataxia, abnormal reflexes, tremors, difficulty in urination, emotional instability, and difficulty in walking, leading to increasing disability. There is no specific treatment; corticosteroids and other drugs are used to treat symptoms. Also called **disseminated multiple sclerosis**.

MUMPS n. an acute viral disease characterized by swelling of the parotid glands, most likely to affect nonimmunized children, but it may occur at any age, sometimes producing a severe illness in adults. After early symptoms of fever, malaise, headache, and low-grade fever, earache, parotid gland swelling, and fever to 104° Fahrenheit (40° Celsius) occur, sometimes with salivary gland enlargement, and, in postpubertal males, swelling and tenderness of the testes. Complications include mumps meningitis, arthritis, and nephritis. Treatment includes rest, drugs to relieve pain and reduce fever. Prevention is by immunization with attenuated live-virus vaccine, routinely given at 15 months of age.

MUNCHAUSEN'S SYNDROME n. condition in which a person pleas for treatment and hospitalization for symptomatic but imaginary illness.

MURINE TYPHUS n. an acute infection caused by *Rickettsia typhi*, transmitted by the bite of an infected flea and characterized by chills, fever, headache, muscle aches, and a dull red rash. Treatment is by *chloramphenicol* or *tetracycline*. Also called **endemic typhus**; **rat typhus**; **urban typhus** (compare *epidemic typhus*, *Rocky Mountain spotted fever*).

MURMUR n. a short, usually soft sound, esp. an abnormal one of the heart or circulation.

MUSCLE n. a kind of vascular, conductive and elastic tissue, composed of fibers that can contract, causing movement of parts and organs. There are three basic kinds of muscle: skeletal muscle, which is striated in appearance, controls voluntary movement, responds quickly to neural stimulation, and is paralyzed if innervation is lost; smooth muscle, which is not striped in appearance, comprises the musculature of all vis-

Smooth or involuntary
muscle

Cardiac or heart muscle

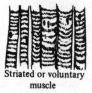

Striated or voluntary
muscle

Types of muscle

ceral organs, responds slowly to stimulation, and controls involuntary movement; and cardiac muscle, which is striped in appearance, but does not respond as quickly as skeletal muscle and which continues to contract if it loses its neural stimuli.

MUSCLE RELAXANT n. a drug that reduces the contractility of muscle fibers by blocking the transmission of nerve impulses at neuromuscular junctions, by increasing the time between contractions of fibers, by decreasing the excitability of the motor end plate, by interfering with nerve synapses in the central nervous system, or by interfering with calcium release from muscle or by other actions; the drugs are used to treat muscle spasm and as adjuncts to anesthesia for certain surgical procedures.

MUSCULAR adj. pert. to *muscle*.

MUSCULAR DYSTROPHY n. any of a group of hereditary diseases of the muscular system characterized by weakness and wasting of groups of skeletal muscles, leading to increasing disability. The various forms differ in age of onset, rate of progression, and mode of genetic transmission; the most common is Duchenne's muscular dystrophy.
Duchenne's muscular dystrophy n. the most common of the muscular dystrophies (approximately 50%), it is an X-linked recessive disease (affecting only males) with symptoms first appearing around the age of 4. Progressive wasting of leg and pelvic muscles produces a waddling gait and abnormal curvature of the spine, progressing to inability to walk and confinement to a wheelchair (usually by age 12), often accompanied by progressive weakening of cardiac muscle. There is no specific treatment and death, usually from heart dis-

orders, often results by age 20; also: **pseudohypertrophic dystrophy**.
myotonic muscular dystrophy n. a severe form of muscular dystrophy characterized by drooping eyelids, facial weakness, difficulty with speech, and weakness of the hands and feet spreading to arms, shoulders, legs and hips; also: **myotonia atrophica**; **Steinert's disease**
limb-girdle muscular dystrophy n. a form of muscular dystrophy (*autosmonal recessive disease*) characterized by progressive muscular weakness beginning in either the shoulder or pelvic girdle.

MUSCULO- comb. form indicating an association with muscles (e.g., **musculocutaneous**, pert. to muscles and skin).

MUSCULOSKELETAL adj. pert. to the muscles and skeleton.

MUSCULOSKELETAL SYSTEM n. the network of bones, muscles, ligaments, tendons, joints, and associated tissues (e.g., ligaments and tendons) of the body involved in the maintenance of body form and movement.

MUSHROOM POISONING a toxic condition caused by the ingestion of certain species of mushrooms, esp. *Amanita* species. Symptoms include tearing, salivation, abdominal cramps, diarrhea, difficulty in breathing, and, in severe cases, liver and kidney damage, convulsions, coma, and sometimes death. Treatment depends on the species of mushroom eaten; it often involves gastric lavage.

MUTAGEN n. an agent, physical or environmental, that induces a genetic mutation or increases the mutation rate.   adj. **mutagenic**

MUTAGENESIS n. the induction of a *mutation*, or change, in a *gene*.

MUSCLES

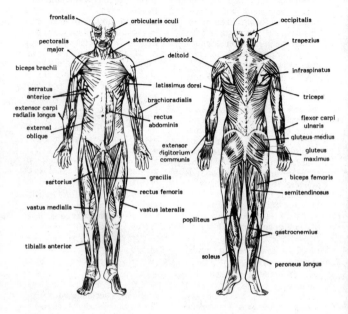

frontalis
orbicularis oculi
pectoralis major
sternocleidomastoid
biceps brachii
deltoid
serratus anterior
latissimus dorsi
extensor carpi radialis longus
brachioradialis
external oblique
rectus abdominis
extensor digitorium communis
sartorius
gracilis
rectus femoris
vastus medialis
vastus lateralis
tibialis anterior

occipitalis
trapezius
infraspinatus
triceps
flexor carpi ulnaris
gluteus medius
gluteus maximus
biceps femoris
semitendinosus
popliteus
gastrocnemius
soleus
peroneus longus

MUTAMYCIN n. trade name for the antineoplastic *mitomycin*.

MUTANT GENE n. a gene that has changed, affecting the normal transmission and expression of a trait.

MUTATION n. a change in the genetic structure; it may occur spontaneously or be induced (e.g., by radiation or certain mutagenic chemicals).

MUTISM n. the inability or refusal to speak. It may be innate, the result of being deaf-mute from birth; acquired through brain damage (aphasia), or the result of severe psychological disorder.

MUTON n. the smallest unit of the hereditary material—DNA—in which a change can produce a *mutation*.

MY-, MYO- comb. form indicating an association with muscle (e.g., **myovascular**, pert. to muscles and blood circulation).

MYALGIA n. diffuse muscle pain, occurring in many infectious (e.g., influenza, measles, rheumatic fever, toxoplasmosis) and other disorders (e.g., fibrositis, Guillain Barre Syndrome, muscle tumor), and sometimes as the result of certain drugs.

MYASTEHENIA n. abnormal muscle weakness, the result of disease, as in myasthenia gravis, or inadequate blood circulation to a given area.

MYASTHENIA GRAVIS n. a

disease characterized by chronic fatiguability and weakness of muscles, esp. in the face and neck region, but also affecting the muscles of the trunk and limbs. Onset is gradual, usually with drooping eyelids and facial muscle weakness, and the course of the disease variable, sometimes mild with many remissions, in other cases progressing to affect the respiratory muscles and cause respiratory distress. It is caused by deficiency of acetylcholine at the neuromuscular junctions. Treatment involves rest, restricted physical activity, and the use of anticholinesterase drugs (*neostigmine* or *pyridostigmine*).

MYC-, MYCET-, MYCO- comb. form indicating an association with fungus (e.g., **mycetogenic**, caused by a fungus)

MYCHEL n. trade name for the antibacterial *chloramphenicol*.

MYCIFRADIN n. trade name for the antibacterial *neomycin*.

MYCITRACIN n. trade name for a topical, fixed-combination drug containing the antibacterials *polymyxin* and *neomycin*.

MYCOLOG n. trade name for a topical fixed-combination drug containing two antibacterials (*gramicidin* and *neomycin*), an antifungal (*nystatin*) and a glucocorticoid; it is used to treat skin and mucous membrane infections and irritations.

MYCOLOGY n. the study of fungi and fungus-caused diseases.

MYCOPLASMA n. a group of very small organisms, the smallest free-living organisms known, some of which produce disease in humans (e.g., *mycoplasma pneumonia*); also called **pleuropneumonialike organism**.

MYCOPLASMA PNEUMONIA n. a contagious disease, primarily of children and young adults, caused by *Mycoplasma pneumoniae* and characterized by cough, fever, and other signs of upper respiratory infection. Treatment is by *erythromycin* or *tetracyclines*.

MYCOSIS n. any fungus-caused disease.

MYCOSTATIN n. trade name for the antifungal *nystatin*.

MYDRIASIS n. dilation of the pupil of the eye, caused by muscle action pulling the iris outward and enlarging the pupil; it occurs in response to a decrease in light or the action of certain drugs (compare *miosis*).

MYDRIATIC n. a drug (e.g., atropine) that causes the pupil of the eye to dilate; used to aid examination of the eye and to treat certain eye disorders.

MYELATELIA n. any developmental defect of the spinal cord.

MYELIN n. a complex material, containing phospholipids and proteins, that forms a sheath around the axons of certain nerve fibers, called myelinated (or medullated) nerve fibers. The myelin is produced by Schwaan cells along the axon. Myelinated nerve fibers conduct impulses more rapidly than do unmyelinated fibers.

MYELINATED adj. having a *myelin* sheath.

MYELINIZATION n. the development of a *myelin* sheath around a nerve fiber.

MYELIN SHEATH n. the segmented, fatty covering composed of *myelin* that covers the axons of some nerve fibers.

MYELITIS n. inflammation of the *spinal cord*.

MYELOBLAST n. a precursor of the granulocytic leukocytes (eosinophils, basophils, and neutrophils) that normally occurs in bone marrow but increases in number in peripheral circulation in certain diseases, esp. *myeloblastic leukemia*.

MYELOBLASTIC LEUKEMIA n. a malignant neoplasm of blood-forming tissues characterized by numerous *myeloblasts* in the circulating blood.

MYELOCELE n. a saclike protrusion of the spinal cord through a congenital defect in the vertebral column; (see also *myelomeningocele*).

MYELOCYSTOCELE n. a protrusion of a cyst containing spinal cord material through a developmental defect in the vertebral column; (see also *myelomeningocele*).

MYELOCYTE n. an immature granulocytic leukocyte (eosinophil, basophil, or neutrophil) normally found in bone marrow and present in the circulating blood in certain diseases, esp. *myelocytic leukemia*.

MYELOCYTIC LEUKEMIA n. a malignant neoplasm of blood forming tissues characterized by proliferation of *myelocytes* and their presence in circulating blood; also called **granulocytic leukemia**.

MYELOGRAM n. an X ray of the spinal cord, spinal nerve roots, and subarachnoid space.

MYELOGRAPHY n. an X-ray procedure in which the spinal cord and subarachnoid space are photographed (myelogram) after injection of a contrast medium into the subarachnoid space; it is used to examine the spinal cord and detect possible lesions.

MYELOID adj. pert. to bone marrow; 2. pert. to the spinal cord.

MYELOID LEUKEMIA see *acute myelocytic leukemia*; *chronic myelocytic leukemia*.

MYELOMA n. a bone-destroying malignant neoplasm of bone marrow tissue that occurs most often in the vertebrae, ribs, pelvis, and skull bones; symptoms include spontaneous bone fractures and bone pain. It may develop in several areas simultaneously (*multiple myeloma*). Treatment of local lesions is by radiotherapy.

MYELOMALACIA n. softening of the spinal cord, often due to inadequate blood supply.

MYELOMENINGOCELE n. a congenital defect of the central nervous system in which a sac containing a part of the spinal cord and its meninges and cerebrospinal fluid protrudes through an opening in the vertebral column; it is due to a failure of the neural tube to close during embryonic development or to its reopening after closure. It most commonly occurs in the lower thoracic, lumbar, or sacral areas. The extent of neurological dysfunction depends on the location of the anomaly and the amount of spinal tissue involved; lower extremity paralysis and bladder and anal sphincter problems are common, frequently accompanied by hydrocephalus and mental retardation. Immediate treatment includes the prevention of infection and an assessment of the probable extent of neurological damage to determine if surgery to correct the defect is indicated.

MYESTHESIA n. perception of a sensation (e.g., touch, pressure) by a muscle.

MYIASIS n. infection or infestation with the larvae of flies, most often through a wound or other opening.

MYOCARDIAL INFARCTION n. a heart attack; the death of an area of heart muscle due to interruption of its blood supply through occlusion of the *coronary arteries* by *atherosclerosis* or an *embolus*. Typical signs include crushing, viselike pain in the chest that may radiate to the arm, esp. the left arm, and neck region; shortness of breath; faintness; anxiety; and an ashen appearance; there is also often irregularities of heart rhythm, demonstrable on an electrocardiogram; weak pulse; and low blood pressure. Treatment involves cardiopulmonary resuscitation, if necessary; oxygen, if necessary; and drugs to control heart rhythm, anticoagulants, sedatives, and analgesics; close monitoring to guard against complications and prevent ventricular fibrillation or cardiac arrest is essential. Prognosis depends on the extent of heart damage, but in most cases, patients are able to return to normal life with some limitations regarding diet, activity, and stress.

MYOCARDIOPATHY n. any disease of the heart muscle; also: **cardiomyopathy**.

MYOCARDITIS n. an inflammation of the *myocardium* (heart muscle); it may be caused by viral, bacterial, or fungal infection; by rheumatic fever; or as a complication of another disease. Treatment depends on the cause.

MYOCARDIUM n. the thick, muscular middle layer of the heart wall, composed almost entirely of cardiac muscle. (The other layers being the outer *epicardium* and inner *endocardium*.) adj. **myocardial**

MYOCHRYSINE n. trade name for a gold preparation sometimes used to treat arthritis.

MYOCLONUS n. a sudden spasm of muscles, occurring in some forms of epilepsy and in certain progressive neurological disorders. adj. **myoclonic**

MYOGLOBIN n. an iron-containing pigment responsible for the red color of muscle and its ability to store oxygen.

MYOFIBRIL n. one of many contractile filaments that make up a fiber of a *striated muscle*.

MYOGENIC adj. originating in *muscle*.

MYOGLOBINURIA n. the presence of *myoglobin* in the urine.

MYOGRAM n. a recording of muscle activity (see *electromyography*).

MYOMA n. a benign muscle tumor, esp. one of the uterine muscle.

MYOMENINGOCELE n. an abnormal saclike protrusion through the spine of the *spinal cord* and associated *meninges* due to a failure of neural tube closure during embryonic development. It most commonly occurs in the lumbosacral region, less commonly in other areas of the spine. The extent of neurological impairment depends on the level of protrusion; it may include paralysis, incontinence, skeletal and muscular abnormalities, ulceration; hydrocephalus and mental retardation are commonly associated. Treatment is by placement of myomeningocele tissues back in the spinal column and closure, but neurological damage sustained cannot be corrected (compare *meningocele*).

MYOMETRITIS n. inflammation or infection of the myometrium, the muscular wall of the uterus.

MYOMETRIUM n. the muscular layer of the uterine wall, surrounding the endometrium; it is made up of smooth muscle that has small spontaneous contractions during certain phases of the menstrual cycle and during pregnancy in response to the hormones *estrogen*, *progesterone*, and *oxytocin*.

MYONECROSIS n. the death of muscle cell fibers, sometimes seen in infections of deep wounds.

MYONEURAL JUNCTION see *neuromuscular junction*.

MYOPATHY n. any disease of the muscles, not caused by nerve dysfunction; symptoms depend on the specific disease but generally include muscle weakness and wasting. adj. **myopathic**

MYOPE n. a person who has *myopia*.

MYOPIA n. nearsightedness; a defect in vision caused by elongation of the eyeball or an error in refraction so that the image comes to a focus in front of the *retina*; it can be corrected by concave lenses (compare *hyperopia*).

Normal Eye

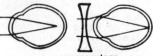

Myopia (nearsighted)

concave lens

In the normal eye, the image comes to a focus on the retina. In myopia, the image comes to a focus in front of the retina. The defect can be corrected by concave lenses.

MYORRHEXIS n. the breaking apart of a muscle.

MYOSARCOMA n. a malignant tumor of muscle tissue.

MYOSIN n. a protein in muscle that, along with actin, makes up the contractile elements of muscles.

MYOSITIS n. inflammation of muscle tissue, usually voluntary muscle, most often caused by infection, parasite infestation, trauma, or degenerative muscle diseases (see also *polymyositis*).
MYOSITIS OSSIFICANS n. a rare, inherited disease in which muscle tissue is replaced by bone, leading to stiffness and impaired mobility.
MYOSITIS TRICHINOSA see *trichinosis*.

MYOTOMY n. surgical division of a muscle.

MYOTONIA n. a condition in which a muscle or group of muscles has abnormally prolonged contractions, not readily relaxing after contraction. adj. **myotonic**

myotonia atrophica see *myotonic muscular dystrophy* under *muscular dystrophy*.
myotonia congenita n. a rare and mild form of myotonia usually manifested only by muscle stiffness; also: **Thomsen's disease**.

MYRINGA see *tympanic membrane*.

MYRINGECTOMY n. surgical removal of the *tympanic membrane* (eardrum).

MYRINGITIS n. inflammation of the *tympanic membrane* (eardrum).

MYRINGO- comb. form indicating a relationship with the tympanic membrane (e.g., **myringomycosis**, a fungal infection of the eardrum).

MYRINGOPLASTY n. surgical repair of perforations of the eardrum with a tissue graft to help correct hearing loss.

MYRINGOTOMY n. surgical incision into the eardrum to relieve pressure and release pus from the middle ear.

MYX-, MYXO- comb. form indicating an association with *mucus* (e.g., **myxadenitis**, mucus gland inflammation).

MYXEDEMA n. a syndrome, caused by deficiency of thyroid hormone in adults (hypothyroidism), including cold intolerance, fatigue, sluggishness, skin coarsening, weight gain, mental dullness, and in women menstrual irregularities.

MYXOMA n. a usually benign, jellylike tumor of connective tissue that may grow to large size. Symptoms depend on the location of the tumor and result from pressure on or interference with the function of an adjacent or underlying organ.

MYXOVIRUS n. any of a group of medium-sized RNA viruses including those that cause mumps and influenza.

n

N chemical symbol for the element *nitrogen* (see Table of Elements).

NA chemical symbol for the element *sodium* (see Table of Elements).

NABOTHIAN CYST n. a usually benign cyst that forms in the *Nabothian glands* of the *cervix* of the *uterus*.

NABOTHIAN GLAND n. one of many small, mucus-secreting glands of the *cervix* of the *uterus*.

NACTISOL n. trade name for a fixed combination drug, containing the antispasmodic poldine and the barbiturate butabarbital, sometimes used to treat *peptic ulcer*.

NADOLOL n. a beta-adrenergic blocking agent used to treat *hypertension* and angina. Adverse effects include cardiac arrhythmias, gastrointestinal disturbances, and allergic reactions.

NAFCILLIN n. an antibacterial, known under the trade name Nafcil, used to treat infections caused by penicillin-resistant strains of staphylococci. Adverse effects include allergic reactions and gastrointestinal upsets.

NAGELE'S RULE n. a method for calculating expected delivery date. Three months are subtracted from the first day of the last menstrual period and seven days added to that date.

NAIL n. a flattened, horny structure, made of keratin from *epidermis*, at the end of each finger and toe. Each nail is composed of a root, body, and free edge. The root fits into a groove in the skin and is closely molded to the skin of the finger or toe with the nail fold overlying the root. The body of the nail lies over the nail bed; the white crescent-shaped structure at the base of the body is the lunula. Nails grow longer as cells in the stratum germinativum of the root proliferate; also: **unguis**.

NALDECON n. trade name for a fixed-combination drug, containing two adrenergics (phenylpropanolamine and phenylephrine) and two antihistamines (chlorpheniramine and phenyltoloxamine); used to treat cough and nasal congestion associated with the common cold, bronchitis, influenza, and similar diseases.

NALFON n. trade name for the antiinflammatory agent *fenoprofen*, used in the treatment of arthritis and other inflammatory conditions.

NALIDIXIC ACID n. an antibacterial, known under the trade name NegGram, used to treat certain infections of the urinary tract. Adverse effects include neurological and gastrointestinal disturbances, and the possibility of seizures, convulsions, and increased intracranial pressure.

NALLINE n. trade name for the narcotic antagonist *nalorphine*.

NALORPHINE n. narcotic antagonist, used to reverse the effects of narcotics, esp. morphine, and to stimulate breathing and restore consciousness.

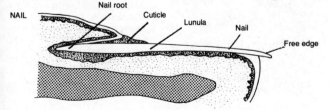

NAIL — Nail root — Cuticle — Lunula — Nail — Free edge

NANDROLONE n. an androgen, known under the trade names Durabolin and Kabolin, used to treat testosterone deficiency, breast cancer in women, and osteoporosis; it also stimulates growth and weight gain. Adverse effects include liver toxicity, electrolyte imbalance, and endocrine disturbances.

NANO- comb. form indicating extreme smallness (e.g., **nanocephaly**, an abnormally small head).

NANISM n. abnormal smallness, dwarfism.

NANOPHTHALMOS n. a condition in which one or both eyes are abnormally small, but other eye defects are not present.

NANUS n. a dwarf.

NAPE n. the back of the neck.

NAPEX n. the area just below the bump (occiput) at the back of the head.

NAPHAZOLINE n. a vasoconstrictor, used in eye drops and nasal sprays, under the trade names Privine and 4-way, used to treat nasal congestion and eye irritation. Adverse effects arise from systemic absorption and include sedation and cardiovascular effects.

NAPHTHALENE POISONING n. a toxic condition caused by ingestion or inhalation of naphthalene and related compounds, commonly found in moth balls and some agricultural insecticides; symptoms include nausea, vomiting, abdominal pain, muscle spasm, and convulsions. Treatment includes induced vomiting, gastric lavage, the use of cathartics and, in some cases, the use of *diazepam* to relieve muscle spasm.

NAPRAPATHY n. a system of medicine based on the idea that many diseases are due to displacement of connective tissues (e.g., ligaments, tendons) and that manipulation of these tissues will bring relief.

NAPROXEN. n. a nonsteroid, antiinflammatory agent, known under the trade names Naprosyn and Anaprox, used in the treatment of arthritis, musculoskeletal inflammation, and moderate pain. Adverse effects include headache, dizziness, gastrointestinal disturbances, and skin eruptions; the drug interacts with many others.

NAQUA n. trade name for the diuretic trichlormethiazide, used to treat *hypertension* and, as an adjunct, congestive heart failure and other conditions.

NAQUIVAL n. trade name for a fixed-combination drug, containing the diuretic trichlormethiazide and the antihypertensive *reserpine*; it is used to treat *hypertension*.

NARCISSISM n. an abnormal interest in oneself, esp. one's body; self-love; in psychoanalytic theory, sexual self-interest, normal in young children but abnormal in adults.   adj. **narcissistic**

NARCISSISTIC PERSONALITY n. a personality characterized by excessive self-love and self-absorption, unrealistic views about one's own attributes, and little regard for others. In some cases there is an exaggerated need for attention, preoccupation with grooming, and self-consciousness. Treatment involves psychotherapy, depending on the severity of the condition.

NARCOLEPSY n. a syndrome characterized by the uncontrollable desire to sleep, sudden sleep attacks lasting from a few minutes to a few hours, episodes of momentary loss of muscle tone (cataplexy) and occasionally visual hallucinations before sleep. The condition usually begins in adolescence and lasts for life; no organic cause is known. Stimulant drugs are sometimes used to prevent attacks.   adj. **narcoleptic**

NARCOLEPTIC n. 1. a substance that produces an uncontrollable desire to sleep; 2. a person with *narcolepsy*.

NARCOSIS n. state of stupor caused by *narcotic* drugs.

NARCOTIC n. a drug, derived from *opium* or produced synthetically, that relieves pain, induces euphoria and other mood changes, decreases respiration and peristalsis, constricts the pupils, and produces sleep. Narcotic drugs are addictive, producing drug addiction after repeated use. Narcotic drugs used for pain relief include *morphine* and *meperidine* (Demerol) and *codeine*; *heroin* and other narcotics are common street drugs. See also *drug addiction*.

NARCOTIC ANTAGONIST n. a drug that such as naloxone and nalorphine used to counter the effects of narcotics, esp. respiratory depression.

NARDIL n. trade name for the antidepressant *phenelzine*.

NARES n. openings in the nose that allow the passage of air into the pharynx. The paired anterior openings are the **anterior nares**, or nostrils; the paired posterior openings at the back of the nasal cavity, leading to the *nasopharynx*, are the **posterior nares**.

NASAL adj. pert. to the *nose* or *nasal cavity*.

NASAL CAVITY n. either of the pair of cavities that open on the face to allow the passage of air into the pharynx.

NASAL DECONGESTANT n. a drug that provides temporary relief of nasal symptoms associated with the common cold, rhinitis, and upper respiratory infections. Most contain an antihistamine and vasoconstrictor, and many are sold without prescription.

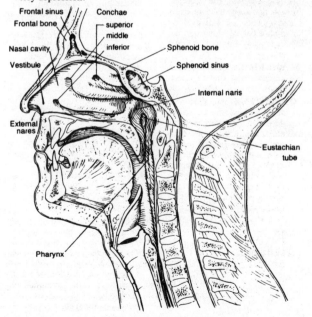

NASAL SEPTUM n. mucous membrane-covered bone and cartilage partition dividing the nostrils.

NASAL SINUS n. any of numerous cavities in the skull lined with a mucous membrane continuous with the nasal membrane; among the nasal sinuses are the frontal sinuses, ethmoidal sinuses, and maxillary sinuses.

NASCENT adj. just born; beginning to exist.

NASION n. depression at the bridge of the nose that indicates the point where the frontal and nasal bones of the skull meet.

NASO- comb. form indicating a relationship with the nose (e.g., **nasolacrimal**, pert. to the nose and *lacrimal apparatus*).

NASOGASTRIC FEEDING n. the process of delivering nutrients in liquid form through a tube passed into the stomach through the nose; used in cases where the person can digest food but cannot eat, as, for example, in some cases of mouth or throat surgery.

NASOLACRIMAL DUCT n. duct that carries tears from the lacrimal sac to the nasal cavity.

NASOPHARYNX n. a region of the throat behind the nose, extending from the posterior nares to the soft palate region and containing the pharyngeal *tonsils* (compare *laryngopharynx*; *oropharynx*) adj. **nasopharyngeal**

NASOTRACHEAL TUBE n. tube inserted into the trachea through the nose and pharynx; it is used to deliver oxygen and respiratory therapy.

NATAL adj. 1. pert. to birth 2. pert. to the *nates*.

NATES n. the buttocks; the fleshy protuberances containing fat and the gluteal muscles at the lower posterior part of the trunk of the body. adj. **natal**

NATRIURESIS n. the excretion of abnormally large amounts of sodium in the urine, usually the result of diuretic drug intake or certain metabolic disorders. adj. **natriuretic**

NATURAL CHILDBIRTH n. labor and childbirth with little or no medical intervention and the mother given minimal or no drugs to relieve pain or aid the birth process. It is considered the safest for the baby, but certain conditions (e.g., inadequate birth canal, fetal distress, illness in the mother) may make it impossible. (See also *Bradley method of childbirth*; *Lamaze method of childbirth*; *Read method of childbirth*).

NATURAL FAMILY PLANNING n. any of several methods of family planning that do not involve the use of drugs (e.g., oral contraceptives), devices (e.g., diaphragm or intrauterine device), or surgical intervention (sterilization). In natural family planning methods several ways are used to determine the time of *ovulation* and thus the fertile period in a woman's *menstrual cycle* and that information used to increase or decrease the chances of conception by avoiding or engaging in coitus at the fertile time (see *basal body temperature method of family planning*; *calendar method of family planning*; *ovulation*; *rhythm*) (see also *contraception*).

NATURAL IMMUNITY n. the stage of being innately resistant to or insusceptible to a particular disease; innate immunity.

NATURAL SELECTION n. the natural process by which those organisms best suited to a particular environment by virtue of their adaptations tend to survive and propagate others with their characteristics, while those less well adapted have less chance for survival and propagation.

NATUROPATHY n. a system of medicine that uses only natural substances (e.g., herbs, water, sunlight, fresh air) to cure illnesses and rid the body of "unnatural" substances.

NAUSEA n. feeling that one is going to vomit; it occurs in motion sickness, early pregnancy, at times of extreme stress, and in many illnesses (e.g., gallbladder disease, gastrointestinal viral infections).

NAVANE n. trade name for the tranquilizer *thiothixene*, used in treatment of certain psychotic disorders.

NAVEL n. the depression in the abdomen at the insertion of the umbilical cord in the fetus; umbilicus; colloquial: **bellybutton**.

NEAR-SIGHTEDNESS see *myopia*.

NEBCIN n. trade name for the antibacterial *tobramycin*.

NEBULA n. a faint opacity or scar on the *cornea*; it seldom interferes with vision.

NECK n. 1. area of the body between the head and the trunk; 2. a constricted section of a body organ, as the neck of the femur (thighbone).

NECRO- comb. form indicating an association with death (e.g., **necrogenic**, causing death).

NECROBIOSIS LIPOIDICA n. a skin disease, occurring most often in people with *diabetes mellitus*, esp. women, in which there is degeneration of skin structure and the development of thin, shiny patches on the skin, esp. in the shin and forearm area.

NECROLOGY n. the study of death.

NECROLYSIS n. disintegration of dead tissue.

NECROPSY see *autopsy*.

NECROPHILIA n. morbid liking or desire for dead bodies, esp. the desire to have sexual contact with a dead body.

NECROSIS n. the death of some or all of the cells in a tissue; usually caused by disease, inadequate blood supply to the tissue, or injury.

NECROTIZING ENTERITIS n. acute inflammation of the small and large intestine, caused by infection with the bacterium *Clostridium perfringens*; it is characterized by bloody diarrhea, severe abdominal pain, and vomiting.

NECROTIZING ENTEROCOLITIS (NEC) n. an acute inflammatory condition of the intestine, occurring in premature or low-birth-weight infants, believed due to a defect or immaturity of natural defenses with microorganisms normally present in the gastrointestinal tract producing infection. Symptoms include abdominal distension, decreased bowel sounds, vomiting, bloody diarrhea, lethargy, poor feeding, and often low body temperature. Necrosis of intestinal tissue due to inadequate blood supply, hyperbilirubinemia, edema, abdominal tenderness, and other abnormalities may follow, sometimes leading to perforation of the gastrointestinal lining, peritonitis, respiratory failure, or death. Treatment depends on the severity of the disease but includes *nasogastric feeding, antibiotics*, and, if perforation of the intestinal wall occurs, surgery.

NEEDLE BIOPSY n. removal of a segment of tissue for microscopic analysis by inserting a hollow needle through the skin or external surface of an organ and twisting it around to obtain a sample of underlying cells.

NEGATIVISM n. a pattern of behavior characterized by opposition, resistance to suggestion, unwillingness to cooperate, and a tendency to act in a contrary way; it may be passive, as in a rigid, immobile position; or active, with belligerent acts.

NEGGRAM n. trade name for the antibacterial *nalidixic acid* used to treat some urinary tract infections.

NEMATO- comb. form indicating a relationship with nematodes (e.g., **nematocide**, an agent that kills nematodes) or with thread (e.g., **nematoid**, like a thread).

NEMATODE n. any of a large group (phylum Nematoda) of unsegmented worms, tapered at both ends, including roundworms, pinworms, and hookworms; many species infest humans, producing disease.

NEMBUTAL n. trade name for the barbiturate *pentobarbital* commonly used as an adjunct to anesthesia.

NEO- prefix meaning "new" (e.g., **neoblastic**, pert. to a new tissue).

NEOBIOTIC n. trade name for the antibacterial *neomycin*.

NEOLOGISM n. in psychiatry, the invention of a new word that has meaning only to the person who coined it; it is normal in early childhood, but usually a sign of mental illness (e.g., schizophrenia) in an adult.

NEOMYCIN n. an antibacterial drug, known under the trade name Neobiotic, used orally to treat intestinal infections and topically to treat eye and skin infections. Adverse effects include gastrointestinal upsets, the danger of suprainfection, and, with prolonged use, damage to ears and kidneys.

NEONATAL adj. pert. to a *neonate* or to the first month of life.

NEONATAL DEATH n. death of a live-born infant within the first 28 days of life.

NEONATAL INTENSIVE CARE UNIT (NICU) n. a hospital unit designed with special equipment and devices for the care of the seriously ill, premature, or very low birth weight newborn.

NEONATAL MORTALITY n. the number of infant deaths, during the first 28 days of life, per unit of population (e.g., per 1,000 live births) in a given institution, geographic area, or period of time.

NEONATAL PERIOD n. the first 28 days of life.

NEONATE n. an infant from birth to four weeks (28 days) of life. adj. **neonatal**

NEONATOLOGY n. that branch of medicine concerned with the newborn, specifically the diagnosis and treatment of neonates.

NEOPLASIA n. new and abnormal development of a cell; it may be benign or malignant. adj. **neoplastic**

NEOPLASM n. any abnormal growth of new tissue, benign or malignant.

NEOSPORIN n. trade name for a fixed-combination topical drug containing the antibacterials *polymixin*, *neomycin*, and *bacitracin*; used in ointment form for skin irritations and minor skin infections and in eye drop form for minor eye infections.

NEOSTIGMINE n. a cholinergic used to treat *myasthenia gravis*. Adverse effects include intestinal pain and cramping, excess salivation, and respiratory depression.

NEOTHYLLINE n. trade name for the smooth muscle relaxant dyphylline, used to treat bronchial asthma and bronchospasm associated with acute bronchitis and emphysema.

NEPHR-, NEPHRO- comb. form indicating an association with the kidneys (e.g., **nephropathy**, any disorder of the kidney).

NEPHRALGIA n. pain in the kidney, usually felt in the loin.

NEPHRECTOMY n. surgical removal of a kidney, performed to remove a tumor, drain an abscess, or treat other kidney disorder.

NEPHRITIS n. inflammation of the kidney (see also *glomerulonephritis*).

NEPHROANGIOSCLEROSIS n. death of cells of the kidney arterioles associated with hypertension; symptoms include, in addition to high blood pressure, headache, blurred vision, and often an enlarged heart; if hypertension cannot be controlled, it can lead to kidney failure and heart failure (see *malignant hypertension*).

NEPHROBLASTOMA see *Wilms' tumor*.

NEPHROCALCINOSIS n. a condition in which calcium deposits form in the kidney, often at the site of previous inflammation leading to diminished kidney function, infection, and blood in the urine; it may be associated with excess calcium in the blood or kidney malfunction.

NEPHROGENIC DIABETES INSIPIDUS n. an unusual form of *diabetes insipidus* caused by lack of response to normal levels of *antidiuretic hormone* (ADH) by the kidney, leading to excessive production of dilute urine and extreme thirst.

NEPHROLITH n. a calculus (stone) formed in the kidney.

NEPHROLITHIASIS n. a disorder characterized by the presence of stones in the kidney. There may be no symptoms or pain and blood in the urine may occur. If urinary blockage, severe pain, or infection occur, surgical removal of the stones and/or kidney is indicated (see also *urinary calculus*).

NEPHROLOGY n. the study of the kidney, its development, anatomy, and physiology and the diagnosis and treatment of disorders affecting it.

NEPHRON n. the structural and functional unit of the kidney; there are more than one million nephrons in each kidney. Each nephron consists of a renal corpuscle, containing a *glomerulus* enclosed in Bowman's capsule; renal tubules; and the loop of Henle.

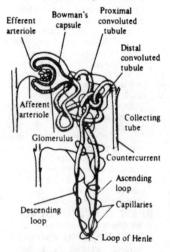

The kidney includes many nephrons

NEPHROPTOSIS n. abnormal downward placement of the kidney.

NEPHROSCLEROSIS see *nephroangiosclerosis*.

NEPHROSIS n. a disease of the kidney, esp. a degenerative, noninflammatory disease.

NEPHROTIC SYNDROME n. an abnormal condition, marked by edema, the presence of large amounts of protein in the urine and lower than normal levels of albumin in the blood, often with nausea, weakness, and loss of appetite; it is usually associated with disease of the glomerulus (*glomerulonephritis*) or kidney veins or occurs as a complication of many systemic diseases (e.g., *multiple myeloma*, *diabetes mellitus*, *systemic lupus erythematosus*).

NEPHROTOMY n. incision into the kidney, usually performed to remove a stone.

NEPHROTOXIC adj. toxic to a kidney, as some drugs.

NERVE n. one or more bundles of fibers that connect the brain and spinal cord (central nervous system) with the rest of the body. **Sensory nerves** transmit impulses (afferent impulses) from the sense organs and other organs of the body to the brain and spinal cord. **Motor nerves** transmit impulses (efferent impulses) from the brain and spinal cord to the glands, muscles, and other organs of the body. A nerve consists of an *epineurium* enclosing bundles (fasciculi) of fibers; each fasciculus contains microscopic nerve fibers, each enclosed in a *neurolemmal sheath*. (See also *nervous system*; *neuron*).

NERVE BLOCK ANESTHESIA see *conduction anesthesia*.

NERVE COMPRESSION n. harmful pressure on a nerve, causing nerve damage and muscle weakness; nerves over rigid prominences are particularly vulnerable. Rest and alteration of any causal activities often heals the damage (compare *nerve entrapment*).

NERVE ENTRAPMENT n. an abnormal condition in which a nerve is subject to repeated or long-term compression, resulting in nerve damage, often with symptoms of pain and muscle weakness. It most commonly involves nerves located near joints subject to inflammation or swelling as in arthritis or pregnancy. *Carpal tunnel syndrome* is a type of nerve entrapment (compare *nerve compression*).

NERVOUS BREAKDOWN n. colloquial for a mental condition that disrupts normal functioning.

NERVOUS SYSTEM n. the extensive network of cells specialized to conduct information in the form of impulses that controls, regulates, and coordinates all functions of the body. It is divided into the central nervous system, made up of the brain and spinal cord, and the peripheral nervous system, which includes the cranial nerves, spinal nerves, and the *autonomic nervous system*. The basic unit of the nervous system is the *neuron*, or nerve cell.

NEUR-, NEURO- comb. forms indicating an association with a nerve or the nervous system (e.g., **neuroblast**, a cell in the embryo that develops into a nerve cell.

NEURAL adj. pert. to nerves or the nervous system.

NEURALGIA n. severe, often burning, pain along the course of a nerve.

NEURAL TUBE n. in the embryo, a tube of ectodermal tissue from which the brain and spinal cord develop.

NEURAL TUBE DEFECT n. any of a group of congenital defects involving the brain and spinal cord and resulting from failure of the neural tube to close normally during embryonic development or occasionally from a reopening of the tube after it has closed. The defects range from total absence of the skull to protrusions of the brain material (e.g., *meningoencephalocele, cranial meningocele*) to more common protrusions of spinal cord material (with or without meninges) through an incomplete closure of the vertebral column (e.g., *meningocele, myelomeningocele, spina bifida*). The amount and extent of mental impairment, neurological dysfunction, and other abnormalities depend on the location and site of the defect. In some cases surgical intervention is undertaken. Many

Central   Peripheral   Autonomic

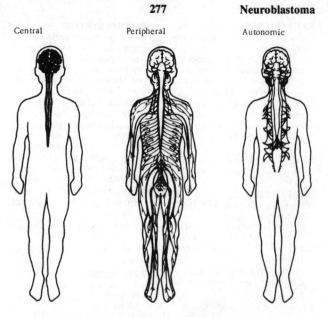

The nervous system is divided into central, peripheral, and autonomic divisions

neural tube defects can be determined before birth through analysis of *amniotic fluid*; an elevated level of *alpha-fetoprotein* usually indicates a neural tube defect.

NEURASTHENIA n. an abnormal condition characterized by many physical and psychological symptoms, including fatigue, intolerance to noise, and irritability; it is associated with depression and other abnormal psychological conditions; severe stress; occasionally organic disease. adj. **neurasthenic**

NEURILEMMA n. a thin membranous sheath enclosing a nerve fiber; also: **neurolemma**

NEURILEMOMA see *neurofibroma*.

NEURECTOMY n. surgical removal of all or part of a nerve.

NEURINOMA n. a tumor, usually benign, of the sheath surrounding a nerve.

NEURITIS n. inflammation of a nerve, producing pain, loss of sensation, defective reflexes, and muscular atrophy. It can result from many causes. (See also *retrobulbar neuritis*).

NEUROANATOMY n. the study of the structure of the nervous system, including its gross and microscopic structure.

NEUROBLAST n. an embryonic cell that develops into a neuron.

NEUROBLASTOMA n. a malignant tumor containing embryonic nerve cells; it most commonly develops in the adrenal medulla in children, but may arise in any part of the *sympathetic nervous system*. Neuroblastomas typically metastasize quickly, spreading to the lymph nodes, liver, lungs, and other organs.

NEURODERMATITIS n. a skin disease in which localized areas, esp. the forearm, back of the neck, or outer part of the ankle, itch persistently and become thickened because of constant scratching. The cause is unknown.

NEUROENDOCRINE adj. pert. to the endocrine and nervous systems, esp. as they function together to control the activities of the body.

NEUROEPITHELIOMA n. a neoplasm of the *neuroepithelium*.

NEUROEPITHELIUM n. epithelium associated with special sense organs and containing sensory nerve endings; it is found in the *retina*, inner ear, nasal cavity, and taste buds. adj. **neuroepithelial**

NEUROFIBROMA n. a tumor of the fibrous coverings of a *peripheral nerve*.

NEUROFIBROMATOSIS n. a congenital disease (*autosomal dominant disease*) characterized by numerous tumors of the fibrous covering the nerves (*neurofibromas*), by cafe-au-lait spots on the skin, and often by developmental abnormalities of bone, muscle, and internal organs.

NEUROGENESIS n. the development of nerve tissue.

NEUROGENIC adj. 1. arising in nervous tissue; 2. caused by nervous stimulation.

NEUROGENIC BLADDER n. a urinary bladder that functions abnormally because of a nervous system lesion (see *flaccid bladder*; *spastic bladder*).

NEUROGLIA n. a type of cell, including astrocytes, microglia, and oligodendroglia, found in the nervous system; neuroglia serve as support and nourishment for the neurons, the cells involved in nerve impulse transmission (compare *neuron*).

NEUROHORMONE n. a hormone secreted by nerve endings, as, for example, *vasopressin* released from nerve endings in the *hypothalamus* and released into the bloodstream from the *posterior pituitary gland*.

NEUROHUMOR n. a chemical transmitted by a *neuron* and essential for the activity of adjacent neurons, muscles, or other organs. Important neurohumors are *acetylcholine*, *serotonin*, *dopamine*, and *epinephrine*. adj. **neurohumoral**

NEUROHYPOPHYSEAL adj. pert. to the neurohypophysis (the *posterior pituitary gland*).

NEUROHYPOPHYSIS n. the *posterior pituitary gland*.

NEUROLEMMA see *neurilemma*.

NEUROLEPSIS n. an altered state of consciousness marked by indifference to the surroundings; quiescence.

NEUROLEPTIC n. a drug that produces neurolepsis.

NEUROLOGY n. that branch of medicine concerned with the structure, function, and diseases of the nervous system. adj. **neurologic**

NEUROMA n. a neoplasm consisting chiefly of *neurons* and *nerve fibers*.

NEUROMUSCULAR adj. pert. to the nerves and muscles.

NEUROMUSCULAR BLOCKING AGENT n. a substance that interferes with the transmission or reception of impulses from motor neurons to skeletal muscles; used to induce muscle relaxation during surgery and in the treatment of tetanus, poliomyelitis, and certain other disorders.

NEUROMUSCULAR JUNCTION n. the area of contact between a nerve fiber and the muscle it supplies. A neurotransmitter passes across the small gap (synapse) between the *motor end plate* of the motor nerve and the muscle, triggering contraction of the muscle; also **myoneural junction**.

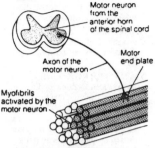

Motor neuron from the anterior horn of the spinal cord

Axon of the motor neuron

Motor end plate

Myofibrils activated by the motor neuron

NEUROMUSCULAR JUNCTION

Impulses travel from the spinal cord through the axon of a motor neuron to the motor end plate, where myofibrils of a muscle are activated.

NEURON n. a nerve cell; the basic structural and functional unit of the nervous system; neurons are specialized to carry information in the form of electrochemical impulses from one part of the body to another. Each neuron is composed of a cell body containing a nucleus and one or more processes: dendrites that carry impulses toward the cell body and axons that carry impulses away from the cell body. **Sensory neurons** transmit impulses from sense organs to the brain and spinal cord; **motor neurons** transmit impulses from the brain and spinal cord to muscles and glands.   adj. **neuronal**

NEUROPATHY n. any abnormal condition of the peripheral nerves. adj. **neuropathic**

NEUROSARCOMA n. a malignant neoplasm made up of nerve tissue, fibrous tissue, and connective tissue; also: **malignant neuroma**.

NEUROSIS n. an inefficient way of thinking or behaving, that may be manifested by depression, anxiety, defense mechanisms, compulsion, phobias, or obsessions and which produce psychological pain or discomfort. The perception of reality is usually not impaired and behavior remains within socially accepted limits (compare *psychosis*).

NEUROSYPHILIS n. infection of the central nervous system by the organism causing *syphilis*.

NEUROSURGERY n. any surgery involving the brain, spinal cord, or peripheral nerves.

NEUROTOXIC adj. poisonous or harmful to *nerves* and *nerve cells*.

NEUROTOXIN n. a toxin, found in the venom of certain snakes, in some fish, shellfish, and bacteria, and in certain other organisms that is toxic to nervous tissue.

NEUROTRANSMITTER n. a chemical that affects or modifies the transmission of an impulse across a *snyapse* between nerves or between a nerve and a muscle. Important neurotransmitters are *acetylcholine*, and *norepinephrine*.

NEUTROPENIA n. an abnormal decrease in the number of *neutrophils* (a type of white blood cell) in the blood; it is associated with infection, rheumatoid arthritis, leukemia, and certain vitamin deficiencies.

NEUTROPHIL n. a granular leukocyte (white blood cell). Neutrophils are phagocytes, engulfing bacteria and cellular debris. An increase in the number of neutrophils occurs in acute infections, certain malignant neoplastic diseases, and some other disorders.

NEVUS n. a congenital discoloration of the skin; a birthmark (see also *mole*; *port-wine stain*).

NEWBORN n. an infant recently born; neonate.

NEXUS n. a connection or link.

NGU abbreviation for *nongonococcal urethritis*.

NIACIN n. a vitamin of the B complex group. It is essential for normal function of the nervous system and gastrointestinal tract. Rich sources are meats, fish, eggs, nuts, and wheat germ. Symptoms of deficiency include fatigue, muscle weakness, loss of appetite, mouth sores, nausea, vomiting, and depression; Severe deficiency leads to *pellagra* (see Table of Vitamins).

NICONYL n. trade name for the antibacterial *isoniazid*.

NICOTINE n. a poisonous alkaloid found in tobacco, thought responsible for the dependence of regular smokers on tobacco. In small doses nicotine stimulates the nervous system, causing an increase in pulse rate, a rise in blood pressure, and a decrease in appetite. In large doses, it is a depressant, slowing the heartbeat and leading to respiratory depression.

NICOTINE POISONING n. a toxic condition caused by the ingestion or inhalation of large amounts of nicotine. Nicotine poisoning is characterized at first by nervous system stimulation, followed by depression, leading, if untreated, to respiratory failure.

NICOTINIC ACID see *niacin*.

NICU abbreviation for *neonatal intensive care unit*.

NIDATION n. implantation of the conceptus in the endometrial layer of the *uterus*.

NIDUS n. point of origin of a disease.

NIEMANN-PICK DISEASE n. an inherited disease of lipid metabolism, in which phospholipids accumulate in the bone marrow, spleen, and lymph nodes. Symptoms, which begin in early childhood, include an enlarged spleen and liver, anemia, and progressive mental and physical deterioration, usually leading to death within a few years. The disease is largely confined to people of Jewish descent.

NIGHT BLINDNESS n. an abnormal reduction in vision in darkness, due to deficiency of vitamin A or retinal disorder.

NIGHTMARE n. a dream that arouses feelings of fear, terror, panic or anxiety (compare *night terror*).

NIGHT TERROR n. an episode, most often occurring in young children, in which the person awakens in terror, with a panicky scream, feelings of fear, anxiety, and total inability to recall any dream or incident provoking the feelings; the person typically does not recall the event the next morning (compare *nightmare*).

NIHILISM n. in psychiatry, a delusion that certain things or everything, including the self, does not exist; associated with some forms of *schizophrenia*.

NIPPLE n. a small pigmented structure that projects from the breast and is surrounded by the pigmented *areola*. In women the nipple contains the openings of the *lactiferous ducts* that transport milk from the milk-producing glands in the breast.

NIPPLE DISCHARGE n. spontaneous release of material from the nipple; it may be normal, as in the release of *colostrum* during *pregnancy*; or it may be a sign of endocrine or infectious disease or neoplasm.

NIPPLE SHIELD n. a rubber or plastic device to protect the nipples of nursing women, esp. cracked or sore nipples and to allow them to heal.

NITROFURANTOIN n. an antibacterial, known under the trade name Macrodantin, used to treat urinary tract infections. Adverse effects include gastrointestinal disturbances, fever, and hypersensitivity reactions.

NITROGEN n. a nonmetallic element that is a component of all protein and many organic compounds. Nitrogen compounds are essential parts of all organisms, present in nucleic acids, proteins, and other biologically important compounds, (see Table of Elements).

NITROGLYCERIN n. a coronary *vasodilator* used in the treatment of *angina pectoris*. Adverse effects include headache, flushing, and low blood pressure.

NITROSPAN n. trade name for *nitroglycerin*.

NITROSTAT n. trade name for *nitroglycerin*.

NITROUS OXIDE n. a gas used as an anesthetic. Nitrous oxide produces light anesthesia and is used in minor surgery, childbirth, and dentistry, but not alone for major surgery. In small doses it sometimes produces exhilaration and is called **laughing gas**.

NOCTURIA n. excessive urination at night; it may be due to excessive fluid intake before bedtime, to renal disorder, or in older men, to prostatic disease (compare *enuresis*).

NOCTURNAL EMISSION n. involuntary emission of semen during sleep, usually associated with an erotic dream; colloquial: **wet dream**.

NODE n. 1. a small rounded knot of tissue; 2. a lymph node.

NODE OF RANVIER n. a gap, occurring at regular intervals, in the *myelin* sheath of a *nerve*.

NODULE n. a small node.

NOMA n. an acute ulceration of mucous membranes of the mouth or genitals, most often seen in undernourished children; it often leads to destruction of underlying bone and connective tissue.

NONDISJUNCTION n. the failure of homologous pairs of chromosomes to separate during the processes of nuclear division, resulting in an abnormal number of chromosomes in the daughter cells.

NONGONOCOCCAL URETHRITIS (NGU) n. an infectious disease of the *urethra*, usually caused by the *Chlamydia trachomatis* parasite and sexually transmitted. Symptoms are painful urination and discharge from the *penis* in males, and erosion of the *cervix* in women. An infant passing through the birth canal of an infected mother may develop infection of the nasopharnyx and eyes. Treatment is by tetracyclines or erythromycin.

NONINVASIVE adj. in medicine, pert. to a diagnostic or therapeutic technique that does not involve puncturing the skin or entering the body cavity or organ.

NONRAPID EYE MOVEMENT (NREM) n. a period of sleep representing about 75% of normal sleep time, during which dreaming and rapid eye muscle contractions do not occur. NREM sleep periods alternate with short REM (dreaming) sleep periods during normal sleep. Most NREM sleep occurs in four stages: stage 1 characterized by *theta brain wave patterns*; stage 2 characterized by distinctive sleep patterns; stages 3 and 4 characterized by *delta brain wave patterns* (compare *rapid eye movement* (see also *sleep*).

NONSPECIFIC URETHRITIS (NSU) n. inflammation of the *urethra* not known to be caused by a specific organism. There are often no symptoms in women; in men urethral discharge.

NOONAN'S SYNDROME n. a disorder, occurring only in males, characterized by short stature, low-set ears, and often decreased fertility.

NOREPINEPHRINE n. 1. a hormone secreted by the adrenal medulla and a neurotransmitter released at nerve endings. It constricts small blood vessels, raises blood pressure, slows heart rate, increases the rate of breathing, and relaxes the smooth muscles of the intestinal tract; 2. a drug used to treat cardiac arrest and to maintain blood pressure.

NORETHINDRONE n. a progestin compound used in oral contraceptives and to treat endometriosis and abnormal uterine bleeding. Adverse effects include gastrointestinal upsets, breast changes, and irregular uterine bleeding.

NORGESTREL n. a *progestin* used in oral contraceptives.

NORINYL n. trade name for an oral contraceptive containing *norethindrone* and *mestranol*.

NORLESTRIN n. trade name for an oral contraceptive containing *estradiol* and *norethindrone*.

NORLUTIN n. trade name for *norethindrone*.

NORMOTENSIVE adj. pert. to the conditon of having normal blood pressure (compare *hypertensive*; *hypotensive*).

NOR-Q-D n. trade name for oral contraceptive containing *norethindrone*.

NORTRIPTYLINE n. an antidepressant. Adverse effects include sedation, gastrointestinal, cardiovascular and neurological reactions, and the possibility of drug interaction if taken with other drugs.

NOSE n. the structure on the face that serves as a passageway for air into and out of the lungs and as an organ of smell.

NOSEBLEED n. hemorrhage from the nose; it may be caused by injury or associated with hypertension or blood disorders; also: **epistaxis.**

NOSO- comb. form indicating an association with disease (e.g.,

nosology, the classifying of diseases).

NOSOCOMIAL adj. pert. to a hospital.

NOSOCOMIAL INFECTION n. an infection acquired during a hospital stay.

NOSTRILS see *nares.*

NOTCH n. a small indentation, as on a bone (e.g., the **mandibular notch,** the depression in the middle of the lower jawbone).

NOTOCHORD n. the rodlike structure in the embryo that in humans and other vertebrates is replaced by the *vertebral column.*

NOTOMELUS n. congenital abnormality in which one or more accessory limbs are attached to the back.

NOURISH v. to supply foods and nutrients to maintain life. n. **nourishment**

NOVOCAIN n. trade name for the local anethetic *procaine.*

NREM abbreviation for *nonrapid eye movement.*

NUCHA n. the nape, or back of the neck. adj. **nuchal**

NUCHAL CORD n. the condition in which the umbilical cord is wrapped around the neck of the fetus or of the baby as it is being born. It most cases it can be slipped over the child's head or cut without harm to the child.

NUCLE-, NUCLEO- comb. form indicating a relationship to the nucleus (e.g., **nucleosis,** the production of an abnormal number of cell nuclei).

NUCLEAR adj. pert. to a *nucleus.*

NUCLEAR MAGNETIC RESONANCE (NMR) n. diagnostic technique in which an electromagnetic field stimulates atomic nuclei within the patient's body, causing those nuclei to release energy that is recorded with sensitive receivers. The technique is much more accurate than x-ray films for showing certain abnormalities in the body.

NUCLEIC ACID n. a compound composed of nucleotides, each of which is made up of a phosphate group, a ribose or deoxyribose sugar, and a purine or pyrimidine base. Nucleic acids are involved in the determination of hereditary characteristics and in energy storage. See also *deoxyribonucleic acid*; *ribonucleic acid*.

NUCLEOLUS n. a small structure, composed mostly of *ribonucleic acid*, found in the *nucleus* of cells and involved in the formation of *ribosomes*.

NUCLEOPLASM n. the protoplasm of the *nucleus* (compare *cytoplasm*).

NUCLEOTIDE n. a compound containing a base (a purine or pyrimidine), a sugar, and a phosphate group. Nucleic acids (e.g., DNA, RNA) are composed of chains of linked nucleotides.

NUCLEUS n. a usually spherical structure, enclosed in a membrane (the nuclear membrane), and is contained within a cell and that controls the cell and its functions. It contains the genetic information for the maintenance, growth and reproduction of the organism; 2. a group of cells, esp. in the central nervous system, having a distinct function, as, for example, the auditory center in the brain.

NULLIPARA n. a woman who has never given birth to a viable infant.   adj. **nulliparous**

NUMBNESS n. partial or total lack of sensation in a part of the body, often accompanied by tingling. It may be caused by minor nerve damage or more serious nerve injury or dysfunction.

NUTATION n. the act of nodding the head, esp. uncontrolled nodding.

NUTRIENT n. a substance that must be supplied by the diet to provide for normal health of the body, and for energy supplies and materials for growth. Nutrients include proteins, fats, carbohydrates, vitamins, and minerals.

NUTRITION n. 1. nourishment; 2. all of the chemical and physical processes involved in the ingestion, digestion, absorption, assimilation, and excretion of nutrients; 3. the study of food and drink as related to the needs of the body.

NYCTALOPIA   see *night blindness*.

NYCTOPHOBIA n. an irrational fear of darkness.

NYCTURIA   see *nocturia*.

NYDRAZID n. trade name for the antibacterial *isoniazid*.

NYMPHOMANIA n. a psychosexual disorder of women characterized by an insatiable desire for sexual gratification (compare *satyriasis*).   n. **nyphomaniac** adj. **nymphomaniacal**

NYSTAGMUS n. involuntary rhythmic eyeball movement; it may be congenital or result from brain or other disorder.

NYSTAN n. trade name for *nystatin*.

NYSTATIN n. an antifungal and antibacterial, known under the trade name Nystan; it is available as a topical cream, as a suppository, in eyedrops, and for oral administration; it is used to treat gastrointestinal, skin, and vaginal infections.

O

O symbol for oxygen (see Table of Elements).

OAT CELL CARCINOMA n. a malignant neoplasm consisting of small epithelial cells that do not typically form masses but spread through the lymphatics; more than 25% of lung cancers are oat cell carcinomas. Surgery is usually not possible; chemotherapy and radiation often ineffective.

OB abbreviation for *obstetrics*.

OBESITY n. overweight; an increase in the amount of fat in the subcutaneous tissues of the body.

OBLIGATE adj. surviving only in a particular environment, as an obligate parasite cannot survive without a particular host.

OBLIGATE AEROBE n. an organism that cannot grow in the absence of oxygen.

OBLIGATE ANAEROBE n. an organism that cannot grow in the presence of oxygen (e.g., *Clostridium botulinum*)

OBSESSION n. an abnormally persistent focus on a single idea.

OBSESSIVE-COMPULSIVE adj. characterized by the tendency to repeat certain acts or rituals (e.g., washing the hands more than is necessary, usually to relieve anxiety).

OBSESSIVE-COMPULSIVE PERSONALITY n. a person who has an uncontrollable need to repeat certain acts or rituals; it may be mild or serious, involving irrational acts that interfere with normal social relationships and behavior.

OBSTETRICS n. that branch of medicine concerned with the care of women during pregnancy, childbirth, and the immediate postpartum period; it is often practiced in conjunction with *gynecology*   adj. **obstetric; obstetrical**

OBSTIPATION n. extreme constipation, caused by obstruction in the intestinal system.

OBSTRUCTION n. a blockage; something that blocks or prevents passage.

OBTUND v. to blunt or deaden sensitivity, as to pain by use of an anesthetic agent.

OBTURATOR n. a device used to close or cover an opening, as a device implanted to cover the opening in the roof of the mouth in *cleft palate*.

OCCIPITAL adj. pert. to the *occiput*, or back part of the head, as the occipital lobe of the brain.

OCCIPITAL BONE n. one of the bones of the skull; the saucer-shaped skull bone that forms the back and part of the base of the cranium, articulating with the first vertebra of the backbone.

OCCIPITAL LOBE n. one of the five lobes of each cerebral hemisphere.

OCCIPITO- comb. form indicating an association with the back of the head (*occiput*) (e.g., **occipitocervical,** pert. to the back of the head and the neck).

OCCIPUT n. the back part of the head.   adj. **occipital**

OCCLUSION n. 1. a blockage or closing off of a vessel or passageway in the body, as in a clot occluding a blood vessel; 2. the manner in which the teeth in the opposing jaws meet in biting.   v. **occlude**   adj. **occlusive**

OCCULT adj. hidden, difficult to observe, as, for example, an occult fracture that is at first not observable on an X ray.

OCCULT BLOOD n. a very small or hidden amount of blood, not observable and usually only detected by chemical tests or microscopic analysis (e.g., occult blood in the stool of someone with an intestinal disorder).

OCCUPATIONAL DISEASE n. an illness or disability resulting from employment, usually from long-term exposure to noxious substances (e.g., to asbestos) or from continuous repetition of certain acts.

OCCUPATIONAL HAZARD n. any condition of a job, such as exposure to radiation or chemicals, that can result in injury or illness.

OCCUPATIONAL THERAPY n. a division of physical therapy in which handicapped or convalescing people learn and use, under the direction of a trained therapist, skills for daily life activities and for specific occupations with the goal of providing recreation and exercise and maximizing the capabilities of the person.

OCHRONOSIS n. the condition marked by the accumulation of brown-black pigment in cartilage and other connective tissue, usually due to the disease alkaptonuria or phenol poisoning.

OCULAR adj. pert. to the eye; n. the eyepiece of an optical instrument.

OCULIST see *ophthalmologist*

OCULO- comb. form indicating an association with the eye (e.g., **oculomycosis,** any fungus-caused disease of the eye).

OCULOMOTOR NERVE n. either of a pair of cranial nerves essential for eye movement; the third cranial nerve.

OCULUS n. the eye, usually designated **oculus dexter** (O.D.), the right eye; **oculus sinister** (O.S.) the left eye. pl. **oculi** adj. **ocular**

ODONT-, ODONTO- comb. form indicating an association with teeth (e.g., **odontitis,** inflammation of the pulp of a tooth).

ODONTALGIA n. *toothache.*

ODONTIASIS n. the process of cutting teeth; teething.

ODONTOLOGY n. the study of the anatomy and physiology of teeth and the surrounding structures in the mouth.

ODOR n. a scent or smell.

ODYNOPHAGIA n. severe burning, squeezing pain on swallowing, due to disorder of the *esophagus* (e.g., gastroesophageal reflux, tumor, chemical irritation of the mucous membrane lining, or infection).

OEDIPUS COMPLEX n. in psychoanalysis, repressed sexual feeling of a child toward the parent of the opposite sex and feelings of competition with the parent of the same sex, esp. a boy's sexual feelings toward his mother and sense of competition with his father. adj. **oedipal**

-OID suffix meaning "resembling" (e.g., **mastoid,** like a breast or breast-shaped).

OINTMENT n. a semisolid preparation, usually containing a drug, applied externally, as, for example an anesthetic or antibacterial ointment applied to a skin irritation.

OLECRANON n. the projection of the *ulna* (one of the lower arm bones) that forms the outer bump of the elbow and fits into the fossa of the *humerus* (upper arm bone) when the arm is extended; also: **olecranon process.**

OLFACTION n. the sense of smell. Special sensory cells in the mucous membrane lining of the nasal cavity respond to the presence of chemical particles (odors) dissolved in the mucus and transmit the impulses along the *olfactory nerve* to the brain for interpretation.

OLFACTORY adj. pert. to olfaction, or the sense of smell.

OLFACTORY CENTER n. a group of neurons in the brain, located near the junction of the parietal and temporal lobes, concerned with the interpretation of odors.

OLFACTORY NERVE n. either of a pair of cranial nerves that transmit impulses from the mucous membranes of the nasal cavity to the *olfactory center* in the brain; the first cranial nerve.

OLIG-, OLIGO- comb. form meaning "few" "little" "insufficient amount" (e.g., **oligodipsia,** a condition in which the sense of thirst is abnormally reduced or absent).

OLIGODACTYLY n. a congenital condition characterized by the absence of one or more fingers or toes.

OLIGODENDROCYTE n. a *glia* cell of the nervous system.

OLIGODONTIA n. a congenital condition in which some of the teeth are missing.

OLIGOMENORRHEA n. abnormally light or infrequent *menstruation*.

OLIGOSPERMIA n. insufficient number of spermatozoa in the *semen*.

OLIGURIA n. the production of an abnormally small amount of urine; it may be due to kidney disease, urinary tract obstruction, edema, imbalance in fluid and electrolytes in the body, or occasionally profuse sweating.

OMENTUM n. a fold of peritoneal tissue attaching and supporting the stomach and adjacent organs. pl. **omenta** adj. **omental**

GREATER OMENTUM n. tissue that covers the intestine; it is rich in fat and acts as a heat insulator and prevents friction between abdominal organs.

LESSER OMENTUM n. tissue that links the stomach, the liver, and the first part of the small intestine.

OMO- comb. form indicating an association with the shoulder (e.g., **omoclavicular,** pert. to the shoulder and clavicle (collarbone).

OMPHAL-, OMPHALO- comb. form indicating an association with the navel (e.g., **omphalorrhagia,** a flow of lymph from the navel).

OMPHALOCELE n. a congenital defect in which abdominal organs protrude through the umbilical region; umbilical hernia; it is usually treated surgically.

OMPHALUS n. the navel; umbilicus adj. **omphalic**

ONCHOCERCIASIS n. a disease common in Central and South America and Africa in which the bite of black fleas transmits filariae under the skin, causing subcutaneous nodules, an itchy rash, and eye lesions. Treatment involves surgical incision of nodules to remove the worms and the use of anthelmintics (diethylcarbamazine); also called **river blindness.**

ONCO- comb. form indicating an association with a tumor or mass (e.g., **oncogenesis,** the process of *neoplasm* formation.

ONCOLOGY n. that branch of medicine concerned with the study of tumors.

ONCOVIN n. trade name for the antineoplastic drug *vincristine* used to treat certain cancers.

ONEIRISM n. day-dreaming. It is a normal phenomenon, but if engaged in to excess, is often a sign of *autism* or other problem in functioning normally.

ONEIRO- comb. form indicating an association with a dream or dreaming (e.g., **oneirology,** the study of dreams and dreaming).

ONOMATOMANIA n. an abnormal condition in which a person repeatedly uses a specific word or name or it intrudes into the consciousness; usually a form of obsession or other abnormal mental state.

ONTOGENY n. the development of an organism from fertilized egg through developmental and growth stages to maturity. adj. **ontogenic**

ONYCH-, ONYCHO- comb. form indicating an association with a nail or the nails (e.g., **onychauxis,** a condition in which the nails are thickened).

ONYCHOLYSIS n. separation of the nail from its normal attachment to the nail bed; associated with trauma, certain infections, and other disorders of the skin.

ONYCHOSIS n. any disease or disorder of the nails.

ONYXIS n. an ingrown nail.

OO- comb. form indicating an association with an *ovum* (egg) (e.g., **oogonium,** the precursor cell from which an oocyte develops in the female fetus during embryonic development).

OOCYTE n. the cell from which a mature *ovum* develops.

OOGENESIS n. the development of ova, female reproductive cells. During the reproductive years of a woman's life, at roughly monthly intervals, one (sometimes two) oocytes present in the ovary since birth undergo a series of meiotic divisions that lead to the formation of a mature ovum (ova). The mature ovum has the haploid chromosome number and is released from the graafian follicle at the time of *ovulation*, ready for fertilization (compare *spermatogenesis*).

OOPHOR-, OOPHORO- comb. form indicating an association with the *ovary* (e.g., **oophorocytosis,** cyst formation in an ovary).

OOPHORECTOMY n. the surgical removal of one or both ovaries, usually performed to remove an ovarian tumor or cyst, to treat an ovarian abscess, to treat endometriosis, or to remove the source of estrogen in some cases of cancer (e.g., breast cancer). If both ovaries are removed, sterility results and menopause occurs; also: **ovariectomy.**

OOPHORITIS n. inflammation of one or both ovaries, often occurring with *salpingitis* (inflammation of the *Fallopian tubes*).

OOPHOROSALPINGECTOMY n. the surgical removal of one or both ovaries and the corresponding oviducts (Fallopian tubes); performed to remove a cyst, tumor, or abscess or to treat endometriosis (see also *oophorectomy*).

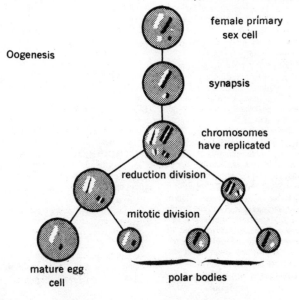

Oogenesis

female primary sex cell

synapsis

chromosomes have replicated

reduction division

mitotic division

mature egg cell

polar bodies

OOTID n. mature *ovum* after penetration by the spermatozoon but before fusion of the pronuclei (genetic material) to form a *zygote*.

OPACIFICATION n. a clouding of a part or loss of transparency, esp. of the *cornea* or *lens* of the eye.

OPEN FRACTURE see *compound fracture* under *fracture*.

OPERANT CONDITIONING n. in behavioral therapy, a form of learning in which a person is rewarded for the desired response and punished for the undesired response; used to break harmful habits and reinforce desirable behavior.

OPERATING MICROSCOPE n. a binocular microscope used in surgery to enable the surgeon to view clearly small and inaccessible parts of the body, as, for example, parts of the eye or ear (see also *microsurgery*).

OPERATING ROOM (O.R.) n. a room in a health care facility where surgical procedures requiring anesthesia are performed.

OPERATION n. any surgical procedure   adj. **operative**

OPERATOR GENE n. a segment of DNA (the hereditary material) that regulates the transcription of structural genes in its operon and acts with a *repressor gene* to control the activity of structural genes (see also *regulatory gene*).

OPERCULUM n. a lid, covering, or plug, as the mucous plug that closes the *uterus* during *pregnancy*.   pl.   **opercula**   adj. **opercular**

OPERON n. a segment of DNA (the genetic material) containing several structural genes that determine related functions and an *operator gene* and *regulatory gene* that control the function of the structural genes.

OPHIDISM n. poisoning by snake venom.   adj.**ophidic**

OPHTHALM-, OPHTHALMO- comb. form indicating an association with the eye (e.g., **ophthalmovascular,** pert. to the blood vessels of the eye).

OPHTHALMECTOMY n. surgical removal of an eye.

OPHTHALMIA NEONATORUM n. a type of *conjunctivitis* occurring in newborns, who contact the disease passing through the birth canal; the most serious form is gonococcal. Routine administration of silver nitrate drops or topical antibiotics in the eyes of newborns largely prevents the disease; if it occurs, antibiotic therapy is indicated.

OPHTHALMIC adj. pert. to the eye.

OPHTHALMOLOGIST n. a specialist in *ophthalmology;* oculist (compare *optometrist*).

OPHTHALMOLOGY n. the study of the eye, its development, structure, functions, defects, diseases, and treatment.   adj. **ophthalmologic**

OPHTHALMOPLEGIA n. an abnormal condition characterized by paralysis of the motor nerves of the eyes; sometimes occurring in *myasthenia gravis, botulism, thiamine* deficiency, and disorders of the nerves of the cranial area.

OPHTHALMOSCOPE n. a device that allows clear visualization of the structures of the interior of the eye.

OPHTHOCHLOR n. trade name for ophthalmic preparation containing *chloramphenicol*.

OPHTHOCORT n. trade name for a fixed-combination ophthalmic preparation containing hydrocortisone and the antibacterials *chloramphenicol* and *polymixin*.

OPIATE n. a drug that contains *opium*, is derived from opium, or is produced synthetically and has opiatelike characteristics. Opiates are central nervous system depressants: they relieve pain and suppress cough. Included among them are *morphine, codeine,* and *heroin.*

OPISTHORCHIASIS n. infestation of the liver and bile ducts with flukes of the genus *Ophisthorchia,* obtained from eating raw or inadequately cooked fish; common in eastern Asia. Symptoms include gastrointestinal disturbances and weight loss, often leading to damage to tissues of the liver and bile duct; and sometimes to cancer of the liver.

OPISTHOTONOS n. a severe muscle spasm, sometimes occurring in the final stages of *tetany,* in which the back arches, the head bends back, and the heels are flexed toward the back.

OPIUM n. a substance derived from poppy plants (*Papaver* species) that contains morphine, codeine, papaverine and other narcotic substances used to relieve pain.

OPPORTUNISTIC INFECTION n. an infection caused by a microorganism that does not normally produce disease in humans; it occurs in those with abnormally functioning immune systems, as, for example, those with *acquired immune deficiency syndrome* and those receiving immunosuppressive drugs (e.g., transplant patients).

OPSONIN n. a component of serum that attaches to foreign particles (e.g., invading microorganism or other antigen) making them more vulnerable to *phagocytosis* by *leukocytes.*

OPSONIZATION n. the process by which opsonins make an invading microorganism more susceptible to *phagocytosis.*

OPTIC adj. pert. to the eye or to sight.

OPTIC DISK n. a small spot on the *retina,* insensitive to light; blind spot.

OPTICIAN n. a person who grinds and fits eyeglasses and contact lens by prescription (compare *ophthalmologist*).

OPTIC NERVE n. either of a pair of cranial nerves that arise in the *retina* and transmit visual impulses from the eye to the visual cortex of the brain; second cranial nerve.

OPTO- comb. form indicating an association with sight (e.g., **optoblast,** a large nerve cell in the *retina*).

OPTOMETRIST n. one who practices *optometry.*

OPTOMETRY n. the practice of testing the eyes for visual acuity and prescribing corrective lenses or other visual aids (compare *ophthalmology*).

ORAL adj. pert. to the mouth.

ORAL PHASE n. in psychoanalytic theory, the first stage in a person's development, from birth through the first year, in which sucking and biting are prime sources of pleasure (compare *anal phase; phallic phase*).

ORAL CANCER n. a malignant neoplasm of the lips or mouth, most commonly occurring in men over the age of 60, often associated with tobacco use, esp, pipe smoking; alcoholism; syphilis; and poor oral hygiene. Premalignant *leukoplakia* or lip or mouth lesions may occur. Treatment depends on the size and location of the neoplasm and may include surgery, irradiation, and the use of chemotherapeutic agents.

ORAL CONTRACEPTIVE n. a pill containing a combination of estrogen and progestin preparations that inhibits ovulation and thus prevents conception. It is a highly effective contraceptive if taken as directed and is generally acceptable to users and has several useful side effects, including relief of dysmenorrhea, the regularization of menstrual cycles, and the relief of acne. However, oral contraceptives have been associated with side effects, some serious, that make them unadvised for some women. Serious adverse effects include an increased tendency to develop thromboembolus disorders (e.g., a stroke); less serious side effects experienced by many women include weight gain, breakthrough bleeding, breast tenderness, and depression. The use of oral contraceptives is generally not recommended for women with a history of breast or pelvic cancer, undiagnosed vaginal bleeding, cardiovascular disease, liver disease, renal disease, thyroid disorders, diabetes, and generally in women over 35 who smoke; also called **the pill.**

ORAL POLIOVIRUS VACCINE (OPV) n. see *Sabin vaccine.*

ORASONE n. trade name for *prednisone.*

ORBIT n. either of a pair of bony cavities in the skull that house the eyeball and associated structures; the eyeball socket. adj. **orbital**

ORBITO- comb. form indicating an association with the orbit, or eye socket (e.g., **orbitonasal,** pert. to the eye socket and the nose).

ORCHI-, ORCHIO- comb. form indicating an association with the *testis* or testes (e.g., **orchidoptosis,** abnormally low-slung testes).

ORCHIDALGIA n. pain in the testes; it may be caused by a hernia in the groin, by a calculus in the lower ureter, or by disease of the testis itself.

ORCHIDECTOMY n. surgical removal of one or both testes, usually performed to treat cancer of the testes or serious injury to the testes or to control cancer of another organ (e.g., prostate) by removing the source of androgenic hormones. Removal of both testes results in *sterility.*

ORCHIOPEXY n. surgical procedure to bring an undescended testis into the *scrotum* and attach it so that it will not retract.

ORCHIS see *testis.*

ORCHITIS n. inflammation of one or both testes, characterized by pain and swelling; it occurs in mumps, syphilis, and certain other diseases.

ORCHITOMY n. surgical incision into the testis to obtain material for microscopic analysis, as, for example, in cases of abnormally low sperm count in *semen.*

ORETON n. trade name for a *testosterone* preparation.

OREXIGENIC adj. pert. to a substance that increases appetite.

ORF n. a viral infection of sheep that can be transmitted to humans, causing a painless skin eruption that crusts and heals spontaneously.

ORGAN n. a part of the body that forms a structural unit concerned with a specific function; it is often made up of more than one kind of tissue. An example is the lungs, organs that are responsible for the exchange of carbon dioxide and oxygen.

ORGANELLE n. a specialized part of a cell, as, for example, the *mitochondrion, ribosome,* or *Golgi apparatus.*

ORGANIC adj. 1. pert. to an organ or to organs of the body; 2. a chemical compound containing carbon; 3. pert. to a disorder caused by a structural or detectable change in an organ (compare *functional disorder*).

ORGANIC BRAIN SYNDROME n. any mental abnormality resulting from transient or permanent disturbance of the structure or function of the brain; it may result from cerebral atherosclerosis; the effects of aging, drugs, or poisonous chemicals (e.g., lead); a tumor; or other conditions.

ORGANISM n. an individual animal, plant, microorganism, or cell capable of carrying on life functions.

ORGANO- comb. form indicating an association with an organ (e.g., **organogenesis,** the formation of organs and organ systems during embryonic development).

ORGASM n. sexual climax, usually involving strong involuntary contractions of the genital musculature, perceived as pleasurable.

ORIENTAL SORE n. the cutaneous form of *leishmaniasis;* a skin disorder caused by the *Leishmania tropica* parasite, occurring in Africa, Asia, and areas around the Mediterranean Sea; it is characterized by ulcerative skin lesions. Treatment usually involves the use of antimony preparations; also called **Old World leishmaniasis; tropical sore; Aleppo boil.**

ORIENTATION n. a person's awareness of self with regard to position, time, place, and personal relationships.

ORIFICE n. an opening to a body cavity or chamber (e.g., the **aortic orifice,** the opening from the lower left heart chamber to the *aorta*).

ORINASE n. trade name for the oral antidiabetic *tolbutamide.*

ORNADE n. trade name for a fixed-combination drug containing a decongestant (*phenylpropanolamine*), an antihistamine (*chlorpheniramine*) and an anticholinergic (*isopropamide*); used to relieve symptoms of upper respiratory infection.

ORO- comb. form indicating an association with the mouth (e.g., **orolingual,** pert. to the mouth and tongue).

OROPHARYNX n. part of the pharynx extending from the soft palate at the back of the mouth to the hyoid bone region and containing the palatine and lingual tonsils (compare *nasopharynx; laryngopharynx*). adj. **oropharyngeal**

ORPHENADRINE n. a skeletal muscle relaxant used in several forms to treat severe muscle strain and parkinsonism. Adverse effects include allergic reactions, rapid heartbeat, and dry mouth.

ORTHO- comb. form indicating an association with straightening, normality, or appropriateness (e.g., **orthostatic,** pert. to an erect, correct stance).

ORTHODONTICS n. that branch of dentistry concerned with *malocclusion* and irregularities of the teeth and their correction. adj. **orthodontic**

ORTHOPEDICS n. that branch of medicine concerned with the musculoskeletal system (bones, joints, muscles, ligaments, tendons) and the treatment of disorders affecting it.

ORTHOPEDIST n. a specialist in *orthopedics.*

ORTHOPNEA n. an abnormal condition in which the person can breathe normally or comfortably only when sitting erect or standing; it is associated with *asthma, emphysema, angina pectoris,* and many other respiratory and heart disorders. adj. **orthopneic**

ORTHOPTIC adj. pert. to normal binocular vision.

ORTHOPTICS n. the practice of using nonsurgical measures, esp. eye exercises, to treat abnormalities of vision and coordinated eye movement, such as *strabismus* and *amblyopia.*

ORTHOPTIST n. a specialist in *orthoptics.*

ORTHOSTATIC adj. pert. to an upright position. For example, **orthostatic hypotension** is low blood pressure occurring in some people when they stand up.

OS n. 1. a bone; pl. **ossa** 2. a mouth or mouthlike part (e.g., external os of the uterus) (compare *oro-*) pl. **ora**

OSCHE- comb. form indicating an association with the *scrotum* (e.g., **oschecele,** a swelling of the scrotum).

OSCULUM n. a small opening.

-OSIS a suffix indicating a condition, esp. a diseased condition (e.g., *nephrosis*), or an increase or excess (e.g., *leukocytosis*).

OSMOSIS n. the movement of a solvent through a membrane from a place of higher concentration to a place of lower concentration until the concentration on both sides equalize. adj. **osmotic**

OSMORECEPTOR n. a group of cells in the *hypothalamus* that monitor blood concentration and influence the release of *vasopressin* from the *posterior pituitary gland.*

OSSEO- comb. form indicating an association with bone (e.g., **osseocartilaginous,** pert. to bone and cartilage).

OSSEOUS adj. bony; of bone

OSSICLE n. a small bone. The **auditory ossicles** are the three small bones (incus, stapes, and malleus) of the middle ear that transmit sound vibrations from the *tympanic membrane* to the inner ear.

OSSIFICATION n. the process of bone development.

OSTEITIS n. inflammation of a bone, caused by trauma, degeneration, or infection (see also *osteomyelitis; Paget's disease*).

OSTEITIS DEFORMANS see *Paget's disease.*

OSTEO- comb. form indicating an association with bone (e.g., **osteocampsia,** a bending of bone resulting from disease or nutritional deficiency)

OSTEOARTHRITIS n. the most common form of arthritis, occurring mostly in the elderly, characterized by degenerative changes in the joints. Symptoms of pain after exercise or use, joint stiffness, and swelling develop, causing more disability when they affect the hip, spine, or knee. The cause is unknown but may involve many factors, sometimes aggravated by stress. Treatment includes rest, heat, antiinflammatory and pain-relieving drugs, injection of corticosteroids into the joint areas, and, if severe, surgery (compare *rheumatoid arthritis*).

OSTEOBLAST n. a cell that functions in the formation of *bone* tissue.

OSTEOBLASTOMA n. a benign tumor of bone and fibrous tissue, occurring in the vertebrae, femur, tibia, or arm bones, esp. in young adults. Symptoms include pain and resorption of normal bone tissue. Treatment is by surgical excision.

OSTEOCHONDROMA a benign tumor of bone and cartilage.

OSTEOCLASIA n. destruction of bony tissue by *osteoclasts.*

OSTEOCLASIS n. intentional fracture of a bone to correct a deformity.

OSTEOCLAST n. a cell that functions in the breakdown and resorption of bone tissue.

OSTEOCYTE n. a mature bone cell.

OSTEODYSTROPHY n. a defect in bone development, usually due to renal disease or disturbances in phosphorus and calcium metabolism.

OSTEOGENESIS IMPERFECTA n. a genetic disorder (*autosomal dominant disorder*) of connective tissue characterized by abnormally brittle bones that are fractured by the slightest trauma. The disease varies from extreme, in which the child is born with multiple fractures and is deformed and usually dies shortly after birth, through milder forms that typically manifest themselves after the child begins to walk and may ameliorate after puberty. In addition to bones that fracture easily, symptoms include translucent skin, blue sclerae, a tendency to bruise easily, and hyperextensibility of the ligaments. There is no cure; treatment involves measures to minimize the likelihood of fractures, esp. in young children.

OSTEOLYSIS n. degeneration and dissolution of bone, by disease, inadequate blood supply, or infection.

OSTEOMA n. a tumor of bone tissue.

OSTEOMALACIA n. abnormal softening of bone, due to loss of calcification resulting from a deficiency of phosphorus, calcium, or vitamin D, by a metabolic disorder causing malabsorption of these nutrients, or as a complication of another disease. Treatment involves administration of needed minerals and vitamins and correction of any underlying disorder.

OSTEOMYELITIS n. infection of bone and bone marrow, usually caused by bacteria (esp. staphylococci) introduced by trauma or surgery or by extension of another infection. Symptoms include; bone pain, tenderness, fever, and muscle spasm in the affected region. Treatment is by rest of the affected area, pain-relieving drugs, antibiotics, and surgery to remove necrotic tissue, if necessary.

OSTEOPATHY n. a treatment system that uses all the usual forms of medical therapy, including drugs and surgery, but places greater emphasis on the relationship of organs and the musculoskeletal system, using manipulation to correct structural problems.

OSTEOPETROSIS n. an inherited disorder characterized by an increase in bone density, ranging from a mild form marked by short stature, fragile bones, and a tendency to develop *osteomyelitis* to a severe form in which the bone marrow cavity is obliterated and severe anemia, skull abnormalities, and cranial nerve pressure results, often leading to death. also: **Albers Schonberg disease; marble bones.** adj. **osteopetrotic**

OSTEOPOROSIS n. abnormal loss of bony tissue causing fragile bones that fracture easily; pain, esp. in the back; and loss of stature. The condition is common in postmenopausal women and also occurs in those immobilized or given steroid therapy for a long period and as a result of some endocrine disorders. Postmenopausal osteoporosis is sometimes treated with *estrogen* preparations.

OSTEOSARCOMA n. a malignant bone tumor, most common in children and young adults in whom it often affects the femur, but also occurring in older adults and affecting other body sites. Pain and swelling typically mark the tumor site. Treatment is by surgery, usually amputation of the limb, followed by *chemotherapy*.

OSTEOSCLEROSIS n. an abnormal increase in bone density, resulting from a variety of diseases, including tumor formation, inadequate blood supply, or chronic infection (compare *osteopetrosis*) adj. **osteosclerotic**

OSTIUM n. an opening, as, for example, the ostium appendicis vermiformis, the opening between the appendix and the large intestine (see also *os; stoma*) pl. **ostia** adj. **ostial**

OSTOMY n. a surgical procedure in which an opening is made to allow the passage of urine from the bladder or feces from the intestines (see *colostomy; cystostomy; ileostomy*).

OT-, OTO- comb. form indicating an association with the ear (e.g., **otopharyngeal,** pert. to the ear and pharynx).

OTALGIA n. earache.

OTIC adj. pert. to the ear; also: **auricular.**

OTITIS n. inflammation of the ear, either *otitis externa, otitis media,* or otitis interna (*labyrinthitis*)

OTITIS EXTERNA n. inflammation of the auricle of the external ear leading to the tympanic membrane (eardrum). It may be caused by infection (bacterial, viral, or fungi); allergic reaction to earrings, cosmetics, or drugs; and other factors. Treatment depends on the cause.

OTITIS INTERNA see *labyrinthitis*.

OTITIS MEDIA n. inflammation or infection of the middle ear, a common disorder of children, often occurring as an upper respiratory infection spreads through the *eustachian tube*. Pain, diminished hearing, and fever typically occur. Treatment is by antimicrobials, pain relievers, and decongestants.

OTORRHEA n. a discharge from the external ear.

OTOSCLEROSIS n. a hereditary condition in which ossification in the *labyrinth* of the inner ear causes tinnitus and eventually deafness. Surgery to remove the *stapes* (one of the middle ear bones) is usually successful.

OTOSCOPE n. an instrument to examine the outer ear, tympanic membrane, and middle ear.

OTOTOXIC adj. harmful to the organs of hearing or balance or to the auditory nerve, as some drugs.

OVARI-, OVARIO- comb. form indicating an association with an *ovary* or the ovaries (e.g., **ovari-**

otubal, pert. to the ovaries and Fallopian tubes).

OVARIAN adj. pert. to the **ovary.**

OVARIAN CANCER n. a malignant neoplasm of the ovary, occurring most often between the ages of 40 and 60. Symptoms, which often do not appear until the disease is advanced, include abdominal discomfort, vaginal bleeding, irregular or excessive menstrual bleeding, constipation, and urinary problems. Treatment is by surgery, irradiation, and chemotherapy.

OVARIAN CYST n. a sac, often filled with fluid or semisolid material, that develops in or on the ovary. It may be transient and functional or a sign of pathology.

OVARIECTOMY see *oophorectomy*.

OVARY n. one of a pair of female gonads, or sex organs, located in the lower abdomen. Under the influence of follicle-stimulating hormone (FSH) and luteinizing hormone (LH) from the pituitary gland an ovum is released from a follicle on the surface of the ovary at roughly monthly intervals during a woman's reproductive life. The ovum then enters the Fallopian tube (oviduct) for possible fertilization and for passage to the uterus. adj. **ovarian**

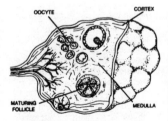

A typical ovary, showing internal maturation of ova

OVCON n. trade name for an *oral contraceptive* containing *estradiol* and *norethindrone*.

OVERBITE n. a condition in which the upper teeth extend abnormally over the lower teeth (see *malocclusion*).

OVERCOMPENSATION n. a conscious or unconscious exaggerated attempt to overcome or neutralize a real or imagined defect or unwanted characteristic (see also *compensation*).

OVER-THE-COUNTER adj. pert. to a drug that is sold without a prescription.

OVI-, OVO- comb. form indicating an association with an *ovum* or with ova (e.g., **oviferous,** capable of producing eggs).

OVIDUCT see *Fallopian tube*.

OVOTESTIS n. a hermaphroditic gonad, containing both ovarian and testicular tissue.

OVRAL n. trade name for an oral contraceptive containing *estradiol* and *norgestrel*.

OVRETTE n. trade name for an *oral contraceptive* containing *norgestrel*.

OVULATION n. the expulsion of an *ovum* (egg) from the ovary after the rupture of a *Graafian follicle* in the ovary under the influence of pituitary and ovarian hormones. Ovulation typically occurs midway in the *menstrual cycle,* 14 days after the first day of the last menstrual period, and is sometimes marked by a sharp pain in the lower abdomen on the side of the ovulating ovary.

OVULATION METHOD OF FAMILY PLANNING. n. a method of family planning that uses observation of changes in the character and quantity of cervical mucus to determine the time of ovulation and thus the time during the woman's menstrual cycle when conception is most likely to occur. After several days of scanty mucus discharge, the time around ovulation is marked by an increase in mucus that becomes sticky, then clearer, slippery and elastic, before again decreasing and becoming whitish and sticky before menstruation begins. This method is often combined with the *basal body temperature method of family planning* (see also *calendar method of family planning; contraception*).

OVULEN n. trade name for an oral contraceptive containing the estrogen compound *mestranol* and a *progestin* compound.

OVUM n. 1. the female germ cell produced in the *ovary* that on uniting with a *spermatozoon* in *fertilization* begins the formation of an embryo; 2. an egg cell

OXACILLIN n. an antibiotic of the *penicillin* family that is resistant to penicillinase, the penicillin-destroying enzyme released by some bacteria, esp. staphylococci. It is used to treat severe infections caused by penicillinase-producing staphylococci. Adverse effects include allergic reactions and gastrointestinal disturbances.

OXAZEPAM n. a minor tranquilizer, known under the trade name Serax, used to treat anxiety. Adverse effects include fatigue and dizziness.

OXYGEN n. a colorless, odorless gas essential for respiration and metabolism (see Table of Elements).

OXYGEN DEFICIT n. a condition existing in cells during a period of temporary oxygen shortage, as, for example, during strenuous exercise when energy is obtained through the breakdown of glucose in the absence of oxygen and waste products, chiefly lactic acid, accumulate in the muscles and other tissues, creating a need for oxygen to rid the body of those waste products.

OXYHEMOGLOBIN n. the complex of hemoglobin and oxygen that is the form in which oxygen is transported from the lungs to the cells of the body.

OXYOPIA n. unusually sharp vision.

OXYPHENBUTAZONE n. a nonsteroid antiinflammatory and antirheumatic drug, known under the trade name Tandearil, used to treat bursitis, arthritis, and other inflammations. Adverse effects include fluid retention, gastrointestinal upsets, blood disorders, and interaction with other drugs.

OXYPHENCYCLIMINE n. an anticholinergic drug, known under the trade name Daricon, used in the treatment of peptic ulcer. Adverse effects include dry mouth, urinary retention, and severe hypersensitivity reactions.

OXYTETRACYCLINE a *tetracycline* antibiotic, known under the trade name Terramycin, used to treat various bacterial and rickettsial infections. Adverse effects include gastrointestinal upsets, allergic reactions, the danger of superinfection, and discoloration of the teeth in young children.

OXYTOCIC n. a drug that induces or accelerates labor by stimulating contractions of the muscles of the *uterus*.

OXYTOCIN n. a hormone released by the *posterior pituitary gland* that causes contractions of the smooth muscles of the pregnant uterus and the release of milk from the breasts of lactating women. Preparations of oxytocin are sometimes used to induce or augment labor or to contract uterine musculature after childbirth to prevent hemorrhage.

OZENA n. a condition of the nose, sometimes following chronic inflammation of the nasal mucosa, characterized by a nasal discharge, an offensive odor, and crusting of nasal secretions.

OZONE n. a form of oxygen containing three atoms of oxygen per molecule (not the usual two), found in the upper atmosphere where it shields out ultraviolet radiation from the sun.

OZONE SICKNESS n. an abnormal condition, occurring among those exposed to ozone in high altitude aircraft, characterized by sleepiness, headache, chest pains and itchiness.

p

PABA abbreviation for *para-aminobenzoic acid*.

PABULUM n. any food or nutrient.

PACEMAKER n. 1. an electrical (battery operated) device used to maintain a normal heart rhythm by stimulating the heart muscle to contract. Some pacemakers stimulate the heart at a fixed rate; others stimulate the heart muscle on demand, sensing when heart contractions fall below a minimum rate; 2. the *sinoatrial node* of the heart, that part of the heart that regulates heartbeat.

PACHY- comb. form meaning "thick" (e.g., **pachycheilia,** abnormal thickness of the lips)

PACHYDERMA n. abnormal skin thickness.

PACINIAN CORPUSCLES n. small, bulblike sensory end organs attached to the end of nerve fibers in subcutaneous and submucous areas, esp. in the palms, soles, joints, and genitals.

PACK n. to treat the body or any part of it by wrapping it (e.g., with blankets or sheets), applying compresses to it, or stuffing it (e.g., gauze in a wound or tampon in a body opening) to provide cover or containment, to provide therapy (e.g., cold ointment), or to absorb blood.

PACKED CELLS n. a preparation of blood cells separated from the liquid plasma, used in the treatment of some cases of severe anemia to restore adequate levels of *erythrocytes* without overloading the circulatory system with too much fluid.

PAGET'S DISEASE n. a disease of bone, common in the middle aged and elderly, in which there is excessive bone destruction and disorganized bone structure, sometimes leading to bone pain, frequent fractures, and skeletal deformities.

PAIN n. a subjective unpleasant sensation resulting from stimulation of sensory nerve endings by injury, disease, or other harmful factor. Pain may be mild, severe, chronic, acute, burning, lancinating, sharp, or dull; it may precisely located, diffuse or referred (see also *referred pain*).

PAINT v. to apply a medicated solution (e.g., antiseptic or germicide) to the skin.

PAIN THRESHOLD n. the point at which a stimulus activates pain receptors to produce a feeling of pain. Individuals differ in pain threshold, some experiencing pain sooner than others with a higher pain threshold.

PALATAL adj. pert. to the *palate*.

PALATE n. the structure that is the roof of the mouth and floor of the nasal cavity; it is divided into the *hard palate* and the *soft palate*. adj. **palatal, palantine**

PALATINE BONE n. either of a pair of roughly L-shaped bones of the skull that form the posterior part of the hard palate, part of the floor of the orbit, and part of the nasal cavity.

PALATO- comb. form indicating an association with the palate (e.g., **palatoglossal**, pert. to the palate and tongue).

PALEO- comb. form indicating an association with old, ancient, or primitive (e.g., **paleocerebellum**, the anterior lobe of the cerebellum which in evolutionary terms was one of the earliest parts of the hindbrain to develop in mammals).

PALILALIA n. an abnormal condition in which a word is rapidly and involuntarily repeated; associated with Gilles de la Tourette syndrome and with some brain disorders.

PALLIATIVE adj. bringing relief, but not curing, as in drugs that provide relief from pain and other symptoms of a disease but do not cure the disease.

PALLIUM n. the outer part of the cerebral hemispheres; the *cerebral cortex*.

PALLOR n. abnormal paleness of the skin.

PALM n. the lower side of the hand between the wrist and the fingers.

PALMATURE n. an abnormal condition in which the fingers are webbed.

PALPABLE adj. perceivable by touch.

PALPATION n. a technique of examination in which the examiner feels the firmness, texture, size, shape, or location of body parts. v. **palpate**

PALPEBRA n. eyelid. pl. **palpebrae**

PALPEBRATION n. winking, esp. if uncontrolled and persistent. v. **palpebrate**

PALPITATION n. rapid, strong beating of the heart, associated with emotional arousal and certain heart abnormalities.

PALSY n. a condition associated with paralysis, as, e.g., *Bell's palsy* or *cerebral palsy*.

PAN- comb. form meaning ''all'' (e.g., **pansinusitis**, inflammation of all the sinuses at the front of the head).

PANACEA n. a substance said to be a universal remedy.

PANADOL trade name for the over-the-counter pain reliever *acetaminophen*.

PANCARDITIS n. inflammation of the entire heart, including the *epicardium,* the *myocardium,* and the *endocardium.*

PANCREAS n. a compound gland, about 6 inches (15 centimeters) long, lying behind the stomach. It is both an *exocrine gland,* secreting pancreatic juice, which contains several digestive enzymes, into the pancreatic duct that unites with the common bile duct opening into the *duodenum;* and an *endocrine gland,* secreting the hormones *insulin* and *glucagon* from its islets of Langerhans directly into the bloodstream.

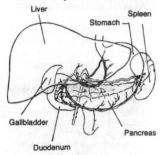

PANCREATECTOMY n. surgical removal of all or part of the *pancreas,* performed to remove a tumor, repair injury, or treat disease affecting the pancreas.

PANCREATIC DUCT n. pancreatic-juice-carrying duct leading from the *pancreas* and joining with the *common bile duct* to empty its secretions into the duodenal part of the small intestine.

PANCREATIC JUICE n. fluid secretion of the *pancreas,* containing water, salts, and enzymes, including trypsin and chymotrypsin; it is essential for the breakdown of starches, proteins, and fats.

PANCREATICO-, **PANCREATO-** comb. form indicating an association with the *pancreas* (e.g., **pancreaticoduodenal,** pert. to the pancreas and duodenum).

PANCREATIN n. an extract from the pancreas, containing pancreatic enzymes; used to treat conditions (e.g., *pancreatitis*) characterized by insufficient pancreas secretion.

PANCREATITIS n. inflammation of the pancreas, usually marked by abdominal pain, often radiating to the back, nausea and vomiting. It may occur in an acute or chronic form, often associated with alcoholism, injury to the biliary tract, trauma, or infection. Treatment depends on the cause and severity; it may include surgical removal of all or part of the pancreas and administration of pain-relieving drugs and pancreatin.

PANCYTOPENIA n. an abnormal condition in which there is a marked decrease in all cells (red blood cells, white blood cells, and platelets) of the blood, usually associated with *aplastic anemia* or bone marrow tumor.

PANDEMIC n. a widespread epidemic, occurring throughout a country, geographic area, or the world.   adj. **pandemic**

PANDICULATION n. yawning and stretching actions, as when first awakening.

PANENCEPHALITIS n. inflammation of the entire brain marked by progressive deterioration of mental and motor skills.

SUBACUTE **SCLEROSING PANENCEPHALITIS** n. a rare, often fatal, form of pancephalitis occurring as a complication of *measles.*

RUBELLA PANENCEPHALITIS n. a rare, chronic deterioration of mental and physical skills, occurring in adolescents and associated with the rubella virus.

PANHYSTERECTOMY n. surgical removal of the uterus including the cervix, the Fallopian tubes, and ovaries.

PANIC n. intense, overwhelming fear, producing terror, physiological changes and often immobility or hysterical behavior.

PANMYCIN n. trade name for a *tetracycline* antibacterial.

PANNICULUS n. a membrane layer. pl. **panniculi**

PANNUS n. an abnormal vascular membrane growing from the conjunctiva and covering the cornea of the eye; it is usually associated with inflammation of the cornea or conjunctiva.

PANTOTHENIC ACID n. a member of the Vitamin B complex (see Table of Vitamins).

PAPANICOLAOU TEST n. a method of examining stained cells shed by mucous membranes, esp. that of the cervix, used for early diagnosis of cancer and precancerous changes in cells. In its most common use, a smear of cervical cells is obtained during a routine pelvic examination; also called **pap test.**

PAPAVERINE n. a smooth muscle relaxant used to treat cardiovascular or visceral spasm. Adverse effects include jaundice.

PAPILLA n. a small nipplelike projection, as, e.g., the **lacrimal papilla** at the inner angle of the eye. pl. **papillae** adj. **papillary**

PAPILLARY MUSCLE n. any of several muscles associated with the *atrioventricular valve* of the heart.

PAPILLEDEMA n. a swelling of the *optic disc,* the beginning of the optic nerve, usually associated with increased intracranial pressure.

PAPILLIFORM adj. shaped like a *papilla.*

PAPILLOMA n. a benign growth on the skin or mucous membrane.

PAP SMEAR see *Papanicolaou test.*

PAP TEST see *Papanicolaou test.*

PAPULE n. a small, firm raised skin lesion, as in chickenpox. adj. **papular**

-PARA suffix meaning ''a woman who has given birth in a number of pregnancies'' (e.g., **bipara,** a woman who has given birth to a child after two separate pregnancies) (compare *-gravida*).

PARA- prefix meaning near ''beside'' (e.g., **paranasal,** near the nasal cavity) or indicating an abnormality (e.g., **paracusis,** abnormal hearing).

PARA-AMINOBENZOIC ACID n. a part of *folic acid,* one of the members of the vitamin B complex (see Table of Vitamins); a drug used as a sunscreen in many lotions and creams.

PARACENTESIS n. a procedure in which fluid is withdrawn from a body cavity, most often the abdomen, through a hollow needle; it is performed for therapeutic (e.g., to remove excess fluid from the abdomen) or diagnostic (e.g., to obtain a sample for analysis) purposes.

PARACERVICAL BLOCK n. a type of *regional anesthesia* in which a local anesthetic agent is injected on each side of the cervix to achieve anesthesia during labor and childbirth.

PARAFON FORTE n. trade name for fixed-combination drug, containing the analgesic *acetaminophen* and the skeletal muscle relaxant chlorzoxazone; used to treat musculoskeletal abnormalities associated with pain.

PARAINFLUENZA VIRUS n. a virus causing upper respiratory infections, including the common cold, bronchiolitis, croup, and other disorders, most commonly in children.

PARAL n. trade name for the sedative *paraldehyde.*

PARALDEHYDE n. a colorless, strong-smelling liquid, known under the trade name Paral, used to induce hypnotic states or sedation; it is also used as a solvent.

PARALYSIS n. an abnormal condition characterized by loss of sensation or loss of muscle function; it may be congenital or result from injury, disease, or poisoning (see also *flaccid paralysis; paraplegia; quadriplegia; spastic paralysis*). pl. **paralyses** adj. **paralytic**

PARAMEDICAL adj. pert. to health-related activities or personnel supplemental to physicians and nurses and their activities; for example, ambulance attendants are paramedical personnel.

PARAMETHADIONE n. an anticonvulsant, known under the trade name Paradione, used in the treatment of petit mal epilepsy. Adverse effects include dermatitis, sedation, blood disorders, disturbances of vision, and hepatitis.

PARAMETRITIS n. inflammation of the tissues around the *uterus*.

PARAMYXOVIRUS n. any of a family of viruses, including the parainfluenza viruses and the viruses responsible for measles and mumps.

PARANASAL SINUS n. any of several air cavities in bones around the nose.

PARANOIA n. a rare mental disorder characterized by delusions of persecution, often organized into an elaborate and logical system of thinking and often centered on a specific theme, such as job persecution or a financial matter. Suspiciousness, hostility, and resistance to therapy are often characteristic of the paranoic person. adj. **paranoid**

PARANOID adj. pert. to *paranoia*.

PARANOID SCHIZOPHRENIA see under *schizophrenia*.

PARAPARESIS n. weakness of both legs.

PARAPHILIA n. abnormal sexual activity. Kinds of paraphilia include exhibitionism, fetishism, pedophilia, voyeurism and zoophilia.

PARAPLEGIA n. paralysis of the lower limbs, sometimes accompanied by loss of sensory and/or motor function in the back and abdominal region below the level of the injury; it most often occurs as a result of trauma (e.g., automobile accident or sports accident), but may also be congenital (e.g., spina bifida) or acquired as a result of alcoholism, syphilis, or disease affecting the spinal cord or associated nerves. Treatment depends on the cause and extent of damage; it may include surgery (e.g., laminectomy); use of special immobilization devices; and the administration of pain-relieving drugs and drugs to prevent infection, esp. of the bladder (see also *quadriplegia*). adj. **paraplegic**

PARAPSYCHOLOGY n. the study of psychic phenomenon, such as extrasensory perception, clairvoyance, and mental telepathy.

PARAQUAT POISONING n. toxic condition resulting from the ingestion of the pesticide paraquat characterized by progressive damage to the esophagus, kidneys, and liver, often leading to death.

PARASITE n. an organism that lives in or on another organism—the host—obtaining nourishment from it. adj. **parasitic**

PARASITEMIA n. the presence of parasites in the blood.

PARASYMPATHETIC NERVOUS SYSTEM n. one of the two divisions of the *autonomic nervous system* (the other being the *sympathetic nervous* *system*), consisting of nerve fibers that leave the brain and sacral portion of the spinal cord, extend to nerve cell clusters (ganglia) at specific sites, from which fibers are distributed to blood vessels, glands, and other internal organs. In general parasympathetic nerves slow the heart rate, stimulate peristalsis, induce the secretion of bile, insulin and digestive juices, dilate peripheral blood vessels, and contract the bronchioles, pupils, and esophagus. The system works in balance with the sympathetic nervous system, often opposing its actions.

PARASYMPATHOMIMETIC adj. having an effect (as from a drug) similar to that caused by stimulation of the *parasympathetic nervous system* (e.g., slowing heart rate).

PARATHION POISONING n. a toxic condition caused by the inhalation or ingestion of the insecticide parathion. Symptoms include abdominal pain, nausea, vomiting, headache, convulsions, difficulty in breathing, sweating, and signs of stimulation of the *parasympathetic nervous system*.

PARATHYROID GLAND n. one of four small endocrine glands attached to the *thyroid gland* in the neck that secretes *parathyroid hormone*, which acts to maintain normal levels of calcium in the blood and normal neuromuscular function. Decreased activity of the parathyroid glands can result in *tetany*.

PARATHYROID HORMONE n. a hormone synthesized and released into the bloodstream by the parathyroid glands. It regulates calcium and phosphorus distribution in the body and functions in neuromuscular excitation and blood clotting; also: **parathormone.**

PAREGORIC n. an opium derivative used to treat diarrhea and to relieve pain. Adverse effects include constipation.

PARENCHYMA n. the functional part of an organ, apart from supporting or connective tissue (compare *stroma*).

PARENTERAL adj. pert. to administration of a substance (e.g., a drug) not through the digestive system, as, for example, by injection under the skin.

PARENTERAL NUTRITION n. the administration of nutrients by a route other than the digestive system, say, for example, by intravenous administration of fluids.

PARESIS n. slight or partial paralysis. adj. **paretic**

PARESTHESIA n. an abnormal sensation, as tingling or pins and needles; usually associated with partial damage to a peripheral nerve.

PARIES n. the wall of an organ or body cavity. pl. **parietes** adj. **parietal**

PARIETAL adj. 1. pert. to the inner walls of a body cavity as opposed to the contents (viscera); 2. pert. to the *parietal bone*.

PARIETAL BONE n. either of two skull bones forming the top and sides of the cranium.

PARIETAL LOBE n. one of the main divisions of each hemisphere of cerebral cortex, located beneath the crown of the head and concerned with sensory and associative nerve functions.

PARIETO- comb. form indicating an association with the parietal bone (e.g., **parietofrontal**, pert. to the parietal and frontal bones of the skull).

PARITY n. in obstetrics, the classification of a woman based on the number of live-born children she has delivered; for example, a woman who is classified as para 3 has delivered three live children (compare *gravida*).

PARKINSONISM n. a slowly progressive neurological disorder characterized by resting tremor, shuffling gait, stooped posture, rolling motions of the fingers, drooling, and muscle weakness, sometimes wih emotional instability. It most often occurs after the age of 60 and its cause is unknown, but it may occur in young people as a result of encephalitis, syphilis, or certain other diseases. Treatment is by *levodopa*, and occasionally in severe cases, by surgery; also called **Parkinson's disease.**

PARONYCHIA n. infection of the skin fold at the margin of a nail. adj. **paronychial**

PAROSMIA n. a disorder of the sense of smell.

PAROTID GLAND n. either of a pair of large *salivary glands,* located at the side of the face below and in front of the ear, that release saliva through the parotid ducts into the mouth.

PAROTITIS n. inflammation of one or both parotid glands, as in *mumps.*

PAROUS adj. having given birth to at least one child.

PAROXYSM n. 1. a sudden, violent attack, esp. a seizure or convulsion; 2. a marked increase in symptoms. adj. **paroxysmal**

PARROT FEVER see *psittacosis.*

PARS n. a part of an organ, as, for example, the pars nervosa of the pituitary gland pl. **partes**

PARTHENOGENESIS n. a type of reproduction in which an unfertilized ovum develops into a complete organism; it occurs in certain insects and other invertebrate animals. adj. **parthenogenetic**

PARTURITION n. the process of giving birth.

PASSIVE adj. not active; not initiated by the self (e.g., **passive movement,** movement of body parts by a therapist or other agent and not by the efforts of the person).

PASSIVE IMMUNITY n. a type of *acquired immunity* in which antibodies against a particular disease or against several diseases are transmitted naturally, through the placenta to an unborn child or through colostrum to a nursing infant; or artificially, through the administration (usually by injection) of antiserum. Passive immunity is not permanent (compare *active immunity*).

PASSIVE TRANSPORT n. the movement of small molecules across a cell membrane by *diffusion;* it does not require the expenditure of energy (compare *active transport*).

PASTEURIZATION n. the process of applying heat (e.g., to temperatures of 140° Fahrenheit [60° Celsius]) for a specified time (e.g., 60 minutes) to kill or retard the development of disease-causing microorganisms, esp. bacteria, in milk and other products.

PATCH TEST n. a skin test for identifying an *allergen.* A paper or cloth patch containing suspected allergens (e.g., pollen, animal hair) is applied to the skin; the appearance of a red, swollen skin or any rash when the patch is removed—usually 1 or 2 days later—usually indicates allergy to that particular substance.

PATELLA n. flat, triangular bone at the front of the knee joint; also: **sesamoid bone** colloquial: **kneecap.** adj. **patellar**

PATELLAR REFLEX n. a deep tendon reflex in which tapping the tendon below the *patella* causes a contraction of the quadriceps muscle of the thigh and extension (kicking) of the lower leg; used diagnostically to test nerve function; also called **knee-jerk reflex.**

PATENT adj. open, as a tube or passageway

PATENT DUCTUS ARTERIOSUS see *ductus arteriosus.*

PATENT MEDICINE n. a drug or other therapeutic substance that carries a specific trademark and is available without a prescription.

PATERNITY TEST n. a comparison of blood types among mother, child, and a man suspected of being the father of the child in an effort to determine the father of the child. If the child's blood group could not have resulted from the combination of the man's blood group in combination with that of the woman, then the man is definitely not the father of the child. However, other findings are not conclusive, since a finding that the man could be the father does not prove that he is necessarily the father.

PATHOGEN n. a microorganism capable of producing disease. adj. **pathogenic**

PATHOGENESIS n. the production of a disease, esp. the development of a disease from a specific cause or source.

PATHOGNOMONIC adj. describing a sign or symptom that is specific to or characteristic of a particular disease (e.g., Koplik's spots on the mucous membranes of the mouth are pathognomonic for *measles*).

PATHOLOGIC adj. pert. to or arising from disease (e.g., **pathologic fracture** is a fracture arising from bone disease, not from injury).

PATHOLOGY n. the study of disease, its causes and effects, esp. the observable effects of disease on body tissues. adj. **pathological**

-PATHY suffix indicating disease or abnormal state (e.g., **craniopathy,** a skull disease).

PAVABID n. trade name for the smooth muscle relaxant *papaverine*.

PAVACAP n. trade name for the smooth muscle relaxant *papaverine*.

PAVARINE n. trade name for the smooth muscle relaxant *papaverine*.

PAVOR NOCTURNUS see *sleep terror*.

PCP abbreviation for *phencyclidine hydrochloride*.

PEAK n. the highest value of a measurement or recording, as the top temperature of a patient's fever period or the sharp elevation during an electrocardiographic tracing (compare *spike*).

PECTIN n. a gelatinous substance found in fruits and used in jams and jellies.

PECTINATE adj. comb-shaped.

PECTINEAL adj. pert. to the *pubic bone*.

PECTORAL adj. pert. to the chest.

PECTORALIS MAJOR n. the large fan-shaped muscle of the upper chest wall that acts on the shoulder, flexing and rotating the arm.

PECTORALIS MINOR n. a thin, triangular shaped muscle of the upper chest, beneath the *pectoralis major*, that functions to draw the shoulder down and forward.

PECTUS n. the chest. adj. **pectoral**

PEDERASTY n. homosexual anal intercourse, esp. that between a man and a young boy who is the passive partner.

PEDIATRICS n. that branch of medicine concerned with the development of children and the diagnosis and treatment of diseases and disorders affecting children.

PEDIAMYCIN n. trade name for the antibacterial *erythromycin*.

PEDICLE n. a narrow stemlike part of an organ.

PEDICULICIDE n. an agent that kills *lice*.

PEDICULOSIS n. infestation with lice. Symptoms include intense itching, which often produces skin irritation that become secondarily infected. Treatment is by pediculidides.

pediculicides capitis n. infestation of the scalp with lice; head lice.

pediculicides corporis n. infestation of body skin with lice.

pediculicides pubis n. infestation of pubic hair with lice; also called **crab louse.**

PEDOPHILIA n. sexual activity, either homosexual or heterosexual, of an adult with a child.

PEDUNCLE n. a stalklike connection. adj. **peduncular**

PELAGE n. all the body hair.

PELLAGRA n. a disease caused by deficiency of *niacin* or *tryptophan* in the diet or by a defect in the metabolic conversion of tryptophan to niacin; it is characterized by dermatitis, inflammation of the tongue, diarrhea, and emotional and mental symptoms including depression, disorientation, and confusion. Treatment includes the administration of niacin and tryptophan and a well-balanced diet containing other vitamins.

PELVI-, PELVO- comb. form indicating an association with the *pelvis* [e.g., **pelvifemoral,** pert. to the hip area where the pelvis and femur (upper leg bone) meet].

PELVIC adj. pert. to the *pelvis*.

PELVIC GIRDLE n. the bony structure, made up of the left and right hipbones, the sacrum and coccyx, to which the bones of the legs are attached.

PELVIC INFLAMMATORY DISEASE (PID) n. inflammatory condition of the female pelvic organs, often associated with bacterial infection. Symptoms include lower abdominal pain, fever, and foul-smelling vaginal discharge. Treatment is by antibiotics; pain relieving drugs, if necessary; and, if an abscess develops, surgical drainage. Severe or recurrent attacks often lead to scarring of *Fallopian tubes,* sometimes leading to *infertility.*

PELVIMETRY n. measurement of the dimensions of the bony birth canal done to determine if a vaginal birth is possible.

PELVIS n. the lower part of the trunk of the body, composed of the right and left hip bones (the innominate bone, made up of the ilium, ischium, and pubis), the sacrum and the coccyx; it protects the lower abdominal organs and provides for the attachment of the legs. The pelvis is usually lighter and wider in females than in males. adj. **pelvic.**

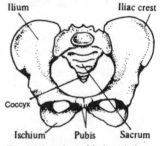

The pelvis is made up of the innominate, or hip, bone (the ilium, ischium, and pubis), the sacrum, and the coccyx.

PEMPHIGOID n. any condition characterized by the appearance of bullae, often on reddish macules; treatment is by corticosteroids, but there may be spontaneous remission (compare *pemphigus*).

PEMPHIGUS n. a disease of the skin, characterized by thin-walled bullae arising from normal skin or mucous membrane; the bullae frequently rupture, leaving raw patches that often become infected. Treatment is by corticosteroids.

PEN A n. trade name for the antibacterial *ampicillin*.

PENAPAR VK n. trade name for a *penicillin* antibacterial.

PENBRITIN n. trade name for the antibacterial *ampicillin*.

-PENIA suffix indicating a deficiency or amount below normal (e.g., **erythropenia,** a deficiency of red blood cells).

PENICILLAMINE n. a drug, known under the trade name Cuprimine, used in the treatment of heavy metal poisoning, Wilson's disease, and severe arthritis. Adverse effects include blood abnormalities, rash, and fever.

PENICILLIN n. any of a group of antibiotics, including ampicillin, oxacillin, penicillin G, and penicillin V, known under many trade names (e.g., Penabar, Pen-Vee K, Pentids) derived from *Penicillium* fungus or produced synthetically, which are used to treat a wide variety of bacterial infections. Some members of the penicillin family are effective administered orally; others must be given by injection. Some forms are inactivated by the enzyme pencillinase produced by certain bacteria; others, including cloxacillin and oxacillin, are penicillinase-resistant. Hypersensitivity reactions, manifested by rash, fever, bronchospasm, and other symptoms occur in some people given penicillin and a small number develop a serious reaction leading to *anaphylactic shock*.

PENICILLINASE n. an enzyme produced by certain bacteria, esp. staphylococci strains, that inactivates *penicillin* and causes resistance to the antibiotic.

PENICILLINASE-RESISTANT ANTIBIOTIC n. an antibiotic that is not rendered inactive by penicillinase; included are nafcillin, cloxacillin, oxacillin, and certain other semisynthetic penicillins.

PENIS n. the external reproductive organ of the male that contains the *urethra* through which urine and semen pass. Most of the organ is composed of erectile tissue that becomes engorged under conditions of sexual excitement, causing the penis to become erect; it is then capable of entering the vagina during *coitus* and discharging semen in ejaculation. Urination occurs without erection. adj. **penile**

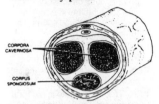

CORPORA CAVERNOSA

CORPUS SPONGIOSUM

Cross section of the penis, showing three columns or erectile tissue

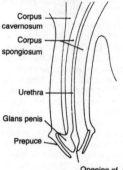

Corpus cavernosum

Corpus spongiosum

Urethra

Glans penis

Prepuce

Opening of urethra

PENTAERYTHRITOL n. a coronary vasodilator, known under the trade name Peritrate, used to treat *angina pectoris*. Adverse effects include headache, low blood pressure, and allergic responses.

PENTAZOCINE n. an analgesic, known under the trade name Talwin, used to treat moderate to severe pain. Adverse effects include nausea, dizziness, gastrointestinal upsets, and in high doses respiratory and circulatory depression; withdrawal symptoms after prolonged use may also occur.

PENTIDS n. trade name for the antibacterial *penicillin* G.

PENTOBARBITAL n. a sedative drug, known under the trade name Nembutal, used as a preoperative sedative, to control convulsions, and to treat insomnia and agitation. Adverse effects include respiratory and circulatory depression and withdrawal symptoms on discontinuance and the potential for addiction.

PENTOTHAL n. trade name for the barbiturate *thiopental*.

PEN-VEE trade name for the antibacterial *penicillin* V.

PEN-VEE K n. trade name for the antibacterial *penicillin* V.

PEPSIN n. an enzyme secreted by the stomach that catalyzes the breakdown of proteins.

PEPTIC adj. pert. to digestion or the enzymes of digestion.

PEPTIC ULCER n. a circumscribed erosion in or loss of the mucous membrane lining of the gastrointestinal tract. It may occur in the esophagus (esophageal ulcer), stomach (*gastric ulcer*), duodenum (duodenal ulcer), or jejunum (jejunal ulcer), the stomach and duodenum being the most common sites. It may result from excess acid production or from a breakdown in the normal mechanisms protecting the mucous membranes and is often associated with stress, the intake of certain drugs (e.g., corticosteroids and certain antiinflammatory agents). Symptoms include gnawing pain, often worse when the stomach is empty, after eating certain foods, or when the patient is under stress. Treatment includes avoidance of tobacco, alcohol, and irritating foods; drugs to decrease acidity (e.g., cimetidine); and a diet of small, frequent meals; if the ulcer perforates the wall of the gastrointestinal tract and hemorrhage occurs, surgery is usually required.

PEPTIDE n. a compound formed of two or more amino acids linked by peptide bonds. Proteins are made up of chains of polypeptides.

PERCEPTION n. the process by which information received by the senses is recognized, interpreted and analyzed to become meaningful. adj. **perceptive**

PERCEPTUAL DEFECT n. any abnormality that interferes with the recognition and interpretation of sensory stimuli; it may occur in organic brain disorders and certain other disorders.

PERCODAN n. trade name for the narcotic *analgesic* oxycodone used to treat moderate to severe pain.

PERCOGESIC n. trade name for a fixed-combination drug, containing the *antihistamine* phenyltoloxamine and the analgesic *acetaminophen;* used in the treatment of certain respiratory disorders.

PERCUSSION n. a technique of physical examination in which the fingers or a small tool (percussor) are used to tap parts of the body in an attempt to determine the size and outline of internal organs and to detect the presence of fluid.

PERCUTANEOUS adj. through the skin.

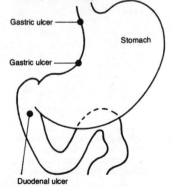

Peptic ulcers may occur in the stomach (gastric ulcers) or in the first part of the small intestine (duodenal ulcer).

Gastric ulcer

Stomach

Gastric ulcer

Duodenal ulcer

PERFORATE v. to pierce or otherwise make a hole. n. **perforation**

PERFORATED EARDRUM n. a puncture in the tympanic membrane (eardrum), resulting from trauma or other causes; it can interfere with normal hearing and cause other ear problems.

PERGONAL n. trade name for a preparation of gonadotropins extracted from the urine of menopausal women and used to induce *ovulation* in some cases of *infertility*.

PERI- comb. form meaning "around" (e.g., **periocular**, around the eye).

PERIACTIN n. trade name for the *antihistamine* and antipruritic cyproheptadine used in the treatment of certain allergic reactions.

PERIANAL adj. around the *anus*.

PERIAPICAL n. pert. to tissues around the apex of a tooth, as in **periapical abscess**, an infection around the root of a tooth.

PERIARTERITIS n. inflammation of the outer coats of one or more arteries.

PERIARTERITIS NODOSA n. a progressive disease of connective tissue characterized by nodules (often large) along arteries that may cause blockage of the artery and resulting inadequate circulation to the affected area. Symptoms include visceral pain, fever, and, as the disease progresses, signs of lung, kidney and intestinal damage. Treatment is by corticosteroids; also: **polyarteritis nodosa**.

PERICARDITIS n. inflammation of the *pericardium*, the double-layered sac that surrounds the heart and the major blood vessels around it. It may be due to infection, trauma, neoplastic disease, or myocardial infarction; or it may result from unknown causes. Symptoms include fever, dry cough, difficulty in breathing, pain below the sternum (breastbone) often radiating upward, rapid pulse, and increasing anxiety and fatigue; untreated, it can lead to restricted heart action due to effusion. Treatment depends on the cause; it may include antibiotics, analgesics, removal of accumulated fluid, oxygen, and steps to lower fever.

PERICARDIUM n. the double-layered sac surrounding the heart and large vessels entering and leaving the heart. The inner serous pericardium contains a layer that adheres to the surface of the heart and a layer that lines the inside of the outer fibrous pericardium. The fibrous pericardium is tough and comparatively inelastic; it protects the heart and inner membranes. Between the two layers is the **pericardial space**, containing pericardial fluid that lubricates the membrane surfaces and allows easier heart movement. adj. **pericardial**

PERILYMPH n. clear fluid in the inner ear, separating the osseous and membranous labyrinth.

PERINATAL adj. pert. to the time and just before and after birth.

PERINATOLOGY n. that branch of medicine concerned with the anatomy, physiology, and diagnosis and treatment of disorders of the mother and fetus or newborn child during late pregnancy, childbirth, and the puerperium.

PERINEAL adj. pert. to the *perineum*.

PERINEOTOMY n. surgical incision into the *perineum*.

PERINEUM n. the region between the urethral opening and the anus, including the skin and underlying tissues. (In females it contains the vaginal opening). adj. **perineal**

PERINEURIUM n. connective tissue covering around bundles of nerve fibers. adj. **perineural**

PERIOD n. colloquial, the *menses*.

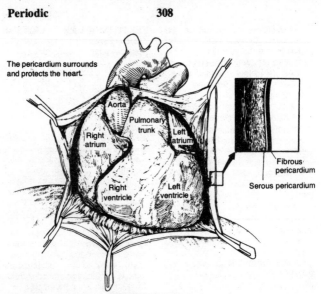

The pericardium surrounds and protects the heart.

Aorta

Pulmonary trunk

Right atrium

Left atrium

Right ventricle

Left ventricle

Fibrous pericardium

Serous pericardium

HEART AND PERICARDIUM

PERIODIC adj. occurring at intervals.

PERIODIC APNEA OF THE NEWBORN n. a condition of newborn infants characterized by an irregular breathing pattern with periods of rapid breathing followed by brief periods of not breathing (apnea); it is normal in most infants, often associated with REM sleep. Frequent episodes of apnea, not associated with REM sleep or periodic breathing patterns, may be a sign of neural, respiratory, circulatory or other disorder and are thought to be associated with *sudden infant death syndrome*.

PERIODIC BREATHING see *Cheyne-Stokes respiration*

PERIODONTAL adj. pert. to the area around a tooth.

PERIODONTAL DISEASE n. disease of the tissues around a tooth, often leading to damage to the bony sockets of the teeth.

PERIODONTICS n. that branch of dentistry concerned with the diagnosis and treatment of diseases of the tissues surrounding the teeth.

PERIOSTEUM n. the vascular membrane covering bones, except at the extremities where bones articulate with other bones; it contains nerves and blood vessels that nourish and innervate the enclosed bone.

PERIPHERAL adj. pert. to the outside, surface, or area away from the center of an organ or of the body.

PERIPHERAL NERVOUS SYSTEM n. the sensory and motor nerves outside the brain and spinal cord; it consists of 12 pairs of cranial nerves and 31 pairs of spinal nerves and the branches of these nerves that innervate the organs of the body. Sensory, or afferent, peripheral nerves transmit impulses to the central nervous system (the brain and spinal cord); motor, or efferent, peripheral nerves transmit impulses from the central nervous system to the muscles and organs of the body. Peripheral nerves that regulate respiratory, endocrine cardiovascular and other automatic functions make up the *autonomic nervous system.*

PERIPHERAL VASCULAR DISEASE n. any abnormal condition including *atherosclerosis* and *Buerger's disease,* affecting blood vessels outside of the heart.

PERISTALSIS n. rhythmic, wavelike contractions of the smooth musculature of the digestive tract that force food through the tube and wastes toward the anus. adj. **peristaltic**

PERITHELIUM n. the tissue layer around small blood vessels. adj. **perithelial**

PERITONEUM n. serous membrane that covers the entire abdominal wall (parietal peritoneum) and envelopes the organs contained in the abdomen (visceral peritoneum) adj. **peritoneal**

PERITONITIS n. inflammation of the *peritoneum* caused by bacteria or irritating substances (e.g., digestive enzymes) introduced into the abdominal cavity by a puncture wound, by surgery, by a ruptured abdominal organ, or through the bloodstream. A ruptured appendix is the most frequent cause, but peritonitis can also result from perforated peptic ulcer or rupture of the spleen or Fallopian tubes (as in ectopic pregnancy), or from other conditions. Symptoms include abdominal distension and pain, nausea, vomiting, rebound tenderness, chills, fever, rapid heart rhythm, and if untreated, electrolyte imbalance, shock, and heart failure. Treatment involves control of the infection, usually with antibiotics; repair of any perforation; withdrawal of fluid from the abdominal cavity, if necessary; and maintenance of fluid and electrolyte balance.

PERITONSILLAR ABSCESS see *quinsy.*

PERLECHE see *cheilosis.*

PERMANENT TOOTH n. any of the set of 32 teeth that appear during and after childhood and last until old age. In each jaw there are four incisors, two canines, four premolars, and six molars. They replace the 20 deciduous (milk) teeth of early childhood, usually starting to erupt in the sixth year and continuing to erupt until the 18th to 25th year with the eruption of the third molars (wisdom teeth).

PERNICIOUS adj. dangerous or likely to lead to death, as a pernicious disease.

PERNICIOUS ANEMIA n. a type of anemia characterized by defective red blood cell production, the presence of megaloblasts in the bone marrow, and deterioration of nerve tissue in the spinal cord. It is caused by a lack of intrinsic factor essential for the absorption of vitamin B_{12} or to a deficiency of vitamin B_{12} in the diet. Symptoms include pallor, anorexia, weight loss, fever, weakness, and tingling of the extremities. Treatment includes the administration of vitamin B_{12}, folic acid, and iron.

PERNIO see *chilblain.*

PERONEAL adj. pert. to the outer part of the leg, over the peroneal nerve.

PERONEUS n. either of two (peroneus brevis and peroneus longus) muscles of the lower leg, involved in movement of the foot.

PERPHENAZINE n. a tranquilizer and antidepressant known under the trade name Triavil, used to treat some types of depression, anxiety, and agitation; it is also an antiemetic, used to treat nausea and vomiting in adults. Adverse effects include extrapyramidal signs (e.g., ataxia, dyskinesia) blood abnormalities, and hypersensitivity reactions.

PERSONA n. in psychology, the personality role that a person assumes and presents to the world (compare *anima*).

PERSONALITY n. the composite of a person's behavior and attitudes; a tendency to feel and behave in a certain way.

PERSONALITY DISORDER n. any of a group of mental disorders characterized by maladaptive and usually rigid patterns of behavior.

PERSPIRATION n. 1. sweat, the moisture passing through the sweat glands in the skin that functions to maintain body temperature (a cooling mechanism) and to rid the body of wastes; 2. the act of sweating.

PERTUSSIS an acute, contagious, respiratory disease, occurring most commonly in nonimmunized young children and characterized by attacks of coughing ending in inspiration with a loud whooping sound. It is caused by *Bordetella pertussis* bacteria; transmitted directly (via contact with infectious particles spread by coughing or sneezing) or indirectly (through contaminated articles); and has a 1 to 2 week incubation period; and typically lasts 6 to 8 weeks. The disease starts with sneezing, runny nose, dry cough, loss of appetite, and slight fever—the catarrhal stage. About 10 days later paroxysms of coughing with the characteristic whoop on inspiration begin, often accompanied by marked facial redness and signs of distress, the expulsion of large amounts of mucus, and frequently vomiting, after choking on mucus; this stage, the paroxysmal stage, lasts about 4 to 6 weeks. The convalescent stage, of about two weeks, is characterized by a persistent cough. Treatment includes rest; adequate fluid intake; oxygen, if necessary; and sometimes antibacterials to pre-

vent secondary infection. One attack usually confers immunity. The disease can be prevented by pertussis vaccine, usually given along with diphtheria and tetanus toxoids (DPT) in a series of injections in early childhood. Also called **whooping cough.**

PERVERSION n. an action considered unnatural or abnormal, esp. a sexual activity deviating from what is considered normal.

PES n. the foot or a footlike part.

PES CAVUS n. deformity of the foot characterized by an abnormally high arch and hyperextension of the toes, giving the foot a clawlike appearance. Treatment depends on the severity of the condition; it may involve surgery; also **clawfoot**

PES PLANUS   see *flatfoot.*

PESSARY n. a plastic or metal device, usually ring-shaped, inserted into the vagina to correct the position of the uterus or to provide support in cases of uterine prolapse; it is usually used in cases where surgery to correct the problem is unwise, as, for example, because of the advanced age or general poor health of the woman.

PESTICIDE POISONING n. a toxic condition brought on by ingestion or inhalation of a pesticide (see *malathion poisoning; parathion poisoning*).

PET abbreviation for *positron emission tomography.*

PETECHIA n. tiny reddish or purplish flat spot appearing on the skin as the result of tiny hemorrhages within the skin or subcutaneous layers.   pl. **petechiae** adj. **petechial**

PETIT MAL n. a form of epilepsy characterized by brief (usually momentary) episodes of unconsciousness, sometimes accompanied by muscular spasm, twitching, or loss of muscle tone. Treatment to prevent attacks includes anticonvulsants (compare grand mal).

PETRISSAGE n. a massage technique in which the skin is gently lifted and squeezed; used to promote circulation and muscle relaxation.

PEYER'S PATCHES n. a group of lymph nodes near the junction of the *ileum* and *colon;* in typhoid fever and certain other infectious diseases, they typically become enlarged and sometimes ulcerated.

PEYOTE n. cactus from which the hallucinogen *mescaline* is derived.

PFIZER-E n. trade name for the antibacterial *erythromycin*.

PFIZERPEN-AS n. trade name for a *penicillin* G preparation.

PFIZERPEN G n. trade name for a *penicillin* G preparation.

PFIZERPEN VK n. trade name for a *penicillin* V preparation.

pH n. a measure of the acidity or alkalinity of a solution. A pH of 7 is neutral, below 7 acid, above 7 alkaline (see also *acid-base balance*).

PHACO- comb. form indicating an association with the lens of the eye (e.g., **phacocele,** protrusion of the lens).

PHAGE n. *bacteriophage.*

-PHAGIA, -PHAGY suffix indicating eating or an abnormality of appetite (e.g., **coprophagia,** the eating of feces).

PHAGO- comb. form indicating an association with eating or ingesting (e.g., **phagomania,** persistent concentration on food or an abnormal desire for food).

PHAGOCYTE n. a cell that surrounds, engulfs and digests microorganisms and cellular debris. Fixed phagocytes, including macrophages, do not circulate in the blood but are found in the liver, bone marrow, spleen, and other areas. Free phagocytes, such as leukocytes, circulate in the blood.   adj. **phagocytic**

PHAGOCYTOSIS n. the process by which certain cells (phagocytes) engulf and digest microorganisms and cellular debris.

PHALANGES n. the bones of the fingers and toes; the digits. The thumb and big toe each have two phalanges; the other fingers and toes each have three, for a total of 14 on each hand or foot.   sing. **phalanx**   adj. **phalangeal**

PHALANGITIS n. inflammation of a finger or toe.

PHALANX n. any of the 14 bones of the fingers of one hand or a like number in the toes of one foot. pl. **phalanges**

PHALLIC PHASE n. in psychoanalytic theory, the period in psychosexual development, usually between the ages of 2 and 6, when awareness of or self-manipulation of the genitals is a prime source of pleasure (compare anal phase; oral phase).

PHALLO- comb. form indicating an association with the *penis* (e.g., **phalloncus,** tumor of the penis).

PHALLOPLASTY n. surgical repair or reconstruction of the penis done to treat congenital abnormality or injury.

PHALLUS n. the *penis*   adj. **phallic**

PHANTOM LIMB SYNDROME n. a sense of pain, discomfort, or other sensation at a site where an arm or leg has been amputated.

PHARMACEUTICAL adj. pert. to drugs, esp. those used in medical treatment, or to a pharmacy.

PHARMACIST n. a specialist in formulating and dispensing drugs.

PHARMACOKINETICS n. the study of the action of drugs in the body, including the method and rate of absorption and excretion, the duration of effect, and other factors.

PHARMACOLOGY n. the study of the preparation, properties, uses, and effects of drugs.

PHARMACOPOEIA n. a book containing a list of all drugs used in medicine and including their preparation, formula, doses, and standards of purity.

PHARMACY n. the study of the preparation and dispensing of drugs.

PHARYNGEAL REFLEX see *gag reflex*.

PHARYNGEAL TONSIL n. either of two masses of lymph tissue at the back of the nasopharynx behind the posterior nares.

PHARYNGITIS n. inflammation or infection of the pharynx, usually producing a sore throat; it may be caused by bacterial or viral infection. Treatment depends on the cause.

PHARYNGO- comb. form indicating an association with the pharynx (e.g., **pharyngodynia,** pharyngeal pain).

PHARYNX n. the throat; muscular tube extending from the base of the skull to the esophagus that serves as a passageway for food from the mouth to the esophagus and for air from the nose and mouth to the larynx. It is divided into the nasopharynx, oropharynx, and laryngopharynx, and it connects with the Eustachian tubes, the posterior nares, the mouth, the larynx, and the esophagus. adj. **pharyngeal**

PHENACETIN n. an *analgesic* and *antipyretic* drug, known under many trade names, used to relieve pain and reduce fever. Adverse effects include skin rashes, and, with prolonged use, the possibility of kidney damage.

PHENAZOPYRIDINE n. an analgesic drug known under the trade name Gantrisin used to relieve pain associated with urinary tract inflammation, including cystitis and urethritis. Adverse effects include gastrointestinal disturbances.

PHENCYCLIDINE HYDROCHLORIDE (PCP) n. a hallucinogenic drug now rarely used in medicine; street name: **angel dust.**

PHENELZINE n. a monoamine oxidase inhibitor (MAO inhibitor), known under the trade name Nardil, used to treat some forms of depression. Adverse effects include vertigo, constipation, dry mouth, and interaction with many foods and drugs, sometimes producing serious effects.

PHENAPHEN n. trade name for the analgesic and antipyretic *acetaminophen.*

PHENIRAMINE n. an antihistamine, found in many preparations for allergies and respiratory infections, used to treat rhinitis, skin rashes, and pruritis. Adverse effects include sedation, dry mouth, and rapid heart rate.

PHENOBARBITAL n. a barbiturate used as a sedative to treat anxiety and as an anticonvulsant to treat some forms of epilepsy. Adverse effects include drowsiness, skin reactions, interaction with many other drugs, and possible development of dependence.

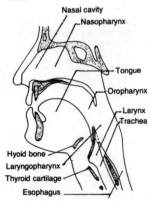

Nasal cavity
Nasopharynx
Tongue
Oropharynx
Larynx
Trachea
Hyoid bone
Laryngopharynx
Thyroid cartilage
Esophagus

PHENOL a disinfectant used to clean wounds and in various lotions and ointments used to treat inflammations; it is poisonous if taken internally.

PHENOLPHTHALEIN a *laxative,* found in many preparations under a variety of trade names. Adverse effects include abdominal cramps and possible allergic reactions.

PHENOMENON n. an observable event, which, in medicine, may be specific to a particular disease and therefore of diagnostic significance.

PHENOTHIAZINE n. any of a large group of drugs, many of which are used as tranquilizers, antiemetics, antihistamines, and adjuncts to anesthesia.

PHENOTYPE n. the observable characteristics of an organism that are the result of genetic makeup and environmental factors (compare *genotype*) adj. **phenotypic**

PHENSUXIMIDE n. an anticonvulsant, known under the trade name Milontin, used to treat petit mal epilepsy. Adverse effects include gastrointestinal upsets, drowsiness and other signs of central nervous system depression, and blood abnormalities

PHENYLALANINE n. an amino acid essential for growth in children and for protein metabolism in children and adults; it is abundant in milk and eggs (see also *phenylketonuria*).

PHENYLBUTAZONE n. a nonsteroid antiinflammatory agent, known under the trade name Butazolidin and Zolaphin, used to treat bursitis, rheumatoid arthritis, and other inflammatory conditions. Adverse effects include nausea and other gastrointestinal upsets, fluid retention, and blood abnormalities.

PHENYLEPHRINE a drug that constricts blood vessels, raising blood pressure; dilates the pupils of the eyes; and relieves nasal congestion. It is given by injection to raise blood pressure and is combined with other drugs in many nasal sprays and eye drop preparations (under many trade names, including Neosynephrine, Sinex, Dimetapp, and Histatapp) to relieve symptoms of allergy and the common cold (e.g. runny nose).

PHENYLKETONURIA n. a genetic disorder in which the absence of or a deficiency in the enzyme necessary for conversion of the amino acid phenylalanine into tyrosine causes the accumulation of phenylalanine and its metabolites in the body and in the urine. Symptoms include eczema, a mousy odor to the urine, and progressive mental retardation. Treatment includes a diet low in free of phenylalanine. Most states routinely tests newborns for the defect.

PHENYLPROPANOLAMINE n. a drug used in many preparations to relieve the symptoms of allergic reactions, the common cold, and other respiratory infections. Adverse effects include nervousness, increased blood pressure, and loss of appetite.

PHENYTOIN n. an anticonvulsant, known under the trade name Dilantin, used to treat *grand mal* epilepsy and other seizure disorders and to restore normal cardiac rhythm in cases of digitalis-induced arrhythmia. Adverse effects include ataxia, hypersensitivity reactions, and interaction with many other drugs.

PHEOCHROMOCYTOMA n. a vascular tumor of the *adrenal gland* that causes hypersecretion of epinephrine and norepinephrine, resulting in intermittent hypertension and symptoms of headache, palpitations, sweating, and nervousness. Treatment is usually surgical removal of the tumor.

PHIMOSIS n. a condition in which the foreskin of the *penis* is abnormally tight, preventing retraction over the *glans;* it may be congenital or the result of infection. Treatment is usually by *circumcision.*

PHLEB-, PHLEBO- comb. form indicating an association with a vein or veins (e.g., **phlebangioma,** a saclike swelling of a vein).

PHLEBECTOMY n. surgical removal of all or part of a vein, sometimes done to treat severe varicose veins.

PHLEBITIS n. inflammation of the wall of a vein, most often occurring in the legs. Thrombosis commonly develops (see *thrombophlebitis*). Treatment includes rest and support of the area (e.g., by elastic stockings), antiinflammatory drugs, and analgesics.

PHLEBOTHROMBOSIS n. an abnormal condition marked by the formation of a clot within a vein without prior inflammation of the wall of the vein; it is associated with prolonged bed rest, surgery, pregnancy, and other conditions in which blood flow becomes sluggish or the blood coagulates more quickly than normal. The affected area, usually the leg, may become swollen and tender. The danger is that the clot may become dislodged and travel to the lungs (pulmonary embolus).

PHLEBOTOMY n. incision of a vein for letting of blood, as in collecting blood from a donor or as treatment of polycythemia; also called venesection

PHLEGM n. thick mucus of the respiratory passages.

PHOBIA an anxiety disorder characterized by irrational and intense fear of an object (e.g., a dog), an activity (e.g., leaving the house), or physical conditions (e.g., height). The intense fear usually causes tremor, panic, palpitations, nausea, and other physical signs. Types of phobia include *agoraphobia, claustrophobia, zoophobia,* and *pyrophobia.* Treatment includes desensitization therapy and other techniques of behavior therapy.

-PHOBIA comb. form meaning "abnormal fear" (e.g., **zoophobia,** an abnormal fear of animals).

PHOCOMELIA n. a developmental abnormality marked by the absence of the upper portion of the arm or leg so that the hands and/or feet are attached to the trunk of the body by short stumps; it is a rare anomaly, occurring as an effect of *thalidomide* taken during pregnancy; also called **seal limbs** (compare *phocomelia*).

PHON-, PHONO- comb. form indicating an association with sound, esp. the sound of the voice (e.g., **phonasthenia,** a weakness or difficulty in speaking).

PHOSPHATASE n. an enzyme that acts as a catalyst in reactions involving phosphorus.

PHOSPHOLIPID n. any of a class of compounds containing a nitrogenous base, phosphoric acid, and fatty acids. Phospholipids are found in many cells.

PHOSPHORUS n. a nonmetallic element essential in the body for calcium, protein, and glucose metabolism and for the production of *adenosine triphosphate* (ATP) (see Table of Elements).

PHOT-, PHOTO- comb. form indicating an association with light (e.g., **photolysis,** the breakdown of substances in light).

PHOTALGIA n. pain in the eye caused by bright light.

PHOTOCOAGULATION n. the destruction of tissue by an intense beam of light; used to destroy diseased retinal tissue or to create scar tissue to bind the *retina* in cases of *detached retina.*

PHOTOMICROGRAPH n. photographic record of an object in a microscopic field taken by attaching a camera to a microscope.

PHOTOPHOBIA n. abnormal intolerance to light, often associated with albinism, drug-induced pupil dilation, migraine, encephalitis, measles, and other diseases.

PHOTOPSIA n. the sensation of flashing lights caused by irritation of the *retina*.

PHOTORETINITIS n. damage to the *retina* caused by looking at the sun without adequate protection.

PHOTOSENSITIVITY n. abnormal sensitivity of the skin to the sun caused by a disorder (e.g., albinism) or the result of certain drugs (e.g., tetracycline, phenothiazines). adj. **photosensitive**

PHOTOTHERAPY n. the use of strong light to treat disorders such as *acne* and *hyperbilirubinemia of the newborn*.

PHRENIC adj. 1. pert. to the *diaphragm;* 2. pert. to the mind.

PHRENIC NERVE n. one of a pair of nerves, arising from cervical spinal roots and passing down the thorax to innervate the diaphragm and help control its movements during breathing.

PHYCOMYCOSIS n. any infection caused by fungi of the order Phycomycetes. These fungi inhabit soil and do not usually produce disease in humans but may cause opportunistic infections.

PHYSICAL adj. in medicine, pert. to the body, not the mind.

PHYSICAL MEDICINE n. that branch of medicine concerned with the rehabilitation of patients with disabilities.

PHYSICAL THERAPY n. the treatment of disorders with methods such as massage, manipulation, cold, heat, diathermy, hydrotherapy and light to restore normal function following an accident or injury or illness.

PHYSIOTHERAPY   see *physical therapy*.

PHYSOSTIGMINE n. parasympathomimetic drug used to constrict the pupil and reduce pressure in the eye in cases of *glaucoma*. Adverse effects include bronchospasm, digestive upsets, and excess salivation.

PIA MATER n. the innermost of the three meninges covering the brain and spinal cord (the other two being the *dura mater* and *arachnoid*); it is highly vascularized and closely applied to the brain and spinal cord, nourishing the nerve cells.

PIAN   see *yaws*.

PICA n. the eating of nonfood substances, such as clay, chalk, hair, or glue; it occurs in some cases of nutritional deficiency, pregnancy, and some mental disorders.

PICK'S DISEASE n. a form of presenile dementia occurring in middle aged people, characterized by degeneration in the frontal and temporal lobes of the brain (not diffuse throughout the brain as in *Alzheimer's disease*) and manifested by changes in behavior and deterioration of intellectual abilities.

PICKWICKIAN SYNDROME n. an abnormal condition in which there is extreme obesity, often with decreased lung function and sleepiness.

PICORNAVIRUS n. any of a group of small, RNA viruses, including the coxsackie virus and rhinoviruses.

PIEBALD adj. having patches of nonpigmented hair or skin due to the absence of melanocytes in those areas (compare *albinism; vitiligo*).

PIGEON BREAST n. a congenital condition in which there is abnormal forward projection of the sternum (breastbone); it is usually harmless and requires no treatment; also called **pigeon chest.**

PIGEON TOES n. abnormal posture in which the toes are turned inward; often associated with knock-knee.

PIGMENT n. a substance giving color, including blood pigments (e.g., hemoglobin), retinal pigments (e.g., rhodopsin) and melanin found in the skin and iris of the eye.

PILAR CYST see *wen.*

PILES see *hemorrhoids.*

PILO- comb. form indicating an association with hair (e.g., **pilosis,** excessive development of hair).

PILOCARPINE n. a cholinergic agent used in eyedrops to treat glaucoma. Adverse effects include difficulty in breathing, excess salivation, and muscle tremors.

PILOMOTOR REFLEX n. erection of the hairs of skin in response to emotional stress, skin irritation, or cold; also called **gooseflesh.**

PILONIDAL FISTULA n. an abnormal tract containing hairs extending from an opening in the skin, usually near the cleft at the top of the buttocks; also called **pilonidae sinus.**

PILOSEBACEOUS adj. pert. to a hair follicle and its sebaceous gland.

PILUS n. a hair   pl. **pili**   adj. **pilar**

PIMPLE a small, inflamed, pus-containing swelling on the skin usually due to infection of a pore obstructed with sebaceous secretions.

PIN n. in orthopedics, a rodlike metal device used to secure fragments of a bone.

PINEAL GLAND n. a small, cone-shaped gland in the brain thought to secrete melatonin; also called **pineal body; epiphysis.**

PINEALOMA n. a neoplasm of the *pineal gland,* usually causing headache, nausea, vomiting, and hydrocephalus.

PINKEYE see *conjunctivitis.*

PINNA n. that part of the outer ear seen outside the head; auricle.

PINOCYTOSIS n. the process by which certain cells (e.g., some leukocytes) engulf and take in droplets of fluid (compare *phagocytosis*).

PINTA n. a skin infection caused by the *Treponema carateum* spirochete and common in Central and South America; it is characterized by a slowly enlarging papule, followed by a generalized rash, and later by depigmentation of affected areas. Treatment is by penicillin.

PIPERAZINE n. an anthelmintic used to treat infestations with pinworms and roundworms. Adverse effects include fever, vertigo, abdominal discomfort, and diarrhea.

PITOCIN n. trade name for *oxytocin,* used to stimulate labor.

PITRESSIN n. trade name for the antidiuretic hormone *vasopressin.*

PITTING n. 1. small, depressed scars on the skin following severe acne or other disorder; 2. temporary indentation in the skin following pressure on edematous tissue.

PITUITARY DWARF n. a dwarf whose small size is due to lack of growth hormone from the anterior pituitary; the body is typically normally proportioned with no deformities, and mental and sexual development is normal.

PITUITARY GLAND n. a small endocrine gland attached to the *hypothalamus* that releases many hormones controlling many body activities and influencing the activity of many other endocrine glands. It is divided into anterior and posterior portions, each with separate functions (see *anterior pituitary gland; posterior pituitary gland*).

PITYRIASIS n. any of several skin disorders

pityriasis alba n. a common skin disorder, occurring most often in children and young adults, characterized by circumscribed round or oval patches of depigmentation or less than normal pigmentation.

pityriasis rosea n. a skin disease in which a mildly itchy rash develops over the trunk of the body several days after a single localized patch—a herald patch.

PIVOT JOINT n. a synovial joint in which movement is limited to rotation; the articulation of the radius and ulna is a pivot joint.

PKU abbreviation for *phenylketonuria*.

PLACEBO n. an inactive substance (e.g., distilled water or sugar) or less-than-effective dose of a harmless substance prescribed and administered as if it were an effective dose of a needed drug; used as a control in tests of drug efficacy and to treat certain patients who do not need or should not be given a drug they request.

PLACEBO EFFECT n. a change, usually beneficial, occurring after a substance (a placebo) is taken that is not the result of any property of that substance but usually reflects the faith or expectations the person has in the substance.

PLACENTA n. highly vascular fetal organ through which the fetus absorbs oxygen, nutrients, and other substances from the mother and excretes carbon dioxide and other wastes. It forms around the eighth day of gestation as the *blastocyst* becomes implanted in

the wall of the *uterus*. At the end of pregnancy the placenta weighs about one sixth the weight of the infant. Its maternal side is rough, divided into lobules, and has fingerlike chorionic villi that project into the uterine wall. The fetal side is smooth, covered with the fetal membranes. The placenta is expelled after the birth of the child in the third stage of labor. Also called **afterbirth.**   adj. **placental**

PLACENTA PREVIA n. a condition of pregnancy in which the placenta is implanted abnormally in the uterus so that it partially or completely covers the outlet from the uterus to the vagina; it is a common cause of bleeding in late pregnancy. If severe hemorrhage occurs immediate Cesarean section is required to save the mother's life. If the placenta is next to, but not blocking, the uterine outlet, vaginal delivery may be attempted.

PLACIDYL n. trade name for the sedative ethchlorvynol.

PLAGIOCEPHALY n. congenital malformation of the skull.

PLAGUE n. 1. an infectious disease caused by the bite of rat fleas infected with *Yersinia pestis* (see *bubonic plague*); 2. any epidemic disease with a high death rate.

PLANO- comb. form meaning "flat" (e.g., **planocellular,** having flat cells).

PLANTAR adj. pert. to the undersurface (sole) of the foot.

PLANTAR REFLEX n. reflex in which drawing a blunt instrument or firmly stroking the outer part of the sole from the heel toward the little toe causes the toes to bunch and curl downward. In those over the age of $1\frac{1}{2}$–2 years. an upward movement of the big toe after this stimulus is usually a sign of neurological damage, the Babinski sign.

PLANTAR WART n. a wart occurring on the sole that, because of pressure, develops a callus ring around its soft center and becomes painful. Treatment includes cryosurgery, electrodesiccation, and application of topical acids.

PLANTIGRADE adj. pert. to walking on the entire sole of the foot, as in the human gait.

PLAQUE n. 1. a flat, raised patch on the skin or mucous membrane; 2. a deposit of atherosclerosis; 3. a deposit of saliva and bacteria found on teeth that encourages the development of *caries*.

PLASMA n. acellular, colorless, fluid part of blood and lymph which contains water, electrolytes, glucose, fats, proteins, and bile and in which erythrocytes, leukocytes, and platelets are suspended. In addition to carrying the cellular elements, plasma helps maintain the fluid-electrolyte and the acid-base balances of the body and helps transport wastes (compare *serum*).

PLASMA CELL n. a lymphocyte-like cell found in bone marrow and sometimes in the blood that functions in immune responses; large numbers of plasma cells are found in *multiple myeloma*.

PLASMACYTOMA n. a neoplasm of plasma cells, occurring in bone marrow usually in association with multiple myeloma, or less commonly occurring in soft tissues, esp. those of the upper respiratory tract.

PLASMAPHERESIS n. a method of removing plasma from the blood. Blood is withdrawn from the body and the cellular elements separated and transfused back to the patient. The technique has been used to identify and analyze plasma proteins for diagnostic purposes and has been tried experimentally in the treatment of certain diseases.

PLASMA PROTEIN n. any of various proteins in blood plasma, including fibrinogen and prothrombin, important for blood coagulation and gamma globulins, which are important in immune responses.

PLASMID n. a small cellular inclusion consisting of DNA, capable of self-replicating, and involved in certain metabolic functions.

PLASMO- comb. form indicating an association with plasma (e.g., **plasmocyte,** a plasma cell).

PLASMODIUM n. genus of parasites that includes the malaria-causing organisms

PLASTIC SURGERY n. that branch of surgery concerned with the alteration, reconstruction, and replacement of body parts to correct a structural or cosmetic defect. Common plastic surgery procedures include the repair of cleft lips and cleft palate, *rhinoplasty,* the reconstruction of body parts destroyed by injury, and skin grafting.

-PLASTY comb. form indicating plastic surgery on a specific body part (e.g., **otoplasty,** plastic surgery on the ear).

PLATE n. 1. a flat structure or part, as the neural plate in the embryo that develops into the neural tube; 2. a denture.

PLATELET n. a disc-shaped small cellular element in the blood, essential for blood clotting. Normally 200,000 to 300,000 platelets are found in one cubic centimeter of blood.

PLATY- comb. form indicating broadness or flatness (e.g., **platyopia,** a broad face).

PLATYSMA n. a broad muscle, on each side of the neck, extending from the lower jaw to the region of the clavicle and involved in mouth and jaw movement.

PLAY THERAPY n. a form of psychotherapy for children in which play with games and toys is used to gain insight into the child's feelings and thoughts and to help treat conflicts and psychological problems.

PLEASURE PRINCIPLE n. in psychoanalytic theory, the tendency to pursue actions or objects that provide immediate gratification of instinctual drives and to avoid discomfort and pain (compare reality principle).

-PLEGIA suffix indicating paralysis (e.g., **hemiplegia,** paralysis of one side of the body).

PLETHORA n. an excess of blood or other body fluid. adj. **plethoric**

PLEUR-, PLEURO- comb. form indicating an association with the *pleura* (e.g., **pleurobronchitis,** inflammation of the pleura and bronchi).

PLEURA n. the delicate membrane covering the lungs; it is divided into the visceral pleura that covers the lungs and the parietal pleura that lines the chest wall and covers the *diaphragm.* Between the two layers of the pleura is a small space (pleural space) containing fluid that acts as a lubricant. pl. **pleurae** adj. **pleural**

PLEURAL CAVITY n. the cavity in the thorax that contains the lungs.

PLEURAL SPACE n. the small space between the visceral and parietal layers of the *pleura.*

PLEURISY n. inflammation of the *pleura,* esp. the parietal layer of the pleura, marked by difficulty in breathing and sharp pain. Causes include pneumonia, tuberculosis, and cancer of bronchi. Treatment depends on the cause.

PLEURODYNIA n. acute inflammation of the muscles between the ribs, causing pain, tenderness, and often fever.

PLEUROPNEUMONIA n. pleurisy and pneumonia.

PLEUROPNEUMONIALIKE ORGANISM (PPLO) see *mycoplasma.*

PLEXUS n. a network of intersecting nerves, blood vessels, or lymph vessels (e.g., the *brachial plexus*).

PLICA n. a fold of tissue (e.g., the plica vocalis, the vocal cord). pl. **plicae** adj. **plical**

PLUMBISM see *lead poisoning.*

PLURI- comb. form indicating more than one (e.g., **pluriglandular,** pert. to more than one gland).

-PNEA comb. form indicating an association with breathing (e.g., *dyspnea,* difficult breathing).

PNEUMA-, PNEUMATO- comb. form indicating an association with air or gas (e.g., **pneumarthrosis,** gas in the joints).

PNEUMO-, PNEUMONO- comb. form indicating an association with the *lungs* (e.g., **pneumogastric,** pert. to the lungs and stomach).

PNEUMOCOCCAL pert. to bacteria of the genus *Pneumococcus.*

PNEUMOCOCCAL VACCINE n. an active immunizing agent effective against many strains of *Pneumococcus* associated with most cases of pneumococcal pneumonia.

PNEUMOCONIOSIS n. any lung disease caused by chronic inhalation of dust, usually of occupational origin; types of pneumoconiosis includes *asbestosis, anthracosis,* and *silicosis.*

PNEUMOCYTOSIS n. infection with the parasite *Pneumocystis carinii,* usually occurring only in infants or immunosuppressed people (e.g., those with acquired immune deficiency syndrome); it is characterized by fever, cough, rapid breathing, and cyanosis and is difficult to treat; also called **interstitial plasma cell pneumonia**

PNEUMOENCEPHALOGRA-PHY n. a technique for X-ray visualization of some brain tissues that involves the injection of oxygen or other gas into the ventricles of the brain to displace *cerebrospinal fluid* and provide a contrast medium.

PNEUMONECTOMY n. surgical removal of a lung, usually to treat cancer.

PNEUMONIA n. inflammation of the lungs, usually caused by infection with bacteria, (esp. pneumococcus), viruses, fungi, or rickettsiae. Symptoms include fever, chills, headache, cough, chest pain, and, as the disease progresses, difficult and painful breathing, the production of thick, purulent sputum, rapid pulse, and sometimes gastrointestinal complications. Treatment depends on the cause; it often includes antibiotics, analgesics, expectorants, rest, fluids, and oxygen (see also *bronchopneumonia*).

PNEUMONITIS n. inflammation of the lung, caused by a virus or allergic reaction. Treatment includes removal of the offending agent, if possible, and corticosteroids.

PNEUMOTHORAX n. a collection of air or gas in the pleural cavity causing the lung to collapse. It may occur spontaneously but usually results from injury to the chest that allows the entrance of air. Symptoms include sudden, sharp chest pain, difficulty in breathing, rapid heart beat, weakness, and low blood pressure. Treatment involves aspiration of the air from the pleural cavity and the administration of oxygen and pain relievers.

POD-, PODO- comb. form indicating an association with the foot (e.g., **podalgia,** foot pain).

PODIATRY n. that medical specialty concerned with the diagnosis and treatment of diseases and disorders of the feet.

-POIESIS comb. form meaning "the production of" (e.g., **erythropoiesis,** red blood cell production).

POISON n. a substance that when inhaled, ingested, or absorbed impairs health or causes death.

POISON IVY see *rhus dermatitis*

POISON OAK see *rhus dermatitis*

POISON SUMAC see *rhus dermatitis*

POLIO- comb. form indicating an association with the gray matter of the brain and/or spinal cord (e.g., **polioencephalitis,** inflammation of the gray matter of the brain caused by a virus).

POLIOMYELITIS n. an infectious disease that affects the central nervous system. It is caused by the poliovirus and was once epidemic in many parts of the world, but now is largely prevented by vaccination with Salk or Sabin vaccines. Many infections are asymptomatic; some produce only mild symptoms of fever, malaise, headache, and gastrointestinal upsets; others cause paralysis, most often of the lower limbs. Treatment is largely symptomatic. Also: **polio; infantile paralysis**

POLIOSIS n. depigmentation of the hair.

POLIOVIRUS n. an organism that causes *poliomyelitis*.

POLIOVIRUS VACCINE n. a vaccine prepared from poliovirus to provide immunity to poliomyelitis. The live oral form of the vaccine, called the Sabin vaccine, is routinely given to children under the age of 18; inactivated polio vaccine, known as the Salk vaccine, is given subcutaneously, usually to infants and unvaccinated adults.

POLLEX n. the thumb.

POLLINOSIS n. *hay fever*

POLY- comb. form indicating many or a large amount (e.g., **polycystic,** having many cysts).

POLYARTERITIS n. inflammation of several arteries.

POLYARTERITIS NODOSA see *periarteritis nodosa*.

POLYCILLIN n. trade name for the antibacterial *ampicillin*.

POLYCYSTIC KIDNEY DISEASE (PKD) n. an abnormal condition in which the kidneys are enlarged and contain many cysts. It occurs in childhood and adult forms and often leads to kidney failure.

POLYCYTHEMIA n. an abnormal increase in the number of *erythrocytes* in the blood, often associated with pulmonary or heart disease, or exposure to high altitudes for a long period, but in many cases of unknown cause.

POLYDACTYLY n. a congenital abnormality characterized by the presence of more than the normal number of fingers or toes; it is usually corrected by surgery; also: **hyperdactyly.**

POLYDIPSIA n. excessive thirst, often associated with *diabetes mellitus, diabetes insipidus* or kidney dysfunction.

POLYMORPHISM n. the state of existing or occurring in several forms.

POLYMORPHONUCLEAR adj. having a nucleus with multiple lobules, as some leukocytes.

POLYMOX n. trade name for the antibacterial *amoxicillin*.

POLYMYOSITIS n. inflammation of many muscles.

POLYMYXIN n. an antibiotic, used to treat certain bacterial infections. Adverse effects include allergic skin reactions and kidney damage.

POLYNEURITIC PSYCHOSIS see *Korsakoff's psychosis*.

POLYNEURITIS n. inflamma-

tion of all or most of the peripheral nerves.

POLYP n. a growth or nodule, usually benign, most commonly arising from a mucous membrane (e.g., in the nose, ear or uterus).

POLYPEPTIDE n. a molecule consisting of three or more amino acids; proteins are polypeptides.

POLYPHARMACY n. the act of prescribing or administering more than one drug to a patient. The possibility of drug interaction must be considered in these cases.

POLYSACCHARIDE n. a complex carbohydrate, such as starch, that can be broken down into simpler monosaccharides like sugar.

POLYSOMY n. the presence of one or more extra chromosomes in somatic cells as a result of nondisjunction of chromosomes during gamete formation. It is usually associated with congenital defects.

POLYSPORIN n. trade name for a fixed-combination, topical ophthalmic drug, containing the antibacterials *polymixin* and *bacitracin;* used to treat eye infections.

POLYURIA n. the production of large volumes of usually dilute and pale urine; it is often associated with *diabetes mellitus, diabetes insipidus,* renal disorder, or the intake of large amounts of fluid.

POLY-VI-FLOR n. trade name for an oral, pediatric, fixed combination of vitamins and minerals, including sodium fluoride.

PONS n. any bridgelike part connecting two parts, esp. the **pons Varolii** (Varolius), between the medulla oblongata and the midbrain, which contains white matter and the nuclei of several cranial nerves.

PONSTEL n. trade name for the antiinflammatory and analgesic agent mefenamic acid used to treat mild to moderate pain.

PONTO- comb. form indicating an association with the *pons* of the brain (e.g., **pontocerebellar,** pert. to the pons and cerebellum).

POPLITEAL adj. pert. to the area behind the knee.

POPLITEAL ARTERY n. artery extending from the femoral artery and branching to supply the legs and foot.

PORE n. a small opening, as the openings of the sweat glands in the skin.   adj. **porous**

PORPHYRIA n. any of several inherited disorders characterized by disturbance of the metabolism of porphyrins, affecting primarily the liver or bone marrow. The affected person excretes large amounts of porphyrins in the urine and has photosensivity, neuritis, and mental disturbances.

PORPHYRIN n. any of a number of pigments widely distributed in living tissue (in, e.g., hemoglobin, myoglobin, and cytochromes) and important in many oxidation reactions.

PORTA n. an opening or entry, esp. one through which blood vessels pass into an organ (e.g.,

porta hepatis, the opening through which major blood vessels enter and leave the liver).

PORTACAVAL SHUNT n. communication surgically created between the portal vein and the inferior *vena cava* so that blood drained from abdominal organs bypasses the liver and is channeled directly to the inferior vena cava for movement to the heart; it is used to decrease portal hypertension.

PORTAL adj. pert. to the *portal system*.

PORTAL HYPERTENSION n. an increase in pressure within the veins of the *portal system,* caused by obstruction in the portal (hepatic) blood system, often associated with alcoholic cirrhosis of the liver. It causes enlargement of the spleen and collateral veins, and, if severe and untreated, systemic *hypertension*.

PORTAL SYSTEM n. a system of veins that drains blood from abdominal organs (the digestive organs, pancreas, spleen, and gallbladder) and transports it to the liver.

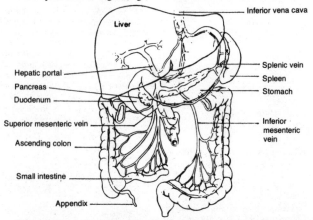

In the portal system deoxygenated blood from the intestines, spleen, and other organs passes into the hepatic portal vein that carries it into the liver. After the blood is detoxified and nutrients in it modified, it passes into the inferior vena cava, thus returning to the systemic circulation.

PORTAL VEIN n. a short vein that receives branches from many veins leading from abdominal organs, including the splenic vein from the spleen and pancreas and the mesenteric vein from the intestine, and enters the liver, ramifying there and ending in capillarylike sinusoids where the nutrients from the blood pass into liver cells. The blood then passes through the hepatic vein to the inferior *vena cava*.

PORT-WINE STAIN n. a flat birthmark, varying from pale pinkish red to deep purple; also: **nevus flammeus.**

POSITRON EMISSION TOMOGRAPHY (PET) n. a computerized radiographic technique that allows examination of the metabolic activity of various tissues, esp. brain tissue. Radioactively tagged substances (usually glucose) taken by the patient give off positively charged particles (positrons) that interact with certain cells, esp. neurons in the brain, giving off gamma rays, which are detected by special devices and converted through computer analysis into colorcoded images that reveal the metabolic activity of the organ involved. It is wisely used in the diagnosis of brain disorders.

POST- comb. form meaning "after" "behind" (e.g., **postadolescence,** the time in a person's life after adolescence).

POSTERIOR adj. pert. to, situated in, or toward the back or the back part of a structure.

POSTERIOR NARES see *nares.*

POSTERIOR PITUITARY GLAND n. the posterior lobe of the pituitary gland that secretes two hormones: antidiuretic hormone, or vasopressin, that acts on the kidney to reduce urine production; and oxytocin, that produces contractions of the pregnant uterus and causes milk to flow from the breasts of lactating women; also: **neurohypophysis.**

POSTERO- comb. form indicating a posterior position (e.g., **posteroanterior,** from the back to the front).

POSTHITIS n. inflammation, usually due to bacterial infection, of the foreskin of the *penis*, causing redness, swelling, and pain; often associated with inflammation of the glans. Treatment is by antibiotics (see also *balanitis*).

POSTHUMOUS BIRTH n. 1. the birth of a child by Cesaerean section after the death of the mother; 2. the birth of a child after the father's death.

POSTICTAL adj. pert. to period following a convulsion.

POSTMATURE INFANT n. an infant born after 42 weeks gestation and usually showing signs of placental insufficiency. The child usually has dry, peeling skin, skin folds, long nails, and is prone to electrolyte imbalance and hypoglycemia and may have lost weight the last few days in utero.

POSTMENOPAUSAL adj. pert. to the time after menopause.

POSTNASAL DRIP n. the discharge of nasal mucus into the pharynx, caused by rhinitis, sinusitis, or hypersecretion of mucus and usually associated with a feeling of nasal and throat obstruction and unpleasant taste and odor. Treatment includes agents to constrict nasal vessels; the irrigation of sinuses, if necessary; the surgical correction of nasal polyps or deviated septum, if indicated; allergy treatment and/or antibiotics.

POSTOPERATIVE adj. pert. to the period following surgery, including the emergence from anesthesia and the abatement of the acute signs of anesthesia and surgery.

POSTPARTUM adj. pert. to the few days following childbirth.

POSTURAL HYPOTENSION see *orthostatic hypotension*.

POTASSIUM n. a metallic element, essential to life. It is the major intracellular ion, functioning in nerve and muscle activity (see Table of Elements).

POTASSIUM CHLORIDE n. a salt of potassium used to treat potassium deficiency, which is usually the result of diuretic intake.

POTENCY n. 1. strength or power, as of a drug; 2. the ability of a male to achieve and maintain an erection and thus engage in coitus (see also *impotence*).

POTENTIATION n. a synergistic effect in which the effect of two drugs given simultaneously is greater than the effect of the drugs given separately.

POTT'S DISEASE n. tuberculosis of the spine; it is rare and untreated leads to bone destruction and skeletal deformity.

POUCH n. a saclike part.

POULTICE n. a preparation of hot, moist material applied to any part of the body to increase local circulation, alleviate pain, or soften and lubricate the skin.

POX n. any of several diseases, usually viral, in which the skin breaks out in pustules or vescicles (small blisters) (see *chickenpox; smallpox*).

PPLO abbreviation for pleuropneumonialike organism (see *mycoplasma*).

PRANDIAL adj. pert. to a meal.

PRAZOSIN n. an antihypertensive drug, known under the trade name Minipress. Adverse effects include rapid heartbeat, fainting and a sudden drop in blood pressure.

PRE- prefix meaning ''before'' (e.g., **premenopausal,** pert. to the time before menopause).

PRECANCEROUS adj. pert. to a growth that is not malignant but probably will become so if left untreated.

PRECIPITIN n. an antibody that combines with its antigen to form a complex that settles out of solution as a precipitate. This reaction is used to identify an unknown antigen or to establish the presence of antibodies to a known antigen.

PRECOCIOUS adj. pert. to earlier-than-expected development of physical or mental abilities (e.g., **precocious dentition,** the eruption of deciduous or permanent teeth at an age earlier than expected).

PRECORDIAL adj. pert. to the region of the chest over the heart (the precordium).

PREDISPOSITION n. a tendency to be affected by a particular disease or to develop or react in a certain way; it may be genetic or the result of environmental factors (e.g., nutritional factors).

PREDNISOLONE n. a glucocorticoid, known under the trade name Prednis, used to treat inflammatory conditions. Adverse effects include those associated with most of the corticosteroids, including fluid and electrolyte imbalances and gastrointestinal and endocrine disturbances.

PREDNISONE n. a glucocorticoid used to treat rheumatoid arthritis, allergic reactions, and inflammatory conditions.

PREECLAMPSIA n. an abnormal condition of pregnancy characterized by hypertension, edema, and the presence of protein in the urine. Abnormal metabolic functioning, ocular disorders, and other complications frequently occur in the pregnant woman; fetal malnutrition and lowered birth weight in the child. Untreated severe preeclampsia can lead to eclampsia and convulsions that threaten the life of both the mother and fetus.

PREFRONTAL LOBE n. the region of the brain at the front part of each cerebral hemisphere; it is concerned with learning, memory, emotions and behavior.

PREGNANCY n. gestation; the period during which a woman carries a developing fetus in the uterus, from the time of conception to the birth of the child. Pregnancy lasts 266 days from the day of fertilization but is usually calculated as 280 days from the first day of the last menstrual period. The fertilized ovum, or zygote, implants in the wall of the uterus and undergoes growth and development, nourished and protected by the placenta that forms from embryonic and maternal tissue in the uterus. Pregnancy involves changes in virtually every system of a woman's body, including an increase in total blood volume and cardiac output, an increase in kidney filtration and increased urination; enlargement of the breasts and changes in the color of the nipple area as the breasts prepare to provide milk for an infant; skin changes, sometimes including chloasma; gastrointestinal changes, often manifested as heartburn, nausea, vomiting and constipation; increased nutritional needs and weight gain (20 to 25 pounds or more); and numerous endocrine changes, including increased thyroid and adrenal function and the release of hormones from the placenta. adj. **pregnant**

PREGNANEDIOL n. a compound found in the urine of pregnant women and in the urine of women during certain phases of the menstrual cycle.

PREINVASIVE CANCER see *carcinoma in situ*.

PREMARIN n. trade name for an *estrogen* compound.

PREMATURE adj. occurring before the normal time; not fully developed, esp. a premature infant, one born before 37 weeks of gestation.

PREMATURE EJACULATION n. emission of semen and loss of erection during early stages of sexual excitement before or immediatley after insertion of the penis in the vagina. Numerous behavioral techniques are used to extend the time between erection and ejaculation.

PREMATURE INFANT n. an infant born prior to 37 weeks gestation regardless of birth weight. Premature infants are usually of low birth weight, have incompletely developed organ systems and appear scrawny with little subcutaneous fat and a large head and pinkish translucent skin. The cause of prematurity is unknown in many cases, but in some is associated with toxemia, multiple pregnancy, chronic disease, trauma, or poor nutrition. The prognosis depends on the maturity of the various organ systems of the infant's body and on the postnatal care given, with the best care being provided in *intensive care neonatal units*. Treatment involves maintenance of stable body temperature and respiration, provision for adequate fluid and nutrient intake, and prevention of infection.

PREMATURE LABOR n. labor beginning before the 37th or 38th week of gestation or before the fetus has reached a weight of 2,000 grams. Premature labor may occur spontaneously without apparent cause or it may result from trauma, chronic disease, infection in the mother, placental problems, or other factors; predisposing factors are poor nutrition, low weight gain, smoking, and multiple pregnancies. In some cases labor can be inhibited and the pregnancy prolonged to allow further development of the fetus.

PREMATURE VENTRICULAR CONTRACTION (PVC) n. an irregularity of cardiac rhythm. Isolated PVC's may not be significant but frequent recurrent PVC's usually indicate heart abnormality and may be a precursor of *ventricular fibrillation* and inadequate cardiac output.

PREMENSTRUAL TENSION (PMT) n. a poorly understood syndrome of tension, irritability, edema, headache, mastalgia, bloating, appetite changes, and changes in muscular coordination occurring in many women several days before the onset of the menstrual flow.

PREMOLAR n. any of eight teeth in adult dentition, two on each side of each jaw, situated behind the canines and in front of the molars, also called **bicuspids.**

PRENATAL adj. prior to birth; used in reference to the pregnant woman or the growth and development of the fetus; also: **antenatal**

PRENATAL DEVELOPMENT n. the process of growth, differentiation, development, and maturation between fertilization and birth. The fertilized egg immediately begins dividing in the process of *cleavage,* passes through stages of *morula, blastocyst, gastrula;* the three primary germ layers are laid down and differentiation of the tissues, organs, and organ systems of the body occurs. By fourteen weeks all the major organs and systems of the body have been formed; from then on there is further growth and maturation, so that at birth, the average fetus is about 20 inches (50 centimeters) long and weighs between 7 and 8 pounds (approx. 3.2–3.6 kilograms). See accompanying illustrations.

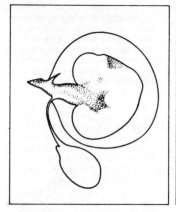

A human embryo approximately 5 weeks after fertilization, surounded by its amnion. The smaller yolk sac attached to the embryo will become incorporated into the umbilical cord. Rudimentary eyes and limbs are visible on the embryo.

A 7-week embryo showing attachment of the developing umbilical cord to the placenta.

PRENATAL DIAGNOSIS n. any of various diagnostic procedures to determine if the fetus has a genetic or other abnormality. The procedures involve X rays and ultrasonography (sonograms), which can reveal structural abnormalities and allow growth to be followed; *amniocentesis* in which amniotic fluid is withdrawn for analysis and identification of *chromosome* and metabolic defects, and *fetoscopy* in which fetal blood can be withdrawn and analyzed (see also *genetic counseling*).

PREOPERATIVE adj. pert. to the period prior to surgery, when the patient is prepared for surgery by limitations on food and fluids by mouth, by removal of body hair on the area to be incised, by premedication, and/or by other procedures.

PREPRANDIAL adj. before a meal.

PREPUBERTY n. period of about 2 years immediately before puberty when growth and changes leading to sexual maturity occur. adj. **prepubertal**

PREPUCE n. the fold of skin that is a retractable cover over the *glans* of the *penis* or the fold around the *clitoris;* also: **foreskin.**

PRESAMINE n. trade name for the antidepressant *imipramine.*

PRESBYOPIA n. farsightedness developing with advancing age as the lens of the eye becomes less elastic. adj. **presbyopic**

PRESCRIPTION n. a written order for medication, therapy or a device given by a properly authorized medical practitioner, esp. a written order for a drug given by a physician to a pharmacist.

PRESCRIPTION DRUG n. a drug that can only be dispensed to the public with a prescription (compare *over-the-counter drug*).

PRESENILE DEMENTIA see *Alzheimer's disease.*

PRESENTATION n. the position of the baby in the uterus with reference to the part of the baby directed toward the birth canal. Normally the head appears first (cephalic presentation), but in some cases the buttocks, feet, shoulder, or side may present first. Abnormal presentations may cause difficulty in childbirth and attempts to turn the baby may be made, or if normal delivery is deemed hazardous a Cesarean section performed.

PRESSOR adj. acting to increase blood pressure.

PRESSURE n. force or stress applied to a surface.

PRESSURE POINT n. point over an artery where pulse can be felt and where pressure on the point may stop hemorrhage distal to that point.

PRESSURE SORE see *decubitus ulcer.*

PRETERM INFANT see *premature infant.*

PREVALENCE n. in epidemiology, the number of occurrences of a disease or event during a particular period of time; it is usually expressed as a ratio, the number of events occurring per the population at risk for the occurrence.

PREVENTIVE MEDICINE n. that branch of medicine concerned primarily with the prevention of disease; it concerns itself with immunization, the eradication of disease carriers (e.g., malaria-carrying mosquitoes), screening programs, and other factors.

PRIAPISM n. an abnormal condition in which the *penis* is constantly erect, often with pain and seldom with sexual arousal; it may be caused by lesion in the central nervous system or the penis itself or be associated with certain systemic diseases.

PRICKLY HEAT see *miliaria.*

PRIMAQUINE n. a drug used to treat *malaria*. High doses may cause gastrointestinal upsets and blood disorders.

PRIMARY n. 1. first in occurrence, importance, or development; 2. not derived from any other source, as the original condition in a disease process.

PRIMARY AMENORRHEA see *amenorrhea*.

PRIMARY HEALTH CARE n. he2lth care provided by a physician, nurse, or other health care professional in the first contact of the patient with health care. It may involve a private internist, family physician, pediatrician, an ambulatory health care facility, or a hospital emergency room.

PRIMIDONE n. an anticonvulsant used to treat *grand mal epilepsy* and other seizure disorders. Adverse effects include drowsiness, dizziness, ataxia, and blood disorders.

PRIMIGRAVIDA n. a woman pregnant for the first time.

PRIMIPARA n. a woman who has been delivered of a child (or children, as in twins or triplets) for the first time. adj. **primiparous**

PRIMITIVE adj. undeveloped, undifferentiated, rudimentary.

PRIMORDIAL adj. pert. to undeveloped or primitive state; first or original.

PRIMORDIAL DWARF n. a very short person with normal proportion of body parts and normal mental and sexual development; also called **normal dwarf; true dwarf; hypoplastic dwarf.**

PRIMORDIUM n. the first recognizable stage in the differentiation and development of a particular organ or structure. pl. **primordia** adj. **primordial**

P.R.N. in prescriptions, an abbreviation for "*pro re nata,*" meaning "as needed."

PRO- prefix meaning "before" "in front of" "preceding" (e.g., **proenzyme,** a precursor of an enzyme, as pepsinogen is the precursor of *pepsin*).

PROBENECID n. a drug that reduces the level of uric acid in the blood and is used in the treatment of *gout.* Adverse effects include urinary frequency, headache, skin rashes, and stomach upsets.

PROCAINE n. a local anesthetic agent, known under the trade name Novocaine used for epidural, caudal, and other regional anesthesia; it is not used topically. Adverse effects include neurological and cardiovascular reactions.

PROCARBAZINE n. an antineoplastic used to treat *Hodgkin's disease* and other neoplasms. Adverse effects include bone marrow depression, nausea, and vomiting.

PROCESS n. in anatomy, a thin projection or prominence, as on the vertebrae.

PROCHLORPERAZINE n. an antipsychotic and antiemetic used in the treatment of schizophrenia and certain other mental disorders and to combat nausea and vomiting. Adverse effects include drowsiness, abnormal muscle movements, low blood pressure, liver toxicity, and blood abnormalities

PROCT-, PROCTO- comb. form indicating an association with the *rectum* (e.g., **proctalgia,** pain in the rectum).

PROCTITIS n. inflammation of the *rectum* characterized by blood in the stool, frequent urge to defecate but inability to do so, and sometimes diarrhea. It may be associated with *ulcerative colitis,* or *Crohn's disease,* or it may be caused by trauma, infection, or radiation.

PROCTOCELE n. protrusion of the *rectum,* usually into the *vagina* in cases of uterine prolapse.

PROCTOLOGIST n. a physician who specializes in *proctology*.

PROCTOLOGY n. that branch of medicine concerned with the diagnosis and treatment of disorders of the colon, rectum, and anus.

PROCTOSCOPE n. an instrument (a type of endoscope) used to examine the rectum and the end portion of the *colon*.

PROCYCLIDINE n. a drug used to reduce tremor in *parkinsonism*. Adverse effects include dry mouth, blurred vision, rapid heartbeat, and decreased sweating.

PRODROME n. the earliest sign of a disease or a developing condition. adj. **prodromal**

PROGENITOR n. a parent or ancestor.

PROGENY n. offspring.

PROGERIA n. a rare, abnormal condition characterized by premature aging and the appearance of gray hair, wrinkled skin, and the posture of an aged person in a child or adolescent.

PROGESTERONE n. hormone produced by the *corpus luteum* of the ovary, the *placenta* during pregnancy, and in small amounts by the adrenal cortex; it prepares the uterus for a fertilized egg. Natural and synthetic progesterones and progestational compounds (e.g., norethindrone) are used in *oral contraceptives* and in drugs to treat abnormal uterine bleeding.

PROGESTIN (progestogen) n. any natural or synthetic progestational hormone.

PROGNOSIS n. prediction of the probable outcome of a disease based on what is known about the usual course of the disease and on the age and general health of the patient.

PROGRESSIVE adj. increasing, worsening, as a progressive muscular disease.

PROGYNON n. trade name for an estradiol preparation.

PROJECTION n. 1. a protuberance, something that juts out; 2. in psychology, an unconscious defense mechanism in which a person attributes his/her own unacceptable ideas and attitudes to another person.

PROKARYOTE n. a cell without a nucleus, the nuclear material being scattered throughout the cell. Bacteria, blue-green algae, and certain other microorganisms are prokaryotes. (compare *eukaryote*)

PROLACTIN n. a hormone produced in and secreted by the *anterior pituitary gland* that stimulates growth and development of mammary glands in females and the production of milk after parturition; also: **lactogenic hormone; luteotropin.**

PROLAPSE n. the dropping or falling of an organ from its normal position, as in the prolapse of the *uterus* into the vagina.

PROMETHAZINE n. an antihistamine, sold under the trade name product Phenergan, used to treat allergies and to induce sedation; it is also an antiemetic, effective in treating nausea, esp. that of motion sickness. Adverse effects include drowsiness and dry mouth.

PRONATION n. the action of lying face downward or turning the hand so that the palm is downward.

PRONE adj. having the face and abdomen downward while in a lying position.

PRONUCLEUS n. the nucleus of the *ovum* or the *spermatozoon* after *fertilization* but before fusion of the pronuclei to form the nucleus of the *zygote*. Each pronucleus contains the *haploid chromosome number*. pl. **pronuclei**

PROPANTHELINE n. a drug, known under the trade name Probanthine, that decreases smooth muscle activity and is used to treat *peptic ulcer* and certain other gastrointestinal disorders. Adverse effects include rapid heart rate, dry mouth, allergic reactions, and central nervous system disturbances.

PROPHASE the first of the four major phases of nuclear division (*mitosis* and *meiosis*) in which the nuclear membrane disappears and the chromosomes become recognizable individually and start to move toward the midplane of the developing spindle.

PROPHYLACTIC adj. preventing the spread of disease, as a prophylactic agent; n. an agent that prevents disease.

PROPHYLAXIS n. the prevention of disease. adj. **prophylactic**

PROPOXYPHENE n. a mild narcotic analgesic, known under the trade name Darvon, used to relieve mild to moderate pain. Adverse effects include liver disorders and oversedation.

PROPRANOLOL n. a beta-adrenergic blocking agent, known under the trade name Inderal, used in the treatment of hypertension, angina pectoris, and other heart ailments. Adverse effects include cardiac and gastrointestinal disturbances and hypersensitivity reactions.

PROPRIOCEPTOR n. a sensory nerve ending, located in muscles, tendons, and other organs, that responds to internal stimuli regarding body position and movement.

PROSENCEPHALON see *forebrain*

PROSTAGLANDIN n. any of a group of hormonelike fatty acids produced in small amounts in many body tissues, including the *uterus*, brain, kidneys, and semen, and acting on target organs to produce wide ranging effects. Prostaglandins affect capillary action, endocrine and nervous system function, smooth muscle, and many other body functions, including contractions of the uterus and lowering of blood pressure. Aspirin and certain other analgesics are believed to act by reducing the effect of prostaglandins at the site of inflammation.

PROSTATE n. firm, chestnut-sized gland in males at the neck of the *urethra* that produces a secretion that is the fluid part of semen. adj. **prostatic**

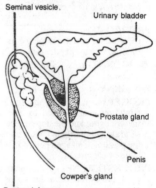

PROSTATECTOMY n. surgical removal of all or part of the *prostate gland* performed to treat benign overgrowth or a malignant neoplasm. adj. **prostatic**

PROSTATITIS n. inflammation of the prostate gland, usually the result of infection. Symptoms include pain, frequency, burning, fever, and chills. Treatment is by antibiotics.

PROSTATORRHEA n. discharge from the prostate, usually the result of prostate infection.

PROSTHESIS n. an artificial device attached to the body to aid its function or replace a missing part; included among prostheses are artificial limbs, hearing aids, and implanted pacemakers.

PROSTRATION n. a state of exhaustion (see also *heat prostration*).

PROTEIN n. any of a large group of complex compounds, containing carbon, hydrogen, oxygen, nitrogen, and sometimes phosphorus and sulfur, and consisting of chains of amino acids joined by peptide bonds. Proteins form the structural part of most organs, and make up enzymes and hormones that regulate body function. They are synthesized in the body from their constituent amino acids obtained in the diet.

PROTEINURIA n. the presence of abnormally large amounts of protein, chiefly albumin, in the urine; it is usually associated with kidney disorder but can also result from fever or other causes.

PROTEOLYSIS n. the breakdown of complex proteins into their constituent amino acids through the action of proteolytic enzymes.   adj. **proteolytic**

PROTHROMBIN n. a plasma protein that is a precursor of thrombin, the first step in blood coagulation; also called **Factor II.**

PROTOPLASM n. the essential substance of all cells, including cytoplasm and nucleus.   adj. **protoplasmic**

PROTOZOA n. a single-celled, animal-like microorganism, some of whom produce disease in humans.   sing. **protozoon.**

PROTOZOAL INFECTION n. any disease, such as malaria, caused by a protozoon.

PROTRIPTYLINE n. a tricyclic antidepressant used to treat depression. Adverse effects include dry mouth, gastrointestinal and cardiovascular disturbances, and the possibility of interaction with many other drugs.

PROTUBERANCE n. a projecting part, esp. a rounded projection, as the mental protuberance, the projecting part of the chin.

PROVERA n. trade name of a *progestin*.

PROVITAMIN n. a substance that in the body may be converted into a *vitamin;* a vitamin precursor.

PROXIMAL adj. nearer to or toward an axis or center, as the trunk of the body (compare *distal*).

PRURIGO n. any of a group of skin inflammations characterized by multiple blister-capped papules that are itchy and may become hardened and crusted as a result of repeated scratching. Causes include allergies, drug reactions, and endocrine imbalances. Treatment depends on the cause.

PRURITUS n. itching. Causes include allergies, lymphoma, jaundice, infection, and other factors. Treatment depends on the cause but relief of the itching may be obtained by antihistamines, corticosteroids, cool applications, or alcohol applications.
pruritus ani n. a common and chronic itchiness of the skin around the anus, often caused by contact dermatitus, pinworms, candida infections, or hemorrhoids.
pruritus vulvae n. persistent itching of the external female genitalia, often associated with candida infection, trichomoniasis, or contact dermatitis.

PSAMMOMA n. a small tumor containing sandlike particles occurring in the meninges, ovaries, and certain other organs; also called **sand tumor.**

PSEUDO- comb. form meaning "false" (e.g., **pseudojaundice,** yellowing of the skin not caused by excess bilirubin but usually the result of excessive ingestion of carotene-containing foods).

PSEUDOCYESIS n. false pregnancy; a condition in which a woman experiences symptoms of pregnancy, including cessation of menstruation, enlargement of the breasts and abdomen, and weight gain, but is not pregnant; it is usually linked to hormonal changes brought about by emotional stress.

PSEUDOHERMAPHRODITISM n. a congenital condition in which either a male or a female has external genitalia resembling those of the opposite sex (e.g., a woman with an enlarged clitoris and labia resembling the penis and scrotum). adj. **pseudohermaphroditic**

PSEUDOMEMBRANE n. a false membrane, consisting of an exudate forming on skin or mucous membrane (e.g., the false membrane occurring in the throat in diphtheria).

PSITTACOSIS n. a infectious disease, caused by the bacterium *Chlamydia psittaci*, transmitted to humans by infected birds, esp. parrots; it is characterized by pneumonialike symptoms, including fever, headache, and cough. Treatment is by tetracyclines. Also called **parrot fever; ornithosis.**

PSOAS n. either of two muscles of the abdomen and pelvis that flex the trunk and rotate the thigh.

PSORIASIS n. a chronic skin disorder characterized by periods of remissions and exacerbations of dry, scale-covered red patches; occurring esp. on the scalp, ears, genitalia, and skin over bony prominences; a type of arthritis may occur with the skin disorder. Treatment includes corticosteroids, ultraviolet light treatments, and the use of medicated creams and shampoos.

PSORIATIC ARTHRITIS n. a form of rheumatoid arthritis, most often affecting small distal joints (esp. in the fingers and toes), occurring in association with psoriasis.

PSYCH-, PSYCHO- comb. form indicating an association with the mind (e.g., **psychopharmacology,** the study of the effects of drugs on the mind and on the treatment of mental disorders).

PSYCHE n. the mind, including conscious and unconscious processes; in psychoanalysis, the total of the id, ego, superego, and all conscious and unconscious processes.

PSYCHEDELIC adj. 1. describing a mental state with hallucinations, altered perceptions, and usually strong emotions; 2. pert. to a drug that produces these effects.

PSYCHIATRY n. that branch of medicine concerned with the study of the mind and the diagnosis, treatment, and prevention of mental, emotional, and behavioral disorders. adj. **psychiatric**

PSYCHOANALYSIS n. a branch of psychiatry, founded by Sigmund Freud, in which the processes of the mind are studied through techniques such as dream interpretation and free association to bring repressed conflicts into the consciousness, analyze them, and adjust behavioral patterns related to them. adj. **psychoanalytic**

PSYCHOGENIC adj. originating in the mind, not in the body; referring esp. to symptoms or diseases of psychological, not physical, origin.

PSYCHOLOGY n. the study of mental activity, esp. as it relates to behavior. adj. **psychologic; psychological**

PSYCHOMETRICS n. the measurement of individual differences in psychological functions, such as intelligence, by means of standardized tests.

PSYCHOMOTOR adj. pert. to mental and motor activities, esp. in reference to disorders in which muscular activity is affected by brain disorder.

PSYCHOMOTOR DEVELOP-MENT n. the gradual and progressive acquisition and attainment of skills involving both mental and motor activity, as a child of 5 or 6 months learning to sit up, a child of 1 to 1½ years learning to walk and a child of 3 years being able to feed himself.

PSYCHOPATH n. a person with a personality disorder in which behavior is antisocial, and in the extreme, may be criminal; also; **sociopath.** adj. **psychopathic**

PSYCHOPATHOLOGY n. the study of the causes and manifestations of mental disorders.

PSYCHOPATHY n. any disease of the mind; it may be congenital or acquired.

PSYCHOPHYSIOLOGY n. that branch of psychology that observes and records physiological changes and how they relate to mental activities.

PSYCHOSEXUAL adj. pert. to the psychological aspects of sex.

PSYCHOSEXUAL DEVELOP-MENT n. in psychoanalytic theory, the process during childhood and adolescence by which personality and mature sexual behavior emerge. The process is divided into stages, each characterized by sexual interest and gratification centered on a particular part of the body; the stages are the oral stage, anal stage, phallic stage, latency stage, and genital stage.

PSYCHOSIS n. a major mental disorder in which the person is usually detached from reality and has impaired perceptions, thinking, responses, and interpersonal relationships. Most people with a psychosis require hospitalization; treatment involves the use of psychoactive drugs and psychotherapy (compare *neurosis*).

PSYCHOSOMATIC adj. pert. to the interaction of the mind and the body.

PSYCHOSOMATIC MEDI-CINE n. that branch of medicine concerned with the relationship of mental and emotional reactions with body processes, esp. how emotional conflicts affect physical symptoms.

PSYCHOSURGERY n. surgery of the brain, usually involving interruption of certain nerve pathways, to relieve severe abnormal psychological symptoms; the procedure is now rarely employed, only when other treatments (e.g., psychotherapy and drugs) have proved ineffective. Marked changes in personality and also often in cognitive and other mental processes occur.

PSYCHOTHERAPY n. the treatment of mental disorders by psychological, not physical, techniques. There are many approaches to psychotherapy, including *behavior modification, psychoanalysis,* and *group therapy.*

PSYCHOTIC adj. pert. to a psychosis.

PSYCHOTROPIC adj. pert. to drugs that affect mood, such as tranquilizers and antidepressants.

PTERYGIUM n. a thick flap of tissue extending from the nasal border of the cornea to the inner corner of the eye.

PTOSIS n. a drooping of one or both upper eyelids; it may be congenital or result from damage to the oculomotor nerve, myasthenia gravis, or other disorder.

-PTOSIS comb. form indicating a drop or prolapse of an organ from its normal position (e.g., **metroptosis,** a dropping of the uterus).

PTYALIN n. an enzyme present in the mouth that starts the digestion of starches.

PTYALISM n. excessive salivation, sometimes occurring in pregnancy, certain poisonings, and neurological disorders.

PTYALITH n. a stone (calculus) in a salivary gland.

PTYALO- comb. form indicating an association with saliva (e.g., **ptyalocele,** a saliva-containing tumor).

PUBERTY n. the time at which sexual maturity occurs and reproductive function becomes possible. It is characterized by the development of secondary sexual characteristics, such as breast development in girls and deepening voice in males, and by the start of menstruation in girls. The changes are brought about by pituitary gland-stimulated increases in sex hormones.   adj. pubertal

PUBES n. hair-covered surface covering the *pubis* at the front of the pelvis.

PUBIC BONE   see *pubis*

PUBIS n. one of the three bones that make up the innominate (hip) bone on each side of the body (the other two bones being the ilium and ischium); the two pubes meet at the front of the pelvis.   pl. **pubes**   adj. **pubic**

PUDENDAL BLOCK n. a form of regional anesthesia in which a local anesthetic agent is used to anesthetize the pudendal nerves in the region of the *vulva,* labia majora, and perirectal area to ease discomfort during childbirth.

PUDENDUM n. the external genitalia, esp. that of a woman and including the mons veneris, the *labia majora,* labia minora, and opening of the *vagina.* (In males it includes the penis, scrotum, and testes).   pl. **pudenda**   adj. **pudendal**

PUERILE adj. pert. to children or childhood.

PUERPERA n. a woman who has just delivered a baby.

PUERPERAL adj. pert. to the period just after childbirth or to the woman who has just given birth.

PUERPERAL FEVER n. bacterial infection and septicemia occurring in a woman following childbirth, usually due to unsanitary conditions. Symptoms include inflammation of the uterus, fever, rapid heartbeat, and foul lochia, followed, if untreated, by prostration, renal failure, shock, and death. The condition is now uncommon; when it occurs it is treated with antibiotics. Also called **childbed fever.**

PUERPERIUM n. the time following childbirth during which the anatomic and functional changes of pregnancy resolve (e.g., the uterus shrinks).

PULMO-, PULMONO- comb. form indicating an association with the *lungs* (e.g., **pulmogram,** an X-ray film of the lungs).

PULMONARY adj. pert. to the lungs or respiratory system.

PULMONARY ARTERY n. the artery that carries deoxygenated blood from the right ventricle of the heart to the lungs for oxygenation. The artery leaves the heart and passes upward before dividing, one branch going to each lung (see also *pulmonary circulation*).

PULMONARY CIRCULATION n. the system of blood vessels transporting blood between the heart and the lungs. Deoxygenated blood leaves the right ventricle by way of the *pulmonary artery,* which divides, sending branches to each lung. The deoxygenated blood gives off its carbon dioxide and takes in oxygen in the alveoli of the lungs. The freshly oxygenated blood is then transported by the *pulmonary vein* to the left atrium of the heart where it enters the systemic circulation for transport throughout the body.

PULMONARY EMBOLISM n. the blockage of a *pulmonary artery* by foreign matter or a thrombus (blood clot); it is characterized by difficult breathing, sharp chest pain shock, and bluish discoloration of the skin, and, if untreated, by pleural effusion, heart rhythm abnormalities, and frequently death. Predisposing factors include prolonged immobilization, esp. associated with surgery or childbirth; blood vessel wall damage; and factors increasing the tendency of the blood to clot. Treatment is by removal of the embolus, oxygen, cardiac massage, and the use of anticoagulants.

PULMONARY VALVE   see *semilunar valve*.

PULMONARY VEIN n. either of two blood vessels, one leaving each lung, that return oxygenated blood to the left atrium of the heart.

PULP n. 1. soft, spongy tissue, found in the spleen and certain other parts of the body; 2. connective tissue containing nerves and blood vessels that is at the center of a tooth under the *dentine*.

PULSE n. regular, rhythmic beating of an artery resulting from the pumping action of the heart. The pulse is easily detected on superficial arteries (e.g., the radial artery) and corresponds to each beat of the heart. The average adult pulse at rest is 60 to 80 beats per minute, but this may change with illness, emotional stress, exercise, or other factors.

PULSELESS DISEASE   see *Takayasu's arteritis*.

PUNCTUM n. in anatomy, a small area or point, as the punctum lacrimale, tiny opening of the tear ducts in the inner corners of the eyelids.

PUNCTURE v. to pierce with a sharp instrument; n. a wound made by a sharp instrument; it may be made accidentally as a result of trauma or deliberately as in a diagnostic procedure to withdraw fluid for examination.

PUPIL n. the circular opening in the center of the *iris*, lying behind the anterior chamber and *cornea* and in front of the *lens*, through which light passes to the lens and *retina*. The diameter of the pupil changes with muscle action of the iris in response to changes in light and other stimulation.

PUPILLARY REFLEX n. reflex changes in the size of the pupil triggered by the amount of light entering the eye. Bright light stimulates the pupil to contract; dim light stimulates the pupil to widen.

PUPILLO- comb. form indicating an association with the pupil (e.g., **pupillomotor**, pert to pupil movement).

PURGATIVE n. a *cathartic*.

PURINE n. any of a group of nitrogen-containing compounds; some (adenine and guanine) are part of DNA and RNA structure; some result from the digestion of proteins, and some are synthesized in the body.

PURKINJE NETWORK n. the network of muscle fibers that carries the cardiac impulse from the *atrioventricular node* to the ventricles of the heart, causing them to contract.

PURPURA n. any of several disorders in which the escape of blood into tissues below the skin causes reddish or purplish spots (petechiae); it may be due to a defect in capillaries (nonthrobocytopenic purpura) or to a deficiency of platelets (thrombocytopenic purpura).

PURULENT adj. producing or containing *pus*.

PUS n. thick yellowish or greenish fluid, containing dead white blood cells, bacteria, and dead tissue, formed at an infection site.

PUSTULE n. a small, pus-containing elevation on the skin. adj. **pustular**

PUTREFACTION n. the breakdown of proteins by bacteria, usually causing an unpleasant odor.

PYELOGRAM n. an X ray of the *kidney* and *ureters*. In an intravenous pyelogram (IVP) a radiopaque dye that shows the outline of the kidney and associated structures is injected into the patient; the procedure is used to detect tumors, kidney stones, and other abnormalities of the urinary tract.

PYELONEPHRITIS n. an infection, usually bacterial, of the kidney. **Acute polynephritis,** usually resulting from the spread of a bladder infection, causes chills, fever, pain in the flank region, and urinary frequency. **Chronic polynephritis,** often associated with a stone or narrowing of the urinary passageways, develops more slowly and may, if untreated, lead to renal failure. Treatment involves antimicrobial drugs and removal of any obstruction.

PYEMIA n. blood poisoning by pus-forming bacteria released from an abscess; abscesses may develop in various parts of the body. adj. **pyemic**

PYLORIC SPHINCTER n. muscular ring in the stomach separating the *stomach* from the *duodenum;* also: **pyloric valve**

PYLORIC STENOSIS n. a narrowing of the pyloric sphincter blocking the passage of food into the duodenum from the stomach and often causing projectile vomiting. It may be *congenital* or in adults result from an ulcer or neoplasm. Treatment is usually by surgery.

PYLORUS n. tubular portion of the stomach, encircled by the *pyloric sphincter,* leading into the *duodenum*.

PYOGENIC adj. producing pus.

PYORRHEA n. 1. discharge of pus; 2. purulent inflammation of tissues surrounding the teeth.

PYRAMIDAL TRACT n. a pathway in the *medulla oblongata* where nerve fibers pass from the brain to the spinal cord. In this area the fibers from one side of the brain cross to the opposite side of the spinal cord, giving the region a pyramid-shaped structure.

PYREXIA see *fever*.

PYRECTIC adj. having fever; n. a substance that produces fever.

PYRIDOXINE n. a water-soluble vitamin, part of the B complex group; it functions as a coenzyme in many metabolic processes; also called vitamin B_6 (See Table of Vitamins).

PYRILAMINE n. an antihistamine used to treat many allergic reactions including *rhinitis* and *pruritus*. Adverse effects include drowsiness, dry mouth, and skin rashes.

PYRIMIDINE n. any of several nitrogen-containing compounds, including cytosine, thymine, and uracil, important in the structure of *DNA* and *RNA*.

PYROGEN n. a substance (e.g., bacterial toxin) that produces an increase in body temperature.

PYROMANIA n. an uncontrollable urge to set fires.

PYROSIS n. a burning feeling in the substernal or epigastric area, often associated with eructation of stomach contents; also called **heartburn.**

PYURIA n. the presence of leukocytes in the urine, usually a sign of urinary tract infection.

q

Q FEVER n. an acute illness, caused by the rickettsia *Coxiella burnetti* transmitted to humans through contact with infected animals, esp. sheep, goats, and cattle; symptoms include high fever and signs of respiratory illness. Treatment is by *tetracycline* antibiotics.

QUAALUDE n. trade name for the sedative *methaqualone*.

QUADRANTANOPIA n. a condition characterized by loss of one fourth of a person's visual field.

QUADRI- comb. form indicating "four" (e.g., **quadricuspid**, a tooth having four points on its surface).

QUADRICEPS n. one of the extensor muscles of the legs.

QUADRIPARA n. a woman who has given birth to a viable infant after each of four pregnancies.

QUADRIPLEGIA n. paralysis affecting all four limbs and the trunk of the body below the level of spinal cord injury. Trauma is the usual cause.

QUADRUPLET n. any of four offspring born at the same time from the same pregnancy.

QUARANTINE n. isolation of people with communicable diseases or people exposed to communicable diseases during the period of contagion in an effort to prevent the spread of the disease.

QUARTAN adj. occurring every fourth day, or about every 72 hours, as the fever and weakness of quartan *malaria*.

QUECKENSTEDT'S TEST n. a test to determine if there is a blockage in the spinal canal or whether cerebrospinal fluid can flow freely.

QUELLUNG REACTION n. swelling of the capsule surrounding a bacterium after it is exposed to specific antibodies or antisera; the reaction forms the basis of some tests to identify microorganisms.

QUICKENING n. a pregnant woman's first awareness of the movement of the fetus, usually occurring about the 16th week of pregnancy but sometimes earlier.

QUIESCENT adj. inactive.

QUINACRINE n. an anthelmintic and antimalarial used to treat certain worm infestations (e.g., cestodiasis) and malaria. Adverse effects include skin eruptions, nausea, vomiting, jaundice, liver dysfunction, and *aplastic anemia*.

QUINIDEX n. trade name for *quinidine*.

QUINIDINE n. a drug, known under the trade name Quinidex, used to treat certain heart arrhythmias. Adverse effects include gastrointestinal upsets, high blood pressure, and cardiac arrhythmia.

QUININE n. an antimalarial with antipyretic and analgesic properties. Adverse effects include tinnitus, deafness, visual disturbances, gastrointestinal upsets, blood disorders, and hypersensitivity reactions.

QUINORA n. trade name for the cardiac drug *quinidine*.

QUINSY n. a pus-filled inflammation of the *tonsils* and *palate*, usually a complication of *tonsillitis*. Incision of the abscess is usually necessary; also: **peritonsillar abscess.**

QUINTIPARA n. a woman who has given birth to a viable infant after each of five pregnancies.

QUINTUPLET n. any one of five offspring born at the same time from the same pregnancy.

r

Ra symbol for the element radium (see Table of Elements).

RABBIT FEVER see *tularemia*.

RABIES n. an acute, often fatal, viral disease affecting the brain and spinal cord, transmitted to humans by the bite of infected animals, esp. dogs, skunks, bats, foxes, and raccoons. After an incubation period that may range from a few days to one year, symptoms of fever, malaise, headache, and muscle pain are followed after a few days by severe and painful muscle spasms, esp. of the throat, delirium, difficulty in breathing, paralysis, coma, and death. The disease may be prevented in those bitten by an animal suspected of being rabid by a series of very painful injections of rabies vaccine often used in combination with rabies immune globulin. A less painful treatment is under investigation.

RACEMOSE adj. resembling a cluster of grapes, as, for example, certain glands consisting of a number of small sacs.

RACHI-, RACHIO- comb. form indicating an association with the spine (e.g., **rachialgia**, spinal column pain).

RACHIS n. *backbone*.

RACHISCHISIS see *spina bifida*.

RACHITIC adj. pert. to *rickets*.

RACHITIS n. 1. *rickets*; 2. inflammation of the vertebral column.

RACIAL IMMUNITY n. a type of natural immunity shared by members of a race.

RADIAL ARTERY n. branch of the brachial artery that starts at the elbow, extends through the forearm, wraps around the wrist and extends into the hand, sending branches into the fingers.

RADIAL adj. pert. to the *radius*, one of the lower arm bones.

RADIAL KERATOTOMY n. a minor surgical procedure that corrects *myopia*; shallow incisions are made in the *cornea*, making it bulge.

RADIAL NERVE n. the largest branch of the brachial plexus, the nerve supplying the arm.

RADIAL PULSE n. the pulse of the *radial artery*, palpated at the wrist; it is the pulse commonly taken.

RADIATE v. to spread from a focus or point of origin.

RADIATION n. electromagnetic energy emitted in the form of rays or particles, including gamma rays, X rays, ultraviolet rays, visible light and infrared radiation. Some of these radiation forms are used in medicine for diagnosis (e.g., X rays) and treatment (e.g., use of radioactive elements, such as radium, in cancer treatment).

RADIATION SICKNESS n. an abnormal condition caused by exposure to ionizing radiation, as, for example, from exposure to nuclear bomb explosions or from exposure to radioactive chemicals in the workplace. Symptoms and prognosis depend on the amount of radiation, the exposure time, and the part of the body affected. Low-to-moderate dose causes nausea, vomiting, headache, and diarrhea, sometimes followed by hair loss and bleeding. Severe exposure causes sterility, damage to the fetus in pregnant women and in many cases the development of cataracts, some forms of cancer, and other diseases. Severe exposure can cause death within hours.

RADIATION SYNDROME see *radiation sickness*.

RADIATION THERAPY see *radiotherapy*.

RADICAL MASTECTOMY see under *mastectomy*.

RADICULITIS n. inflammation of the root (radicle) of a nerve.

RADIO- comb. form indicating an association with the emission of *radiation* (e.g., **radiobiology**, that branch of science dealing with the effects of radiation of living systems).

RADIOACTIVE adj. emitting radiation, as some elements.

RADIOACTIVE IODINE EXCRETION TEST n. an evaluation of thyroid function. The patient is given orally a tracer dose of radioactive iodine-131 and the amount excreted in the urine and the amount accumulated in the thyroid gland (detected by a special device placed over the neck region) are measured to indicate normal, under, or over activity of the thyroid gland. In the related **radioactive iodine uptake (RAIU) test** the amount of radioactive iodine taken up by the thyroid is measured.

RADIOACTIVITY n. the emission of radiation (in the form of particles or waves) as a result of the disintegration (decay) of the nucleus of certain naturally occurring radioactive elements (e.g., uranium, radium) or of artificially produced radioactive isotopes (e.g., iodine-131).

RADIOGRAPHY n. the use of ionizing radiation, esp. X rays, to produce images on photographic plates or fluorescent screens (fluoroscopy); it is used to detect broken bones and the presence of ulcers, stones, or tumors in internal body organs, and many other disorders.

RADIOIMMUNOASSAY n. a method of determining the concentration of a protein in the serum by monitoring any reaction produced by the injection of a radioactively labelled substance known to react in a particular way with the protein being studied.

RADIOISOTOPE n. a radioactive isotope of an element used in medicine for diagnostic and therapeutic purposes.

RADIOLOGY n. that branch of medicine concerned with radioactive substances and their use in diagnosis and treatment.

RADIOPAQUE adj. not allowing the passage of X rays or other forms of radiation (e.g., lead used as a shield around radioactive equipment, or radiopaque iodine isotopes used as contrast media in producing X-ray images).

RADIOPAQUE DYE n. a chemical that does not permit the passage of X rays; used to outline the interior of certain organs during X ray and fluoroscopic procedures.

RADIOSENSITIVE adj. susceptible to radiation, as certain cancer cells that can be treated with radiotherapy.

RADIOTHERAPY n. the treatment of disease, esp. certain forms of cancer, by the use of radiation given off by special machines or by radioactive isotopes. The radiation interferes with the division (mitosis) of cells and the synthesis of DNA in the cells. Many cancer cells are destroyed by radiation; the major disadvantage is possible damage to cells and tissues in nearby areas.

RADIUM n. a radioactive metallic element used in *radiotherapy* (see Table of Elements).

RADIUS n. the outer part and shorter of the two forearm bones that partially revolves around the ulna (the other lower arm bone; the radius articulates with the humerus (upper arm bone) at the elbow and with the ulna and carpal bones at the wrist.

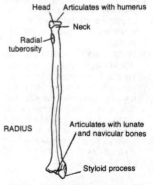

Head   Articulates with humerus

Neck

Radial tuberosity

RADIUS

Articulates with lunate and navicular bones

Styloid process

Courtesy Carolina Biological Supply Co.

RADIX   see *root*.   adj. **radical.**

RADON n. a radioactive, gaseous, nonmetallic element, used in radiotherapy (see Table of Elements).

RALE n. an abnormal chest sound, usually a bubbling noise on inspiration, heard through the stethoscope; it is associated with pneumonia, tuberculosis, congestive heart failure, and some other respiratory disorders.

RAMOSE adj. branched.

RAMSAY HUNT'S SYNDROME n. an abnormal condition, caused by the varicellazoster virus (the virus that causes chicken pox and shingles), characterized by ear pain, vertigo, facial nerve paralysis (sometimes permanent), and often hearing loss. Treatment is by corticosteroids.

RAMUS n. a small branch, esp. of a nerve or blood vessel; 2. a thin process projecting from a bone. pl. **rami**   v. **ramify**   n. **ramification**

RANGE OF MOTION n. the full measure that a limb or other body part can be moved.

RANULA n. a cyst on the underside of the tongue, usually due to obstruction of a mucous or salivary gland.   adj. **ranulae**

RAPHE n. a line, ridge, or seam showing the union of two parts (e.g., the **palatine raphe**, the seam at the center of the hard palate).

RAPID EYE MOVEMENT (REM) n. a period of sleep characterized by rapid eye muscle contractions, detectable by electrodes placed over the skin near the eyes, and during which dreaming occurs. REM sleep periods, lasting from a few minutes to about 30 minutes, alternate with *nonrapid eye movement* (NREM) periods during sleep.

RAPTUS n. 1. intense excitement; ecstasy; 2. a sudden seizure or attack (e.g., **raptus hemorrhagicus**, a sudden, profuse hemorrhage).

RASH n. a skin eruption, usually characterized by red spots or generalized reddening; rashes occur with chickenpox, measles, and rubella; in cases of local irritation and/or infection (e.g., diaper rash), and in certain other diseases (e.g., butterfly rash of *systemic lupus erythematosus*).

RATBITE FEVER n. either of two infectious diseases transmitted to humans by the bite of a rat or mouse; general symptoms include fever, headache, malaise, nausea, vomiting, and skin eruption. In the United States, the disease (also called Haverhill fever) is usually caused by *Streptobacillus moniliformis* and characterized by a rash on the palms and soles, painful joints, and a short (about two weeks) duration. In the Far East, the disease (also called *sodoku*) is usually caused by *Spirillum minus*, characterized by a rash on the extremities, lymph node enlargement, relapsing fever and a longer duration. Treatment by penicillin is effective for both forms.

RATE n. the incidence or frequency of an event per unit of time (e.g., the heart rate is the number of beats per minute) or per number of possible occurrences (e.g., one illness per 100 people exposed to the illness) (see also *heart rate*; *sedimentation rate*; *mortality rate*).

RATIONAL adj. capable of, derived from, or using reason.

RATIONALIZATION n. in psychiatry, a defense mechanism in which a person justifies behavior or occurrences by giving reasonable, but not true, explanations.

RATTLE n. an abnormal sound heard through a stethoscope in some types of respiratory disorders; it usually results from moisture in the air passages.

RAUDIXIN n. trade name for a rauwolfia *antihypertensive*.

RAU-SED n. trade name for *reserpine*; used to treat *hypertension*.

RAUWOLFIA n. any of several alkaloids, including *reserpine*, from the *Rauwolfia serpentina* shrub of Asia, used chiefly to treat *hypertension*.

RAUZIDE n. trade name for a fixed-combination drug, containing the *diuretic* bendroflumethiazide and a rauwolfia *antihypertensive*, used to treat certain cardiovascular abnormalities.

RAYNAUD'S SIGN see *acrocyanosis*.

RBC abbreviation for red blood cell (see *erythrocyte*).

REACTION n. 1. response to a stimulus, esp. in medicine, a response in opposition to a substance, drug, or treatment (e.g., allergic reaction); 2. in chemistry, the change in a chemical acted on by another chemical.

REACTION FORMATION n. in psychiatry, a defense mechanism in which a person unconsciously develops attitudes and behavior contrary to repressed unacceptable drives and impulses and serving to conceal them (e.g., a strong moral stance that hides an impulse to lust).

REACTION TIME n. the interval between the presentation of a stimulus and the subject's response to it.

REACTIVE DEPRESSION see under *depression*.

REACTIVE SCHIZOPHRENIA see under *schizophrenia*.

READ METHOD OF CHILDBIRTH n. a system of natural childbirth, developed by Grantly Dick-Read, based on the idea that childbirth is a normal physiologic process and that pain during labor and childbirth is largely of psychological origin, the result of fear, ignorance, and tension. The method involves education of the woman on the physiologic process of childbirth, a series of breathing exercises to foster relaxation, and a series of exercises to attain maximal physical conditioning for childbirth (compare *Bradley method of childbirth; Lamaze method of childbirth*) (see also *natural childbirth*).

REAGIN n. an antibody (an IgE immunoglobulin) formed against allergens (e.g., pollen) that attaches to cell membranes, causing the release of *histamine* and other substances responsible for the local inflammation characteristic of an allergy or for systemic anaphylaxis.

REALITY PRINCIPLE n. in psychoanalysis, the modifying influences of environment and life circumstances on the pleasure principle whereby behavior toward the immediate gratification of instinctual pleasures is changed in order to obtain long-term goals.

REBOUND v. to spring back (e.g., to recover from an illness); n. a sudden contraction of a muscle following relaxation, occurring in cases where inhibitory reflexes are disturbed.

REBOUND TENDERNESS n. pain elicited by the sudden release of a hand pressing on the abdomen; usually a sign of peritoneal inflammation.

RECEPTOR n. 1. the endings of a sensory nerve specialized to detect changes and trigger impulses in the sensory nerve (e.g., cells at the end of the olfactory nerve that detect odors in the nasal cavity); 2. a structure or part of a structure or organ that receives, as the configuration on a cell surface for receiving an antigen.

RECESS n. a small hollow cavity, as the pharyngeal recess, a slit-like cavity in the wall of the pharynx.

RECESSIVE GENE n. a member of a pair of genes (an allele) that cannot express itself in the presence of its more dominant allele; it is expressed only in the homozygous state. For example, the gene for blue eyes is recessive and will not manifest itself if the gene for brown eyes (which is dominant) is also present; blue eyes will manifest themselves only if both genes are recessive. (see also *autosomal recessive disease*).

RECIPROCAL INHIBITION n. in behavior therapy, a theory that the simultaneous presence of an anxiety-evoking stimulus and an anxiety-lessening situation will result in the stimulus producing less anxiety. The relaxing technique of deep breathing to decrease the pain and discomfort of childbirth is based on this idea.

RECOMBINANT DNA n. a DNA (*deoxyribonucleic acid*) molecule in which genes have been artificially rearranged and genetic material from another organism, sometimes a member of another species, has been inserted. Replication of the new recombined DNA and its results in genetic changes in the organism. Recombinant DNA technology is being used to produce human insulin and growth hormone and is being investigated for many other medical applications.

RECRUDESCENCE n. the return of symptoms of a disease soon after they had disappeared and recovery appeared to be underway. adj. **recrudescent**

RECTAL REFLEX n. normal response to the presence of *feces* in the *rectum*, allowing defecation; also called **defecation reflex**.

RECTO- comb. form indicating an association with the *rectum* (e.g., **rectourethral**, pert. to the rectum and the urethra).

RECTOCELE n. a protrusion of the rectum and often part of the posterior wall of the vagina into the vagina; it occurs when pelvic muscles have been weakened by childbirth, surgery, or other factor. Pain and difficulty in defecation and painful coitus may occur. Treatment is by surgery; also called **proctocele**.

RECTOSIGMOID adj. pert. to the *sigmoid colon* and the upper part of the *rectum*.

RECTUM n. the last portion of the large intestine, about 5 inches (12-13 centimeters) long, connecting the *sigmoid colon* and the *anus*. Feces are stored in the rectum before defecation.   adj. **rectal**

RECTUS n. any of several straight muscles, as the **rectus abdominis**, a pair of muscles extending the length of the ventral part of the abdomen; adj. indicating a straight or almost straight body part.

RECUMBENT adj. lying down or leaning backward.

RECUPERATION n. recovery, or return to a normal state of health.

RED BLOOD CELL   see *erythrocyte*.

RED MARROW see *bone marrow*.

REDUCE v. in surgery, the return of a dislocated part to its normal position by manipulation or operation, as in *hernia* correction when a displaced part is returned to its normal position in the body.

REDUCTION DIVISION   see *meiosis*.

REFERRED PAIN n. pain felt at a site in the body different from the diseased or injured part where the pain is expected. Angina pectoris, resulting from coronary artery insufficiency, often occurs in the left shoulder, and pain from gallbladder disease is frequently felt in the right shoulder area.

REFLEX n. an involuntary function or movement of a part in response to a particular stimulus (e.g., the knee jerk, or *patellar reflex*).

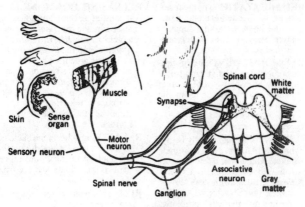

The Reflex Arc

REFLEX ARC n. a nervous circuit involved in a reflex; at its simplest it involves a sensory nerve linked with a motor nerve, supplying a muscle or gland, as in the patellar reflex.

REFLUX n. abnormal backflow, as sometimes occurs with fluids in the esophagus (*gastroesophageal reflux*) or other body parts.

REFRACTION n. the change in direction of light (or other energy) as it passes from one medium to another, as from air into glass; 2. a means for determining the amount of refractive power of the eye and the need for corrective lenses.

REFRACTORY adj. unresponsive, resistant to treatment.

REFRACTORY PERIOD n. in neurology, the period of recovery needed by a neuron following excitation or by a muscle following contraction and during which repolarization of the cell membrane occurs; a stimulus applied during the refractory period will not evoke a response.

REFRACTURE v. to break a bone that, having been broken before, mended in an abnormal way.

REGENERATION n. the replacement of lost tissue by an organism.

REGIONAL ANESTHESIA n. anesthesia of an area of the body through administration of a local anesthetic that blocks a group of sensory nerve fibers. Kinds of regional anesthesia include *epidural anesthesia* and *spinal anesthesia*.

REGIONAL ENTERITIS see *Crohn's disease*.

REGRESSION n. a return to an earlier condition, esp. the retreat of an adult into childlike behavior. adj. **regressive**

REGROTON n. trade name for fixed-combination drug, containing the diuretic chlorthalidone and the antihypertensive *reserpine*, that is used to treat hypertension.

REGULATORY GENE n. a gene that regulates or suppresses the activity of one or more structural genes.

REGURGITATION n. 1. the return of swallowed food into the mouth; 2. the backflow of blood through a defective heart valve.

REHABILITATION n. the restoration of an individual or of a part of the body to normal function after injury, disease, or other abnormal state.

REINFORCEMENT n. in psychology, the strengthening of a particular response or behavioral pattern by rewarding desirable behavior and punishing undesirable behavior.

REITER'S SYNDROME n. a disorder of males, usually beginning with diarrhea and low-grade fever, which after a few weeks is followed by conjunctivitis, *urethritis*, and arthritis, esp. of the ankles and sacroiliac joints. Treatment involves antibiotics (tetracyclines) and antiinflammatory agents, esp. phenylbutazone.

REJECTION n. 1. in medicine, an immunological response whereby substances or organisms that the system recognizes as foreign are not accepted, as in the body's attack against an invading microorganisms (e.g., bacteria) or rejection of a transplanted organ; 2. in psychiatry, denying attention or affection to another person.

RELAPSE v. to show again the signs of a disease from which the patient had appeared to have recovered; n. the recurrence of a disease after apparent recovery.

RELAPSING FEVER n. an infectious disease caused by *Borrelia* microorganisms and transmitted by lice and ticks, most common in South America, Africa and Asia. It is characterized by 2 or 3 day episodes of high fever, chills, headache, muscle pains, and nausea, sometimes with a rash and jaundice, recurring every week or 10 days for a period of several months. Treatment is by antibiotics.

RELAXANT n. a drug or device that reduces muscle tension or relieves anxiety.

RELEASING HORMONE (RH) n. any of several hormones released by the *hypothalamus* into a vein to the *anterior pituitary gland* where they stimulate the release of anterior pituitary hormones. Each releasing factor stimulates the pituitary to secrete a specific hormone (e.g., growth hormone releasing hormone stimulates the release of growth hormone).

RELAXIN n. a hormone secreted by the *corpus luteum* during the last stages of pregnancy that causes the cervix to dilate and prepares the uterus for labor.

REM abbreviation for *rapid eye movement*.

REMISSION n. partial or complete disappearance of or lessening of the severity of the symptoms of a disease; it may be spontaneous or the result of therapy; temporary or permanent.

RENAL adj. pert. to the kidney.

RENAL ARTERY n. either of a pair of arteries arising from the abdominal aorta and supplying the kidneys, adrenal glands, and ureters.

RENAL CALCULUS see *urinary calculus*.

RENAL COLIC n. sharp pain in the lower back radiating to the groin, usually associated with the passage of a calculus (stone) through the *ureter*.

RENAL FAILURE n. the inability of the kidneys to excrete wastes and function in the maintenance of electrolyte balance. **Acute renal failure**, characterized by the inability to produce urine and an accumulation of wastes, is often associated with trauma, burns, acute infection, or obstruction of the urinary tract; its treatment depends on the cause and often includes antibiotics and reduced fluid intake. **Chronic kidney failure**, which may occur as a result of many systemic dis-

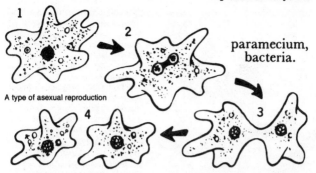

paramecium,
bacteria.

A type of asexual reproduction

orders, causes fatigue and sluggishness, diminished urine output, anemia, and often
complications of *hypertension* and
congestive heart failure; treatment depends on the cause, often
involving the use of diuretics, restricted protein intake, and if it
cannot be otherwise treated, *hemodialysis*.

RENIN n. an enzyme released by
the kidney that affects blood pressure by catalyzing the formation
of the strong pressor angiotensin.

RENNIN n. an enzyme produced
in the stomach that functions in
the digestion of milk.

REPEN-VK n. trade name for a
penicillin antibacterial.

REPLACEMENT n. the substitution of a missing part or substance, as the replacement of lost
blood with a transfusion of donor
blood.

REPLICATION n. the process of
duplication, copying, or reproducing, esp. in genetics, the
process by which deoxyribonucleic acid (DNA) makes a copy
of itself prior to cell division. In
this process the double stranded
molecule of DNA unwinds to become two separate strands, each
of which acts as a template for the
synthesis of a strand complemen-
tary to it. The two new molecules, each with one parental
strand and one new strand, then

rewind to form the characteristic
double helix configuration. See
accompanying illustration.

REPRESSION n. 1. the inhibition
of an action, as that of an enzyme
or gene. 2. in psychoanalysis, an
unconscious defense mechanism
whereby unacceptable thoughts,
feelings, memories, and impulses are pushed from the consciousness into the unconscious
where they are submerged but remain important in influencing behavior and are often the source of
anxiety.

REPRESSOR n. in genetics, a gene
that represses the activity of a
structural gene.

REPRODUCTION n. the process
by which living organisms give
rise to offspring; it may be asexual, involving only one parent that
divides, buds, or otherwise produces an offspring of the same
genetic makeup; or it may be sexual, involving the union of sex
cells, or gametes, from two parents and the recombination of the
genetic material of the parents to
produce an offspring with a new
genetic makeup. Humans and
higher animals reproduce sexually.

REPRODUCTIVE SYSTEM n.
the organs and tissues involved in
the production and maturation of
gametes and in their union and
subsequent development to pro-

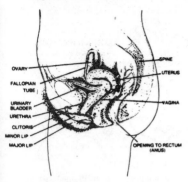

Side view of internal female sexual and reproductive organs

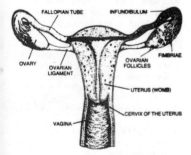

Front view of the female reproductive system

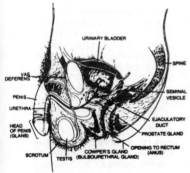

Side view of external and internal male sex organs.

duce offspring. In the male the reproductive system includes the *testes*, vas deferens, *prostate gland*, seminal vesicles, *urethra*, and *penis*. In the female it includes the ovaries, Fallopian tubes, *uterus*, vagina, and vulva. The reproductive system is under the control of numerous hormones secreted by the pituitary gland, the sex organs (ovaries and testes) and the adrenal glands.

RESCINNAMINE n. an antihypertensive. Adverse effects include gastrointestinal and cardiovascular disturbances.

RESECT v. to surgically remove tissue from the body.

RESECTION n. the cutting out of a significant portion of a structure or organ.

RESERPINE n. a drug, extracted from *Rauwolfia* plants, known under the trade name Rau-Sed, used to treat hypertension. Adverse effects include depression, impotence, and gastrointestinal upset, including exacerbation of peptic ulcers.

RESERVE n. potential capacity to respond to maintain vital functions, as in the pulmonary reserve, the extra volume of air that the lungs could inhale or exhale when breathing to the limits of capacity, as in times of stress.

RESIDENT n. a physician (graduate of a medical school) in one of the postgraduate years of clinical training, after the first internship year; the residency period is often concentrated on a particular medical specialty.

RESISTANCE n. the degree of immunity or resistance to a disease that the body possesses; the degree to which a disease-causing microorganism is unaffected by antibiotics or other drugs, as in penicillin-resistant bacteria.

RESOLUTION n. 1. the ability to distinguish fine details, as through a microscope; 2. the period during which disease symptoms (e.g., swelling or other signs of inflammation) decrease or disappear.

RESONANCE n. echolike sound produced by percussion of an organ or cavity during physical examination. adj. **resonant**

RESORCINOL n. drug, used in ointments for acne and certain other disorders and in dandruff shampoos, that causes the skin to peel.

RESPIRATION n. the processes involved in the exchange of gases—oxygen and carbon dioxide—between an organism and the environment, involving both external respiration, or breathing, in which oxygen is taken from the air by alveoli in the lungs and carbon dioxide is released from the blood to be exhaled; and internal respiration whereby the oxygen in the blood is absorbed by cells throughout the body and waste product carbon dioxide is absorbed by the blood to be transported to the lungs.

RESPIRATORY adj. pert. to respiration or the respiratory system.

RESPIRATORY ACIDOSIS n. a form of acidosis (excess hydrogen ion concentration in the blood) in which reduced alveolar function in the lungs, caused by emphysema, pneumonia, chest trauma, or other conditions results in decreased carbon dioxide excretion. The excess carbon dioxide combines with water to form carbonic acid that increases the acidity of the blood, producing acidosis. Headache, hypertension, and rapid heartbeat commonly appear. Treatment involves correction of the underlying cause, if possible; the use of bronchodilators, oxygen, and sodium bicarbonate if indicated, and the restoration and maintenance of normal fluid and electrolyte balances (compare *respiratory alkalosis*).

RESPIRATORY ALKALOSIS n. a form of alkalosis (lower than normal hydrogen ion concentration in the blood) in which there is greater than normal excretion of carbon dioxide, usually caused by hyperventilation associated with extreme anxiety, asthma, or pneumonia, or by aspirin intoxication or metabolic acidosis. Deep rapid breathing, dizziness, lightheadedness, muscular weakness, and cardiac rhythm disturbances commonly occur. Treatment involves correction and treatment of any underlying causes, breathing into a paper bag to inhale carbon dioxide, and the use of sedatives to decrease the breathing rate (compare *respiratory acidosis*).

RESPIRATORY CENTER n. that part of the pons and medulla oblongata of the brain that controls the rate of breathing in response to changes in the levels of oxygen and carbon dioxide in the blood.

RESPIRATORY DISTRESS SYNDROME OF THE NEWBORN n. an acute lung disease of the newborn, esp. a premature newborn, in which the alveoli are airless and the lungs inelastic due to a deficiency of a surfactant substance necessary for normal alveolar function and lung expansion. Symptoms include rapid and shallow breathing, nasal flaring, and often edema of the extremities and the formation of a hyaline membrane in the collapsed alveoli. Treatment involves oxygen and fluid administration and use of a specially designed device to maintain positive airway pressure. Properly treated, the condition resolves and the infant suffers no aftereffects. Also called **hyaline membrane disease**.

RESPIRATORY FAILURE n. inability of the heart and lungs to maintain an adequate level of gaseous exchange. Treatment involves correction of any underlying cardiac or lung disorder,

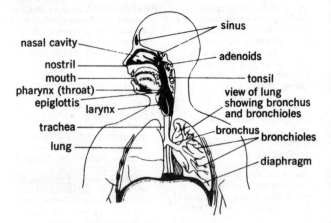

nasal cavity
nostril
mouth
pharynx (throat)
epiglottis
larynx
trachea
lung

sinus
adenoids
tonsil
view of lung
showing bronchus
and bronchioles
bronchus
bronchioles
diaphragm

RESPIRATORY SYSTEM

administration of oxygen, maintenance of clear airways, the use of bronchidilators, and other measures.

RESPIRATORY RATE n. the rate of breathing at rest, about 14 per minute in an adult.

RESPIRATORY SYNCYTIAL VIRUS (RS) n. any of a group of myxoviruses responsible for many respiratory infections (including bronchiolitis, bronchopneumonia, and the common cold), esp. in children.

RESPIRATORY TRACT n. the organs and structures associated with breathing, gaseous exchange, and the entrance of air into the body. It includes the nasal cavity, pharynx, larynx, and trachea (the upper respiratory tract) and the bronchi, bronchioles, and lungs (lower respiratory tract) and associated muscles.

RESPIRATORY TRACT INFECTION n. any infection affecting the respiratory tract.

lower respiratory infection n. infection of the trachea, bronchi, and/or lungs as in bronchitis, pneumonia, or bronchiolitis.

upper respiratory infection n. an infection affecting the nasal cavity or pharynx, as in the common cold, pharyngitis (sore throat), sinusitis, rhinitis or tonsillitis.

RESPONSE n. reaction to a stimulus.

RESTING POTENTIAL n. the electrochemical difference between the two sides of a nerve cell membrane when the cell is not conducting an impulse.

RESTLESS LEGS SYNDROME n. a condition characterized by restless movement, twitching, and unpleasant sensations of the legs, esp. the lower leg; it is sometimes associated with a sleep disturbance. It is relieved by walking or moving the legs.

RESUSCITATION n. the act of reviving a person or returning him/her to consciousness through the use of *cardiopulmonary resuscitation* and similar techniques.

RETARDED adj. abnormally slow, as in development or growth.

RETCH v. to attempt to vomit but without bringing up anything.

RETE n. a net or meshlike structure (e.g., the *rete testes*, a network of tubes carrying sperm from the seminiferous tubules in the testes to the vasa efferentia).

RETENTION n. 1. the holding of something inside a part, cavity or organ, as in urinary retention; 2. the ability to remember information.

RETICULAR adj. having a netlike pattern.

RETICULAR ACTIVATING SYSTEM n. a system of nerve pathways in the brain concerned with the level of consciousness, from sleep and relaxation to full attention and concentration.

RETICULAR FORMATION n. a cluster of nerve cells and nerve fibers in the brainstem connecting nerves to and from the spinal cord, cranial nerves, and areas of the brain; it constantly monitors the state of the body and functions in the control of breathing, heart-rate, level of consciousness, and many other functions.

RETICULOCYTE an immature *erythrocyte* (red blood cell) with a network of threads and particles at the former site of the nucleus; normally making up about 1% of the total red blood cell count. (Mature erythrocytes lack a nucleus).

RETICULOENDOTHELIAL SYSTEM (RES) n. functional unit of the body made up of phagocytic cells (e.g., Kupffer cells of the liver, macrophages, and cells of the spleen and bone marrow) functioning in immune responses to infection and in ridding the body of cellular debris.

RETICULUM n. a network, esp. of blood vessels or tubules.

RETINA n. the multi-layered light-sensitive layer of the eyeball that receives images of objects and transmits visual impulses through the *optic nerve* to the brain for interpretation. The outer part of the retina, next to the *choroid*, contains the pigment *rhodopsin*; the inner layers, continuing to the *vitreous body*, contain *rods* and *cones* (light-sensitive nerve cells) and their associated ganglia and fibers. adj. **retinal**

STRUCTURE OF THE RETINA

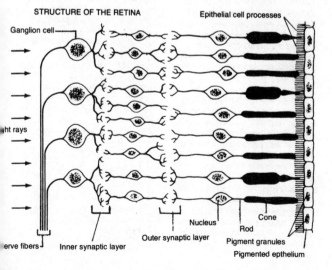

RETINACULUM n. a retaining structure or part that holds an organ or tissue in place, as the **retinaculum unguis**, the band of tissue holding the nail to the nail bed.

RETINAL DETACHMENT see *detached retina*.

RETINITIS n. inflammation of the *retina*.

RETINO- comb. form indicating an association with the *retina* (e.g., **retinomalacia**, a softening of the retina).

RETINOBLASTOMA n. a congenital, hereditary neoplasm of retinal cells, the most common eye malignancy in childhood. Diminished vision, retinal detachment, and abnormal pupillary reflexes are common. Treatment includes removal of the eye.

RETINOL n. a form of vitamin A (see Table of Vitamins).

RETRACTION n. the act of pulling, holding, or drawing a part back, as during surgery.

RETRACTOR n. an instrument used in surgery to hold back the edges of organs to maintain exposure of underlying structures.

RETRO- comb. form indicating a backward position or motion (e.g., **retroperitoneal**, behind the *peritoneum*, as in the space between the peritoneum and the abdominal wall in which the kidneys are located).

RETROBULBAR NEURITIS n. inflammation of the optic nerve behind the eye, usually causing blurred vision; it is a common sign of *multiple sclerosis* but may also result from other causes and heal completely.

RETROFLEXION n. the bending backwards of an organ, esp. the upper part of the *uterus*.

RETROGRADE adj. moving or going backward; moving in a direction opposite to that considered normal.

RETROGRADE AMNESIA n. loss of memory for events occurring before a particular time; it may result from brain injury or disease or from emotional trauma.

RETROGRESSION n. return to a less complex, less differentiated condition.

RETROVERSION n. backward displacement or inclination of an organ, esp. in reference to the *uterus*, the upper part of which may be tilted backward in relation to the lower part, or cervix, which is pointed toward the pubic bone.

REYE'S SYNDROME n. a poorly understood syndrome involving abnormal brain function and fatty infiltration of internal organs, esp. the liver. It occurs chiefly in children following an acute viral infection (esp. viruses associated with influenza and chickenpox); an association with aspirin intake has also been observed. Vomiting and confusion typically occur about a week after the viral infection, sometimes leading to disorientation, seizures, coma, and respiratory arrest. The cause is unknown and there is no specific treatment. Intensive monitoring of all vital functions and correction of any imbalances, along with antibiotics improves the prognosis.

RHABDOMYOSARCOMA n. a highly malignant tumor derived from striated muscle cells. Embryonal forms, occurring mainly in children and adolescents, primarily affect the head, neck, and genitourinary tract; pleomorphic forms affect the limb muscles of older adults. Surgical excision is often impossible, treatment involving chemotherapy and irradiation.

RHAGADES n. cracks in the skin, most common around the mouth.

RHEUMATIC AORTITIS n. inflammation of the *aorta*, occurring in rheumatic fever.

RHEUMATIC FEVER n. an inflammatory disease, occurring primarily in children, as a result of a delayed reaction to an inadequately treated streptococcal infection of the upper respiratory tract (e.g., strep sore throat). Symptoms, appearing several weeks after the acute infection, include fever, abdominal pain, vomiting, arthritis, and consequent pain affecting many joints, and palpitations and chest pain associated with inflammation of the heart; other signs include reddish patches on the skin and abnormal involuntary muscular movements . Treatment includes bed rest, restricted activity, and sometimes antibiotics, steroids, and pain relievers. Most cases resolve within 1 or 2 months, except for the residual effects of carditis (see *rheumatic heart disease*).

RHEUMATIC HEART DISEASE n. damage to the heart muscle and heart valves caused by recurrent episodes of *rheumatic fever*. It is characterized by stenosis or malfunctioning valves, changes in the size of the heart chambers, often with abnormal heart rhythm. Treatment depends on the nature and extent of heart damage and valve damage; it may include digitalis, diuretics, surgery to correct valve abnormalities, prevention of repeat attacks of rheumtic fever by prophylactic use of antibiotics, and other measures.

RHEUMATOID ARTHRITIS n. a chronic, destructive disease characterized by joint inflammation. It usually begins in early middle age, most often in women, and is marked by periods of remission and exacerbation. Symptoms are varied, often including fatigue; low-grade fever; loss of appetite; morning stiffness; tender, painful swelling of two or more joints, most commonly the joints of the fingers, ankles, feet, hips, and shoulders; and small subcutaneous nodules near joints. There is no cure; treatment includes rest, pain-relieving drugs, exercises to maintain joint mobility, and antiinflammatory agents (e.g., indomethacin, phenylbutazone), and, if other measures are not successful, corticosteroids.

RHEUMATOID FACTOR n. antibodies found in the serum of many people (about 70%) with *rheumatoid arthritis*, but also occurring in persons with certain other connective tissue disorders and other diseases.

RHEUMATOLOGY n. the study of disorders characterized by degeneration or inflammation of connective tissues.

Rh FACTOR n. an antigen present in the erythrocytes (red blood cells) of about 85% of people; it is called Rh factor because it was first identified in the blood of rhesus monkeys. Those persons having the factor are designated Rh-positive; those lacking the factor Rh-negative. Blood for transfusions must be classified for Rh factor, as well as for ABO classification, to prevent possible incompatibility reactions. If an Rh-negative person received Rh-positive blood hemolysis and anemia can result; a similar reaction can occur if an Rh-positive fetus (the fetus having inherited the Rh factor from the father) is exposed to antibodies to the factor by an Rh-negative mother (see also *erythroblastosis fetalis*; *Rhogam*).

Rh INCOMPATIBILITY n. lack of compatibility between two blood samples because one contains *Rh factor* and the other does not.

RHIN-, RHINO- comb. form indicating an association with the nose (e.g., **rhinopharyngeal**, pert. to the nose and pharynx).

RHINENCEPHALON n. part of each cerebral hemisphere that contains the *limbic system* and the *olfactory nerve*.

RHINION n. point at the end of the suture between the two nasal bones.

RHINITIS n. inflammation of the mucous membrane lining of the nose, usually associated with a nasal discharge; it may be caused by a viral infection, as in the common cold; or by allergic reaction, as in hay fever; also: **coryza**.

RHINOPATHY n. any disease or malformation of the nose.

RHINOPLASTY n. a plastic surgery technique in which the structure and shape of the nose is altered to correct a deformity, repair the effects of trauma, or most often for cosmetic purposes.

RHINOPHYMA n. a condition, usually associated with *rosacea*, in which there is marked swelling and redness and prominent vascularization of the nose. Treatment includes dermabrasion and plastic surgery.

RHINOSCOPE n. an instrument for examining the nasal passages through the anterior *nares* or through the *nasopharynx*.

RHINORRHEA n. persistent, usually watery, mucus discharge from the nose, as in the common cold.

RHINOSPORIDIOSIS n. fungus (*Rhinosporidium seeberi*) infection of nose, often acquired by swimming in infected waters, characterized by reddish polyps on the mucous membranes of the nose, eyes, throat, and sometimes the genitals. Treatment is by cauterization.

RHINOTOMY n. a surgical procedure in which an incision is made along one side of the nose to drain accumulated pus.

RHINOSTENOSIS n. a narrowing of the passages in the nasal cavity.

RHINOVIRUS n. any of a group of small RNA viruses, responsible for almost one half of all respiratory infections, typically characterized by a scratchy throat, headache, runny nose and other signs of nasal congestion.

RHIZOTOMY n. a surgical procedure in which certain nerve roots are cut at the point where they emerge from the spinal cord; it is performed to relieve severe muscle spasm (posterior roots) or to relieve intractable pain (anterior roots).

RHODOPSIN a purple pigment within the rods of the *retina* of the eye essential for vision in dim light.

RHOGAM n. trade name for Rh immune globulin given to prevent Rh sensitization.

RHOMBOID n. any of several muscles of the upper back that function in the movement of the shoulder blade.

RHONCHUS n. abnormal sounds heard through a stethoscope, usually during expiration, as air passes through narrowed passageways obstructed by mucus, neoplasm, muscle spasm, or pressure. pl. **rhonchi** adj. **rhonchal, rhonchial**

RHUS DERMATITIS n. a type of *contact dermatitis* resulting from contact with plants of the genus *Rhus*, including poison ivy, poison oak, and poison sumac.

RHYTHM METHOD OF FAMILY PLANNING n. a natural family planning method based on determination of the fertile time in a woman's *menstrual cycle* and avoiding coitus at that time to try to prevent conception or engaging in coitus at that time to increase the chances of conception. Determination of the fertile time, the time around ovulation, may be based on the calendar method, on the basal body temperature method, or on changes in cervical mucus that typically occur around ovulation (see *calendar method of family planning*; *basal body* *temperature method of family planning*; *ovulation method of family planning*) (see also *contraception*).

RHYTIDOPLASTY n. a procedure in plastic surgery in which an incision is made near the hairline and excess tissue excised, the face tightened, wrinkles removed, and the skin made to appear firm; also **face lift**.

RIB n. one of the twelve pairs of curved bones that form the skeletal framework of the chest and protect the heart and lungs. In the back, the head of each rib articulates with one of the 12 thoracic vertebrae; in the front, the first seven ribs (the true ribs) attach to the sternum (breastbone); each of the next three ribs (the false ribs) attaches to the rib above it and thus indirectly to the sternum; the last two (the floating ribs) end freely in the musculature; also: **costa** adj. **costal**

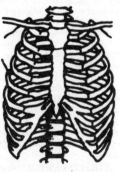

Human rib cage

RIBOFLAVIN n. a water-soluble vitamin, one of the B complex group, important as a coenzyme in metabolic processes; also called **vitamin B$_2$** (see Table of Vitamins).

RIBONUCLEIC ACID (RNA) n. a nucleic acid that in most cells transmits genetic information from the DNA in the nucleus to the cytoplasm and functions in the synthesis of proteins. It is the genetic material of some viruses.

RIBOSOME n. an organelle composed of RNA and found in the cytoplasm of cells where it serves as the site of protein synthesis.

RICKETS n. a condition caused by a deficiency of vitamin D, calcium and/or phosphorus, occurring primarily in children and characterized by abnormal bone formation and resulting skeletal deformities, often accompanied by muscle pain and spleen and liver enlargement. Prevention and treatment include a diet adequate in calcium, phosphorus, and vitamin D and adequate exposure to sunlight (see also Table of Vitamins).

RICKETTSIA n. any of a group of bacterialike microorganisms that live as parasites in ticks, fleas, lice, and mites and are transmitted to humans by these *vectors*. Rickettsia-caused diseases include *Rocky Mountain spotted fever*, *typhus*, and *trench fever*. adj. **rickettsial**

RICKETTSIALPOX n. a mild infectious disease caused by *Rickettsia akari* transmitted to humans by mites. Symptoms include chills, fever, malaise, and chickenpoxlike lesions that dry and form scabs and fall off, leaving no scars. Chloramphenicol or tetracyclines are usually given.

RIDGE n. a projecting edge, crest, or rim, as the pectoral ridge, the crest of the larger tubercle in the bone of the upper part of the arm.

RIFADIN n. trade name for the antibacterial *rifampin*.

RIFAMPIN n. an antibacterial, known under the trade names Rifadin and Rimactane, used in the treatment of tuberculosis. Adverse effects include gastrointestinal upsets, discoloration of urine and sweat, and sometimes an influenzalike syndrome and liver toxicity.

RIFT VALLEY FEVER n. a self-limiting, usually short-lived viral infection of Africa transmitted by mosquitoes or handling of infected animals with symptoms of fever, malaise, headache, and photophobia.

RIGHT ATRIOVENTRICULAR VALVE see *tricuspid valve*.

RIGHT-HANDEDNESS n. a natural tendency to use the right hand in writing and manipulating objects; also **dextrality**.

RIGIDITY n. a condition of inflexibility, hardness, or stiffness. adj. **rigid**

RIGOR n. 1. rigidity of the tissues of the body, as in rigor mortis; 2. sudden attack of shivering.

RIGOR MORTIS n. rigid stiffening of the skeleton and some muscle shortly after death.

RIMA n. a crack, cleft, or opening, as the **rima glottidis**, the space between the vocal cords.

RIMACTANE n. trade name for the antibacterial *rifampin*.

RINGWORM n. any of several fungal infections of the skin often characterized by ringlike skin lesions, including athlete's foot and jock itch (see *tinea*).

RITALIN n. trade name for a central nervous stimulant methylphenidate used in the treatment of *attention deficit syndrome* in children.

RIVER BLINDNESS see *onchocerciasis*.

RNA abbreviation for *ribonucleic acid*.

ROBAXIN n. trade name for skeletal muscle relaxant *methocarbamaol* used to treat muscle spasm associated with many injuries.

ROBICILLIN VK n. trade name for the antibiotic *penicillin V*.

ROBIMYCIN n. trade name for the antibacterial *erythromycin*.

ROCKY MOUNTAIN SPOTTED FEVER n. an infectious disease caused by *Rickettsia rickettsii* and occurring throughout North and South America. It is characterized by fever, headache, muscle pains, mental confusion, and red macules that spread from the wrist and ankles over the trunk of the body; abdominal distension and hemorrhage sometimes occur. Treatment is by chloramphenicol and tetracycline. Also called **mountain fever; spotted fever**.

ROD n. 1. a rhodopsin-containing cylindrical element of the *retina* that functions in detecting low light; 2. a straight cylindrical structure, as the notochord of an embryo.

ROOTING REFLEX n. normal response of newborns in which touching or stroking the side of the mouth and cheek causes the infant to turn toward the stimulated side and begin to suck.

RORSCHACH TEST n. a personality assessment test consisting of ten pictures of inkblots which the subject interprets, the interpretations being used by the examiner to assess personality and the integration of emotional and intellectual factors.

ROSACEAE n. a skin disease of adults, more often women, associated with enlarged blood vessels, esp. of the nose forehead, and cheeks; also called **acne rosaceae**.

ROSEOLA n. any rose-colored rash, as in *measles* or *roseola infantum*.

ROSEOLA INFANTUM n. a benign illness of infants and young children. Characterized by abrupt, high fever; mild sore throat; and a few days later, by a faint macular pinkish rash that lasts for a few hours to a few days. Treatment involves fever-reducing agents (e.g., aspirin, acetaminophen), and, if convulsions occur in association with high fever, anticonvulsants.

ROSTRUM n. a structure that looks like a beak, as the sphenoidal rostrum, a ridge on the lower part of the sphenoid bone of the skull.

ROUNDWORM n. a worm of the phylum Nematoda, including several that produce disease in humans.

-RRHEA suffix indicating a flow or discharge from a body part (e.g., **rhinorrhea**, discharge from the nose).

RUBEFACIENT n. an agent that causes reddening and warming of the skin, used as a counterirritant.

RUBELLA n. a contagious viral disease characterized by fever, mild symptoms of upper respiratory infection, and a diffuse fine red rash lasting for short period, usually three or four days. The disease is usually mild and self-limiting; however, if contracted by a woman in early pregnancy it may cause serious damage to the fetus. There is no treatment; prevention is by rubella vaccine, usually given to children as part of a normal immunization program; the vaccine should not be given to a pregnant woman or one who plans to become pregnant within three months. Also called **three-day measles, German measles**.

RUBIN TEST n. a test that determines the patency of the Fallopian tubes used in tests to determine the causes of infertility. Carbon dioxide gas is introduced into the tubes through a cannula inserted in the cervix and attached to a *manometer*. Increases in pressure shown on the manometer indicate that the tubes are blocked and the gas cannot escape into the abdominal cavity; a drop in pressure indicates open tubes.

RUBOR n. redness, one of the signs of *inflammation*.

RUGA n. a fold or ridge, as ruga of the stomach.   pl. **rugae**

RUMINATION n. regurgitation of small amounts of food after feeding, seen in some infants.

RUPTURE n. 1. a tear or break; 2. a *hernia*.

RUSSELL'S BODIES n. inclusions found in plasma cells in cancer; also called **cancer bodies**.

S

SABIN VACCINE n. an oral vaccine, consisting of live attenuated poliovirus, given to provide immunity to poliomyelitis. It is given as part of the recommended immunization schedule for infants, usually in two or three doses before the age of 6 months with an added dose at 18 months and 4 or 5 years (compare *Salk vaccine*) also: **trivalent live oral poliomyelitis vaccine (TOPV)**.

SAC n. a pouch or baglike organ, as the pericardial sac, the membrane surrounding the heart.

SACCHARIDE n. any of a large group of carbohydrates, including sugars and starches.

SACCHARIN n. a crystalline substance, much sweeter than sugar, used as a substitute for sugar in low-calorie and no-sugar products.

SACCULE n. a small sac or pouch.

SACH'S DISEASE   see *Tay-Sachs disease*.

SACRAL adj. pert. to the *sacrum*.

SACRAL PLEXUS n. a network of motor and sensory nerves, branches of which innervate the pelvic region and lower limbs.

SACRAL VERTEBRA n. any of the five segments of the vertebral column that fuse in the adult to form the *sacrum*.

SACRO- comb. form indicating an association with the *sacrum* (e.g., **sacrococcygeal**, pert. to the *sacrum* and *coccyx*).

SACROILIAC adj. pert. to the joint in the pelvis where the sacrum and iliac bones join.

SACRUM n. the large, triangular bone between the two hip bones at the back of the pelvis. It is formed by the fusion of five sacral vertebrae. Its base connects with the last lumbar vertebra, its apex with the *coccyx*.

SADDLE-BLOCK ANESTHESIA n. a form of regional anesthesia in which those areas of the body that would touch a saddle if the patient were sitting astride one are anesthetized by injecting a local anesthetic agent into the spinal cavity; used sometimes for childbirth and gynecological procedures.

SADISM n. a condition in which pleasure is obtained by inflicting physical or psychological harm and pain on another person, esp. the achievement of sexual pleasure and gratification from inflicting pain or humiliation on another person, who may be a consenting or nonconsenting partner (compare *masochism*). n. **sadist** adj. **sadistic**

SADOMASOCHISM n. an abnormal condition characterized by both *sadism* and *masochism*; in it pleasure is derived from inflicting and receiving physical or psychological pain.

SAFE PERIOD n. that time in a woman's menstrual cycle during which conception is least likely to occur, usually the time immediately before and after a period and not in midcycle when ovulation is likely to occur (see also *calendar method of family planning*).

SAGITTAL adj. pert. to a line from front to back in the midline of an organ or the body.

SALICYLATE n. any of several commonly used drugs derived from salicylic acid, including aspirin (*acetylsalicylic acid*) that have antipyretic, antiinflammatory, and analgesic properties. Methyl salicyclate is a topical drug used as a counterirritant in ointments (see also *salicylate poisoning*).

SALICYLATE POISONING n. a toxic condition caused by the ingestion of aspirin (acetylsalicylic acid) or other salicylates; it is characterized by vomiting, headache, rapid breathing, tinnitus, low blood sugar, electrolyte imbalance, and, in severe cases, by convulsions, respiratory arrest, and death. Treatment is by induced emesis and/or gastric lavage, saline cathartics, and correction of electrolyte imbalances.

SALINE adj. containing a salt, esp. sodium chloride;   n. a solution containing sodium chloride used as a plasma substitute and to correct electrolyte imbalances.

SALIVA n. clear fluid, containing water, mucin, the enzyme ptyalin, and salts, secreted by the salivary glands and mucous glands of the mouth and serving to moisten food, aid in chewing and swallowing, and start the digestion of starches. adj. **salivary**

SALIVARY adj. pert. to *saliva* or its formation.

SALIVARY DUCT n. a duct through which saliva passes from a salivary gland to the mouth.

SALIVARY GLAND n. any of three pairs of glands that secrete saliva into the mouth. The parotid salivary glands secrete a serous fluid; the sublingual salivary glands a mucous fluid; and the submandibular glands a fluid with both serous and mucous components.

SALK VACCINE n. a vaccine consisting of inactivated polio virus injected subcutaneously to provide immunity to poliomyelitis. It is used for infants, children with deficient immune systems, and unvaccinated adults; also: **IPV** (compare *Sabin vaccine*).

SALMONELLA n. a genus of gram-negative rod-shaped bacteria, some of which cause typhoid fever and some forms of gastroenteritis in humans.

SALMONELLOSIS n. a form of food poisoning, produced by eating food contaminated with *Salmonella* bacteria; symptoms include sudden abdominal pain, nausea, vomiting, fever, and diarrhea (sometimes bloody and watery). There is no specific treatment, but dehydration should be prevented.

SALPING-, SALPINGO- comb. form indicating an association with a tube, esp. the *Fallopian tubes* (e.g., **salpingectomy,** surgical removal of one or both Fallopian tubes).

SALPINGITIS n. inflammation or infection of a *Fallopian tube,* usually the result of infection spreading from the *vagina* or *uterus;* if scar tissue forms the tube may become blocked and inability to conceive in that tube result. Treatment is by antibiotics or surgical removal of the tube.

SALPINGOSTOMY n. a surgically created opening in one or both Fallopian tubes to restore patency that has been closed by chronic inflammation or to drain fluid.

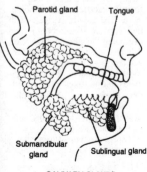

SALIVARY GLANDS

SALPINX n. a tube. pl. **salpinges**

SALT n. a compound formed by the reaction of an acid and a base, esp. sodium chloride, table salt.

SALT DEPLETION n. the loss of salt from the body by vomiting, diarrhea or profuse perspiration or urination without replacement (see *electrolyte imbalance*).

SALT-FREE DIET see *low-sodium diet.*

SALUBRIOUS adj. healthful.

SANDRIL n. trade name for the antihypertensive *reserpine.*

SANGUI-, SANGUINO- comb. form indicating an association with *blood* (e.g., **sanguifacient,** blood-producing).

SANGUINEOUS adj. pert. to blood.

SANGUIS n. blood.

SA NODE see *sinoatrial node.*

SAPHENOUS NERVE n. a branch of the femoral nerve, supplying the inner aspect of the leg.

SAPHENOUS VEIN n. either of two veins of the leg that drain blood from the foot.
 long saphenous vein n. the longest vein in the body; it runs from the foot up the medial side of the leg to the groin, where it joins the femoral vein; also **great saphenous vein.**
 short saphenous vein n. vein running up the back of the lower leg from the foot to the knee.

SAPR-, SAPRO- comb. form indicating decay or putrefaction (e.g., **saprophyte,** an organism that lives on dead tissue).

SARCO- comb. form indicating an association with flesh (e.g., **sarcolysis,** breakdown of flesh).

SARCOID adj. fleshy.

SARCOIDOSIS n. a chronic disease of unknown cause characterized by the formation of nodules in the lungs, liver, lymph glands, and salivary glands. A relationship with tuberculosis is suspected. Recovery is usually complete.

SARCOLEMMA a membrane surrounding a muscle fiber. adj. **sarcolemmic, sarcolemnous**

SARCOMA n. a malignant neoplasm arising in bone, muscle, or other connective tissue (compare *carcinoma*).

SARCOMERE n. a contractile unit of which *skeletal muscle* is composed.

SARCOPLASM n. the cytoplasm of *muscle*.

SARCOPLASMIC RETICULUM n. a network of tubules and sacs that function in muscle contraction and relaxation.

SARTORIUS n. the longest muscle in the body, extending from the pelvis to the calf of the leg; it functions in the movement of the thigh and lower leg.

SATURATED FATTY ACID n. a fatty acid in which all the atoms are joined by single valence bonds; saturated fatty acids are found chiefly in animal fats. (e.g., beef, pork, lamb, veal, milk products). A diet high in saturated fats has been associated with high serum cholesterol levels and in some studies with increased risk of coronary artery disease (compare *unsaturated fatty acid*).

SATYRIASIS n. excessive and uncontrollable sexual desire in a male (compare *nymphomania*).

SCAB see *eschar*.

SCABICIDE n. a drug that destroys the itch mite (*Sarcoptes scabiei*).

SCABIES n. a contagious disease caused by the itch mite (*Sarcoptes scabiei*) and characterized by itching and skin irritation, often leading to secondary infection. Treatment includes scabicides (e.g., sulfur ointments and benzyl benzoate creams) and antihistamines to relieve itching. All contacts and bedding and clothing must be treated to prevent spread and reinfestation.

SCALE n. a flake of dead epidermis shed from the surface of the skin; v. to remove tartar or other encrusted material from the surface of a tooth.

SCALENUS n. any of four pairs of muscles extending from the cervical vertebrae to the second rib and involved in movement of the neck and in breathing movements.

SCALENUS SYNDROME n. symptoms caused by the scalene muscle (esp. scalenus anterior) compressing the subclavian artery and part of the brachial plexus against the bones of upper thoracic or lower cervical vertebrae; loss of sensation, discomfort, and vascular symptoms in the affected shoulder and arm occur (see also *thoracic outlet syndrome*).

SCALP n. the skin covering the head, not including the ears and face.

SCAPHOCEPHALY n. a congenital malformation of the skull in which the skull is abnormally long and narrow; the condition is frequently accompanied by *mental retardation*.

SCAPULA n. either of a pair of large, flat, triangular bones that form the back part of the shoulder girdle. The scapula articulates with the clavicle (collarbone) and overhangs the glenoid fossa (cavity) into which the humerus (upper arm bone) fits and provides for the attachment of many ligaments and muscles; also: **shoulder blade.** pl. **scapulae** adj. **scapular**

SCAPULOHUMERAL adj. pert. to the shoulder blade (scapula) and upper arm bone (humerus).

SCAR see *cicatrix*

SCARLATINA see *scarlet fever*.

SCARLET FEVER n. an acute contagious disease, usually occurring in childhood, caused by a *Streptococcus* bacterium, and characterized by fever, sore throat, enlarged lymph nodes in the neck, and a bright red rash that typically spreads from the armpits and groin to the trunk of the body and limbs. Treatment is by antibiotics. Also: **scarlatina**

SCATO- comb. form indicating an association with *feces* (e.g., **scatophagy,** the eating of feces).

SCHICK TEST n. a skin test to determine immunity to *diphtheria*. A small amount of diphtheria toxin is injected intradermally; the development of redness and swelling at the injection site con-

stitutes a positive reaction and indicates susceptibility to diphtheria. A negative reaction indicates immunity.

SCHISTOSOMIASIS n. infection with the parasite of the genus *Schistosoma*, transmitted to humans by contact with feces-contaminated freshwater or freshwater organisms, esp. snails; it is common in the tropics and Far East, affecting a large percentage of the population in some areas. Symptoms depend on the part of the body infected, often the bladder, intestines, spleen, or blood vessels. Pain, disturbances of organ function, and anemia often result. Treatment is difficult and usually includes use of antimony preparations; also: **bilharziasis**

SCHIZO- comb. form indicating a split or division (e.g., **schizonychia,** a condition in which the nails are split).

SCHIZOPHRENIA n. any of a group of mental disorder characterized by gross distortions of reality, withdrawal from social contacts, and disturbances of thought, language, perception and emotional response. Symptoms are highly varied and may include apathy, catatonia or excessive activity, bizarre actions, hallucinations, delusions, and rambling speech. Some cases are mild; others severe, requiring prolonged or permanent hospitalization. There is no known cause; a combination of hereditary or genetic predisposition factors together with psychological, biochemical, and sociocultural factors is thought to be responsible in many cases. Treatment includes use of tranquilizers, antidepressants, and psychotherapy.

SCHIZOPHRENIC adj. pert. to *schizophrenia;* n. a person with schizophrenia.

SCHWANN CELLS n. cells that lay down the *myelin* sheath around the *axon* of certain nerve fibers.

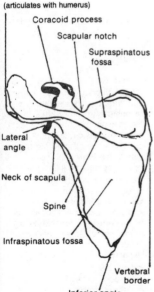

Acromion (articulates with humerus)
Coracoid process
Scapular notch
Supraspinatous fossa
Lateral angle
Neck of scapula
Spine
Infraspinatous fossa
Vertebral border
Inferior angle

Left Scapula (dorsal view)

Courtesy Carolina Biological Supply Co.

SCIATICA n. pain felt in the back and down the back and outer part of the thigh and leg due to compression on sacral spinal nerve roots or the sciatic nerve, often associated with degeneration of an intervertebral disc. Treatment is by rest; intractable cases may require surgery.

SCIATIC NERVE n. the nerve running from the lower spine down the thigh to the knee region, where it divides into two nerves that supply the lower leg.

SCLER-, SCLERO- comb. form indicating hardness (e.g., **scleradonitis,** gland hardening) or the *sclera* of the eye (e.g., **sclerocorneal,** pert. to the sclera and cornea).

SCLERA n. the tough, opaque covering of the posterior part of the eyeball that maintains the size of the eyeball and attaches to muscles involved in eye movement. It is pierced by the *optic nerve*. adj. *scleral*

SCLEREDEMA n. a skin disease in which there is hardening of the tissue, usually beginning on the face and spreading downward, often associated with fluid buildup in the peritoneal and pericardial cavities. There is no known cause or treatment, recovery usually occurring spontaneously.

SCLERODERMA n. an autoimmune disease affecting the blood vessels and connective tissue, most often occurring in middle aged women. Skin changes in the face and fingers and rheumatoid arthritislike symptoms progress to areas where the skin becomes fixed to underlying tissue. Eventually in severe cases the skin of the face may become so taut as to interfere with chewing and swallowing, or there may be pulmonary and cardiac complications leading to death. Other causes remain benign and localized. Treatment includes corticosteroids and analgesics.

SCLEROSIS n. a condition characterized by hardness of tissue, resulting from inflammation, mineral deposits or other causes.

SCOLIOSIS n. an abnormal lateral or sideward curve to the spine; it is common in childhood, caused by congenital malformations, poliomyelitis, unequal limbs, or other factors. Early treatment involving surgery, casts, exercises, and braces may prevent progression of the curvature (compare *kyphosis; lordosis*).

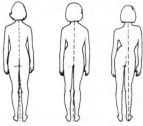

NORMAL SPINE   SCOLIOSIS

In scoliosis there is an abnormal lateral curvature of the spine.

SCOPOLAMINE an anticholinergic drug used to treat nausea and vomiting, as a sedative, and in ophthalmic procedures to dilate the pupils. Adverse effects are blurred vision, dry mouth, decreased sweating, and hypersensitivity reactions.

SCRATCH TEST n. a skin test for identifying an allergen. A small amount of a solution containing a suspected allergen is placed on a scratched skin area; if redness and wheal formation develop, allergy to that particular substance is indicated.

SCROFULA n. a form of *tuberculosis* characterized by abscess formation, usually in the lymph nodes of the neck. adj. **scrofulous**

SCROTUM n. the pouch of skin containing the *testes* and parts of the spermatic cords below the abdomen. It is divided into two lateral portions by a ridge that continues ventrally to the undersurface of the *penis* and dorsally to the perineum. Because it holds the testes away from the abdomen, the scrotum allows the production of sperm at a temperature lower than that of the abdomen. adj. **scrotal**

SCRUB TYPHUS n. a disease of eastern Asia, surrounding islands, and Australia, caused by *Rickesttsia* organisms transmitted to humans by mites. Symptoms include a dark lesion at the site of the bite, lymph node enlargement, fever, muscle ache, rash, and in severe cases cardiovascular and nervous system involvement. Treatment is by antibiotics.

SCURVY n. a condition caused by a lack of ascorbic acid (vitamin C) in the diet and characterized by anemia, weakness, and spongy, bleeding gums. Treatment involves administration of vitamin C and a diet rich in ascorbic acid-containing fruits and vegetables.

SEBACEOUS adj. fatty, greasy, esp. pert. to the *sebaceous glands*.

SEBACEOUS GLAND n. any of numerous *sebum*-secreting organs in the *dermis* throughout the body (except the palms and soles), esp. abundant on the scalp, face, nose, mouth, and ears. In most cases the sebum is secreted into hair follicles but in some places (e.g. the labia minora, lips) it is secreted onto the surface. The sebum oils the hair and skin, helps retain body heat and prevent sweat evaporation.

SEBORRHEA n. any of several conditions in which there is overactivity of the *sebaceous glands* and the skin becomes oily.

SEBORRHEIC DERMATITIS n. a chronic skin disease associated with overactivity of the sebaceous glands and greasy scales on the scalp (*cradle cap* or *dandruff*), eyelids (*blepharitis*), or other parts of the skin. Treatment includes medicated shampoos, corticosteroids, antibiotics, and the treatment of any underlying disorder (e.g., *diabetes mellitus* or allergic reaction) causing the condition.

SEBUM n. the secretion of the sebaceous glands, containing fat and cellular debris. With sweat, it moistens and protects the skin.

SECOBARBITAL n. a sedative, known under the trade name Seconal, used in the treatment of insomnia and convulsions. Adverse effects include respiratory depression, paradoxical excitement, and allergic reactions.

SECONDARY AMENORRHEA see *amenorrhea*.

SECONDARY DYSMENOR-RHEA see *dysmenorrhea*.

SECONDARY SEX CHARACTERISTIC n. any of the physical characteristics associated with sexual maturity but not directly involved in reproductive functioning. In males they include deep voice and facial and pubic hair; in females breast development and pubic hair.

SECRETIN n. a hormone secreted by the small intestine when acidic, partially digested food enters it; it stimulates bile production and pancreatic secretion.

SECRETION n. the process by which substances (e.g., enzymes and hormones) are released from specific organs or the blood for a particular purpose. v. **secrete** adj. **secretory**

SECRETORY PHASE n. that phase of the *menstrual cycle* after *ovulation* during which *progesterone* secreted by the *corpus luteum* stimulates the development and thickening of the *endometrium* in preparation for the implantation of an *embryo*. If fertilization does not occur, the secretory phase ends as the corpus luteum involutes, progesterone levels decrease, and menstrual flow begins; also: **luteal phase** (compare *proliferative phase*).

SECTION n. the act of cutting; v. to cut.

SECUNDI- comb. form meaning second (e.g., **secundigravida,** a woman pregnant for the second time).

SEDATION n. an induced state of reduced activity and excitability; a state of calm and quietness, sometimes with sleep.

SEDATIVE n. an agent that decreases activity and excitability, relieves anxiety, and calms the person. Some sedatives have a general effect; others affect the activities of certain organs (e.g., intestines or vasomotor system).

SEDATIVE-HYPNOTIC n. a drug that depresses central nervous system activity, relieves anxiety, and induces sleep. Barbiturates, minor tranquilizers (e.g., diazepam and chlordiazepoxide), chloral hydrate, and many other drugs act as sedative-hypnotics.

SEIZURE see *convulsion*.

SELF-BREAST EXAMINATION see *breast examination*.

SELF-LIMITED adj. pert. to a disease that tends to end or resolve without treatment.

SEMEN n. the thick, whitish secretion discharged from the *urethra* during ejaculation. It contains spermatozoa and secretions of the *prostate gland,* seminal vesicles, and other glands: also: **seminal fluid** adj. **seminal**

SEMI- prefix meaning "one-half" (e.g., **semicoma,** a stuporous state from which arousal is possible; half a coma)

SEMICIRCULAR CANAL n. any of three, bony, fluid-filled loops in the osseous labyrinth of the inner ear, concerned with the sense and maintenance of balance.

SEMILUNAR VALVE n. a valve with half moon-shaped cusps (semilunar), as the aortic valve also: **tricuspid valve.**

SEMINAL DUCT n. a duct through which *semen* passes, as the *ejaculatory duct*.

SEMINAL FLUID see *semen*.

SEMINAL VESICLE n. either of a pair of accessory male sex glands that produce most of the fluid portion of *semen,* secreting it into the *vas deferens* before it joins the *urethra*.

SEMINIFEROUS TUBULE n. any of numerous, long and convuluted tubes found in the testis; they are the sites of spermatozoa maturation.

SEMINOMA n. a malignant tumor of the *testis,* usually occurring in older men. Treatment is by surgery (orchidectomy).

SEMIPERMEABLE MEMBRANE n. a membrane, such as the cell membrane, that allows the passage of some molecules but not others.

SENILE adj. pert. to or characteristic of old age or aging, esp. deterioration association with aging n. **senility**

SENILE DEMENTIA n. a mental disorder of the aged, resulting from atrophy and degeneration of the brain, with no signs of cerebrovascular disease. Symptoms, which are generally slowly progressive, include loss of memory, periods of confusion and irritability, confabulation, and poor judgment; also **senile psychosis** (compare *Alzheimer's disease*).

SENSATION n. a feeling; the result of the process by which messages from sensory receptors are relayed to the brain and interpreted as information or impressions.

SENSE n. one of the facilities by which information about the external environment is received and interpreted; there are five major senses: sight, hearing, smell, taste, and touch.

SENSE ORGAN n. a collection of specialized cells—receptor cells—capable of responding to a particular stimulus (e.g., an odor) and transmitting that message as an impulse along a sensory nerve to the central nervous system for interpretation.

SENSIBILITY n. the ability to be affected by changes in the environment.

SENSITIVITY the capacity to feel or react to a stimulus   adj. **sensitive**

SENSITIZATION n. an acquired reaction in which antibodies develop in response to an antigen.

SENSORY NERVE n. a nerve that conducts impulses from the periphery of the body (e.g., from sense organs) to the brain or spinal cord (compare *motor nerve*).

SEPSIS n. destruction of tissue by bacterial toxins; contamination; infection (compare *aseptic*).

SEPTAL DEFECT n. a congenital abnormality in the wall (septum) separating the left and right sides of the heart. It may occur between the two atria or between the two ventricles (*ventricular septal defect*). The defect allows abnormal circulation of blood and causes numerous symptoms, depending on the location and size of the defect.

SEPTICEMIA n. an infection in which disease-causing organisms are present in the circulating blood, usually resulting from spread of an infection from a specific site. Symptoms include fever, chills, nausea, diarrhea, headache, and prostration. Treatment is by antibiotics. Also called **blood poisoning.**

SEPTUM n. a partition or dividing wall in an organ (e.g., the septum dividing the left and right sides of the heart and the septum dividing

the nasal cavity).   adj. **septal, septate**

SEQUELA n. abnormality following or resulting from a disease, injury, or treatment (e.g., paralysis following poliomyelitis). pl. **sequelae**

SER-AP-ES n. the trade name for a fixed-combination drug, containing the diuretic *hydrochlorothiazide* and the antihypertensives *reserpine* and *hydralazine;* used to treat *hypertension.*

SERAX n. the trade name for the tranquilizer *oxazepam.*

SERENTIL n., the trade name for a phenothiazine tranquilizer (mesoridazine).

SERO- comb. form indicating an association with *serum* (e.g., **seroglobulin,** a globulin found in serum).

SEROLOGY n. that branch of science concerned with the study of blood serum, esp. the search for evidence of infection and the evaluation of immune reactions. adj. **serologic; serological**

SEROSA   see *serous membrane.*

SEROTONIN n. a chemical widely distributed in the body, esp. in the brain, where it acts as a *neurotransmitter;* in the blood platelets, where, upon an injury, it acts as a *vasoconstrictor;* and in the small intestine, where it stimulates smooth muscle to contract.

SEROUS MEMBRANE n. a smooth, transparent membrane, containing fibrous connective tissue, that lines many large cavities of the body, as the pleura cavity, peritoneal cavity, and the pericardial cavity. These membranes usually consist of two layers: a visceral layer covering the organs and a parietal layer lining the cavity walls. Between the two layers is a small space filled with serous fluid, derived from blood serum, that moistens the structures and allows frictionless movement.

SERPASIL n. trade name for antihypertensive *reserpine*.

SERPASIL-APRESOLINE n. trade name for fixed -combination drug containing two antihypertensives—*reserpine* and *hydralazine;* used to treat *hypertension*.

SERPASIL-ESIDRIX n. trade name for fixed-combination drug containing the diuretic *hydrochlorothiazide* and the antihypertensive *reserpine;* used to treat *hypertension*.

SERRATUS n. any of several muscles with sawlike processes, esp. the **serratus anterior,** the muscle between the ribs and shoulder blade involved in shoulder and arm movement, esp. pushing-type motions.

SERTOLI CELLS n. cells found in the *seminiferous tubules* of the testis where they nourish developing spermatozoa.

SERUM n. clear, thin, sticky fluid of blood; like plasma, it contains no cells or platelets; unlike plasma, it also contains no fibrinogen.

SERUM HEPATITIS see *hepatitis*.

SERUM SICKNESS n. a reaction occurring 1 or 2 weeks after the injection of antiserum (as donor serum containing desired antibodies) and caused by an antibody reaction to an antigen in the donor serum. Symptoms of fever, enlarged spleen, joint pain, and swollen lymph glands occur.

SESAMOID BONE n. any of several small round or oval bones lying within a tendon, such as the patella (knee cap).

SEX n. classification of male or female based on physical, psychological, and behavioral characteristics of an animal that relate to reproduction, esp. in having specific chromosomes (Y in the human male) and producing special gametes (ova in females, sperm in males) and in having anatomical and physiological characteristics associated with femaleness or maleness.

SEX CHROMATIN n. chromatin found only in female cells; it usually occurs as a small object (Barr body) near the nucleus or as a drumstick-shaped appendage to the nucleus of some white cells. The presence or absence of sex chromatin is the basis of sex determination before birth through examination of cells obtained through *amniocentesis*.

SEX CHROMOSOME n. the chromosome responsible for sex determination and which carries certain sex-linked genes. In mammals there are two sex chromosomes: X and Y. Female humans have the XX combination and males the XY combination.

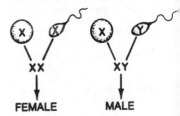

FEMALE   MALE

Pairing of sex chromosomes from the sperm and ovum determine the sex of the offspring at the time of fertilization.

SEX HORMONE n. a steroid hormone responsible for sexual development and reproductive function. The main female sex hormones are estrogens and progesterone; the male sex hormones are androgens (including testosterone).

SEX-LIMITED adj. pert. to a characteristic that is expressed differently in the two sexes.

SEX-LINKED adj. pert. to characteristics the genes for which are carried on the sex chromosomes, specifically on the X chromosome.

SEX-LINKED DISORDER n. a disease or abnormality determined by the sex chromosomes. It may involve an abormality in the number of sex chromosomes (e.g., Turner's syndrome or Kleinfelter's syndrome) or a gene defect on an X-chromosome (e.g., *hemophilia*).

SEXUAL adj. pert. to sex.

SEXUAL INTERCOURSE see *coitus*.

SEXUALLY TRANSMITTED DISEASE n. a *venereal disease*.

SHEATH n. a tubular structure surrounding an organ or body part (e.g., synovial sheath of some tendons).

SHIGELLOSIS n. an acute infection of the intestine with pathogenic *Shigella* bacteria; it is widespread in many lesser developed areas of the world and occurs sporadically in other areas. Symptoms include diarrhea, abdominal discomfort, and fever; also called **bacillary dysentery**

SHIN BONE see *tibia*.

SHINGLES see *herpes zoster*.

SHIRODKAR'S OPERATION n. surgical procedure in which a purse-string suture is used to close the cervix in cases where an incompetent cervix has failed to retain previous pregnancies; also called **purse-string operation.**

SHOCK n. an abnormal state, usually an alarm reaction to trauma, characterized by reduced cardiac output, circulatory insufficiency, low blood pressure, rapid heartbeat, and pallor.

SHORT-ACTING adj. pert. to a drug or other agent that has a short period of effectiveness, usually beginning shortly after administration (compare *long-acting*).

SHORT-TERM MEMORY n. memory of recent events.

SHOULDER BLADE see *scapula*.

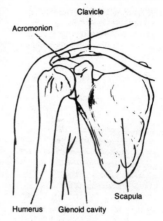

Clavicle
Acromonion
Scapula
Humerus   Glenoid cavity

SHOULDER

SHOULDER JOINT n. a *ball-and-socket joint* in which the *humerus* articulates with the *scapula*.

SHUNT v. to redirect the flow of a body fluid from one vessel to another; n. a device implanted to redirect the flow of a body fluid.

SIAL-, SIALO- comb. form indicating an association with *saliva* or the *salivary glands* (e.g., **sialadenitis,** inflammation of the salivary glands).

SIALOLITH n. a stone formed in a *salivary gland*.

SIAMESE TWINS n. twins born joined together at one or more body parts and often sharing a body part. Most Siamese twins can be separated surgically, the prognosis depending on the site of connection and the extent of shared organs; also: *conjoined twins*.

SIBLING n. one of two or more children who have both parents in common; adj. pert. to a brother or sister.

SICKLE CELL n. an abnormal red blood cell with a crescent shape and abnormal form of hemoglobin.

SICKLE CELL ANEMIA n. a hereditary blood disease, occurring mostly in blacks, in which abnormal hemoglobin (hemoglobin HbS) causes red blood cells to become sickle-shaped, fragile and nonfunctional, leading to anemia. Persons inheriting the trait from only one parent may show few symptoms; those homozygous for the trait (inheriting it from both parents) have chronic anemia, an enlarged spleen, lethargy, weakness, blood clot formation, and joint pain.

SICKLE CELL TRAIT n. heterozygous sickle-cell anemia with both normal and abnormal hemoglobin present. There are usually few or no symptoms, the main concern being possible transmission to offspring (see also *sickle cell anemia*).

SIDEROPENIA n. iron deficiency, caused by inadequate iron intake in the diet or increased loss from the body, as occurs in hemorrhage or chronic bleeding. The major manifestation is anemia, corrected by iron administration.

SIDEROSIS n. a form of *pneumoconiosis* in which iron dust or particles affect the lungs, causing fibrosis; it occurs among welders and other metal workers.

SIDS abbreviation for *sudden infant death syndrome*.

SIGMOID COLON n. that part of the colon extending from the end of the descending colon to the rectum.

SIGMOIDECTOMY n. surgical removal of all or part of the *sigmoid colon*, usually to remove a malignant tumor.

SIGMOIDOSCOPE n. an instrument, consisting of a tube and light, inserted through the anus to allow visualization of the *sigmoid colon*.

SIGN n. an observable indication of a disease (e.g., *Babinski's sign*) (compare *symptom*).

SILICOSIS n. a form of *pneumoconiosis* produced by inhaling silica dust; common among sandblasters, some miners, and others who work with sand.

SILVER n. a metallic element (see Table of Elements).

SILVER NITRATE n. a topical anti-infective agent used on wound dressings and placed in the eyes of newborns to prevent infection.

SIMPLE FRACTURE see under *fracture*

SIMPLE MASTECTOMY see under *mastectomy*.

SINEQUAN n. trade name for the *antidepressant doxepin*.

SINEW n. a *tendon*.

SINGULTUS see *hiccup*.

SINISTRALITY see *left-handedness*.

SINOATRIAL NODE (SA NODE) n. an area of modified cardiac muscle in the right atrium near the entry of the superior *vena cava* that generates impulses that travel through the muscles of both atria, causing them to contract. Cells in the node have an intrinsic rhythm independent of nerve impulse stimulation. Normally the node fires about 70 to 75 beats per minute, with certain hormones and other factors causing faster rate, as during exercise. An artificial pacemaker can be used in cases of a defective sinoatrial node; also: **pacemaker** (compare *antrioventricular node*).

SINUS n.1. an air cavity within a bone, esp. the paranasal sinuses in the bones of the face and skull; 2. a wide channel containing blood (e.g., venous sinuses in the dura mater draining blood from the brain).

SINUSITIS n. inflammation of one of the paranasal sinuses, occurring as a result of an upper respiratory infection, an allergic response, a change in atmospheric pressure, or defect of the nose.

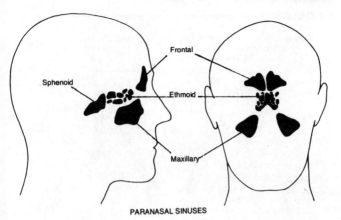

PARANASAL SINUSES

As sinus secretions accumulate, pain, fever, tenderness, and headache develop; serious complications include spread of the infection to the bone or brain. Treatment is by antibiotics (if infection is present), decongestants, steam inhalation, and, in some chronic cases, surgical drainage.

SK-AMPICILLIN n. trade name for the antibacterial *ampicillin*.

SKELETAL adj. pert. to the *skeleton*.

SKELETAL MUSCLE see *striated muscle*.

SKELETON n. the framework of the body, made up of 206 bones that provide structure and form for the body, protect delicate internal organs, provide for the attachment of muscles, produce red blood cells, and serve as blood reservoirs. The skeleton is divided into two major parts: the axial skeleton, which includes the skull, vertebral column, sternum, and ribs; and the appendicular skeleton, which includes the pectoral (shoulder) girdle (clavicle and scapula) and the pelvic (hip) girdle and the upper and lower appendages (arms and legs).

SKIN n. the outer covering of the body, the largest organ of the body. It protects the body from injury and invasion by microorganisms, helps (through hair follicles and sweat glands) maintain body temperature, serves as a sensory network, lubricates and waterproofs the exterior, and serves as an organ of excretion. The skin consists of an outer layer: the epidermis, and an inner layer: the dermis, which contains nerve endings, hair follicles, glands, lymph vessels, and blood vessels; also: **cutis.**

SKIN CANCER n. a neoplasm of the skin. Skin cancer is the most common and most curable malignancy. Treatment depends on the location and extent of the neoplasm; it may involve surgery, radiotherapy and/or chemotherapy.

SKIN GRAFT n. a portion of skin cut and removed from one area of the body and used to cover a part that has lost its skin, due to burns, injury or other cause. A skin graft is usually taken from another part of the body of the same person (autograft), but sometimes from another person (homograft) as a temporary measure.

THE SKELETON

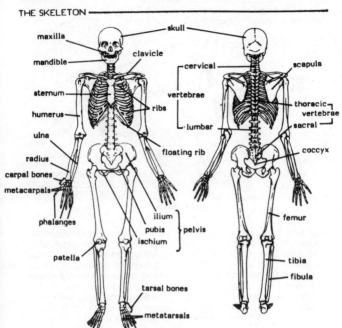

- maxilla
- mandible
- sternum
- humerus
- ulna
- radius
- carpal bones
- metacarpals
- phalanges
- skull
- clavicle
- cervical
- vertebrae
- lumbar
- ribs
- floating rib
- ilium
- pubis
- ischium
- pelvis
- patella
- tarsal bones
- metatarsals
- phalanges
- scapula
- thoracic vertebrae
- sacral
- coccyx
- femur
- tibia
- fibula

Structure of the skin

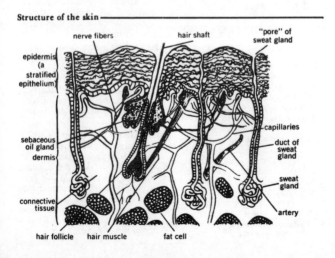

- nerve fibers
- hair shaft
- "pore" of sweat gland
- epidermis (a stratified epithelium)
- sebaceous oil gland
- dermis
- connective tissue
- hair follicle
- hair muscle
- fat cell
- capillaries
- duct of sweat gland
- sweat gland
- artery

SK-PENICILLIN VK n. trade name for a *penicillin* antibacterial.

SKULL n. the bony skeleton of the head, consisting of the *cranium*, made up of 8 bones that contain and protect the brain; and the facial skeleton, consisting of 14 bones.

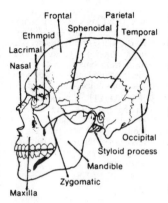

Frontal Parietal
Sphenoidal Temporal
Ethmoid
Lacrimal
Nasal
Occipital
Styloid process
Mandible
Zygomatic
Maxilla

Courtesy Carolina Biological Supply Co.

SLE abbreviation for *systemic lupus erythematosus*.

SLEEP n. a state of reduced consciousness and depressed metabolism occurring normally at regular intervals, ranging from as much as 20 hours a day in some infants to as little as 5 or 6 hours a day in some adults, esp. the aged. Sleep can be divided into two parts: *nonrapid eye movement* sleep, representing about 75% of total sleep and during which dreaming does not occur, and *rapid eye movement sleep* during which dreaming does occur.

SLEEPING PILL colloq. a sedative taken for insomnia or as an aid to sleep.

SLEEPING SICKNESS see *African trypanosomiasis*.

SLEEP TERROR DISORDER n. a disorder of sleep, occurring mostly in children, in which episodes of abrupt awakening with feelings of terror, panic, and anxiety, often with screaming and marked movements, occur without awareness of a frightening dream and with total amnesia of the event afterward; also: **pavor nocturnus.**

SLEEPWALKING see *somnambulism*.

SLIPPED DISC a *herniated intervertebral disc*.

SLOUGH v. to shed or fall away from, as tissue (e.g., skin) that has died and been replaced by new tissue.

SLOW VIRUS n. a virus that remains dormant in the body for a long time, with years elapsing before symptoms may occur. Several human diseases (e.g., kuru) are thought to be caused by slow viruses.

SMALL-FOR-GESTATIONAL-AGE (SGA) INFANT n. an infant whose size and weight are significantly less than the expected for the age of the baby, whether at term or premature. Factors associated with smallness include chronic disease, infection, malnutrition, and smoking in the mother.

SMALL INTESTINE n. the longest part of the digestive tract, about 24 feet (7 meters), extending from the pylorus of the stomach to the ileocecal junction. It is divided into the duodenum, jejunum, and ileum; it is a major site of food digestion and absorption of nutrients.

SMALLPOX n. a highly contagious viral disease characterized by fever, weakness, and a pustular rash. The disease was once widespread, but since 1979 has been eradicated throughout the world as a result of vaccination programs; also: **variola.**

SMEAR n. a thin film of tissue spread on a slide for microscopic examination.

SMEGMA n. white, cheesy secretion of glands of the *foreskin*.

SMOOTH MUSCLE n. one of three major types of muscle in the body (the other two being striated and cardiac), made up of spindle-shaped cells and contracting, under autonomic nervous system control, involuntarily with slow, long-term contractions. Smooth muscle occurs in many organs, including the blood vessels, intestines, and bladder (compare *striated muscle*).

SNARE n. an instrument with a wire hoop used to remove polyps, small tumors, or other growths, esp. in body cavities.

SNEEZE n. an involuntary sudden expulsion of air through the nose and mouth, resulting from irritation of the mucuous membrane of the upper respiratory tract, as from a cold or allergic reaction.

SNELLEN CHART n. a commonly used chart to test visual acuity.

SNOW BLINDNESS n. a temporary and painful disorder caused by excessive exposure to ultraviolet light reflected from snow.

SOCIALIZATION n. the process by which a person learns to adapt to and be productive within the expectations and standards of a group or society.

SODIUM n. a metallic element that is one of the most important elements in the body, essential for acid-base balance, water balance, nerve transmission, and muscle contraction (see Table of Elements).

SODIUM BICARBONATE n. an antacid used in the treatment of indigestion and gastric acidity. Adverse effects include electrolyte imbalance.

SODIUM CHLORIDE n. common table salt, used in the replenishment of fluids and electrolytes and in irrigating mediums and enemas.

SODIUM FLUORIDE n. a salt of sodium used to prevent tooth decay.

SODOMY n. anal intercourse; it is usually homosexual, but may involve an animal or be heterosexual.

SOFT DIET n. a diet containing low residue, easily digested soft foods, such as milk, cheese, custards, strained vegetables, potatoes, rice, breads, and ground meats; advised for those with acute infections or intestinal disorders.

SOFT PALATE n. structure containing muscles and mucous membranes and extending from the back of the hard palate in the posterior of the mouth, part of it hanging between the mouth and pharynx.

SOLAR PLEXUS n. network of nerve fibers and ganglia where sympathetic and parasympathetic nerve fibers combine at the upper part of the back of the abdomen.

SOLEUS n. any of several superficial muscles of the lower leg.

SOMA n. the body, distinguished from the mind (*psyche*).

SOMATIC adj. pert. to the body.

SOMATIC CHROMOSOME n. an *autosome*.

SOMATOTROPIN see *growth hormone*.

SOMN-, SOMNI- SOMNO- comb. form indicating an association with *sleep* (e.g., **somniloquism,** sleep talking).

SOMNAMBULISM n. a condition, occurring primarily in children and often associated with anxiety, fatigue, or stress, in which the person performs motor activity, usually leaving bed and walking around, while sleeping and has no memory of it on awakening.

SOMNOLENT adj. sleepy or drowsy.

SONOGRAM see *ultrasonography*.

SOPORIFIC adj. pert. to a substance or process that causes sleep.

SORE n. a wound or lesion; adj. tender, painful.

SPARINE n. trade name for promazine; used as an antiemetic and antipsychotic.

SPASM n. sudden, involuntary muscle contraction; a sudden constriction of a blood vessel or other hollow organ (see also *bronchospasm*).

SPASMO- comb. form indicating an association with *spasm* (e.g., **spasmolytic**, a drug that relieves smooth muscle spasm).

SPASMODIC adj. occurring in spasms.

SPASTIC adj. pert. to spasm or uncontrolled skeletal muscle contraction.

SPASTIC BLADDER n. a type of neurogenic bladder caused by spinal cord lesion, multiple sclerosis, or trauma and characterized by loss of bladder sensation, incontinence, and interrupted voiding (compare *flaccid bladder*).

SPASTIC COLON see *irritable bowel syndrome*.

SPASTIC PARALYSIS n. loss of muscle function with involuntary spasm or contraction of one or more muscles.

SPECIMEN n. a small sample of something; a part of a whole intended upon analysis to reveal characteristics of the whole (e.g., a urine specimen used for *urinalysis*).

SPECTINOMYCIN n. an antibiotic used to treat gonorrhea and certain other infections. Adverse effects include nausea, fever, dizziness, and rashes.

SPECTROSIN n. trade name for a topical drug containing the antibacterials *neomycin* and *gramicidin*.

SPECULUM n. an instrument inserted into and used to hold open a body cavity (e.g., vagina) for examination.

SPERM see *spermatozoon*.

SPERMATIC CORD n. cord containing arteries, veins, nerves, and lymphatics and extending from the lower abdomen to the testis.

SPERMATID n. a male germ cell that becomes a mature *spermatozoon* in the last stage of sperm formation.

SPERMATOCELE n. a sperm-containing swelling on the epididymis or testis.

SPERMATOCIDE n. a chemical that kills sperm; found in many contraceptive creams, jellies, and foams, also called **spermicide.**

SPERMATOGENESIS n. the process of spermatozoa development from early stages of spermatogonia through other stages leading to spermatids and finally mature spermatozoa.

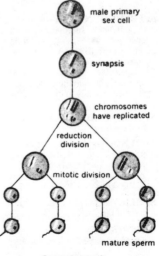

Spermatogenesis

SPERMATOZOON n. the male sex cell that fertilizes an ovum. It develops in the seminiferous tubules of the testis. Tadpolelike, it is tiny (about 1/500 inch) with a head, neck, and tail. pl. **spermatozoa**

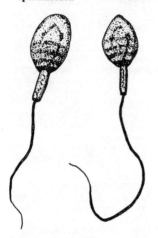

Two typical sperm cells, magnified about 1000x

SPERM COUNT n. estimate of the number of spermatozoa in an ejaculate; used as a indication of male fertility. An ejaculate normally contains between 300,000,000 and 500,000,000 spermatozia; significantly lower numbers usually indicate sterility.

SPERMICIDAL adj. destructive to spermatozoa.

SPHENO- comb. form indicating an association with the *sphenoid bone* (e.g., **sphenofrontal,** pert. to the frontal and sphenoid bones of the skull)

SPHENOID BONE n. bone at the base of the skull.

SPHEROCYTE an abnormal spherical-shaped red blood cell.

SPHINCTER n. a circular band of muscle that constricts or closes an opening in the body, as the *pyloric sphincter*, separating the lower part of the stomach from the *duodenum*.

SPHYGMO- comb. form indicating an association with the *pulse* (e.g., **sphygmogram,** a recording of the strength and rate of the pulse).

SPICULE n. a sharp, needlelike part.

SPIDER ANGIOMA n. dilatation of superficial capillaries with an elevated red dot from which blood vessels radiate.

SPINA BIFIDA n. a relatively common congenital defect in which there is a malformation of a posterior vertebral arch; unless the defect affects a large area or spinal cord material protrudes (*myelomeningocele*), there are few or no symptoms.

SPINAL adj. pert. to the spine, or spinal column.

SPINAL CANAL n. canal within the *vertebral column* through which the *spinal cord* passes.

SPINAL COLUMN see *vertebral column*.

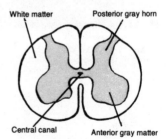

White matter   Posterior gray horn

Central canal   Anterior gray matter

SPINAL CORD

SPINAL CORD n. a major part of the *central nervous system*, that conducts sensory and motor impulses to and from the brain and is a site of reflex activity. It is a cylindrical tube, extending from the base of the brain through the vertebral canal to the upper part of the lumbar region. It has an inner core of gray matter, containing mostly nerve cells, surrounded by white matter with nerve fibers. The entire cord is surrounded by *meninges* (protective membranes). From it arise 31 *spinal nerves*.

SPINAL CURVATURE n. abnormality in curvature of the vertebral column (see *kyphosis; lordosis; scoliosis*).

SPINAL FLUID   see *cerebrospinal fluid*.

SPINAL FUSION n. fixation of an unstable part of the spinal column, usually done surgically by a bone graft, sometimes through traction or immobilization.

SPINAL NERVE n. any of 31 pairs of nerves connected to the spinal cord. Each spinal nerve divides into branches, some serving the voluntary nervous system, others the autonomic nervous system.

SPINAL PUNCTURE   see *lumbar puncture*.

SPINAL TAP   see *lumbar puncture*.

SPINAL TRACT n. any ascending or descending pathway for sensory or motor nerve impulses found in the white matter of the spinal cord.

SPINDLE n. a collection of fibers seen in a dividing cell and which function in chromosome movement in *mitosis* and *meiosis*. The fibers radiate from two poles and meet in the middle at the equator.

SPINAL NERVE DISTRIBUTION

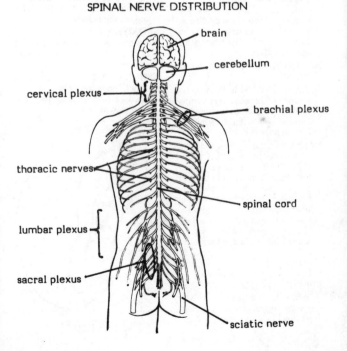

brain

cerebellum

cervical plexus

brachial plexus

thoracic nerves

spinal cord

lumbar plexus

sacral plexus

sciatic nerve

SPINE 1. the *vertebral column;* 2. the process of a bone; adj. **spinal**

SPINOCEREBELLAR DISORDER n. any of several inherited disorders characterized by progressive degeneration of the spinal cord and *cerebellum* and usually marked by increasing spasticity, ataxia, and incoordination.

SPIRILLUM FEVER see *rat-bite fever.*

SPIROCHETE n. a motile, spiral-shaped microorganism, including the causative agents of *syphilis* and *leptospirosis.*

SPIROGRAPH n. an instrument for recording breathing movements; the recording in a **spirogram.**

SPIRONOLACTONE a synthetic corticosteroid, known under the trade name Aldactone, used to treat hypertension and cardiac abnormalities. Adverse effects include headache, gastrointestinal upsets, and sleepiness.

SPLANCHNIC adj. pert. to the internal organs.

SPLANCHNIC NERVE n. any of a series of nerves of the sympathetic part of the *autonomic nervous system,* innervating viscera and blood vessels.

SPLEEN n. large, dark-red, oval organ situated on the left side of the body between the diaphragm and stomach. It is part of the lymphatic and reticuloendothelial systems, functioning to destroy worn out erythrocytes and platelets, to produce leukocytes, lymphocytes, and other cells involved in immune responses; it also stores blood and produces red blood cells before birth; also: **lien** adj. **splenic; lienal**

SPLEN-, SPLENO- comb. form indicating an association with the *spleen* (e.g., **splenitis,** inflammation of the spleen).

SPLENECTOMY n. surgical removal of the *spleen.*

SPLENOMEGALY n. enlargement of the spleen, caused by malaria, certain types of anemia, certain infectious diseases (e.g., *infectious mononucleosis*) and other disorders.

SPLINT n. an orthopedic device to immobilize, support, or restrain an injured part; it may be rigid (plaster, metal) or flexible (leather).

SPONDYL-, SPONDYLO- comb. form indicating an association with the *spinal column* or a *vertebra* (e.g., **spondylarthritis,** arthritis affecting the spinal column).

SPONDYLITIS n. inflammation of a joint of the spinal column, usually characterized by pain and stiffness; it may occur after injury, as the result of rheumatoid arthritis or infection (see also *ankylosing spondylitis*).

SPONDYLOLISTHESIS n. forward dislocation of one vertebrae over the one below it, causing pressure on spinal nerves.

SPONDYLOSIS n. a condition in which vertebral joints become fixed or stiff, causing pain and restricted mobility.

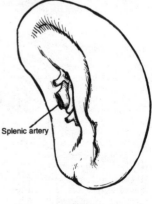

Splenic artery

SPLEEN

SPONTANEOUS adj. occurring without apparent cause, as in spontaneous recovery from a disease.

SPONTANEOUS ABORTION see under *abortion*.

SPORADIC adj. occurring occasionally or in a few isolated situations, as in the sporadic appearance of a disease.

SPOROTRICHOSIS n. a chronic fungal infection of the skin and lymph nodes caused by the fungus *Sporothrix schenckii*, found in soil and decaying vegetation; it causes skin lesions and subcutaneous lymph nodules in lymph channels. Treatment is by antifungal agents.

SPOTTED FEVER see *Rocky Mountain spotted fever*.

SPRAIN n. injury to ligaments around a joint, causing pain, swelling, and skin discoloration. The severity of symptoms and degree of immobility depend on the site of injury and extent of damage to tissues. Treatment includes support, rest, and cold compresses at the time of injury.

SPRUE n. a chronic disorder, occurring in tropical and nontropical forms and affecting both children and adults, characterized by malabsorption of nutrients and symptoms of diarrhea, poor appetite, weight loss, and ulceration of membrane lining of the digestive tract.

SPUTUM n. material usually containing mucus and cellular debris, sometimes pus or blood, coughed up from the lungs and expectorated through the mouth. Differences in the amount, color, and contents of sputum are important in the diagnosis of some respiratory ailments.

SQUINT see *strabismus*.

SQUAMA n. 1. a platelike part; a thin plate of bone; 2. a part resembling a fish scale (e.g.,

squamocellular, having scale-shaped cells).

STAIN n. a pigment or dye, esp. that used to impart color to microorganisms or cell parts for microscopic study.

STAPEDECTOMY n. surgical removal of the *stapes* of the middle ear, performed to restore hearing in cases where the stapes has become ossified and fixed and not able to vibrate in response to sound waves.

STAPES n. one of the three ossicles of the middle ear; it resembles a tiny stirrup and transmits vibrations from the *incus* to the inner ear.

STAPHYLOCOCCAL INFECTION n. infection with pathogenic species of *Staphylococcus* bacteria; usually characterized by abscess formation. Common staphylococcal infections include carbuncles, furuncles, and some forms of food poisoning.

STAPHYLOCOCCUS n. a genus of spherical bacteria typically occurring in grapelike clusters, several species of which are pathogenic to humans, producing boils, some form of food posioning, and other types of infection.

STARTLE REFLEX see *Moro reflex*.

STARVATION n. condition resulting from lack of essential nutrients over a prolonged period and characterized by weight loss, widespread physiologic and metabolic disturbances, and increased susceptibility to infection.

STASIS n. abnormal condition in which the customary flow of a fluid (e.g., blood) is slowed or stopped.

STATIC adj. at rest; in equilibrium; not changing.

STATUS ASTHMATICUS a prolonged, severe asthma attack in which spasm of the bronchi does not respond to treatment; cyanosis and other signs of lack of oxygen may occur, in severe cases leading to unconsciousness. Treatment involves corticosteroids and artificial respiration, if necessary.

STATUS EPILEPTICUS n. a condition in which there are continual attacks of *epilepsy* without intervals of consciousness; it can lead to severe brain damage and death. Therapy includes maintenance of adequate oxygen supply and anticonvulsants.

STEATORRHEA n. greater-than-normal amounts of fat in the *feces* with the feces frothy, foul-smelling, and floating; it is associated with malabsorption syndromes and disorders of fat metabolism.

STENOSIS n. abnormal narrowing or constriction of a passageway or opening, as in *aortic stenosis*.

STERILE adj. 1. pert. to a living organism: unable to reproduce; barren; 2. pert. to a nonliving object: free of disease-causing microorganisms.

STERILITY n. 1. state of being unable to reproduce; 2. state of being free from disease-causing microorganisms.

STERILIZATION n. 1. a surgical procedure in which a woman or man is rendered incapable of reproducing; in males the procedure is a *vasectomy;* in females, a form of *tubal ligation.* 2. a means of rendering objects free of microorganisms that may produce disease by boiling, subjecting to steam in an autoclave, or by use of disinfectants and antiseptics.

STERN-, STERNO- comb. form indicating an association with the *sternum* [e.g., **sternoclavicular,** pert. to the sternum (breastbone) and clavicle (collarbone)].

STERNUM n. the breastbone; an elongated flattened bone forming the middle of the thorax and which articulates with the clavicles and the first seven ribs and serves for the attachment of numerous muscles. It is composed of three parts: upper manubrium; middle body, or gladiolus; and lower xiphoid process.

STERNUTATION n. the act of sneezing.

STETHOSCOPE n. an instrument used for listening to body sounds, such as those of the heart and lungs. A simple stethoscope consists of a bell-shaped structure that is placed on the patient's skin connected by plastic or rubber tubes to earpieces for the examiner.

STILBESTROL see *diethylstilbestrol.*

STILLBIRTH n. birth of a fetus that shows no signs of life (e.g., respiration, heart beat, or movement).

STILL'S DISEASE n. a form of *rheumatoid arthritis,* primarily affecting children, in which large joints become inflamed and bone growth may be affected, causing skeletal deformities. Treatment includes antiinflammatory agents, analgesics, and rest; also called **juvenile rheumatoid arthritis.**

STIMULANT n. an agent, such as a drug, that activates or increases the activity of a body part or system. Amphetamines and caffeine are central nervous system stimulants.

STIMULUS n. anything that causes a reaction or response, as in an odor activating olfactory receptors in the nasal cavity. pl. **stimuli** v. **stimulate** n. **stimulation**

STIRRUP see *stapes.*

STITCH n. 1. suture; 2. a sharply localized pain, a form of cramp, commonly occurring in the abdomen after strenuous exercise, esp. after eating.

STOKES-ADAMS SYNDROME see *Adams-Stokes syndrome.*

STOMA n. an opening or pore on the surface, esp. a surgically created opening of an internal organ on the surface of the body, as in colostomy or tracheostomy.

STOMACH n. an expandble, sac-like organ that forms part of the digestive tract between the *esophagus* and the *duodenum*. It is located below the diaphragm in the right upper part of the abdomen, partly under the liver. The stomach receives partly digested food from the esophagus through the cardiac sphincter. In the stomach the food is churned by muscular layers of the stomach and mixed with the secretions of the gastric glands, chiefly hydrochloric acid and the enzyme pepsin. The semiliquid mass then passes through the pyloric sphincter to the duodenum.

STOMACH

Esophagus
Cardiac sphincter
Cardia
Fundus
Lesser curvature
Pyloric sphincter
Greater curvature
Pylorus

STOMATITIS n. an inflammation of the mouth; it may result from vitamin deficiency, infection, exposure to irritating substances, or systemic diseases.

STOMATO- comb. form indicating an association with the *mouth* (e.g., **stomatogastric,** pert. to the *mouth* and *stomach*).

-STOMY suffix meaning "surgical opening" (e.g., *tracheostomy*).

STONE n. a hard mass (see *gallstone; renal calculus*).

STOOL n. *feces*.

STRABISMUS

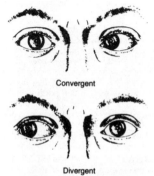

Convergent

Divergent

STRABISMUS n. an abnormal eye condition in which the eyes are not properly aligned. It may be inherited or the result of trauma or injury to the eye or brain; convergent, in which the eyes are directed inward toward each other, or divergent, in which one or both eyes are directed outward. Some forms of strabismus can be corrected in early childhood by the child wearing a patch over the normal eye, forcing the child to use the deviating eye; other types can be corrected surgically but some *amblyopia* will often remain; also called **squint.**

STRAIN n. 1. injury to a muscle, resulting in swelling and pain, usually caused by overuse; 2. a group or line of microorganisms having characteristics that separate them from others of their species.

STRANGULATION n. constriction of a tubular structure that prevents passage of material, as strangulation of the bowel preventing the passage of feces.

STRATUM n. a layer of tissues or cells, as the layers of the skin. pl. **strata**

STRATUM CORNEUM n. the horny, outermost layer of the *epidermis* containing dead cells that slough off; it is thick over the palms and soles, thinner in more protected areas; also called **horny layer.**

STRATUM GERMINATIVUM n. the innermost layer of the *epidermis*, containing dividing cells and melanocytes (pigment cells) that resupply the outer skin layers. The outer part of this layer forms a prickle-cell portion with cells connected by spines or intercellular bridges; the inner part of this layer is the basal layer with dividing cells; also: **stratum basale.**

STRATUM GRANULOSUM n. layer of epidermis just under the *stratum corneum* or, in the area of the palms and soles, just under the *stratum lucidum*; it contains cells with visible granules that die and move to the surface.

STRATUM LUCIDUM n. layer of epidermis just under the *stratum corneum*, most noticeable in the skin of the palms and soles.

STRAWBERRY HEMANGIOMA n. congenital, bright red superficial vascular tumor, resembling a strawberry; it tends to decrease in size and disappear during childhood.

STREAK n. in anatomy, a line or furrow.

STREP THROAT n. infection of the oral pharynx and tonsils with streptococcus, producing fever, sore throat, chills, lymph node enlargement, and occasionally gastrointestinal disturbances. Treatment is by antibiotics, usually penicillin or erythromycin, and analgesics. Complications include sinusitis, ear infection, or if inadequately treated, *rheumatic fever*.

STREPTOCOCCAL SORE THROAT see *strep throat*.

STREPTOCOCCUS n. a genus of bacteria, many species of which produce disease in humans, including tonsillitis, pneumonia, and urinary tract infections. Some strains of Streptococcus bacteria have become resistant to penicillin.

STREPTOKINASE n. an enzyme produced by some strains of *Streptococcus* that liquefies blood clots by converting plasminogen to plasmin; it is used in some cases of myocardial infarction and pulmonary embolism to dissolve the clot blocking the blood vessel and restore normal blood flow. Side effects include hemorrhage, fever, and gastrointestinal upsets.

STREPTOMYCIN n. an antibiotic used to treat tuberculosis and many other bacterial infections. Adverse effects include ear and kidney damage.

STRESS n. any factor—physical (e.g., infection) emotional (e.g., anxiety)—or other—that requires a change in response or affects health in any way, esp. having an adverse effect on the functioning of the body or any of its parts. Continual stress brings about widespread neurological and endocrine responses that over a period of time lead to changes in the functioning of many body organs, often leading to disease (e.g., hypertension and allergic responses).

STRESS FRACTURE see under *fracture*.

STRESS TEST n. test that measures the function of a system when it is subjected to controlled amounts of stress. For example, the treadmill test measures the effect of stress on cardiovascular and respiratory function; the fetal stress test measure the adequacy of fetal-placental function and the condition of the fetus.

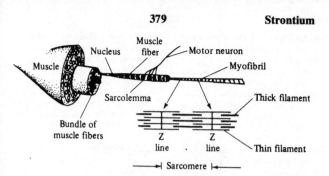

The fine structure of skeletal muscle

STRETCH MARK see *stria*.

STRIA n. a streak or narrow line, often resulting from tension in the skin, as on the skin of abdomen after pregnancy; also: **stretch mark.**

STRIATED MUSCLE n. one of three major types of muscle (the other two are *smooth muscle* and *cardiac muscle*); it makes up the major part of the body's musculature, is called *skeletal muscle* because it is attached to the skeleton, and *voluntary muscle* because it is under voluntary control. Striated muscle is composed of parallel, multinucleur fibers, each made of numerous *myofibrils* that have striations due to the position of *actin* and *myosin* protein filaments. When a muscle contracts, the two sets of filaments slide pass each other, reducing the length of the fibril (compare *smooth muscle*).

STRICTURE n. narrowing of any tubular structure (e.g., esophagus, ureter) caused by inflammation, the presence of a tumor, pressure from an adjacent organ, or muscle spasm.

STRIDOR n. abnormal breathing sound, usually heard on inspiration, occurring when the trachea or larynx is obstructed (e.g., by neoplasm or by inflammation).

STROKE see *cerebrovascular accident*.

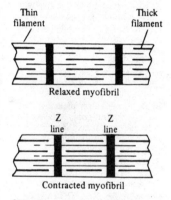

Sliding filament mechanism of muscle contraction

STROMA n. the supporting tissue of an organ, as opposed to its functional tissue (*parenchyma*) pl. **stromata** adj. **stromal**

STRONGYLOIDIASIS n. infection of the intestine with *Strongyloides stercoralis* roundworm, usually acquired as larvae in the soil penetrate the skin and migrate to the intestines, producing symptoms of diarrhea and malabsorption. Treatment is by anthelmintics.

STRONTIUM a metallic element, radioactive isotopes of which are used in diagnostic procedures.

STRYCIN n. trade name for the antibiotic streptomycin.

STUMP n. that part of a limb remaining on the body after amputation of part of the limb.

STUPOR n. a state of unresponsiveness and near unconsciousness, occurring in some neurologic and psychotic disorders. adj. **stuporous**

STUTTER v. to speak with frequent repetitions of words or parts of words.

ST. VITUS DANCE see *Sydenham's chorea*.

STYE n. bacterial (often staphylococcal) infection of a gland at the base of an eyelash, characterized by a pus-filled cyst, redness, pain, and other signs of inflammation; also: **sty.**

STYPTIC n. a substance used as an astringent, often to control bleeding.

SUB- comb. form meaning ''under'' (**sublingual**, under the tongue) or ''almost'' or ''just before'' (e.g., subclinical, not yet showing symptoms).

SUBACUTE adj. less than acute; pert. to a disease present in a person with no symptoms of it.

SUBACUTE BACTERIAL ENDOCARDITIS n. chronic bacterial infection of the valves of the heart, often associated with surgical or dental procedures or drug abuse. Symptoms of fever, heart murmur, enlarged spleen, and abnormal tissue in the heart develop slowly. Treatment involves prolonged administration of an antibiotic; acute episodes are also treated with fever reducers and pain relievers, rest, and adequate fluid intake.

SUBARACHNOID adj. located under the arachnoid layer and above the pia mater layer of the meninges. The subarachnoid space contains cerebrospinal fluid. A type of spinal anesthesia, often used for obsterical and gyneco-logical procedures, is achieved by injecting an anesthetic agent into the subarachnoid space.

SUBCLAVIAN ARTERY n. either of two arteries that supply blood to the neck and arms. The right subclavian artery branches from the innominate artery; the left subclavian artery directly from the *aortic arch*.

SUBCONSCIOUS adj. partially conscious; partially aware and responsive.

SUBCUTANEOUS adj. beneath the skin, as in a subcutaneous injection.

SUBDURAL adj. beneath the *dura mater* and above the *arachnoid* layer of the *meninges*.

SUBLIMATION n. the replacement of a socially unacceptable means of satisfying desires by means that are socially acceptable, esp. the diversion of components of the sex drive to nonsexual goals.

SUBLIMINAL adj. below or outside the range of conscious awareness or sensory perception.

SUBLINGUAL adj. below the tongue.

SUBLINGUAL GLAND n. either of a pair of mucus-secreting salivary glands located on the floor of the mouth below the tongue.

SUBLUXATION n. partial dislocation of a joint, so that the bones are misaligned but still touching.

SUBMANDIBULAR GLAND n. either of a pair of salivary glands located near the lower jaw and secreting mucus and serous fluid components of saliva.

SUBSTRATE n. material acted upon by an enzyme.

SUCCINYLCHOLINE n. a skeletal muscle relaxant used as an adjunct to anesthesia during certain surgical procedures. Adverse effects include respiratory depression and cardiac arrhythmias.

SUCCUSSION n. sound heard when a person with a large amount of fluid in a body cavity moves or is shaken.

SUCKING BLISTERS n. blister-like pads on the lips of newborns that form as the baby begins to suck and which seem to help the seal of the lips around the nipple.

SUCKING REFLEX n. involuntary sucking movement of newborns.

SUCKLE v. to provide nourishment, esp. by breast feeding.

SUCTION CURETTAGE see *vacuum aspiration*.

SUDDEN INFANT DEATH SYNDROME (SIDS) n. unexpected and sudden death of an apparently healthy infant during sleep with no autopsic evidence of disease. It is the leading cause of death in infants between two weeks and one year of age. The cause is unknown, but certain risk factors have been identified: prematurity, low-birth weight, male sex, winter months, and mothers who are very young, smoke, or are addicted to a drug; and recent mild upper respiratory infection. Also called **cot death; crib death.**

SUDO- comb. form indicating an association with sweat (e.g., **sudorific**, producing sweat).

SUDORIFEROUS GLAND n. any of several million small structures in the skin that produce sweat. Most of the glands are eccrine, producing sweat that contains salt and the waste product urea; a few, associated with the hair of the armpits and pubic region, are apocrine, secreting a thicker fluid (see *eccrine gland; apocrine gland*).

SULAMYD n. trade name for a sulfonamide antibacterial (sulfacetamide).

SULCUS n. a small groove or furrow on the surface of an organ, as the sulcus that separates convo-lutions on the surface of the cerebral hemispheres.

SULFACETAMIDE n. a topical sulfonamide most commonly used to prevent infection following injury to the cornea and to treat eye infections. Adverse effects include local irritation.

SULFADIAZONE see *sulfonamide*.

SULFAMETER see *sulfonamide*.

SULFAMETHAZINE see *sulfonamide*.

SULFAMETHIZOLE see *sulfonamide*.

SULFAMETHOXAZOLE see *sulfonamide*.

SULFAMETHOXYPYRIDA-ZINE see *sulfomamide*.

SULFAPYRIDINE see *sulfonamide*.

SULFONAMIDE n. any of a large group of antibacterial drugs; they act by halting the growth and reproduction of bacteria, but they do not kill the bacteria. Sulfonamides are used to treat bacterial urinary tract infections and certain other infections. Adverse effects include jaundice and blood abnormalities; they are not given in pregnancy or to young children, nor to persons with impaired liver or kidney function.

SULFONYLUREA n. any of a group of drugs, including *tolazamide* and *tolbutamide*, that reduce the level of glucose in the blood and are used in the treatment of *diabetes mellitus*.

SULFUR n. a nonmetallic element (see Table of Elements).

SULINDAC n. an antiinflammatory agent used in the treatment of arthritis and ankylosing spondylitis. Adverse effects include tinnitus, dizziness, skin rash, gastrointestinal upsets, and the possibility of drug interactions.

SUMYCIN n. trade name for a *tetracycline* antibiotic.

SUNSTROKE n. a condition of high fever and convulsions caused by exposure to the sun.

SUPEN n. trade name for the antibacterial *ampicillin*.

SUPEREGO n. in psychoanalysis, part of the psyche that functions as a conscience and for the formation of ideals; it forms as parental and societal standards are incorporated in a child's mind (compare *ego; id*).

SUPERFECUNDATION n. the fertilization of two or more ova released during the same menstrual cycle by spermatozoa from separate acts of coitus.

SUPERFETATION n. fertilization of a second ovum after a pregnancy has commenced; this results in two fetuses of different degrees of maturity developing in the uterus at the same time; also: **superimpregnation.**

SUPERFICIAL adj. pert. to the skin or other surface.

SUPERINFECTION n. an infection occurring during treatment with antimicrobials for another infection; it usually is caused by a change in the normal microscopic inhabits of tissue (e.g., a vaginal yeast infection occurring during antibiotic treatment for a bacterial infection).

SUPERIOR VENA CAVA n. vein that returns deoxygenated blood from the upper half of the body to the right atrium of the heart; it is the second longest vein in the body (compare *inferior vena cava*).

SUPINE adj. lying on the back.

SUPPOSITORY n. a mass of material that melts when placed in the vagina, urethra or rectum; it can be used to deliver drugs, esp. in babies or those with vomiting conditions.

SUPPURATE v. to produce pus.

SUPRA- comb. form indicating a position above or over (e.g., **suprapubic,** above the *pubic bone*).

SUPRAINFECTION n. a secondary infection caused by an opportunistic pathogen (e.g., fungus-caused pneumonia occurring in a person debilitated or immunosuppressed because of another illness or treatment).

SURA n. the calf of the leg.

SURFACTANT n. a substance that acts on a surface, esp. certain lipoproteins that alter surface tension of fluids in the lungs and facilitate gaseous exchange in the alveoli; premature infants frequently experience respiratory distress because of a lack of surfactant.

SURGERY n. that branch of medicine concerned with the treatment of injuries and diseases by operations and manipulation. adj. **surgical**

SURROGATE n. a substitute; a person or object replacing another.

SUSCEPTIBILITY n. the condition of being easily affected by a disease-causing organism; the condition of being more than normally vulnerable. adj. **susceptible**

SUTURE n. 1. a natural seam of border in the skull formed by the close joining of bony surfaces; 2. material (e.g., silk, catgut, wire) used for surgical stitches; v. to stitch torn or cut edges together with suture material.

SWEAT see *perspiration*.

SWEAT DUCT n. any tiny tubule conveying sweat from a sudoriferous gland to the skin surface.

SWEAT GLAND see sudoriferous gland.

SYDENHAM'S CHOREA n. a condition, usually of children and associated with rheumatic fever, characterized by involuntary, purposeless movements (chorea) that occur for several weeks and then usually subside; a streptococcal infection of vascular tissue of the brain area is thought to be responsible.

SYMBIOSIS n. in biology, the close association of organisms of two different species, usually to their mutual benefit.

SYMBOLISM n. in psychiatry, the process of representing an object or idea by something else.

SYMPATHECTOMY n. surgical interruption of a nerve pathway in the *sympathetic nervous system;* performed to minimize the effects of sympathetic nervous system function (e.g., to inhibit excess sweating or to improve blood circulation to a particular area as in *Buerger's disease*).

SYMPATHETIC NERVOUS SYSTEM n. one of the two divisions of the autonomic nervous system (the other being the *parasympathetic nervous system*) consisting of fibers that leave the central nervous system, pass through a chain of *ganglia* near the spinal cord, and are distributed to heart, lungs, intestine, blood vessels, and sweat glands. In general sympathetic nerves dilate the pupils, constrict peripheral blood vessels, and increase heart rate. The system works in balance with the parasympathetic nervous system.

SYMPATHOMIMETIC adj. having an effect (as from a drug) similar to that caused by stimulation of the sympathetic nervous system (e.g., dilating the bronchi).

SYMPHYSIS n. a joint in which fibrocartilage unites adjacent bony surfaces.

SYMPTOM n. a subjective indication of a disease; it may or may not be accompanied by an objective sign (compare *sign*).

SYNAPSE n. the tiny gap between two neurons or between a neuron and a muscle across which nerve impulses are transmitted through the action of neurotransmitters (e.g., acetylcholine). When an impulse reaches the end of one neuron it causes the release of a neurotransmitter that diffuses across the gap to trigger an impulse in the other neuron or muscle. adj. **synaptic**

SYNAPSIS n. the pairing of homologous chromosomes during an early stage of *meiosis*.

SYNCOPE n. brief loss of consciousness caused by temporary insufficient flow of blood to the brain; it may be caused by injury, emotional shock, prolonged standing, or other events. In many cases the feeling is preceded by lightheadedness and can be prevented by sitting with the head between the knees; also called **fainting.**

SYNCYTIUM n. mass of protoplasm containing several nuclei, as in muscle fibers.

SYNDACTYLY n. congenital defect characterized by partial or total webbing of some or all of the fingers and toes.

SYNDROME n. a complex of signs and symptoms presenting a clinical picture of a disease or disorder.

SYNECHIA n. an adhesion between the iris and the cornea (anterior synechia) or between the iris and the lens (posterior synechia), developing as a result of trauma or surgery to the eye or as a complication of cataract or glaucoma. Treatment depends on the cause; untreated it can lead to blindness.

SYNERGIST n. a substance that augments the activity of another substance, agent, or organ, as one drug augmenting the effect of another. n. **synergism**

SYNOVIA n. transparent, viscous fluid secreted by synovial membranes and acting as a lubricant for many joints and connective tissues.

SYNOVIAL FLUID see *synovia*.

SYNOVIAL JOINT n. a freely movable joint; types of synovial joints are *ball-and-socket joint, hinge joint, pivot joint,* and *gliding joint*.

SYNOVIAL MEMBRANE n. membrane, secreting synovia, that covers freely movable joints.

SYNOVITIS n. inflammation of the *synovial membrane* lining a joint, resulting in pain and swelling; it may be caused by injury, infection, or rheumatic disease (e.g., rheumatic arthritis). Treatment depends on the cause.

SYNOVIUM see *synovial membrane*.

SYPHILIS n. venereal infection, caused by the *Treponema pallidum* spirochete; it is transmitted by sexual contact or through the placenta (congenital syphilis). Symptoms occur in stages: primary stage: chancre filled with spirochetes, most often in anal or genital region, but can occur elsewhere; secondary stage: malaise, nausea, vomiting, fever, bone and joint pain, rash, and mouth sores; third stage: soft tumors, called gummas, that ulcerate and then heal, leaving scars; they may form anywhere in the body and may or may not be painful. Various parts of the body, including the heart, nervous system and lungs may be damaged, leading to death. These three stages occur over a prolonged period, often stretching 15 or more years before the tertiary stage takes hold. Congenital syphilis may result in the child being born blind or deformed. Treatment is by penicillin, often in very large doses for a prolonged period.

SYRINGE n. a device for withdrawing, injecting, or instilling a fluid. It usually includes a glass or plastic barrel with a close-fitting plunger at one end and a needle at the other end.

SYSTEMIC adj. affecting the body as a whole, rather than individual parts.

SYSTEMIC CIRCULATION n. the system of blood vessels (arteries, veins, and capillaries) that supplies all of the body, except the lungs (see *pulmonary circulation*).

SYSTEMIC LUPUS ERYTHEMATOSUS (SLE) n. a chronic inflammatory disease of unknown cause, affecting women more frequently than men. Symptoms include arthritis, a red rash over the nose and cheeks (butterfly rash), fatigue, and weakness, followed by fever, photosensitivity, and skin lesions starting in the neck region and spreading to mucous membranes and other tissues, damaging the tissues involved. Glomerulonephritis, pericarditis, anemia, and neuritis may develop. Renal failure and neurological abnormalities often occur as the disease progresses. The disease may be controlled by corticosteroids; salicylates and antimalarial drugs are also sometimes used; the patient is warned to avoid fatigue and exposure to the sun. Also: **disseminated lupus erythematosus; lupus erythematosus.**

SYSTOLE n. the contraction of the heart, esp. of the ventricles, driving blood into the aorta and pulmonary artery. adj. **systolic**

SYSTOLIC MURMUR n. a murmur heard during *systole*.

SYSTOLIC PRESSURE see *blood pressure*.

t

TABES DORSALIS n. an abnormal condition, usually associated with *syphilis*, characterized by progressive degeneration of sensory neurons and usually with symptoms of severe stabbing pains in the trunk and legs, unsteady gait, defective reflexes, incontinence, and impotence.

TABLET n. a small solid dosage form of a drug.

TACHI-, TACHO-, TACHY- comb. form indicating an association with speed (e.g., **tachypnea,** rapid breathing).

TACHYCARDIA n. an abnormally rapid heart rate—in an adult over 100 beats per minute. Heart rate normally increases in response to fear and excitement and also when there is a lack of oxygen, as in congestive heart failure, hemorrhage, shock, and other conditions.

TACTILE adj. pert. to the sense of touch.

TAENIA a genus of large parasitic tapeworms, many of which are among the most common parasites affecting humans. Included are the beef tapeworm (*T. saginata*) and the pork tapeworm (*T. solium*).

TAGAMET n. trade name for *cimetidine;* used to treat *peptic ulcer.*

TAKAYASU'S ARTERITIS n. disorder characterized by an absence of pulse in both arms and in the carotid arteries, transient paraplegia, and facial muscle weakness and atrophy caused by progressive occlusion of the left subclavian and left common carotid arteries above the *aortic arch;* also called **pulseless disease.**

TALIPES n. any of several deformities of the foot, including **talipes equinus,** in which the toes are pointed downward, and **talipes calcaneus,** in which the toes are pointed upward so the person walks on the heel of the affected foot.

TALO- comb. form indicating an association with the *ankle* (talus) (e.g., **talofibular,** pert. to the ankle and fibula).

TALUS n. a bone of the ankle; it articulates with the *tibia* and *fibula* of the lower leg and with the *calcaneus* (heelbone) below; also: **astragalus; ankle bone**

TALWIN n. trade name for the analgesic *pentazocine.*

TAMPON a plug of cotton or sponge inserted into a body passage or cavity (e.g., the vagina or nose) to absorb exuded fluids, esp. blood.

TAMPONADE n. cessation of the flow of blood to an organ or part of the body by pressure, as in cardiac tamponade when accumulated fluid compresses the heart.

TANDEARIL n. trade name for the antiinflammatory oxyphenbutazone, used to treat *arthritis* and related disorders.

TANNING n. process by which pigmentation of the skin darkens due to exposure to ultraviolet light.

TAPEWORM INFECTION n. intestinal infection caused by a species of parasitic tapeworm, usually caused by eating raw or undercooked meat or fish that is an intermediate host to the tapeworm or its larva. Symptoms include diarrhea and weight loss; diagnosis is made when worms and eggs are found in the stool.

TAPOTEMENT n. a type of massage, sometimes used on the chest wall of patients with *bronchitis* to loosen mucus, in which the body is tapped rhythmically with the fingers or sides of the hand with short rapid movements.

TARDIVE adj. late-occurring, esp. in reference to symptoms of a disease.

TARDIVE DYSKINDESIA n. abnormal condition characterized by involuntary and repetitious movements of muscles of the face, trunk, and limbs; most often occurring in older people treated with phenothiazine drugs for *parkinsonism.*

TARGET CELL n. 1. an abnormal red blood cell with a ringed appearance; associated with several types of anemia; 2. any cell with a specific receptor for an antigen, antibody, hormone, or other substance.

TARGET ORGAN n. 1. in radiology, the organ intended to receive the greatest therapeutic or diagnostic dose of a radioactive substance; 2. in endocrinology, the organ most affected by a particular hormone, as the thyroid gland is the target organ of thyroid stimulating hormone from the pituitary.

TARSAL adj. pert. to the *tarsus*, or ankle.

TARSAL BONE n. any of seven bones making up the ankle.

TARSAL GLAND n. any of numerous tiny sebaceous glands lining the inner surfaces of the eyelids. Bacterial infection of a tarsal gland produces a *stye;* also: **Meibomian gland.**

TARSITIS n. inflammation of the eyelid.

TARSUS n. 1. the seven bones of the ankle and proximal part of the foot; they articulate proximally with the tibia and fibula (lower leg bones) and with the metatarsals distally; 2. connective tissue that is the basis of each eyelid.

TARTAR n. hard deposit that forms on the teeth and gums.

TASTE n. the sense that occurs in response to the contact of dissolved material with specialized nerve receptors (taste buds) on the tongue; the impulses are then transmitted to taste centers in the brain for interpretation. There are four basic tastes: bitter (detected mostly in the back of the tongue); sour (sides of the tongue); sweet and salty (front of the tongue).

TASTE BUD n. any of numerous special sensory nerve endings located on the tongue and roof of the mouth that respond to dissolved materials, triggering impulses conducted to the taste centers in the brain. There are four basic tastes: bitter, sour, sweet, and salty; all other tastes are a combination of these; also: **gustatory organ**

TAXIS n. in surgery, the restoration by manipulation only of a dislocated organ or part to its normal position.

TAXONOMY n. the science of classifying and naming organisms on the basis of natural relationships.   adj. **taxonomic**

TAY-SACHS DISEASE an inherited disease (*autosomal recessive disease*) characterized by progressive mental and physical degeneration and early death. It is caused by a lack of the enzyme hexosaminidase, which results in an accumulation of sphingolipids in the brain. The disease occurs almost exclusively among Ashkenazic and Sephardic Jews. Symptoms appear by age 6 months, after which there is progressive degneration with blindness, the development of a cherry red spot on the retina, spasticity, dementia, and death before the age of 4. There is no treatment. The disease can be diagnosed prenatally through *amniocentesis*. Also: **amaurotic familial idiocy**

TASTE AREAS OF THE TONGUE

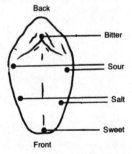

Back

Bitter

Sour

Salt

Sweet

Front

T CELL n. a small circulating *lymphocyte* that matures in the *thymus* and is the chief agent of cell-mediated immunity, involved particularly in transplant rejection and delayed hypersensitivity reactions. Special T cells, called helper T cells and suppressor T cells, affect the production of B cells, the chief agents of the humoral immune reaction.

TEAR DUCT n. a duct, such as the lacrimal duct or the nasolacrimal duct, that transports tears.

TEARING n. watering of the eye resulting from excessive tear production caused by irritation (as from a foreign object), infection, or strong emotion.

TEETHING n. physiological process of the eruption of deciduous (baby) teeth through the gums, usually extending from 4 to 6 months to about 30 months when all 20 milk teeth have appeared. Discomfort in the gum area may occur, and symptoms of drooling, biting of hard objects, and irritability are common.

TELANGIECTASIA n. a localized collection of widened and distended capillaries and small blood vessels, visible as a red spot that typically blanches on pressure. The spots may be found on the skin or mucous membranes.

TELENCEPHALON n. that part of the brain that includes the cerebral hemispheres, basal ganglia, olfactory bulb, and olfactory tracts.

TELEPATHY n. the supposed ability of one person to know the thoughts of another; the communication of thought from one person to another by nonphysical means. adj. **telepathic**

TELOPHASE n. the last of the four main stages of division within a cell nucleus, in which the new daughter chromosomes are at the poles of the division spindle, the nuclear membrane forms around them, the nucleolus reappears, and cytoplasmic division begins (see also *mitosis, meiosis*).

TEMPERATURE n. a measure of the heat associated with the metabolism of the body. Normal temperature taken orally is considered 98.6° Fahrenheit (37° Celsius), but it may vary from person to person—and even in the same person depending on the time of day and level of activity.

TEMPLE n. region of the head in front of and above each ear.

TEMPORAL adj. pert. to the *temple* of the head or the corresponding lobe of the brain.

TEMPORAL ARTERITIS n. inflammation of the cranical arteries, esp. the temporal artery; it occurs most often in elderly women and produces symptoms of headache, chewing difficulty, and sometimes impaired vision.

TEMPORAL ARTERY n. any of three arteries on each side of the head.

TEMPORAL BONE n. one of a pair of skull bones, forming the lower part of the cranium and containing cavities associated with the ear.

TEMPORALIS n. any of several muscles associated with chewing.

TEMPORAL LOBE n. a division of the cerebral cortex, lying at each side within the temple of the skull; it includes parts of the brain associated with speech, sound, and smell.

TEMPORO- comb. form indicating an association with the *temple* (temporal) region of the head (e.g., **temporomandibular,** pert. to the mandible (lower jaw) and temporal bone of the skull).

TENDERNESS n. soreness sensed on being touched; touch sensitivity. adj. **tender**

TENDINITIS n. inflammation of a tendon, usually resulting from strain or injury. Treatment includes rest and corticosteroid injections (see also *tennis elbow*).

TENDON n. one of many whitish, glistening, fibrous bands of tissue that connect muscle to bone; tendons are inelastic and strong and occur in various thicknesses and lengths (compare *ligament*).

TENESMUS n. spasm of the rectum and desire to defecate without the production of significant amounts of *feces*. It is associated with irritable bowel syndrome and other conditions.

TENNIS ELBOW n. a painful inflammation of the tendon at the outer border of the elbow caused by overuse of lower arm muscles. Treatment is by rest and corticosteroid injections.

TENO- comb. form indicating an association with a *tendon* (e.g., **tenodynia,** tendon pain).

TENOSYNOVITIS n. inflammation of the sheath surround a *tendon*, caused by repeated strain, trauma, or certain systemic conditions (e.g., gout, rheumatoid arthritis, or gonorrhea). Treatment includes rest of the affected area, corticosteroid injections, treatment of any underlying cause, and, if severe, surgical intervention.

TENSION n. 1. the condition of being taut or tense, as in muscle tension; 2. a psychophysiological state, usually a response to stress, characterized by an increase in heart rate, muscle tone, and alertness and usually accompanied by irritability, anxiety, and feelings of uneasiness.

TENSION HEADACHE. n. pain, chiefly at the back of the head and often spreading forward, occurring as a result of tensing the body as a response to overwork, strong emotion, or psychological stress.

TENSOR n. any of several muscles of the body that tenses an attached structure [e.g., **tensor tympani,** the muscle that tenses the tympanic membrane (eardrum)].

TENTH NERVE see *vagus nerve*.

TENTORIUM n. a tentlike body part, esp. the tentorium that covers the *cerebellum* and supports the occipital lobes of the cerebrum above.

TEPID adj. moderately warm.

TERAS n. a grossly deformed fetus (monster) that usually does not survive. pl. **terata** adj. **teratic**

TERATO- comb. form indicating an association with a *monster* (e.g., **teratology,** the study of developmental abnormalities).

TERATOGEN n. a substance or agent that interferes with normal embryonic development and causes the development of one or more abnormalities in the *fetus*. The type and extent of the defect is determined by the specific agent and its action, on the stage of embryonic development during which exposure occurs, and on genetic predisposition, and other modifying factors. Among the agents known to be teratogens are X rays and other forms of ionizing radiation; drugs such as thalidomide and alcohol; infectious agents, such as the agents that cause rubella and toxoplasmosis; and various chemicals that may be in the environment. The time of greatest vulnerability for the fetus is between the third and twelfth week of gestation, when most of the major organ systems are laid down. adj. **teratogenic**

TERATOGENESIS n. the development of defects in the embryo.

TERATOMA n. a tumor made up of tissue not normally found at that site, occurring most often in the testes and ovaries; some can become malignant.

TERES n. either of two muscles

(teres major and teres minor) in the shoulder region, responsible for some shoulder and arm movements.

TERM INFANT n. an infant born after the normally expected duration of pregnancy—after the 37th and before the 43rd week—of gestation, regardless of weight (compare *postmature infant; premature infant*).

TERRAMYCIN n. trade name for a *tetracycline* antibiotic (oxytetracycline).

TESTICLE   see *testis*.

TESTICULAR adj. pert. to the *testis*.

TESTICULAR CANCER n. malignant neoplasm of the testis, occurring most often in men between the ages of 20 and 35, often affecting an undescended testis and more frequently the right testis. In its early stages testicular cancer is often asymptomatic, and it may metastasize, later causing urinary and pulmonary symptoms and an abdominal mass. Treatment depends on the nature of the tumor and includes surgery (orchidectomy), radiation and/or chemotherapy.

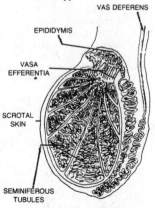

Longitudinal section of a testis, showing sperm-producing and collecting sites

TESTIS either of a pair of male *gonads*, or sex glands, that produces sperm and secretes *androgens*. The adult testes, each about 1½ inches (4 centimeters) long and oval-shaped, are suspended in the *scrotum* below the abdomen. Each testis consists of many hundred seminiferous tubules where sperm develop. The sperm pass from there through efferent ducts to the *epididymis,* after which they pass into the *vas deferens* for movement toward the *penis;* also: **testicle.**   pl. **testes**   adj. **testicular**

TESTOSTERONE n. a male sex hormone, produced chiefly in the testes, but also in small amounts in the adrenal glands and in the ovaries of women. It is responsible for the development of male secondary sex characteristics (e.g., deep voice and facial hair). Preparations of testosterone are used in the treatment of deficiency conditions, breast cancer in women, and certain other conditions. Adverse effects of the use of these preparations include fluid retention, masculinization in women, and acne.

TEST-TUBE BABY n. a baby born as a result of fertilization occurring outside the woman's body. Ova are removed from a woman's body (usually using a laparoscope) and mixed with a sperm in a culture medium. If fertilization occurs and cleavage results, the blastocyst is then implanted in the woman's *uterus* and pregnancy continues.

TETANUS n. an acute and serious infection of the central nervous system caused by an exotoxin produced by the *Clostridium tetani* bacterium. The bacterium, common in the soil, esp. in farm areas, infects wounds with dead tissue, as in a puncture wound laceration, or burn. Symptoms include fever, headache, irritability, and painful spasms of the muscles, causing lockjaw and laryngeal spasm, and, if untreated, leading to muscle spasm of virtually every organ. Prompt and thorough cleaning of wounds is important to prevent the disease. Treatment of the disease includes use of tetanus toxoid and antibiotics, maintenance of an airway if laryngeal spasm occurs, control of muscle spasms, and sedation; also called **lockjaw.**

TETANUS ANTITOXIN a tetanus immune serum given for short-term immunization against *tetanus* in cases of possible exposure to the tetanus organism. Adverse effects include pain at the site of injection and possible allergic reactions.

TETANUS IMMUNE GLOBULIN n. preparation prepared from the globulin of a person immune to tetanus and given to provide short-term protection from tetanus in cases of possible exposure to the tetanus organisms; it is considered safer than tetanus antitoxin, the chief disadvantage being pain at the site of injection.

TETANY n. a disorder, usually caused by a disorder of calcium metabolism, associated with *hypoparathyroidism*, vitamin D deficiency, or alkalosis and characterized by muscular twitching, cramps, and convulsions.

TETRACHEL n. trade name for a *tetracycline* antibiotic.

TETRACHLOROETHYLENE n. an *anthelmintic* used to treat hookworm infestation. Adverse effects include nausea, abdominal cramps, and sometimes liver toxicity.

TETRACYCLINE n. any of a family of antibiotics derived from *Streptomyces* bacteria, including chlortetracycline, oxytetracycline, and doxycycline. They are known under many trade names, and are used to treat a variety of bacterial and rickettsial infections. They are not used during pregnancy nor in young children because they cause discoloration of children's teeth. Other adverse effects include gastrointestinal disturbances, suprainfections, and allergic reactions.

TETRAHYDROCANNABINOL (THC) n. the active principle in hemp plant derivatives such as marihuana, hashish, and ganja. Considered a mild hallucinogen, it causes sensory and perceptual disturbances, euphoria and other mood changes, decreased motor coordination, and various physiological changes including alterations in pulse rate, respiration rate, and pupil size.

TETRALOGY OF FALLOT n. a congenital heart defect characterized by four anomalies: pulmonary stenosis; ventricular septal defect; malposition of the aorta; and hypertrophy of the right ventricle. The infant exhibits cyanosis and other signs of a lack of oxygen; failure to thrive; poor development; and later clubbing of the fingers and toes. Treatment is by surgical repair, usually done when the child is 4 to 5 years old; also called **blue baby.**

TETREX trade name for a *tetracycline* preparation.

THALAMUS n. one of two large, oval-shaped masses of gray matter deep in the *cerebral hemispheres* concerned with relaying sensory impulses to the cerebral cortex and also the site where crude sensations of pain, pressure, and temperature originate. adj. **thalamic**

THALASSEMIA n. a hereditary (autosomal recessive) form of *anemia,* occurring most often in people of Mediterranean origin, characterized by abnormal hemoglobin synthesis. Those homozygous for the trait—**thalassemia major**—are severely affected in childhood with anemia, enlarged

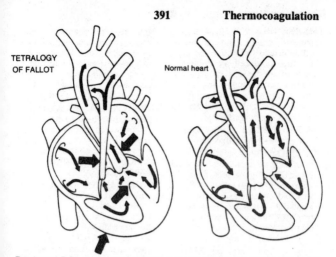

TETRALOGY
OF FALLOT

Normal heart

Tetralogy of Fallot (1) Narrowing of pulmonary artery or valve; (2) defect in the septum separating the ventricles; (3) overriding aorta; (4) hypertrophied right ventricle.

spleen, failure to thrive, iron accumulation in the tissues, respiratory difficulty, and retarded growth and development. There is no cure; treatment involves repeated transfusions. Those heterozygous for the trait, inheriting it from only one parent—**thalassemia minor**—may have few or no symptoms. The disease can be detected prenatally through *amniocentesis*. Also called **Cooley's anemia.**

THALIDOMIDE n. a sedative drug, no longer used, because of its teratogenic properties when taken during pregnancy.

THANATOLOGY n. the study of death and dying.

THC abbreviation for *tetrahydrocannabinol*.

THECA a sheath or capsule covering.

THELARCHE n. the beginning of female breast development, usually occurring between the ages of 9 and 13, before puberty (compare *menarche*).

THENAR n. the palm, esp. the raised fleshy part of the palm at the base of the thumb. adj. **thenal**

THEOBID n. trade name for a fixed-combination drug, containing the smooth muscle relaxant theophylline and the sedative butabarbital; used to treat some respiratory disorders, esp. those marked by spasm of the airways.

THERAPEUTIC ABORTION n. termination of a pregnancy deemed necessary for the physical or psychological health of the woman.

THERAPEUTICS n. that branch of medical science specifically concerned with treatment. adj. **therapeutic**

THERM-, THERMO- comb. form indicating an association with heat (e.g., **thermalgesia,** heat-caused pain).

THERMAL adj. pert to heat or the production of heat.

THERMOCAUTERY n. the destruction of tissue by heat, as by direct flame or electric current.

THERMOCOAGULATION n. congealing of tissue by heat (electric current).

THERMOGRAPHY n. a technique for sensing (by means of an infrared detector) and recording the heat produced by different parts of the body; it is used to study blood flow and detect tumors (which may show as hot spots), esp. those of the breast (*mammothermography*).

THERMOLABILE adj. easily changed or destroyed by heat.

THERMOMETER a device for measuring temperature, usually consisting of glass tube marked with degrees Fahrenheit or Celsius and containing mercury or alcohol that rises or falls as it expands or contracts according to changes in temperature.

THERMOTHERAPY n. the use of heat, as with heating pads, hot compresses, and hot water bottles, to treat a disease or disorder (e.g., to promote circulation in peripheral vascular disease or to relax tense muscles).

THETA RHYTHM n. a brainwave frequency of relatively low frequency and low amplitude; the drowsy waves characteristic of a person who is awake but relaxed and sleepy. It is one of four brain wave patterns (compare *alpha rhythm, beta rhythm, delta rhythm*); also called **theta wave.**

THETA WAVE see *theta rhythm*.

THIAMINE n. a member of the B-complex group of vitamins; essential for functioning of the cardiovascular and nervous systems and for metabolism; also: **thiamin;** also called **vitamin B$_1$, antiberiberi factor.** (see Table of Vitamins).

THIAZIDE n. any of a group of compounds, many of which are commonly used diuretics (see *diuretic*).

THIGH n. section of the leg between the hip and the knee.

THIGH BONE see *femur*.

THIOPENTAL n. a strong, short-acting barbiturate used as anesthesia for very short surgical procedures and as an induction to another anesthetic agent. It depresses respiration and heart activity and may be habit-forming.

THIOGUANINE n. an antineoplastic drug used to treat acute leukemias and other malignant neoplastic diseases. Adverse effects include bone marrow depression and gastrointestinal disturbances.

THIORDIAZINE n. a major tranquilizer, known under the trade name Mellaril, used to treat schizophrenia and many other psychotic disorders. Adverse effects include low blood pressure, liver toxicity, and blood disorders.

THIOSULFIL n. trade name for a *sulfonamide* antibacterial.

THIOTEPA n. an antineoplastic drug used to treat certain malignancies. Adverse effects include nausea, vomiting, and bone marrow depression.

THIURETIC n. trade name for the *diuretic hydrochlorothiazide*.

THORACIC adj. pert. to the thorax.

THORACIC AORTA n. the large upper part of the descending aorta supplying the heart, chest muscles, ribs, and stomach.

THORACIC DUCT n. one of the two major trunks of the lymphatic system; it drains lymph from the abdomen and lower limbs and from the left side of the thorax and head and empties it into the junction of the left subclavian and left internal jugular vein.

THORACIC MEDICINE n. that branch of medicine concerned with diagnosis and treatment of diseases of the chest.

THORACIC NERVES n. the 12 spinal nerves on each side of the thorax distributed to the walls of the thorax and abdomen.

THORACIC OUTLET SYN-DROME n. an abnormal condition characterized by tingling sensation in the fingers and caused by compression on a nerve supplying the arm.

THORACIC VERTEBRAE n. any of 12 vertebrae of the vertebral column, starting (T1) below the seventh cervical vertebra (C7) and extending to the first lumbar vertebra (L1).

THORACO- comb. form indicating an association with the chest (e.g., **thoracocentesis,** draining of fluid through a needle from the chest for diagnostic or therapeutic purposes).

THORAX n. the bone and cartilage cage, formed in the front by the sternum and rib cartilage and in the back by the thoracic vertebrae and dorsal parts of the ribs, that encloses the lungs, heart, esophagus, and other structures; also called **chest.**

THORAZINE n. trade name for *chlorpromazine,* widely used as a *tranquilizer* in the treatment of psychotic disorders.

THREATENED ABORTION see under *abortion.*

THREE-DAY MEASLES see *rubella.*

THRESHOLD n. the minimal point at which a stimulus evokes a response.

THRILL n. a fine vibration that can be felt on placing the hand on the body.

THROB n. a deep, pulsating type of pain or discomfort.

THROMB-, THROMBO- comb. form indicating an association with a blood clot (*thrombus*) (e.g., **thromboclasis,** the breaking up of a clot).

THROMBASTHENIA n. a rare, inherited (autosomal recessive) disease in which platelets do not function normally to produce a clot and hemorrhage ensues. Treatment is by platelet transfusion.

THROMBECTOMY n. surgical removal of a thrombus (blood clot) from a blood vessel to restore circulation to the affected part.

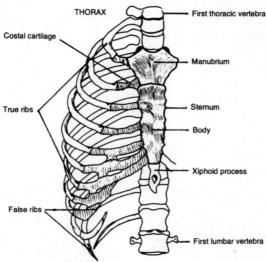

THORAX

Costal cartilage — True ribs — False ribs

First thoracic vertebra — Manubrium — Sternum — Body — Xiphoid process — First lumbar vertebra

Courtesy Carolina Biological Supply Co.

THROMBIN n. a coagulation factor, formed in plasma from prothrombin, calcium, and thromboplastin, that acts to change fibrinogen to fibrin, necessary for a blood clot.

THROMBOANGIITIS OBLITERANS see *Buerger's disease*.

THROMBOCYTE see *platelet*.

THROMBOCYTOPENIA n. an abnormal condition characterized by a lower-than-normal number of platelets and resulting in bleeding and easy bruising. Causes of the reduced platelet level include drug reactions and neoplastic disease of blood forming tissue. Treatment depends on the cause.

THROMBOCYTOPENIC PURPURA n. a bleeding disorder in which *petechiae*, bruises, and bleeding into the tissues occurs because of decreased platelet levels; it may occur as a drug reaction or in association with infectious or toxic disorders.

THROMBOCYTOSIS n. an increase in the number of platelets in the blood, causing an increased tendency for clots to form; it is associated with many chronic infections, neoplasms, and other diseases.

THROMBOEMBOLISM n. a condition in which a blood vessel is blocked by an *embolus* carried in the bloodstream from its site of formation. The area affected by the diminished blood supply may become cyanotic and numb. Treatment includes anticoagulants, rest, warm wet packs, and surgery if the aorta, pulmonary arteries, or other major vessels are obstructed.

THROMBOPHLEBITIS n. inflammation of a vein, usually with clot formation. It occurs as a result to trauma to the blood vessel, prolonged immobilization and consequent venous stasis, hyper-coagulability of the blood, infection, or irritation. Treatment includes rest of the affected area (most often the legs), moist heat, and the use of anticoagulants and agents (e.g., streptokinase) to dissolve clots. Close monitoring to detect signs of pulmonary embolism, myocardial infarction, or other serious complication is essential; also called **phlebitis.**

THROMBOPLASTIN n. a substance found in most tissues and some blood cells that starts the blood coagulation process, converting prothrombin to *thrombin*.

THROMBOSIS n. a condition in which a blood clot (*thrombus*) forms within a blood vessel. Thrombosis in a artery supplying the brain results in a stroke (*cerebrovascular accident*); in an artery supplying the heart in a *myocardial infarction;* in veins *thrombophlebitis*. A thrombus may also move from its site of origin (see *embolism*).

THROMBUS n. a blood clot attached to the interior wall of a vein or artery (compare *embolus*).

THRUSH see *candidiasis*.

THYMIC adj. pert. to the *thymus*.

THYMINE n. a base found in DNA (*deoxyribonucleic acid*).

THYMO- comb. form indicating an association with the *thymus* (e.g., **thymoma,** a tumor, usually benign, of the thymus).

THYMOSIN n. hormone secreted by the thymus, present in greatest amounts in childhood and decreasing in amount throughout life.

THYMUS n. a bi-lobed gland situated below the thyroid gland and behind the sternum and involved in the function of the lymphatic system and the immune system. The gland increases in size until puberty, after which it involutes, becoming smaller and decreasing in functional activity during adulthood.

THYRO- comb. form indicating an association with the *thyroid gland* (e.g., **thyromegaly,** thyroid gland enlargement).

THYROCALCITONIN see *calcitonin.*

THYROID CARTILAGE n. large cartilage of the larynx, forming the Adam's apple.

THYROIDECTOMY n. surgical removal of the thyroid gland, usually done to remove tumors or to treat *hyperthyroidism* that does not respond to other therapies.

THYROID GLAND n. a large *endocrine gland* situated at the base of the neck. It consists of two lobes, one on each side of the *trachea,* connected by an isthmus. Under the influence of thyroid-stimulating hormone (TSH) released from the *anterior pituitary gland,* the thyroid secretes the hormone thyroxin into the bloodstream; it is essential for normal growth and development in children and normal metabolic rates in adults. Disorders of the thyroid include *goiter, myxedema,* and *cretinism.*

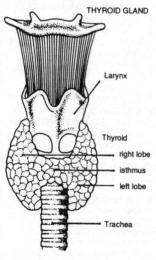

THYROID GLAND

Larynx

Thyroid

right lobe

isthmus

left lobe

Trachea

THYROIDITIS n. inflammation of the thyroid gland. Acute thyroiditis is usually due to bacterial or other infection and is marked by abscess formation and signs of infection; chronic forms include several hereditary conditions (e.g., *Hashimoto disease*) and responses to irradiation of the thyroid.

THYROID - STIMULATING HORMONE (TSH) n. a hormone secreted by the *anterior pituitary gland* that controls the release of thyroid hormone from the thyroid. It is influenced by thyrotropin releasing factor from the *hypothalamus.*

THYROID STORM n. a crisis in uncontrolled hyperthyroidism in which the release of thyroid hormone into the bloodstream causes rapid pulse, fever, respiratory distress, and restlessness, leading to delirium, heart failure, and death. Treatment is by antithyroid drugs.

THYROTOXICOSIS see *Grave's disease.*

THYROTROPIN RELEASING FACTOR (TRF) n. substance released by the *hypothalamus* that controls the release of *thyroid-stimulating hormone* from the *anterior pituitary gland.*

TIBIA n. the inner and larger bone of the lower leg (the second longest bone in the body); it articulates proximally with the femur, forming part of the knee joint, and with the fibula (the other lower leg bone) and talus (ankle bone) distally.

TIBIO- comb. form indicating an association with the *tibia* (e.g., **tibiofemoral,** pert. to the tibia and the femur).

TIC n. a repeated, largely involuntary, spasm or twitch, esp. of part of the face.

TIC DOULOUREUS see *trigeminal neuralgia.*

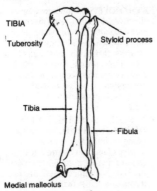

TIBIA

Tuberosity

Styloid process

Tibia

Fibula

Medial malleolus

Courtesy Carolina Biological Supply Co.

TICK n. a blood-sucking parasite, some species of which cause diseases in humans, including *Lyme arthritis*, *Rocky Mountain spotted fever*, and *tularemia*.

TIETZE'S SYNDROME n. a disorder characterized by swelling of rib cartilage causing pain; it may accompany a chronic respiratory disorder, but in many cases the cause is unknown and it resolves without treatment.

TINEA n. any of a group of fungus-caused skin diseases, usually characterized by skin lesions, scaling and itchiness: also called **roundworm**.

TINEA CAPITIS n. contagious fungal infection of the scalp characterized by bald patches, reddening, and crust formation. Treatment is by the antifungal griseofulvin.

TINEA CORPORIS n. fungal infection of nonhairy parts of the skin, most common in warm areas. Treatment is by antifungal agents.

TINEA CRURIS n. fungal infection of the groin, most common in males, and often associated with warmth and local irritation; also called **jock itch.**

TINEA PEDIS n. common fungal infection of the skin of the foot, esp. the skin between the toes. Treatment is by griseofulvin; also called **athlete's foot.**

TINEA UNGUIUM n. fungal infection of the nails that can cause complete crumbling of the nails, esp. the toenails. Treatment is by griseofulvin.

TINE TEST n. a tuberculin skin test in which a disc with several tines bearing tuberculin antigen is used to puncture the skin. The development of hardened skin around the area indicates active disease or previous exposure and the need for further testing.

TINNITUS n. ringing in the ears; it may be a sign of trauma to the ear area, Meniere's disease, or an accumulation of earwax.

TISSUE n. a collection of cells specialized to perform a particular function. The cells may be all of the same type (e.g., in nervous tissue) or of different types (e.g., in connective tissue). An aggregate of tissues with a specific function is an *organ*.

TISSUE TYPING n. a series of tests to determine the compatibility of tissues from a donor and a recipient prior to transplantation.

TOCOPHEROL n. any of a group of fat-soluble compounds with vitamin E activity occurring in many fish, seed, and vegetable oils and functioning as important antioxidants (see Table of Vitamins).

TOE n. a digit of the foot.

TOFRANIL n. trade name for the tricyclic antidepressant *imipramine*.

TOLAZAMIDE n. an antidiabetic used in the treatment of adult-onset, stable *diabetes mellitus*. Adverse effects include nausea, diarrhea, and weakness.

TOLAZOLINE n. a vasodilator used to treat spasms of peripheral blood vessels (e.g., Raynaud's disease).

TOLBUTAMIDE n. an oral antidiabetic used in the treatment of adult *diabetes mellitus*. Adverse effects include low blood sugar and skin reaction.

TOLINASE n. trade name for the antidiabetic *tolazamide*.

TOMOGRAPHY see *computed tomography*

-TOMY suffix meaning a surgical incision into an organ (e.g., **gastromy,** incision into the stomach).

TONE n. normal state of balanced tension and responsiveness of the body, esp. the muscles. also: **tonus** adj. **tonic**

TONGUE n. the mucous-membrane covered, muscular organ attached to the floor of the mouth by the frenulum linguae. The surface is covered with papillae and taste buds. The tongue manipulates food during chewing and swallowing; functions in the production of speech and different sounds; and is the main organ of taste; also: **glossa; lingua.** adj. **lingual**

TONIC adj. pert. to normal muscle tone; 2. marked by tension, as in tonic muscle spasm. n. a substance taken to increase the sense of vigor.

TONICITY n. state of normal muscle tone, ready to contract.

TONOMETER n. an instrument used to measure tension or pressure, esp. intraocular pressure in testing for *glaucoma*.

TONSIL n. mass of lymphoid tissue, esp. one of the paired masses at the back of the mouth (palatine tonsils or lingual tonsils) concerned with response to infection.

TONSILLECTOMY n. surgical removal of the palatine tonsils, usually performed to prevent recurrent streptococcal infections; often performed together with *adenoidectomy*.

TONSILLITIS n. inflammation or infection of a tonsil, esp. the palatine tonsils. Acute tonsillitis, often caused by bacterial, esp. streptococcal, infection, produces sore throat, fever, headache, enlarged lymph glands in the neck region, and difficulty in swallowing. Treatment is by rest, fluids, and antibiotics. Surgery (*tonsillectomy*) is sometimes performed to prevent recurrent streptococcal attacks.

TONUS n. see *tone*.

TOOTH n. any of the hard structures in the mouth used to cut, grind, and process food. Each tooth contains an enamel-covered *crown* above the gum and a neck with a dentin-covered pulp-filled cavity that stretches to the cementum-covered root embedded in the socket of the jaw. Normally two sets of teeth appear during life: a deciduous (milk) set, made up of 20 teeth, that appears during infancy; and a permanent set of 32 teeth that appears gradually during childhood and early adulthood. The 32 adult teeth differ somewhat in their shape and function (see *canine, incisor, molar, premolar*) (see also *deciduous teeth; permanent teeth*).

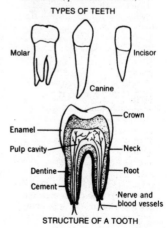

TYPES OF TEETH

Molar — Incisor

Canine

Crown
Enamel
Neck
Pulp cavity
Dentine — Root
Cement

Nerve and blood vessels

STRUCTURE OF A TOOTH

TOPICAL adj. pert. to the surface of a part, as a drug applied to the skin surface.

TOPICAL ANESTHESIA n. surface anesthesia obtained by applying a topical agent, such as benzocaine or lidocaine, to the skin or mucous membrane.

TORPIDITY n. sluggishness. adj. **torpid**

TORPOR n. a state of decreased responsiveness and sluggishness; occurring in some mental disorders, some types of posioning, and some metabolic disorders; also: **torbidity** adj. **torpid**

TORSION n. twisting.

TORTICOLLIS n. abnormal condition in which the head leans to one side due to contraction of the muscles of the neck on that side; it may be congenital or the result of injury. Treatment depends on the cause and severity of the condition; it may include immobilization, pain relievers (if the muscle spasm produces severe pain), and surgical intervention; also called **wryneck.**

TOTACILLIN n. trade name for the antibacterial *ampicillin.*

TOTAL PARENTERAL NUTRITION (TPN) n. administration of a nutritionally adequate solution (containing, e.g., proteins, electrolytes and vitamins) through a catheter into the vena cava; used to provide nutrients in cases of long-term coma, severe burns, and severe gastrointestinal or malabsorption syndromes; also called **hyperalimentation.**

TOURNIQUET n. a device, as a tight bandage or rubber tube, pressed on an artery to stop the flow of blood in a hemorrhage; used only when other measures cannot be used or have not succeeded.

TOX-, TOXI-, TOXICO-, TOXO- comb. form indicating an association with a poison or poisoning

(e.g., **toxicogenic,** producing poisons).

TOXEMIA n. blood poisoning caused by bacterial toxins and characterized by systemic symptoms such as fever and vomiting.

TOXEMIA OF PREGNANCY n. an abnormal condition of pregnancy characterized by high blood pressure, fluid retention and edema, and proteins in the urine. The cause is unknown. Severe cases may lead to *preeclampsia* and *eclampsia.*

TOXIC adj. pert. to a poison; 2. pert. to a disease that is progressive.

TOXICITY n. the extent or degree to which something is poisonous.

TOXICOLOGY n. the study of poisons and their effects on living organisms.

TOXIC SHOCK SYNDROME (TSS) n. a serious acute infection caused by toxin elaborated by certain strains of *Staphylococcus aureus;* it most often occurs in menstruating women using high-absorbency tampons but also occasionally occurs in nonmenstruating women, men, and children. Onset is sudden with fever, headache, reddish skin, sore throat, and gastrointestinal disturbances; low blood pressure and renal and liver abnormalities may follow, leading to death.

TOXIN n. a poison, esp. one produced or occurring in a plant or microorganism.

TOXOID n. a weakened toxin that, when introduced into the body, causes antibody formation and the development of immunity to the specific disease caused by the toxin.

TOXOPLASMOSIS n. a common infection with the parasite *Toxoplasma gondii* transmitted to humans by contact with infected cats or their feces or litter boxes or by eating poorly cooked meat containing cysts of the parasites. The infection often produces only mild illness with few or minimal symptoms, such as malaise, low-grade fever, and swollen lymph glands. However, it is dangerous if contracted by a pregnant woman: it can cause serious damage to the fetus.

TPN abbreviation for *total parenteral nutrition*.

TRABECULA n. mass of connective tissue that divides an organ into parts (e.g., in the penis) or which stabilizes and secures an organ, as with the spleen.   pl. **trabeculae**   adj. **trabecular**

TRACE ELEMENT n. an element necessary to nutrition and normal functioning in minute quantities.

TRACER n. in radiology, a radioactive isotope introduced into the body to allow biological structures to be seen as part of diagnostic X-ray techniques.

TRACHEA n. tube extending from the *larynx* to the bronchi that conveys air to the lungs. It is about 4 inches (11 centimeters) long, covered in the front by the isthmus of the thyroid gland, and in contact in the back with the esophagus; also called **windpipe.**   adj. **tracheal**

TRACHEITIS n. inflammation of the *trachea*, resulting from infection, irritation, or allergic reaction.

TRACHEO- comb. form indicating an association with the *trachea* (e.g., **tracheobronchial,** pert. to the *trachea* and the *bronchi*).

TRACHEOBRONCHITIS n. a common respiratory infection characterized by inflammation of both the trachea and the bronchi.

TRACHEOSTOMY n. a surgically created opening into the *trachea* with a tube inserted to establish an airway when the pharynx is obstructed by tumor, edema, or other cause.

TRACHEOTOMY an incision into the *trachea* through the neck below the larynx performed to gain access to the airway below a blockage and usually to insert an airway tube.

TRACHOMA n. chronic infection of the eye, caused by *Chlamydia trachomatis,* common in many tropical areas, esp. where sanitation is limited; in the United States it occurs primarily in the Southwest, esp. on Amerindian reservations. Early signs of inflammation, pus, and tearing may lead to scar formation, causing blindness. Treatment is by antibiotics.

TRACT n. 1. a group of organs and tissues concerned with a common function or arranged serially (e.g., the digestive tract or the respiratory tract); 2. a group of nerve fibers passing from one part of the central nervous system to another part.

TRACTION n. in orthopedics, to place a bone or limb under tension to immobilize the part, align parts in a particular way, or relieve pressure.

TRAGUS n. a projection of cartilage of the auricle, or outer ear.   pl. **tragi**

TRAIT n. a characteristic, esp. an inherited characteristic.

TRANCE n. a sleeplike state characterized by detachment from one's surroundings, as in deep concentration, or diminished motor activity, as in hypnosis or a cataleptic state.

TRANQUILIZER n. a drug that produces a calming effect, lessening anxiety and tension. Most tranquilizers induce drowsiness and can cause dependence.
major tranquilizer n. a drug, usually a derivative of phenothiazine or butyrophenone, used to treat psychotic conditions in which a calming effect is desired.
minor tranquilizer n. any of several drugs, including diaze-

pam (Valium) and chlordiazepoxide (Librium), used to relieve anxiety, tension, and irritability; many also reduce skeletal muscle spasm.

TRANS- comb. form meaning "across" or "through" (e.g., **transabdominal,** through the wall of the abdomen).

TRANSCRIPTION n. in genetics, the process by which the genetic information contained in DNA (deoxyribonucleic acid) in the nucleus is transferred to messenger RNA (ribonucleic acid), which then leaves the nucleus to direct protein synthesis in the ribosomes.

TRANSFERENCE n. in psychoanalysis, the patient's assignment of qualities, emotions, and attitudes of a person significant in his/her early life, usually a parent, to the therapist; used as a means of understanding and dealing with emotional conflicts.

TRANSFER RNA (tRNA) n. the ribonucleic acid with the function of attaching the correct amino acid to the protein chain being synthesized at the ribosome of a cell, according to the coded directions of messenger RNA (transcribed from the genetic message of DNA in the nucleus).

TRANSFUSION n. the introduction of whole blood or components of blood (e.g., plasma, platelets, or packed erythrocytes) from one person (the donor) or from pooled material into the bloodstream of another (the recipient). Donor and recipient blood must be typed to determine if they are compatible (see also *blood typing*).

TRANSFUSION REACTION n. response by the body to the introduction of blood that is not compatible with its own. Signs of an adverse reaction range from fever, hive formation, and headache to severe asthmatic attacks, deep chest and back pain, diffi-

culty in breathing, vascular collapse, renal failure, shock, and death.

TRANSIENT ISCHEMIC ATTACK (TIA) n. a usually very brief episode in which there is insufficient blood supply to the brain, usually caused by atherosclerotic plaque or embolus. Symptoms depend on the site affected and the size of the blockage and may include dizziness, disturbance of vision, and numbness.

TRANSLATION n. the process by which the genetic information carried in coded form by messenger RNA (after its transcription from DNA in the nucleus) directs the formation of a specific protein at a ribosome in the cytoplasm.

TRANSLOCATION n. in genetics, the rearrangement of genetic material on a chromosome or the transfer of a part of one chromosome to another nonhomologus chromosome. Translocations can result in serious congenital disorders.

TRANSPLACENTAL adj. passing across or through the *placenta,* as nutrients and wastes.

TRANSPLANT v. to transfer an organ or tissue from one person (the donor) to another (the recipient) or from one body part to another to replace a diseased organ or to restore normal function. The organs most commonly transplanted are the skin and kidneys; corneal, bone, cartilage, and vessel transplants also occur; and rarely heart and liver transplants. The major problem with donor-recipient transplants is the tendency of the recipient's body to reject the transplanted tissue as foreign; donor and recipient are carefully matched by blood typing and tissue typing procedures (the best donors are identical twins) to minimize the chances of rejection. n. any organ or tissue transferred from one person to another or from one part of the body to another part.   n. **transplantation**

TRANSPORT n. the movement of materials within the body, esp. across cell membranes (see *active transport; passive transport*).

TRANSPOSITION n. 1. abnormal placement of an organ or part so that it is on the side opposite its normal position; 2. in genetics, the shifting of genetic material from one chromosome to another, often resulting in congenital defects.

TRANSSEXUALISM n. condition in which a person firmly believes and assumes the psychological identity of the sex opposite to his or her biological gender. n. **transsexual**

TRANSUDATION n. the passage of a liquid through a membrane, as into the intercellular space of a tissue or through a capillary wall.

TRANSVERSE adj. situated at right angle to the long axis of the body or organ.

TRANSVERSE COLON n. that part of the colon that extends across the midabdomen from the ascending colon on the right side to the beginning of the descending colon on the left side.

TRANYLCYPROMINE n. an *MAO inhibitor* used to treat *depression*. Adverse effects include headache, vertigo, orthostatic hypotension, and, as with all MAO inhibitors, the possibility of drug or food interactions causing a severe episode of hypertension.

TRAPEZIUM n. a bone of the wrist.

TRAPEZIUS n. the large, flat triangular muscle of the shoulder and upper back region involved in movement of the shoulder and arm.

TRAPEZOID BONE n. the smallest of the wrist bones.

TRAUMA n. 1. physical injury caused by accident, violence, or disruptive action (e.g., a fracture); 2. severe emotional shock. adj. **traumatic**

TRAUMATOLOGY n. that branch of medicine concerned with the surgical repair of wounds and injuries arising from accidents; accident surgery.

TREADMILL TEST n. an exercise device consisting of a moving platform, on which a patient walks while having his/her heart and breathing rates monitored; it is used to determine the effect of exertion on heart function.

TREMATODE n. a parasitic flatworm, some of which cause disease in humans (e.g., shistosomiasis).

TREMOR n. rhythmic, quivering movements from involuntary alternating contraction and relaxation of skeletal muscles; it may occur as a result of age (senile tremor) or disease (e.g., *parkinsonism, multiple sclerosis,* and many degenerative diseases of the nervous system); some forms are hereditary.

TRENCH MOUTH n. infection of the mouth and gums marked by ulcers on the mucous membranes; it often occurs as a secondary infection in malnourished or debilitated people. Treatment depends on the cause, the primary illness, and health of the person.

TREPONEMA n. a genus of spirochetes, some of which produce disease in humans (e.g., *Treponema pallidum,* the cause of *syphilis*).

TRI- prefix meaning "three" (e.g., **trilaminar,** having three layers).

TRIAGE n. a classification process, used in military medicine and in disasters, whereby casualties are sorted according to the severity of their injuries and their need for immediate treatment so that those most likely to survive with treatment will be given medical care first. In many systems, the injured are grouped as those with life threatening injuries that can be saved with immediate treatment; those with serious injuries that should be treated within 1 or 2 hours; and those with noncritical injuries for whom treatment can be delayed until more urgent cases are tended to.

TRIAMCINOLONE n. a synthetic corticosteroid used as an antiinflammatory agent. Adverse effects include gastrointestinal and endocrine disturbances and, if used topically, skin rashes.

TRICEPS adj. three-headed, esp. triceps brachii muscle of the back surface of the upper arm that functions to extend the forearm and adduct the upper arm (compare *biceps*).

TRICHIASIS n. abnormal turning in of the eyelashes that causes irritation of the eyeball; it may result from inflammation of the eyelids.

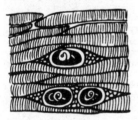

Trichina
(encysted in human muscle)

TRICHINOSIS n. infestation with the parasitic roundworm *Trichinella spiralis*, transmitted by eating undercooked meat, esp. pork. Symptoms vary greatly in severity and include nausea, diarrhea, abdominal pain, and fever, sometimes progressing to muscle pain, tenderness and stiffness as the roundworm larvae migrate from the intestinal tract to the muscles

where they become encysted. There is no specific cure; treatment is aimed at alleviating symptoms. Once all the larvae become encysted completely symptoms usually disappear.

TRICHLORMETHIAZIDE n. a diuretic, known under the trade names Naqua and Ropres, used to treat *hypertension*. Adverse effects include electrolyte imbalances.

TRICHO- comb. form indicating an association with *hair* (e.g., **trichology,** the study of hair).

TRICHOBEZOAR n. a hair ball, sometimes formed in the alimentary canal.

TRICHOMONIASIS n. an infection of the *vagina* (occasionally the urethra in males) caused by the *Trichomonas vaginalis* protozoon and characterized by a foul-smelling, pale yellowish vaginal discharge, burning, and itching. Treatment is by the antimicrobial metronidazole, usually given orally.

TRICHURIASIS n. infestation with the roundworm *Trichuris trichiura,* common in tropical areas, esp. with poor sanitation. Symptoms include diarrhea, nausea, and abdominal pain.

TRICLOFOS n. a sedative-hypnotic related to chloral hydrate, known under the trade name Triclos, used to treat insomnia and produce sedation, esp. in children. Adverse effects include gastrointestinal disturbances and the possibility of drug dependence.

TRICLOS n. trade name for the sedative *triclofos*.

TRICUSPID adj. having three cusps or points.

TRICUSPID VALVE n. a valve with three cusps situated between the right atrium and the right ventricle of the heart, where it allows the passage of blood from the atrium to the ventricle and closes to prevent backflow when the ventricle contracts.

TRIGEMINAL NERVE n. either of the largest pair of cranial nerves; it is involved in facial sensibility, chewing, and other muscular actions of the face; also: **tenth nerve.**

TRIGEMINAL NEURALGIA n. condition resulting from pressure on or degeneration of the trigeminal nerve, causing paroxysms of severe, stabbing pain radiating along a branch of the nerve, usually from the angle of the jaw, also: **tic douloureux.**

TRIGYLCERIDE n. a compound consisting of a fatty acid and glycerol that is the principal lipid in the blood, usually bound to a protein forming a lipoprotein. The amount and proportion of different types of triglycerides in the blood is important in the diagnosis of many diseases, including heart disease and diabetes mellitus.

TRIMESTER n. one of the three periods, each of approximately three months, into which pregnancy is divided.

FIRST TRIMESTER n. that part of pregnancy extending from the first day of the last menstrual period through 12 weeks of gestation.

SECOND TRIMESTER n. that part of pregnancy extending from the 13th through the 27th week of gestation.

THIRD TRIMESTER n. that part of the pregnancy extending from the 28th week until delivery.

TRIMIPRAMINE n. an antidepressant, known under the trade name Surmontil, used to treat depression and anxiety and occasionally insomnia. Adverse effects include symptoms of parkinsonism, rapid heartbeat, hypotension, and increased ocular pressure.

TRIPLET n. any of three off-spring born at the same time from the same pregnancy.

TRIPLOID adj. pert. to an organism or cell that has three complete sets of chromosomes, not the normal two. In humans triploid fetuses are usually spontaneously aborted or stillborn; in the few cases of live birth, they are grossly deformed and die quickly.

TRISMUS n. prolonged spasm of jaw muscles.

TRISOMY n. a condition in which one more than the normal number of chromosomes exists in a cell, or, in other words, there are three, not the normal diploid two, chromosomes in a cell. This chromosomal aberration is associated with many congenital defects, the type and severity of the abnormal condition depending on which chromosome is affected. Trisomy 21, for example, is *Down's syndrome.*

TRI-VI-FLOR n. trade name for an oral, pediatric fixed-combination drug, containing fluorine and vitamins A, C, and D.

tRNA see *transfer RNA.*

TROCHANTER n. one of two bony projections (the greater trochanter and the lesser trochanter) on the proximal end of the femur that serve for the attachment of muscles.

TROCHE n. a lozenge containing a drug.

TROCHLEAR NERVE n. either of the smallest pair of cranial nerves; it is essential for eye sensation and movement; also: **fourth cranial nerve.**

TROPHOBLAST n. the layer of tissue that forms the wall of the *blastocyst* in early development; aids in implantation in the uterine wall; and after implantation, divides into two layers, one becoming the *chorion,* the other the outer layer of the *placenta.* adj. **trophoblastic**

TROPHOBLASTIC CANCER n. a malignant neoplasm of the *uterus* derived from epithelium of the chorion, often associated with *hydatid mole*, sometimes with normal or tubal pregnancy or abortion. Treatment is by hysterectomy and chemotherapy.

TROPICAL MEDICINE n. that branch of medicine concerned with the diagnosis and treatment of diseases, such as shistosomiasis, malaria, and yellow fever, found most commonly in tropical regions.

TROPICAL SORE see *oriental sore*.

TROPICAL SPRUE see *sprue*.

TRUSS n. a device to prevent protrusion of abdominal organs through a weakness in the abdominal wall.

TRYPANOSOMIASIS n. infection with a parasite of the *Trypanosoma* genus. Among these infections are *African trypanosomiasis* and *Chagas' disease*.

TRYPSIN n. an enzyme involved in the digestion of proteins. The inactive form trypsinogen is secreted by the *pancreas* and converted to active trypsin in the *duodenum*.

TRYPTOPHAN n. an amino acid essential for growth and normal metabolism. It is a precursor of niacin.

TSETSE FLY n. insect that carries the parasites that cause *trypanosomiasis*.

TSH abbreviation for *thyroid-stimulating hormone*.

TSS abbreviation for *toxic shock syndrome*.

TUBAL LIGATION n. a sterilization procedure in which both Fallopian tubes are ligated (tied) in two places and the intervening space removed or crushed so that the tube is effectively blocked and conception cannot occur. It is a common method of *contraception*.

TUBAL PREGNANCY n. a type of ectopic pregnancy in which the conceptus implants in the Fallopian tube; it is the most common type of ectopic pregnancy (about 90%), with prior injury to the tube and pelvic infection predisposing factors. Symptoms occur as the embryo grows and ruptures the tube and include sudden sharp pain on one side of the abdomen and bleeding, but diagnosis is often difficult. Treatment is removal of the products of conception and removal or repair of the ruptured tube.

TUBERCLE n. 1. a nodule (e.g., on a bone); 2. a nodule caused by *Mycobacterium tuberculosis*.

TUBERCULIN TEST n. a test to determine past or present infection or exposure to *tuberculosis* based on a skin reaction to the injection, scratching, or puncturing of the skin with tuberculin, a purified protein derivative of the tuberculosis bacterium. Types of tuberculin tests include the Mantoux test and the tine test.

TUBERCULOSIS n. a chronic infection with the *Mytcobacterium tuberculosis*, transmitted by inhalation or ingestion of droplets; it usually affects the lungs but may also affect other organs. Early symptoms include fever, loss of appetite, fatigue, and vague chest pain; later, symptoms of night sweats, difficulty in breathing, production of purulent sputum, and signs of severe lung involvement occur. Treatment is by antituberculosis drugs (e.g., isoniazid) and antibiotics, rest, and proper nutrition (see also *Pott's disease*).

TUBERCULOSIS VACCINE see *bacillus Calmette Guerin*.

TUBULE n. a small tube (e.g., the seminiferous tubules of the *testis*).

TULAREMIA n. an infectious disease of animals, caused by *Pasturella tularensis*, transmitted to humans by insects or direct contact. Symptoms include headache, fever, ulcers on the skin, lymph node enlargement, gastrointestinal symptoms or other manifestations. Treatment is by antibiotics; also called **rabbit fever.**

TUMEFACTION n. the process by which a tissue becomes swollen by accumulation of fluid within it.

TUMESCENCE n. swelling, usually because of the presence of blood or other fluid in the tissue.

TUMOR n. a growth of tissue, characterized by uncontrolled cell proliferation. A tumor may be *benign* or malignant; localized or invasive; also: **neoplasm**

TUNICA n. a covering or layer of an organ.

TUNNEL VISION n. condition in which peripheral sight is diminished and vision is limited to that area in front of the eyes.

TURBIDITY n. the state of being cloudy, as a solution.   adj. **turbid**

TURGID adj. swollen, hard, or full, usually as the result of fluid accumulation.   n. **turgor**

TURNER'S SYNDROME n. a chromosomal abnormality in females in which there is only one X chromosome (instead of the normal two); it is characterized by dwarfism, cardiac abnormalities, underdeveloped reproductive organs, and often varying degrees of mental retardation or learning problems. Treatment is by hormone therapy and surgical correction of cardiovascular or skeletal abnormalities.

TWIN n. either of two offspring born at the same time from the same pregnancy. Twins may result from a single fertilized ovum that divides early in development to form two separate embryos (identical twins) or from two ova fertilized at the same time (*fraternal twins*).

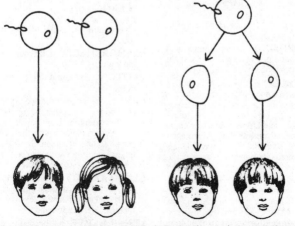

Twinning: Fraternal twins are formed from the fertilization of two ova by two separate sperm. Identical twins are formed from the same fertilized ovum, which divides into two separate cells, each with the same chromosome complement.

TYMPANIC MEMBRANE n. the thin, semitransparent membrane that separates the outer ear from the middle ear. When sound waves enter the outer ear, they cause the membrane to vibrate; these vibrations are transmitted through the ossicles of the middle ear to the inner ear; also: **eardrum.**

TYMPANOPLASTY n. surgical correction or repair of injuries or defects in the *tympanic membrane* or bones of the middle ear to improve hearing.

TYPHOID FEVER n. a serious and sometimes fatal infection with the bacteria *Salmonella typhi*, characterized by high fever, watery diarrhea, delirium, cough, and rosy spots on the abdomen, and an enlarged spleen. Treatment is by antibacterials; Typhoid vaccine provides short short-term prevention.

TYPHUS n. an infection caused by *Rickettsia* organisms and characterized by headache, chills, fever, rash, and malaise.

TYRAMINE n. an amino acid. Persons taking *MAO inhibitors* should avoid foods containing tyramine (e.g., chocolate, cola drinks, beer, some wines, some cheeses).

TYROSINE n. an amino acid, found in most proteins and a precursor of several hormones.

TYROSINEMIA n. a hereditary (autosomal recessive) defect in tyrosine metabolism caused by an enzyme lack and resulting in liver and kidney disturbances and mental retardation. Treatment is by a diet low in tyrosine and phenylalanine.

U

U symbol for the element uranium (see Table of Elements).

ULALGIA n. pain in the gums.

ULCER n. a circumscribed lesion of the skin or mucous membrane of an organ formed by the necrosis of tissue resulting from an infectious, malignant, or inflammatory process. Some types of ulcers are *decubitus ulcers* (bedsores) and *peptic ulcers*. adj. **ulcerative, ulcerous**

ULCERATIVE COLITIS n. a serious and chronic inflammatory disease of the large intestine and rectum characterized by recurrent episodes of abdominal pain, fever, chills, and profuse diarrhea with stools containing pus, blood, and mucus. It affects children, often interfering with their normal growth, and young adults, often preventing many normal life activities. Treatment consists of antiinflammatory agents, including corticosteroids; severe cases may require surgery with removal of parts of the intestinal tract. Complications include arthritis, kidney and liver disease, inflammation of other mucous membranes, and an increased risk of developing cancer of the colon (compare *Crohn's disease*).

ULCERO- comb. form indicating an association with ulcers (e.g., **ulcerogenic**, causing ulcers to form).

ULEMORRHAGIA n. bleeding of the gums.

ULITIS n. inflammation of the gums.

ULNA n. the larger of the two lower arm bones (the other being the *radius*) extending from the elbow where it articulates with the *humerus* to the wrist on the little finger side of the arm; also called **elbow bone.** adj. **ulnar**

ULNAR ARTERY n. large artery that branches from the brachial artery and supplies muscles of the forearm, wrist, and hand.

ULNAR NERVE n. the nerve, a branch of the brachial plexus, that supplies the skin and muscles of the little finger side of the forearm and hand; it is the "funny bone" of the elbow.

ULTRACEF n. trade name for *cephalosporin* antibiotic (cefadroxil).

ULTRACENTRIFUGE n. a high speed centrifuge with rotation fast enough to cause viruses to settle out, even in plasma; used in many forms of biochemical analysis to separate and measure proteins and viruses.

ULTRALENTE ILETIN n. trade name for a long-acting *insulin* zinc preparation.

ULTRASONOGRAPHY n. the process by which the reflection of high frequency sound waves is used to develop an image of a structure; used in medicine to study fetal growth and detect abnormalities, and to study the heart and many other organs.

ULTRASOUND n. sound waves at very high frequencies used in the technique of ultrasonography to aid diagnosis.

ULTRAVIOLET RADIATION n. invisible short wavelength radiation; it is contained in sunlight, but much of it is absorbed by the atmosphere before reaching the earth, where it causes tanning and burning of the skin. Artificial sources of ultraviolet radiation (e.g., iron or mercury vapor arc in ultraviolet lamps) are sometimes used in medicine to treat rickets and certain skin disorders.

UMBILICAL adj. pert. to the *umbilical cord*.

UMBILICAL CORD n. flexible cordlike structure that connects the fetus to the *placenta* during pregnancy. It contains arteries that carry blood to the placenta and a vein that returns blood to the fetus and the remains of the yolk sac and *allantois*. In the newborn it is usually about 24 inches (60 centimeters) long.

UMBILICAL HERNIA n. a protrusion of the intestine and omentum through a weakness in the abdominal wall near the umbulicus; it often closes spontaneously after birth, but large hernias may require surgical closure.

UMBILICUS n. the point on the abdomen where the *umbilical cord* connected to the fetus; in adults it is marked by a depression or occasionally a small protrusion; also called **navel**; **belly button**.

UMBO n. a rounded projection; a knoblike center.   adj. **umbonate**

UNCONDITIONED RESPONSE n. an instinctive, unlearned response to a stimulus; also called **instinctual response**, **instinctive reflex**; **inborn reflex** (compare *conditioned response*).

UNCONSCIOUS adj. unaware of the surroundings; unable to respond to sensory stimuli; n. in psychiatry, part of the mind where thoughts, ideas, and emotions are not subject to ready recall and are outside of awareness.

UNCONSCIOUSNESS n. a state of complete or partial unawareness of the surroundings and lack of response to sensory stimuli. It

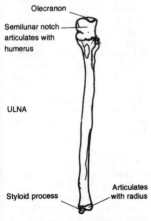

Olecranon

Semilunar notch articulates with humerus

ULNA

Styloid process

Articulates with radius

Courtesy Carolina Biological Supply Co.

may be caused by many conditions, including shock; lack of respiratory efficiency; drugs or poisons; many metabolic disorders, including severe electrolyte imbalance; severe hypoglycemia; and kidney failure; as well as trauma, seizures, tumors, and other causes.

UNCTION n. an ointment.

UNCUS n. a hook-shaped structure, esp. that projecting from the lower surface of the cerebral hemispheres.

UNDESCENDED TESTIS see *cryptorchidism*.

UNDULANT FEVER see *brucellosis*.

UNGUAL adj. pert. to the fingernails or toenails.

UNGUIS n. a fingernail or toenail (see *nail*).

UNI- prefix meaning "one" "single" (e.g., **unicellular**, composed of a single cell).

UNILATERAL adj. affecting only one side (e.g., **unilateral paralysis**).

UNION n. the healing process; the growing together of the edges of a wound or broken bone.

UNIVERSAL DONOR n. a person with type 0, Rh-negative blood; this blood can be used with minimal risk for tranfusion to people of types 0, A, AB, and B blood.

UNSATURATED FATTY ACID n. a fatty acid in which some of the atoms are joined by double or triple valence bonds that are easily split, enabling other substances to join to them. Monounsaturated fatty acids, found in olive oil, chicken, almonds and some other nuts, have one double or triple bond per molecule. Polyunsaturated fatty acids, found in fish, corn, soybean and safflower oil, have more than one double or triple bond per molecule. A diet high in polyunsaturated fatty acids

and low in saturated fatty acids has been linked in some studies to low serum *cholesterol* levels (compare *saturated fatty acids*).

UPPER RESPIRATORY INFECTION see under *respiratory infection*.

UPPER RESPIRATORY TRACT see *respiratory tract*.

URACHUS n. in the fetus, a canal connecting the bladder and the allantois; it remains in the adult as an umbilical ligament. adj. **urachal**

URACIL n. a nitrogen-containing base found in RNA (*ribonucleic acid*).

URAGOGUE n. an agent that increases urinary flow.

URANO- comb. form indicating as association with the roof of the mouth or palate (e.g., **uranoplasty**, surgical correction of a defect in the palate).

URARTHRITIS n. *arthritis* associated with *gout*.

URATEMIA n. the presence of uric acid salts in the blood, occurring in *gout*.

URATURIA n. the presence of uric acid salts in the urine, esp. their presence in abnormally large amounts, as in *gout*.

UREA n. 1. the main breakdown product of proteins and the form in which nitrogen is excreted from the body in the urine; 2. a diuretic preparation used to reduce cerebrospinal and intraocular fluid pressure.

UREMIA n. the presence of excessive amounts of *urea* and other nitrogen-containing wastes in the blood; it occurs in kidney failure, producing symptoms of nausea, vomiting, lethargy, and, if uncorrected, death.

URETER n. either of a pair of thick-walled tubes, about 12 inches (30 centimeters) long, that transport urine from the *kidney* to the *urinary bladder*. adj. **uretal**, **ureteral**, **ureteric**

URETER-, URETERO- comb. form indicating an association with the *ureter* (e.g., **ureterectasis**, a bulging of the ureter).

URETERITIS n. inflammation of the ureter, caused by infection or the passage of a stone.

URETEROCELE n. a prolapse of the end portion of *ureter* into the *bladder*; it may lead to obstructed urine flow and is usually treated by surgery.

URETEROSTENOSIS n. an abnormal narrowing of the *ureter*.

URETHRA n. the small tubular structure that drains urine from the bladder, passing it to the outside. In women it is very short, located behind the pubis between the clitoris and the vaginal opening; in men it is much longer passing from the bladder through the *prostate gland* into the *penis*; in men the urethra also serves as the passageway for *semen* during ejaculation.   adj. **urethral**

URETHRITIS n. inflammation of the *urethra*, usually with symptoms of painful urination. It is most commonly caused by bladder or kidney infection and is treated by antibacterials and pain-relievers.

URETHRO- comb. form indicating an association with the *urethra* (e.g., **urethrophraxis**, obstruction of the urethra).

URETHROCELE n. a herniation or protrusion of the *urethra* into the *vagina*; it may be congenital or acquired, the result of pressure during pregnancy or childbirth, obesity, or poor muscle tone. Treatment depends on the size and location of the hernia and on whether or not it produces symptoms of incontinence and painful urination and coitus. Treatment is usually by surgery.

UREX n. trade name for an antibacterial *methenamine*.

-URIA suffix indicating a characteristic or constituent of *urine*

(e.g., **ammoniuria**, the presence of ammonia in the urine).

URIC ACID n. a product of protein metabolism present in the blood and excreted in urine. Deposits of uric acid and its salts occurs in *gout*.

URICACIDURIA n. greater than normal levels of *uric acid* in the urine, associated with *gout* or urinary system malfunction.

URINALYSIS n. analysis of urine by physical, chemical, or microscopic means to reveal color, turbidity, pH, and the possible presence of microorganisms, blood, pus, or crystals, or abnormal levels of ketones, proteins, sugar, and other compounds. Urinalysis is an important aid in diagnosing urinary system disorders, metabolic disorders, and other conditions.

URINARY adj. pert. to *urine* or the production of urine.

URINARY BLADDER n. muscular sac in the pelvis that stores urine for discharge through the *urethra*. The urine is carried to the bladder through the *ureters* from the *kidneys*.   also: **bladder**

URINARY CALCULUS n. a stone formed in any part of the urinary system (kidney, ureter, bladder); some are small enough to pass in the urine, with or without pain; others must be removed surgically.

URINARY FREQUENCY n. a greater than normal frequency of the urge to void without an increase in the total daily volume of *urine*; it is associated with inflammation of the *bladder* or *urethra* or dysfunction in the bladder and is often accompanied by burning and discomfort. Treatment depends on the cause.

URINARY HESITANCY n. difficulty in beginning the flow of *urine* and decrease in the force of the urine stream. In men it is associated with prostate gland enlargement; in women with narrowing of the opening of the urethra or obstruction between the bladder and urethra; it may also be caused by emotional stress and other causes.

URINARY INCONTINENCE n. inability to control the flow of urine and involuntary passage of urine from the body; it may be caused by central nervous system lesions, multiple sclerosis, neoplasm, trauma, aging, or other factors. Treatment depends on the cause.

URINARY TRACT n. the organs and tubes involved in the production and excretion of urine; it includes the *kidneys*, *ureters*, *urinary bladder*, and *urethra*.

URINARY TRACT INFECTION n. any infection of any of the organs of the urinary system; it is more common in women than in men and is most often caused by bacteria. Symptoms include frequency, burning pain on urination, and sometimes blood or pus in the urine. Treatment is by antibacterials, pain-relievers. Types of urinary tract infections are *cystitis*, *urethritis*, and *pyelonephritis*.

URINATION n. the act of passing urine through the urethral opening to outside the body.

URINE n. fluid secreted by the kidneys, transported through the *ureters* to the bladder, where it is stored until excreted from the body through the *urethra*. Normal urine is straw-colored and slightly acid. Changes in the color, acidity and other characteristics of urine are important clues to many diseases.

URISED n. trade name for a fixed-combination urinary drug, containing the antibacterial methenamine, as well as an antiseptic, antifungal, analgesic, and other drugs; used in the treatment of certain urinary tract infections.

URITONE n. trade name for the urinary antibacterial *methenamine*.

URO-, URONO- comb. form indicating an association with *urine* or the urinary tract (e.g., **urolith**, a urinary stone).

UROBILIN n. a brown pigment found in feces and sometimes in small amounts in urine.

UROBILINOGEN n. a compound formed in the intestine from the breakdown of bilirubin; some is excreted in the feces, some resorbed and excreted in bile or urine.

UROCELE n. a swelling of the *scrotum* from urine that has entered the tissues.

UROCHEZIA n. the discharge of urine from rectum.

URODYNIA n. pain during urination.

UROGENITAL adj. pert. to the urinary and reproductive systems; also: **genitourinary**.

UROKINASE n. an enzyme produced in the kidney that activates fibrinolysis. A urokinase preparation is used in the treatment of pulmonary embolism and some myocardial infarctions to dissolve blood clots.

UROLOGIST n. a specialist in *urology*.

UROLOGY n. that branch of medicine concerned with the anatomy, physiology, disorders and treatment of the urinary tract in both men and women and of the reproductive tract in men.

UROPATHY n. any disease of the *urinary tract*.

URTICARIA n. an itchy skin eruption characterized by well-defined, red-margined, pale-centered transient wheals; it is usually the result of an allergic reaction to drugs, food, or insect bites, but in some cases, esp. chronic diseases, the cause cannot be

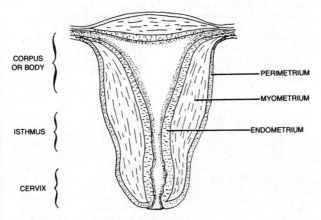

Longitudinal section of the uterus

identified. Treatment is by avoidance of the offending agent, and, when an eruption occurs, antihistamines; also called: **hives.** adj. **urticarial**

UTERINE adj. pert. to the *uterus*.

UTERO- comb. form indicating an association with the *uterus* (e.g., **uteroabdominal**, pert. to the uterus and the abdomen).

UTERUS n. that part of the female reproductive system specialized to allow the implantation, growth and nourishment of a fetus during pregnancy. The non-pregnant uterus is a hollow, pear-shaped organ, about 3 inches (7.5 centimeters) long suspended in the pelvic cavity by ligaments. Its upper end is connected to the Fallopian tubes, its lower end narrows into a neck, or cervix, that opens into the *vagina*. The uterus has an inner mucus layer, the *endometrium*, which undergoes cyclic changes during the menstrual cycle and helps form the placenta in pregnancy; a muscular layer, the myometrium, contractions of which expel a child during labor and childbirth; and an outer connective tissue parametrium that extends into the broad ligament.   adj. **uterine**

UTRICLE n. the larger of two pouches in the membranous labyrinth of the ear; it functions in the maintenance of balance.   adj. **utricular**

UVEA n. layer of the eye containing the *iris, ciliary body,* and *choroid.*   adj. **uveal**

UVEITIS n. inflammation of the *uvea,* characterized by irregular shaped pupil, tearing, pain, pus discharge, and opaqueness. It may be caused by infection, allergic response, or trauma, or it may occur as a complication of certain diseases (e.g., *diabetes mellitus*). Treatment depends on the cause.

UVULA n. small fleshy mass hanging from the soft palate in the mouth.

UVULITIS n. inflammation of the *uvula,* usually caused by allergic reaction or infection.

V

VACCINATION n. the introduction of attenuated (weakened) or killed viruses or microorganisms (or occasionally of substances extracted from these agents) into the body to induce immunity by causing the production of specific antibodies. Vaccination has eradicated smallpox throughout the world; has decreased the incidence of poliomyelitis and diphtheria to very low levels in North America and Europe; and is also available against other diseases, including measles and mumps.   v. **vaccinate**

VACCINE n. a preparation of attenuated or killed disease-producing viruses or microorganisms (or of substances extracted from them) administered orally or by injection to induce active immunity to the specific disease.

VACCINIA   see *cowpox*.

VACUOLE n. a small space in a cell, esp. one containing material taken in by the cell.   adj. **vacuolar**

VACUUM ASPIRATION n. a method of induced *abortion* in which the embryo and placenta are removed by suction applied to the dilated *cervix*. It is performed only in early pregnancy, up to about the 14th week of gestation; also called **suction curettage**.

VAGAL adj. pert. to the *vagus nerve*.

VAGINA n. a muscular tube lined with mucous membrane that forms the lower part of the female reproductive tract, situated behind the bladder and in front of the rectum and extending from the vaginal opening to the cervix of the *uterus*. It receives the penis during coitus, ejaculation of semen usually occurring in the upper vagina, from where the sperm move upward to fertilize an ovum. The vagina is normally sufficiently elastic to allow the passage of a child.   adj. **vaginal**

VAGINAL CANCER n. a malignancy of the *vagina*; it most often results from the spread of cancer from another organ, esp. the uterus

or ovaries, but may occur as a primary neoplasm, esp. in women exposed while in the uterus to diethylstilbestrol (given the mothers to prevent spontaneous abortion). Treatment depends on the size and location of the lesion and the age and health of the women; it may include removal of the vagina, hysterectomy and/or irradiation.

VAGINAL DISCHARGE n. a discharge made up mostly of secretions from cervical glands from the vagina. A clear or whitish discharge is normal, varying in amount and consistency from woman to woman and in each woman during different phases of the menstrual cycle or pregnancy. Inflammation of the vagina and cervix causes the discharge to change in amount, color, and odor.

VAGINISMUS n. contraction of the muscles around the *vagina* causing its opening to close; it usually occurs as a fear or anxiety reaction prior to coitus or pelvic examination; but may also be caused by injury or dryness of the vagina or inflammation of the vagina or bladder.

VAGINITIS n. inflammation of the *vagina*, often producing pain, itchiness, burning on urination, and increased, sometimes foul-smelling discharge. It may be caused by infection (e.g., candidiasis), poor hygiene, dietary deficiency, or local irritation (e.g., from a contraceptive). Treatment depends on the cause.

VAGINO- comb. form indicating as association with the *vagina* (e.g., **vaginoperineal**, pert. to the vagina and perineum).

VAGO- comb. form indicating as association with the *vagus nerve* (e.g., **vagoglossopharyngeal**, pert. to both the vagus and glossopharyngeal nerves).

VAGOTOMY n. the cutting of

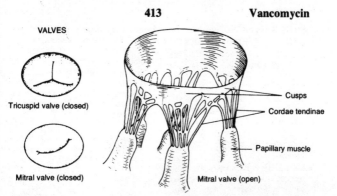

VALVES

Tricuspid valve (closed)

Mitral valve (closed)

Cusps

Cordae tendinae

Papillary muscle

Mitral valve (open)

branches of the *vagus nerve*, usually performed with stomach surgery, to reduce the secretion of gastric juice and thus lessen the chances of ulcer reccurrence.

VAGUS NERVE n. either of the longest pair of cranial nerves; mixed sensory and motor nerves functioning in swallowing, speech, breathing, heart rate and many other body functions; tenth cranial nerve. pl. **vagi** adj. **vagal**

VALGUS n. adj. pert. to a deformity in which part of a limb is turned outward or twisted away from the center of the body (e.g., **talipes valgus**, a deformity in which the foot is twisted outward).

VALINE n. an amino acid needed for growth in children and nitrogen balance in adults.

VALIUM n. trade name for the tranquilizer *diazepam*.

VALLECULA n. a groove or depression on the surface of an organ.

VALLESTRIL n. trade name for an *estrogen* preparation.

VALPROIC ACID n. an anticonvulsant, known under the trade name Depokene, used to prevent some types of seizures. Adverse effects include gastrointestinal disturbances, hair loss, headache, liver damage, and decreased blood clotting ability.

VALVE n. a structure, usually a flap or fold of tissue, found in some tubes and tubular organs that restricts the flow of fluid in them to one direction only. Valves are important structures in the heart, veins, and lymph vessels (see also *mitral valve*; *semilunar valve*; *tricuspid valve*).

VALVOTOMY n. an incision into a *valve* to correct a defect and permit its normal function in opening and closing to control the flow of a fluid.

VALVULAR HEART DISEASE n. a disorder of cardiac valves caused by stenosis and obstructed blood flow or degeneration and blood regurgitation. Major types of valvular heart disease include *aortic stenosis*, *mitral stenosis*, and *tricuspid stenosis*.

VALVULITIS n. inflammtion of a *valve*, esp. a cardiac valve usually resulting from rheumatic fever, sometimes from bacterial endocarditis or syphilis; stenosis and impaired blood flow commonly result.

VANCOCIN n. trade name for the antibacterial *vancomycin*.

VANCOMYCIN n. an antibiotic, known under the trade name Vancocin, used to treat some bacterial infections. Adverse effects include tinnitus, dizziness, and anaphylaxis.

VARICELLA see *chickenpox*.

VARICELLA ZOSTER VIRUS (VZV) n. a member of the herpesvirus family that is responsible for varicella (*chickenpox*) and *herpes zoster* (shingles).

VARICELLIFORM adj. resembling the rash of *chickenpox*.

VARICOCELE n. a dilatation or swelling of blood vessels associated with the spermatic cord in the testes.

VARICOSE VEIN n. a swollen, tortuous vein with abnormally functioning valves. It is a common condition, usually affecting the veins of the legs; it is more common in women than men and often associated with congenitally weak valves, pregnancy, obesity, or thrombophlebitis. Symptoms include pain, muscle cramps, and a feeling of heaviness in the legs. Elevation of the legs and the use of elastic stockings often helps. Severe cases may require surgical intervention.

VARICOSIS n. a condition characterized by one or more varicose veins.

VARICOSITY n. an abnormal condition in which a vein is swollen and tortuous.

VARIOLA n. *smallpox*.

VARIX n. an enlarged and twisted blood vessel or lymph vessel. pl. **varices**

VASAL n. trade name for the smooth muscle relaxant *papaverine*.

VASCULAR adj. pert. to a blood vessel.

VASCULARIZATION n. the process by which body tissue becomes vascular and develops capillaries.

VASCULITIS n. inflammation of a blood vessel, caused by allergic reaction or certain systemic disease.

VAS DEFERENS n. either of a pair of ducts that is the extension of the epididymis of the testis ascending into the abdominal cavity where it passes over the bladder and joins the seminal vesicle. In a vasectomy the vas deferens is severed so that sperm cannot pass from the epididymis to the ejaculatory duct, thus rendering the man sterile.

VASECTOMY n. a surgical procedure to render a male sterile by severing the *vas deferens*. Potency is not affected.

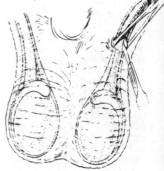

Bilateral incision to expose sheath

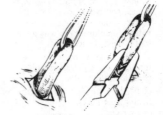

Vas exposed and occluded

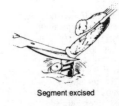

Segment excised

VASECTOMY

VASO- comb. form indicating an association with a vessel or duct (e.g., **vasoconstriction**, narrowing of the opening of a blood vessel).

VASOCONSTRICTOR n. an agent that causes a narrowing of the opening of a blood vessel. Cold, stress, nicotine, epinephrine, norephinephrine, angiotensin, vasopressin, and certain drugs are vasoconstrictors, maintaining or increasing blood pressure.

VASODILATION n. widening of blood vessels, esp. arteries, usually due to certain nerve impulses or drugs that relax the musculature of the arteries.

VASODILATOR n. an agent that dilates or widens blood vessels. Some vasodilators, including nitroglycerine and hydralazine, are used in the treatment of certain heart ailments.

VASOMOTOR adj. pert. to the nerves and muscles that control the diameter of blood vessels.

VASOPRESSIN n. a hormone released by the *posterior pituitary gland* that increases the absorption of water by the kidney, thus preventing excess water loss; it also constricts blood vessels. Also called **antidiuretic hormone**.

VASOPRESSOR n. an agent that causes vasoconstriction and therefore an increase in blood pressure.

VASOVASOSTOMY n. surgical procedure that attempts to restore the function of the vas deferens on either or both sides after the vas has been severed in a vasectomy. In many cases the function of the vas deferens is restored but fertility does not result, usually because antibodies that interfere with sperm production developed after the earlier vasectomy.

VASOVESICULITIS n. inflammation of the *vas deferens* and *seminal vesicles*, usually occurring with prostatitis and causing pain in the scrotum and groin and fever. Treatment is by antibiotics.

VASTUS n. any of three muscles that form part of the quadriceps muscle of the thigh.

V-CILLIN n. trade name for a *penicillin* antibacterial.

VECTOR n. a person, animal, or microorganism that carries and transmits disease. Mosquitoes, for example, are vectors of malaria and yellow fever, carrying disease-producing parasites.

VECTRIN n. trade name for a *tetracylcine* antibiotic.

VEETIDS n. trade name for a penicillin antibacterial.

VEGETARIAN n. a person who restricts his/her diet to foods of vegetable origin, including fruits, grains and nuts.

VEGETATIVE adj. pert. to growth and nutrition, as opposed to reproduction (propagative).

VEIN n. any of many vessels that carry blood to the heart; it may be part of the pulmonary venous system, portal system, or (most veins) the systemic venous system. All veins except the pulmonary vein carry deoxygenated blood from the tissues of the body to the *vena cava* and heart. The walls of veins are thinner and less elastic than the walls of arteries and contain valves that maintain the flow of blood toward the heart (compare *artery*). adj. **venous**

VENA CAVA n. either of two large veins returning deoxygenated blood from the peripheral circulation to the right atrium of the heart.
INFERIOR VENA CAVA n. the large vein, formed by the union of the two iliac veins, that receives blood from parts of the body below the diaphragm and transports it to the heart.
SUPERIOR VENA CAVA n. the large vein that draws blood from the head, neck, chest, and arms and transports it to the heart.

VENEREAL adj. pert. to or caused by sexual intercourse or genital contact, as a venereal disease.

VENEREAL DISEASE (VD) a communicable disease transmitted by sexual intercourse or genital contact. Venereal diseases include gonorrhea, syphilis, and granuloma inguinale.

VENIPUNCTURE n. a procedure in which a vein is punctured through the skin to withdraw blood for analysis, to start an intravenous drip, to instill medication, or to inject a radiopaque dye for a radiographic examination of a part of the body.

VENO- comb. form indicating an association with a *vein* (e.g., **venopressor**, a substance that causes veins to narrow).

VENOGRAM n. an X-ray film of veins injected with a radiopaque contrast medium.

VENOGRAPHY n. the technique of preparing X-ray images of a vein injected with a radiopaque contrast medium.

VENOM n. a toxic fluid secreted by some snakes and other animals and transmitted in their bites or stings. Some venoms produce local irritation and swelling at the site of the bite or sting; other venoms produce systemic sometimes fatal effects, usually focused on the circulatory or nervous system.

VENOUS adj. pert. to a *vein*.

VENOUS BLOOD n. blood found in the veins. Except in the pulmonary vein, venous blood is poor in oxygen and rich in carbon dioxide to be carried to the right side of the heart for transport to the lungs where the carbon dioxide will be given off. (The pulmonary vein carries freshly oxygenated blood from the lungs to the left atrium of the heart.)

VENOUS BLOOD GASES n. the oxygen and carbon dioxide in venous blood.

VENOUS PRESSURE n. the stress exerted by the circulating blood on the walls of the veins.

VENOUS SINUS n. any of several sinuses that collect blood from the *dura mater* covering the brain and drain it into the internal jugular veins.

VENOUS THROMBOSIS n. the presence of a blood clot in a vein in which the wall of the vein is not inflamed. Pain and swelling may occur.

VENTER n. a bellylike part, as the bulging part of a muscle. pl. **ventres**

VENTILATION n. breathing; the process by which gases are moved into and out of the lungs. v. **ventilate**

VENTRAL adj. pert. to or toward the belly side of the body; frontward (compare *dorsal*).

VENTRICLE n. 1. either of the two lower chambers of the *heart*. The left ventricle receives oxygenated blood from the pulmonary vein through the left atrium and pumps it to the *aorta* from which it passes throughout the body. The thinner-walled right ventricle receives deoxygenated blood from the venae cavae through the right atrium and pumps it through the pulmonary artery to the lung for the exchange of gases; 2. any of four fluid-filled cavities in the *brain* containing *cerebrospinal fluid*. adj. **ventricular**

VENTRICULAR adj. pert. to a *ventricle*.

VENTRICULAR ANEURYSM n. a localized dilatation or saccular protrusion on the wall of the left ventricle of the heart, occurring after a myocardial infarction.

VENTRICULR FIBRILLA-TION n. a serious disturbance in cardiac rhythm characterized by disorganized impulse conduction and ventricular contraction. Unconsciousness occurs and death

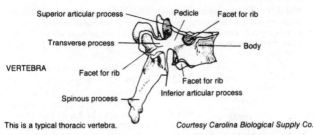

Superior articular process · Pedicle · Facet for rib · Body · Transverse process · VERTEBRA · Facet for rib · Facet for rib · Spinous process · Inferior articular process

This is a typical thoracic vertebra.

Courtesy Carolina Biological Supply Co.

may follow within minutes if defibrillation and other life-saving measures are not immediately provided.

VENTRICULAR SEPTAL DEFECT (VSD) n. the most common congenital heart defect characterized by an abnormal opening in the septum dividing the ventricles which allows blood to pass from the left to the right ventricle. Small openings may cause no symptoms and may heal spontaneously during childhood. Larger openings may cause symptoms of congestive heart failure and rapid breathing and usually require surgical repair of the defect.

VENTRICULO- comb. form indicating an association with a *ventricle* of the heart or brain (e.g., **ventriculoatrial shunt**, a surgically created passageway with plastic tubing leading from the ventricle of the brain to the right atrium of the heart to drain excess fluid from the brain in cases of *hydrocephalus*).

VENULE n. a small vein, esp. one that extends from a capillary network and merges to form a *vein*.

VERACILLIN n. trade name for the antibiotic *dicloxacillin*.

VERMICIDE n. an agent that kills worms, esp. those in the intestines.

VERMIFORM   APPENDIX see *appendix*.

VERMIFUGE n. an agent that causes the evacuation of worms.

VERNIX CASEOSA n. a cheese-like substance that covers the skin of a fetus and newborn, serving as a protective cover.

VERRUCA see *wart*.

VERSION n. changing the position of a fetus in the uterus, usually done to aid delivery.

VERTEBRA n. any of the 33 bones of the spinal column (vertebral column, or backbone), including seven cervical (neck region), 12 thoracic (chest region), 5 lumbar, 5 sacral (fused), and 4 coccygeal (fused). Except for the first two—the *atlas* and *axis*—each vertebra consists of a centrum, or body, from which the neural arch, enclosing a cavity through which the *spinal cord* passes, and processes for the attachment of muscles arise. The vertebrae are connected by ligaments and separated by *intervertebral discs*, which cushion adjacent vertebrae.   adj. **vertebral**

VERTEBRAL COLUMN n. the firm, flexible, bony column that is the longitudinal axis and chief supporting structure of the human body, extending from the base of the skull to the coccyx. It consists of 26 separate bony parts: 7 cervical vertebrae, 12 thoracic vertebrae, 5 lumbar vertebrae, a sacrum (composed of 5 fused sacral vertebrae), and a coccyx (composed of 4 fused coccygeal vertebrae). The vertebrae, which serve for the attachment of muscles, are separated by intervertebral discs. The vertebral column normally has several curves, most visible from a lateral view: a cervical curve, convex ventrally; a thoracic curve, concave ventrally; a lumbar curve, convex ventrally; and a pelvic curve concave ventrally.

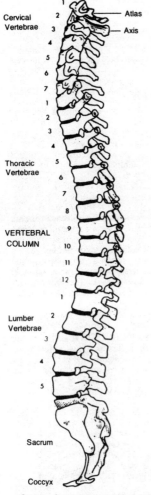

Cervical Vertebrae 1, 2 — Atlas, 3 — Axis, 4, 5, 6, 7

Thoracic Vertebrae 1, 2, 3, 4, 5, 6, 7, 8, 9, 10, 11, 12

VERTEBRAL COLUMN

Lumber Vertebrae 1, 2, 3, 4, 5

Sacrum

Coccyx

Courtesy Carolina Biological Supply Co.

VERTEBRO- comb. form indicating an association with the *vertebral column* or a *vertebra* (e.g., **vertebrocostal**, pert. to a vertebra and a rib).

VERTIGO see *dizziness*.

VESICAL adj. pert. to the *bladder*, esp. the *urinary bladder*.

VESICANT n. an agent, as a drug, that causes blistering of the skin.

VESICLE n. 1. a blister; a small, thin-walled skin lesion containing fluid; 2. a small saclike part (as, e.g., the **seminal vesicle**, which stores semen). adj. **vesicular**

VESICO- comb. form indicating as association with the *urinary bladder* (e.g., **vesicovaginal**, pert. to the urinary bladder and *vagina*).

VESICOCELE n. a bulging of the bladder into another part.

VESICOURETHRAL REFLUX n. abnormal backflow of urine from the bladder to the ureters, caused by congenital defect, obstruction of the bladder outlet, or urinary tract infection. Treatment depends on the cause.

VESICULITIS n. inflammation of the *seminal vesicle*, usually occurring with *prostatitis*.

VESSEL n. a tubelike structure that carries fluids throughout the body. Major body vessels are arteries, veins, and lymph vessels.

VESTIBULAR GLAND n. either of two pairs of glands at the vaginal-vulva junction, the secretions of which lubricate the vagina during coitus. The posterior pair is also called Bartholin's glands.

VESTIBULE n. a space at the entrance to a hollow organ or passageway, as the vestibule of the vagina or the vestibule of the aorta, that part of the left ventricle where the aorta channels off. adj. **vestibular**

VESTIBULOCOCHLEAR NERVE see *auditory nerve*.

VESTIGIAL n. existing in a rudimentary form; pert. to a relatively useless organ that had a function in an earlier stage of life or in a more primitive form of life, as the vermiform appendix in humans.

VIABLE adj. capable of surviving.

VIBRAMYCIN n. trade name for the *tetracycline* antibiotic doxycycline.

VIBRIO n. a genus of comma-shaped bacteria, some members of which produce disease in humans (e.g., *Vibrio cholerae*, the agent that causes cholera).

VIBRISSA n. a stiff coarse hair, esp. that in the front part of the nostrils that helps filter inhaled air.   pl. **vibrissae**

VICARIOUS adj. in medicine, pert. to an action performed by an organ or part of the body not normally involved in that function, as (e.g., **vacarious menstruation**, a rare disease in which monthly bleeding occurs from places other than the vagina, such as the nostrils or sweat glands).

VILLUS n. one of many tiny projections, containing capillaries and a *lacteal,* occurring over the mucous membrane of the small intestine that function in the absorption of nutrients and fluids. pl. **villi**   adj. **villous**

VINBLASTINE n. an antineoplastic drug, known under the trade name Velban, that disrupts cell division and is used to treat many cancers, esp. those of the lymphatic system. Adverse effects include a decrease in white blood cells, nausea, vomiting, and hair loss.

VINCENT'S ANGINA   see *trench mouth.*

VINCRISTINE n. an antineoplastic drug, known under the trade name Oncovin, that disrupts cell division and is used to treat many cancers, esp. those of the lymphatic system. Adverse effects include a decrease in white blood cells, nausea, vomiting, and hair loss.

VIOCIN n. trade name for the antibiotic *viomycin.*

VIOMYCIN n. an antibiotic, known under the trade name Viocin, used to treat *tuberculosis.* Adverse effects include disturbances of kidney and ear function.

VIOSTEROL n. a synthetic vitamin D_2 preparation, used esp. for children (see Table of Vitamins).

VIRAL adj. pert. to a *virus.*

VIRAL HEPATITIS n. a form of *hepatitis*, inflammation of the liver, caused by one of the hepatitis viruses. Symptoms include

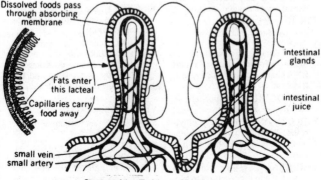

Dissolved foods pass through absorbing membrane

intestinal glands

Fats enter this lacteal

Capillaries carry food away

intestinal juice

small vein
small artery

Structure of the villi of the small intestine

anorexia, headache, fever, pain in the region of the liver, malaise, jaundice, and diarrhea with the stools clay-colored. Treatment includes rest, the avoidance of fatigue, and a low-fat, high-protein diet; the person is usually advised to abstain from alcohol for a year after the attack. Severe infection, esp. with hepatitis B, can cause permanent damage to liver tissue and result in hepatic coma and death.

VIRAL INFECTION n. any disease caused by a *virus* pathogenic to humans. Some viral infections are serious diseases; others are mild, sometimes occurring with few or unnoticed symptoms. Among the common viral infections are measles, mumps, chickenpox, poliomyelitis and some types of hepatitis and pneumonia.

VIRAL PNEUMONIA n. infection of the lung or lungs caused by a virus (see *pneumonia*).

VIREMIA n. the presence of *virus* particles in the blood.

VIRILIZATION n. the process by which secondary male sex characteristics are acquired by a female, usually the result of adrenal malfunction or the intake of certain drugs, esp. hormones; also called **masculinization**.

VIRION n. a virus particle, consisting of a protein coat, called a capsid, and a nucleic acid core.

VIROID n. a tiny particle known to cause some plant diseases and suspected of causing some human diseases. It is much smaller than a virus and consists of a short RNA chain and no protective protein coat.

VIROLOGIST n. a specialist in *virology*.

VIROLOGY n. the study of viruses, their growth, development, and relationship to diseases.

VIRULENCE n. the ability or power of a microorganism to produce disease.   adj. **virulent**

VIRUS n. a small particle that is not living and does not exhibit signs of life but which can reproduce itself within a living cell. A virus particle is called a *virion*; it consists of a nucleic acid (DNA or RNA) core and a protein coat, called a capsid. A virus reproduces by infecting a host cell, and taking over the nucleic acid of that host cell, making more virus nucleic acid and protein. As new virus particles develop, the host cell bursts, releasing the new virus particles. Viruses are responsible for many human diseases (see *viral infection*).

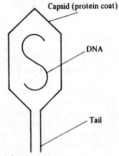

Structure of a virus

VISCERA n. pl. the main internal organs within body cavities, esp. those in the abdominal cavity (e.g., the spleen and stomach). sing. **viscus**   adj. **visceral**

VISCERAL adj. pert. to the internal organs, esp. those of the abdominal cavity.

VISCERO- comb. form indicating an association with the internal organs (e.g., **visceroperitoneal**, pert. to the peritoneum and the internal organs of the abdominal cavity).

VISCID adj. sticky; gluelike.

VISCUS n. a main internal organ. pl. **viscera**

VISION n. the ability to see; the perception of things through the action of light on the eyes and optic centers in the brain.   adj. **visual**

VISTARIL n. trade name for the tranquilizer *hydroxyzine*.

VISUAL ACUITY n. sharpness of vision, most often determined by use of the *Snellen chart*.

VISUAL FIELD n. the area in front of the eye in which an object can be seen without moving the eye.

VISUAL PURPLE n. *rhodopsin*, the pigment in the cones of the *retina*.

VITAL adj. 1. pert. to life or the living state; 2. essential to maintaining life.

VITAL CAPACITY n. the maximum amount of air that can be exhaled after a maximum inhalation; used in determining the status of lung tissue.

VITAL SIGNS n. signs that show the overall health of a person, changes in which are often clues to disease or signs of alteration in a person's health. The vital signs are usually considered to be pulse rate, respiration rate, body temperature, and blood pressure.

VITAL STATISTICS n. data relating to birth, death, disease, marriage and health.

VITAMIN n. any of a group of organic compounds that in very small amounts are essential for normal growth, development, and metabolism. They cannot be synthesized in the body (with a few exceptions) and must be supplied by the diet. Lack of sufficient quantities of any of the vitamins produces a specific deficiency disease. Vitamins are generally classified as water-soluble or fat-soluble. The water-soluble vitamins are the vitamin B complex and vitamin C; the fat-soluble vitamins are vitamins A, D, E, and K (see Table of Vitamins).

VITELLINE CIRCULATION n. the circulation of blood and nutrients between the embryo and yolk sac through the vitelline artery and vitelline vein.

VITELLUS n. the yolk of an *ovum*.

VITILIGO n. an acquired, benign skin disease characterized by irregular patches of unpigmented skin, often surrounded by a hyperpigmented border, occurring most often on exposed areas of the skin. The cause is unknown, and there is no satisfactory treatment. adj. **vitiliginous**

VITREOUS BODY see *vitreous humor*.

VITREOUS HUMOR n. transparent, semigelatinous substance that fills the cavity behind the lens and is closely applied to the *retina*; also: **vitreous body**.

VIVIPAROUS adj. bearing live offspring, not eggs; it is characteristic of most mammals (except monotremes) and also of some fishes and reptiles. n. **viviparity**

VOCAL CORD n. either of two folds of tissue, each containing an elastic tissue known as the vocal ligament, that protrudes from the sides of the larynx forming a narrow slit in the larynx, called the *glottis*. As air is exhaled through the larynx the vocal cords vibrate, producing sound. Movements of the tongue, lips, jaws and accessory mouth structures mold the column of air passing through the glottis, producing sounds of different intensity and pitch.

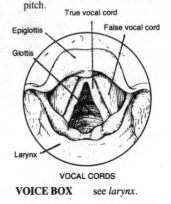

VOCAL CORDS

VOICE BOX see *larynx*.

VOID v. to empty, as urine from the *bladder*.

VOLAR adj. pert. to the palm or sole.

VOLITION n. the act or state of willing or choosing.

VOLUNTARY adj. controlled or accomplished as the result of a person's free will, as a voluntary action.

VOLUNTARY MUSCLE see *striated muscle*.

VOLVULUS n. a twisting of the intestine, most often in the area of the ileum or sigmoid colon, resulting in intestinal obstruction. Severe pain, vomiting, nausea, a tense distended stomach, and the absense of bowel sounds usually occur. If not corrected surgically, the obstruction leads to peritonitis, rupture of the intestines, and death.

VOMER n. the thin bone forming the lower and back part of the nasal septum.

VOMIT v. to expel the contents of the stomach through the esophagus and mouth; n. the contents of the stomach ejected through the mouth, also: **vomitus**.

VOMITING n. reflex action of ejecting the stomach contents through the mouth. Intestinal obstruction, irritation of the stomach, disease-producing organisms in the digestive tract, inner ear disturbances (e.g., in motion sickness), and certain drugs stimulate a special center in the brain that, in turn, produces contractions of the stomach and diaphragm musculature and relaxation of the sphincter muscle at the opening of the stomach, causing the stomach contents to be ejected through the mouth; also: **emesis**

VON RECKLINGHAUSEN'S DISEASE see *neurofibromatosis*.

VOX n. voice.

VOYEURISM n. a disorder in which the person receives sexual excitement and gratification from viewing the naked bodies of others, esp. the genitalia, and from watching the sexual acts of others.

VULVA n. the external genitalia of the female. The *labia majora* and *labia minora* surround the openings of the *vagina* and *urethra* and extend to the *clitoris*. adj. **vulvar**

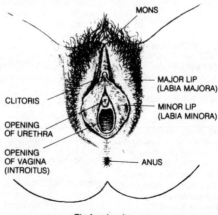

MONS

MAJOR LIP (LABIA MAJORA)

CLITORIS

MINOR LIP (LABIA MINORA)

OPENING OF URETHRA

OPENING OF VAGINA (INTROITUS)

ANUS

The female vulva

VULVECTOMY n. surgical removal of all or part of the *vulva*, usually done to treat malignant or premalignant neoplastic disease.

VULVITIS n. inflammation of the *vulva*, usually producing a burning sensation and intense itching. It may be caused by infection (e.g., candidiasis) or by local irritation (e.g., from poorly fitting underwear).

VULVO- comb. form indicating an association with the *vulva* (e.g., **vulvorectal**, pert. to the vulva and rectum).

VULVOVAGINITIS n. inflammation of the *vulva* and the *vagina*.

W

WALKER n. a light metal apparatus, about waist high with four sturdy legs, used as aid in walking; often used by a person who has had a stroke.

WALKING PNEUMONIA see *mycoplasma pneumonia*.

WALL n. a confining, limiting, or enclosing part, esp. a broad surface, as the wall of the abdominal cavity.

WALLEYE n. abnormal condition in which one or both eyes are off center and point outward; divergent *strabismus*.

WARFARIN n. an anticoagulant, known under the trade name Coumadin, used to prevent and treat thrombosis and embolism. Adverse effects include hemorrhage and the possibility of interaction with many other drugs.

WART n. a small, benign, often hard, growth in the skin, caused by a virus, and more common in children and young adults. Warts frequently disappear spontaneously but may be treated by cryosurgery (usually using liquid nitrogen), electrodesiccation, application of certain chemicals (e.g., salicylic acid), and removal by curette; also **verruca**.

COMMON WART n. benign growth, often with a rough surface.

JUVENILE WART n. benign, small growth, usually on the face and hands of children.

PLANTAR WART n. small, benign growth on the sole, where subject to pressure, it often becomes covered with a callus.

VENERAL WART n. small benign growth on or around the genitalia and anus.

WASSERMANN TEST n. a blood test to detect *syphilis*. A sample of blood is tested, using the complement fixation method, for antibodies to the syphilis organism *Treponema pallidum*; a positive reaction indicates the pesence of antibodies and therefore syphilis infection. A "false positive" reaction also occurs in certain other diseases.

WASTING n. process of deterioration in which there is weight loss and decreased strength, appetite, and activity.

WATERHOUSE - FRIDERICH-SEN SYNDROME n. severe bacteremia (bacteria in the blood) characterized by sudden high fever, bluish skin discoloration, petechiae, adrenal hemorrhage, and collapse. Treatment should be immediate and usually includes antibiotics, vasopressor drugs, plasma, and the maintenance of fluid and electrolyte balance.

WAX see *cerumen*.

WBC abbreviation for white blood cell (see *leukocyte*).

WEAN v. to induce a child to give up breast-feeding, or, more generally, to detach a person from something he or she is dependent on.

WEIL'S DISEASE n. a serious form of *leptospirosis*, characterized by jaundice and liver and kidney damage.

WEN n. a small epidermal cyst of the scalp; also: **pilar cyst**.

WERDNIG-HOFFMAN DISEASE n. a genetic disease (*autosomal recessive disease*) in which degeneration of spinal and brain nerve cells leads to progressive atrophy of skeletal muscles. Symptoms include flaccid paralysis, lack of sucking ability in the infant, lack of muscle tone, and absence of normal reflexes. Death from respiratory complications usually occurs in early childhood.

WERNICKE'S ENCEPHALOPATHY n. an inflammatory, degenerative disease of the brain, characterized by double vision, lack of muscular coordination, and decreased mental function. It is caused by thiamine deficiency, usually associated with *alcoholism*, occasionally with gastrointestinal disorder (compare *Korsakoff's psychosis*).

WET DREAM see *nocturnal emission*.

WET LUNG n. an abnormal condition, characterized by cough and rales in the lung, occurring among those exposed to irritants such as ammonia, chlorine, and corrosive chemical vapors. Treatment involves removal of the irritants and treatment of any possible lung damage.

WHEAL n. an individual lesion, usually with a red margin and pale center, of an itchy skin eruption; characteristic of many allergic reactions.

WHEEZE n. an abnormal high-pitched sound heard through a stethoscope in an airway blocked with mucus, neoplasm, muscle spasm, or pressure. It occurs in asthma, chronic bronchitis and unilaterally when there is a foreign body or neoplasm in the airway.

WHIPLASH n. colloquial for an injury to the cervical (neck) vertebrae and their associated ligaments and muscles, causing pain and stiffness; often the result of rapid accleration or deceleration, as in a car accident.

WHITE BLOOD CELL see *leukocyte*.

WHITE CORPUSCLE see *leukocyte*.

WHITEHEAD see *milia*.

WHITE MATTER n. nerve tissue of the spinal cord, surrounding the gray matter and made up mostly of myelinated and unmyelinated nerve fibers in a network of neuroglia cells. It is divided in each half of the spinal cord into columns containing tracts of closely related nerve fibers.

WHOLE BLOOD n. blood that has not been modified or altered, except for the addition of an anticoagulant; used in blood transfusions. Various components of whole blood may be separated out and used to replace a missing or deficient factor in the blood of those persons with certain diseases (e.g., certain clotting factors separated out and given to those with *hemophilia*).

WHOOPING COUGH see *pertussis*.

WIDAL TEST n. a test to detect *typhoid fever* and other salmonella infections.

WILMS' TUMOR n. a malignant neoplasm of the kidney, occurring in young children; symptoms include hypertension, followed by pain, blood in the urine, and presence of a palpable mass. Treatment includes surgery, irradiation, and chemotherapy.

WILSON'S DISEASE n. a rare, inherited disorder of copper metabolism in which copper accumulates in the liver and then in the erythrocytes (red blood cells) and brain, leading to anemia, tremors, dementia and other symptoms. Treatment includes a diet low in copper and use of drugs to bind copper; also called **hepatolenticular degeneration**.

WINDPIPE   see *trachea*.

WISDOM TOOTH n. any of the four last teeth on each side of the upper and lower jaws. They are the last teeth to erupt, usually between the ages of 16 and 21, and often cause pain and dental problems.

WITCH'S MILK n. milklike substance secreted from the breast of a newborn, caused by lactating hormones circulating in the maternal circulation.

WITHDRAWAL n. 1. a response to extreme stress or danger, characterized by apathy, depression, and, in extreme cases, sometimes associated with schizophrenia; 2. removal of the *penis* from the *vagina* in coitus before *ejaculation* as a means of trying to prevent conception; also: **coitus interruptus**.

WITHDRAWAL SYMPTOMS n. unpleasant and sometimes life-threatening physiological changes that occur when a drug (e.g., narcotic, barbiturate, alcohol, stimulant) is withdrawn after the person became addicted to it during prolonged use. (See also *delirium tremens*.)

WOMB   see *uterus*.

WORD SALAD n. words combined in a way that has no meaning as in the speech of some with *schizophrenia*.

WORMIAN BONES n. any of several tiny soft bones, found along the edges of the sutures between the cranial bones.

WOUND n. an injury or break in the skin, usually caused by accident, not disease.

WRIST n. the joint between the forearm and the hand, formed of eight carpal bones; also: **carpus**

WRITER'S CRAMP n. see *graphospasm*.

WRYNECK   see *torticollis*

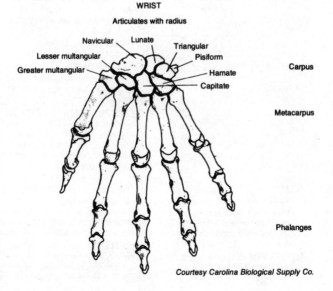

WRIST

Articulates with radius

Navicular — Lunate

Lesser multangular — Triangular — Pisiform

Greater multangular — Hamate — Capitate

Carpus

Metacarpus

Phalanges

Courtesy Carolina Biological Supply Co.

X

XANTHELASMA n. a condition marked by the formation of yellowish fatty deposits around the eyes, occurring chiefly in the elderly.

XANTHEMIA see *carotenemia*.

XANTHINE n. a byproduct of the metabolism of nucleoproteins, found in muscles, liver, and spleen. adj. **xanthic**

XANTHO- comb. form meaning "yellow" or "yellowish" (e.g., **xanthochromia**, a yellowish discoloration, as of the skin or cerebrospinal fluid).

XANTHOMA n. a benign, fatty, yellowish plaque, nodule, or tumor in the subcutaneous layers of the skin, usually due to accumulation of cholesterol and related compounds.

XANTHOMA DISSEMINATUM n. chronic condition in which orange or brownish papules develop on many surfaces of the body, esp. in the region of the mouth, upper respiratory tract, and on skin folds.

XANTHOMATOSIS n. abnormal condition in which a disorder of lipid metabolism leads to the formation of yellowish fatty deposits in the skin and internal organs.

XANTHOPSIA n. an abnormality of vision in which objects appear to have a yellowish hue; sometimes occurring in jaundice or drug toxicity.

XANTHOSARCOMA n. a malignant neoplasm of tendon sheaths and aponeuroses, containing *xanthoma* cells.

XANTHOSIS n. abnormal yellowish discoloration.

XANTHOSIS CUTIS n. yellow or orange-yellow coloring of the skin, usually resulting from consumption of excessive amounts of carotene-containing foods (yellow vegetables).

XANTHOSIS DIABETICA n. yellowish tinge to the skin occurring in some persons with *diabetes mellitus* due to an excess of lipids in the blood.

XANTHOUS adj. yellowish.

X CHROMOSOME n. sex *chromosome* that in humans is present in both sexes—singly in males, in duplicate in females. The X chromosome is carried by all female gametes (ova) and by half of male gametes (sperm); it is larger than the Y chromosome and is associated with many sex-linked disorders (e.g., hemophilia, Hunter's syndrome).

XENO- comb. form meaning "strange" "foreign" (e.g., **xenomenia**, menstruation that occurs vicariously, as in bleeding from the nose).

XENOGRAFT see *heterograft*.

XENOPHOBIA n. an irrational fear of strangers or unfamiliar situations. adj. **xenophobic**

XER-, XERO- comb. form indicating an association with dryness (e.g., **xerocheilia**, dryness of the lips).

XERODERMA n. abnormal dryness and roughness of the skin; also: **xerodermia**

XEROMA n. an abnormally dry condition of the *conjunctiva* of the eye.

XEROPHTHALMIA n. dryness and inflammation of the *conjunctiva*, producing a dull appearance of the eyeball; it is usually associated with vitamin A deficiency.

XERORADIOGRAPHY n. a photoelectric process for producing an X-ray image that uses lower radiation and shorter exposure time than conventional X-ray techniques; it is used chiefly to detect breast tumors.

XEROSTOMIA n. dryness of the mouth caused by decreased saliva secretion; it may be a drug reaction or be caused by disease.

XIPHOID PROCESS n. the smallest of the three parts of the sternum (breastbone) articulating with the body of the sternum and with the seventh rib.

X-LINKED adj. pert. to genes, characteristics, or conditions carried on the *X chromosome*.

X-LINKED DOMINANT INHERITANCE n. a hereditary pattern in which a dominant gene on the X chromosome causes a characteristic to be manifested. All of the daughters of an affected male will be affected; but none of the sons; half of all of the offspring of an affected female will be affected.

X-LINKED RECESSIVE INHERITANCE n. a hereditary pattern in which a recessive gene on the X chromosome results in the manifestation of characteristics of the given condition in males and a carrier state in females.

X RAY n. 1. electromagnetic radiation of short wavelength that is used to penetrate tissues and record densities on film; 2. the film produced by an X ray procedure.

XX in genetics, the normal sex chromosome complement in a female.

XXX in genetics, a chromosomal aberration in which there are three X chromosomes (not the normal two) and an abnormal total chromosome number of 47 (not the normal 46). Affected persons are female with little or no symptoms, except usually some degree of mental retardation.

XXY in genetics, an abnormal sex chromosome complement in males in which more than the normal single X chromosome is present and the total chromosome number of the body cells is abnormal (see *Kleinfelter's syndrome*).

XY in genetics, the normal sex chromosome complement in a male.

XYLOCAINE n. trade name for the local anesthetic *lidocaine*.

XYY in genetics, an abnormal sex chromosome complement in males in which there is more than the normal Y chromosome and an increased total chromosome complement. The condition is usually associated with tall stature and often with abnormal mental effects.

y

YATOBYO   see *tularemia*.

YAWNING n. a reflex, usually triggered by boredom, fatigue, drowsiness, or seeing someone yawn; the mouth is opened wide and air is drawn in and released slowly.

YAWS n. an infection caused by the spirochete *Treponema pertenue* transmitted by direct contact, chiefly among children, living in unsanitary conditions in tropical and subtropical areas. It is characterized by ulcerating sores on the body, leading to destruction of underlying tissue. Treatment is by penicillin (see also *bejel*; *syphilis*).

Y CHROMOSOME n. the sex chromosome that in humans is present only in males, appearing singly (along with a single X chromosome). It is carried by one half of male gametes (sperm), none of the female gametes (ova). It is smaller than the X chromosome and is not associated with many known sex-linked disorders.

YELLOW FEVER n. a virus-caused disease, transmitted by mosquitoes, chiefly female *Aëdes aegypti* mosquitoes, found in tropical Africa and northern South America. Symptoms include fever, headache, pains in the back and limbs, reduced urine output, jaundice, and degeneration of liver and kidney tissue. There is no specific treatment but the disease can be prevented by vaccination (which is advised for all who travel to areas where yellow fever is endemic), and recovery from one attack usually confers subsequent immunity.

YELLOW MARROW see *bone marrow*.

YOLK n. nutritive material, rich in protein and fats, found within the *ovum* to supply nourishment for the developing embryo. It is nearly absent in the ova of humans and other mammals, in whom the embryo receives nourishment from the mother, through the placenta.

YOLK MEMBRANE see *vitelline membrane*.

YOLK SAC n. membranous sac that develops in the early embryo providing part of the primitive gut, a site of blood cell formation, and a means for transporting nutrients to the early embryo. In humans it disappears in early embryonic development.

YOLK STALK n. the narrow duct that connects the yolk sac and mid area of embryonic gut during early development, usually disappearing in early embryonic growth.

YTTRIUM n. a metallic element, radioactive isotopes of which are used in cancer therapy.

Z

ZARONTIN n. trade name for the anticonvulsant ethosuximide used to treat petit mal *epilepsy*.

ZINC n. a metallic element essential to normal body metabolism. Zinc compounds (e.g., zinc sulfate, zinc oxide) are also widely used as astringents in creams, ointments, and powders for skin irritations and minor wounds.

ZINC DEFICIENCY n. a condition caused by inadequate zinc intake in the diet or by liver disease, cystic fibrosis, or certain other diseases that lead to inadequate zinc levels; symptoms include fatigue, mental dullness, poor appetite and susceptibility to infection. Rich sources include meat, eggs, nuts, milk, peanut butter and whole grains.

ZOANTHROPY n. the delusion that one has assumed the form of an animal.

ZOLLINGER-ELLISON SYNDROME n. a condition in which excess gastric juice secretion leads to severe and recurrent peptic ulcers; it is usually caused by a tumor (often malignant) of the pancreas. Treatment may involve removal of the tumor, if possible; gastrectomy; and the use of antiulcer drugs (e.g., cimetidine).

ZOMAX n. trade name for the analgesic *zomepirac*.

ZOMEPIRAC n. an analgesic and antiinflammatory agent, known under the trade name Zomax, used to treat mild to moderate pain. Adverse effects include gastrointestinal bleeding, skin rashes, and palpitations.

ZONA n. a bandlike area around a part or organ. pl.**zonae** adj. **zonal**

ZONA PELLUCIDA n. a thick membrane enclosing the mammalian ovum; it can be penetrated by one sperm in the fertilization process, and usually remains around the fertilized egg until its implantation in the wall of the uterus.

ZONULE n. a small bandlike area, as, for example, the **zonule of Zinn** (zona ciliaris), the ligament holding the lens of the eye in place.

ZOO- comb. form indicating an association with nonhuman animals (e.g., **zoograft**, tissue from an animal transplanted to a person, as in the use of pig tissue to replace a damaged heart valve in a human).

ZOONOSIS n. a disease of animals that can be transmitted to humans (e.g., brucellosis, leptospirosis, rabies).

ZOOPHILISM n. an abnormal fondness for animals, esp. sexual attraction to animals (see also *bestiality*).   adj. **zoophilic**

ZOOPHOBIA n. an irrational and excessive fear of animals.   adj. **zoophobic**

ZOOPSIA n. visual hallucination of animals, sometimes occurring in *delirium tremens*.

ZOOTOXIN n. a poisonous substance from an animal, as snake venom.

ZORANE n. trade name for an *oral contraceptive* containing *estradiol* and *norethindrone*.

ZYGOMATIC adj. pert. to the cheek region of the face.

ZYGOMATIC BONE n. one of a pair of skull bones that form the lower part of the eye socket and prominence of the cheek.

ZYGOTE n. the fertilized *ovum*.

ZYLOPRIM n. trade name for *allopurinol*, used to treat *gout*.

ZYMOID adj. like an enzyme.

ZYMOSIS n. the process of fermentation.

TABLE OF IMPORTANT ELEMENTS

A chemical *element* is any one of over 100 fundamental substances whose atoms are of a single type. An element cannot be broken down to a simpler substance by ordinary chemical means. Most elements combine with other elements to form *compounds*. Elements of one *family* have similar properties (e.g., fluorine, chlorine, bromine, and iodine are members of the halogen family and have similar properties).

Common Name	Chemical Symbol	Atomic No.	Medical/Physiological Significance
aluminum	Al	13	Most abundant metal on earth's outer layer; used in compounds to treat excessive stomach acidity and as a disinfectant
arsenic	As	33	Used in compounds as a poison and for treating skin diseases (e.g., yaws)
barium	Ba	56	Compounds used for removing hair; as insoluble barium sulfate in contrast substances to show the form or action of intestinal parts on X-ray film
boron	B	5	An element believed necessary in trace amounts for cell-wall formation and in the production and breakdown of pectin. Common compounds are borax and boric acid
bromine	Br	35	Compounds (bromides) used as sedatives
calcium	Ca	20	An essential constituent of most animals and plants; a mineral nutrient; needed for formation and maintenance of bone and teeth; exchanges with sodium in some cell actions, as in retinal rod cells during vision (see also *tetany*)
carbon	C	6	Chief element (in combination with hydrogen and oxygen) in organic compounds and, hence, all life forms (e.g., in forming glucose, an important sugar that fuels the cell)
chlorine	Cl	17	Used as a disinfectant in water purification and in insecticides
cobalt	Co	27	An essential trace element in animal and plant metabolism; needed for formation of specific body chemicals; cobalt-60, a radioactive isotope used in treatment of cancer

Common Name	Chemical Symbol	Atomic No.	Medical/Physiological Significance
copper	Cu	29	An important trace element in animal and plant metabolism; needed in the synthesis of hemoglobin; involved in enzyme reactions
fluorine	F	9	Occurs in small amounts in bones and teeth; compounds used in dentifrices and added (one part per million) to drinking water to prevent decay of teeth (dental caries)
gold	Au	79	Formerly used in dental prostheses because of its inertness; used experimentally in compounds to treat arthritis
hydrogen	H	1	Needed in formation of carbohydrates and thus essential to life forms; essential in metabolism and respiration cycles
iodine	I	53	Needed for thyroid gland to work normally; used in antiseptics and in treating goiter and cretinism
iron	Fe	26	Vital in helping to carry oxygen to cells; used in formation of hemoglobin and respiratory enzymes
lead	Pb	82	Used in shielding against radioactivity; a cumulative poison not excreted from the body; children often affected by eating dried paint containing one or more lead compounds
lithium	L	3	Increases serotonin release in parts of the brain; compounds used in treating mental depression and mania
magnesium	Mg	12	Essential component of many enzymes; essential in photosynthesis; abundant in plants and animals (bones, chlorophyll); compounds used as antacids and mild laxatives (Epsom salts, milk of magnesia); needed for formation of bones, teeth
manganese	Mn	25	Trace element in plants and animals; involved in enzyme reactions

Common Name	Chemical Symbol	Atomic No.	Medical/Physiological Significance
mercury	Hg	80	The only common metal that is liquid at normal temperatures; used in blood-pressure apparatuses and in mercury thermometers and as an amalgam in dentistry; implicated in environmental poisonings, esp. as a cumulative poison in fish
molybdenum	Mo	42	Essential trace element involved in enzyme actions
nitrogen	N	7	Makes up about 78% of atmosphere; important in forming proteins and nucleic acids; essential for all living cells and important in antibiotics; important to plant (food) growth through the nitrogen cycle
oxygen	O	8	Essential in respiration and in forming carbohydrates and proteins; most abundant of earth's elements in a free gas form in atmosphere and in combined forms in water and in inorganic and organic (e.g., proteins, carbohydrates) forms
phosphorus	P	15	Essential for formation of bones, teeth; needed by all living cells; used in fertilizers, detergents, toxic nerve gases, rodent and insect poisons; a component of proteins and nucleic acids; found in blood, muscles and nerves
plutonium	Pu	94	Artificially produced radioactive element manufactured in nuclear reactors; said to be the deadliest poison; collects in the bones; interferes with production of white blood cells
potassium	K	19	Essential to nervous system function; principal intracellular positively charged ion of most body tissues; likely plays a role in protein synthesis
radium	Ra	88	Radioactive; used in treatment of cancer and in radiography
silicon	Si	14	Second most abundant element in earth's outer layer (see oxygen); important in electronics (transistors) and silicone rubber implants

Common Name	Chemical Symbol	Atomic No.	Medical/Physiological Significance
sodium	Na	11	Found in animals and most plants; sodium-ion pump is essential in transport of substances across cell membranes; compounds used in diuretics, function tests, detergents, antacids, gargles, anticoagulants; implicated as one cause of high blood pressure
sulfur	S	16	Important in forming proteins; used in fungicides, insecticides, and in compounds for treating skin diseases
zinc	Zn	30	Trace element in plants and animals; essential component of certain enzymes; low levels implicated in causing abnormalities in taste and smell functions

TABLE OF VITAMINS

Common Designation	Scientific Name (or Description)	Physiological Action	Source(s)
A	(either of 2 fat-soluble substances, vitamins A_1, A_2)	prevents drying and horny development (keratinization) of epithelial tissues; essential for normal vision and to prevent "drying" of retina (xeropthalmia); prevents night blindness	liver oils, egg yolk, dairy products, yellow fruits and vegetables, leafy green vegetables
A_1	retinol		
A_2	dehydroretinol		
provitamin A	carotene	converts to vitamin A in the liver	
B complex	(originally thought to be one substance but now separated into several water-soluble "B" vitamins)		
B_1	thiamine	prevents beriberi (inflammation and degeneration of nerves with paralysis and muscle wasting); maintains appetite and growth	seed coats of cereal grains; meats (esp. pork); peas, beans, egg yolks
B_2	riboflavin	prevents skin lesions and weight loss	animal and plant tissue; milk
pellagra-preventing vitamin (PP)	niacin (nicotinic acid)	prevents pellagra (loss of vitality, diarrhea, mental disturbances); essential for proper enzyme function	yeast, veal, liver, pork, milk, eggs, whole wheat
B_6	pyridoxine, pyridoxal, pyridoxamine	needed in proper metabolism of amino acids and of starch (glycogen) to sugar (glucose)	most foods, but esp. vegetables, liver, eggs, whole-grain cereals
B_{12}	cyanocobalamin	effective in curing pernicious anemia	eggs, fish, liver
B_c	(see vitamin M)		

Common Designation	Scientific Name (or Description)	Physiological Action	Source(s)
C	ascorbic acid (water-soluble substance)	prevents scurvy (weakness, joint swelling, gum bleeding)	fresh fruit and vegetables, esp. citrus fruits (vitamin is rapidly destroyed by cooking)
D	calciferol (fat-soluble substance)	prevents rickets (bowed legs, crooked bones); essential for normal use of calcium and phosphorus in the body and for normal bone formation	fish liver oil; egg yolk, butter, and exposure to sunlight
E	tocopherol (fat-soluble substance)	needed for normal reproduction, muscle development, and other functions	wheat-germ oil, egg yolk, beef liver, cereals
G	riboflavin (see vitamin B₂)		
H	biotin (also: coenzyme R)	prevents paralysis and baldness in experimental animals	egg yolk, liver, tomatoes, yeast
K	a group of fat-soluble substances	helps clot blood, increases prothrombin production in liver; prevents hemorrhages; used to treat jaundice; sometimes given to persons undergoing surgery	spinach, cabbage, egg yolk, liver
M	folic acid	may be essential for preventing anemia and to prevent an excess of iron deposits in the body (hemochromatosis)	yeast

COMMON ABBREVIATIONS USED IN MEDICINE

Abbreviation	Latin Derivation	Meaning
ā		before
aa	ana	of each
ac	ante cibum	before meals
AD	auris dextra	right ear
A and D		admission and discharge
ad	addi	let them be added
ad effect	ad effectum	until it is effective
ad lib	ad libitum	as desired, as much as patient desires
agit	agita	shake
AI		aortic insufficiency
ama		against medical advice
amb		ambulatory
amt		amount
AP	ante partum	before childbirth
ap	ante prandium	before dinner
APC		aspirin, phenacetin, caffeine
approx		approximately
aq	aqua	water
ARD		acute respiratory disease
AS	auris sinistra	left ear
AU	auris unitas	both ears
AV		arteriovenous, audiovisual
av		average
awa		as well as
B		black (race)
BCG		Bacillus Calmette-Guerin
bid	bis in die	twice each day
BMR		basal metabolism rate
BP		blood pressure
c̄		with
Ca		cancer, carcinoma
CBC		complete blood count
clin		clinical
CNS		central nervous system
CPR		cardiopulmonary resuscitation
CV		cardiovascular
CVA		cerebrovascular accident
dbl		double
DNA		deoxyribonucleic acid
DOA		dead on arrival
DT	delirium tremens	severe tremors
D/W		dextrose in water
Dx		diagnosis
ea		each
ECG		electrocardiogram
EEG		electroencephalogram
EENT		ear, eye, nose and throat
EKG		electrocardiogram
EM		electron microscope
EMG		electromyogram

Abbreviation	Latin Derivation	Meaning
ENT		ear, nose, and throat
ER		emergency room
EST		electroshock therapy
et al	et alii	and others
F		female
FACP		Fellow, American College of Physicians
FACS		Fellow, American College of Surgeons
FICS		Fellow, International College of Surgeons
FRCOG		Fellow, Royal College of Obstetricians and Gynecologists
FRCP		Fellow, Royal College of Physicians
FRCP(C)		Fellow, Royal College of Physicians of Canada
FRCP(E)		Fellow, Royal College of Physicians of Edinburgh
FRCP(I)		Fellow, Royal College of Physicians of Ireland
GI		gastrointestinal
GP		general practitioner
GSW		gunshot wound
GTT		glucose tolerance test
GU		genitourinary
Gyn		gynecology
GRAS		General Regarded As Safe by FDA
h		height
HG		hemoglobin
hct		hematocrit
Hgb		hemoglobin
HID		headache, insomnia, and depression
HP		high power (microscope)
HPN		hypertension
HR		heart rate
hs	hora somni	at bedtime
HVL		half value layer
Hx		history
I and D		incision and drainage
I&O		intake and output
ID		identification
id	idem	the same
	in diem	during the day
IM		intramuscular
		internal medicine
IOP		intraocular pressure
IQ		intelligence quotient
IST		insulin shock therapy
IUD		intrauterine (contraceptive) device
IV		intravenous
IVP		intravenous pyelogram
IVU		intravenous urogram
JND		just noticeable difference
k		constant
KUB		kidney, ureter, bladder

Abbreviation	Latin Derivation	Meaning
L		left
lab		laboratory
LD		lethal dose
LD_{50}		lethal dose in which 50% of the group survive
LE		lupus erythematosus
liq		liquid
LKS		liver, kidney, spleen
LM		light microscope
loc cit	loco citato	in the place cited
LP		low power, lumbar puncture, latent period
LPN		licensed practical nurse
M		male
MA		mental age
MAO		monoamine oxidase
mb	misce bene	mix well
MD	Medicinae Doctor	doctor of medicine
		muscular dystrophy
MDR		minimum daily requirement
MED		minimum effective dose
mEq		milliequivalent
M:F		male to female ratio
MFT		muscle function test
MI		mitral insufficiency
		myocardial infarction
mm Hg		millimeters of mercury (measure of blood pressure)
MS		multiple sclerosis
N		normal
		number
NA		not applicable
npo		nothing by mouth
NSA		no significant abnormality
$\bar{o}$		no
Ob-Gyn		obstetrics-gynecology
OBS		organic brain syndrome
OD	oculus dexter	right eye
		overdose
OR		operating room
OS	oculus sinister	left eye
OU	oculus uterque	each, both eyes
P		probability
$\bar{p}$		after
p		pulse
Pap		Papanicolaou
PBI		protein-bound iodine
pCO_2		carbon dioxide pressure, tension
PE		physical examination
PI		present illness
PM	post mortem	after death
pO_2		oxygen tension, pressure
po	per os	by mouth

Abbreviation	Latin Derivation	Meaning
prn	pro re nata	as circumstances may require
PT		physical therapy
		prothrombin time
pt		patient
Px		prognosis
qd	quaque die	every day
qh	quaque hora	every hour
qid	quater in die	four times each day
qq	quaque	each, every
qv	quantum vis	as much as you want
R		respiration
		response
r		roentgen
RBC		red blood cell
RES		reticuloendothelial system
RNA		ribonucleic acid
RU		rat unit
Rx	recipe	prescription
		therapy
r̄		without
S		subject
S/S		signs and symptoms
sed		sedimentation (rate)
seq	sequela(e)	that which follows
SI		Systeme Internationale (metric units)
sig	signa	label
S-O-R		stimulus-organism-response
sp		species (singular)
sp g		specific gravity
spp		species (plural)
S-R		stimulus-response
Ss		subjects
STAT	statim	immediately
STP		standard temperature and pressure
sum	sumat	let it be taken
T		temperature
t		time
T&A		tonsillectomy and adenoidectomy
TB		tuberculosis
tid	ter in die	three times each day
tinc		tincture
TLC		tender loving care
TPR		temperature, pulse, respiration
U		unit
UCS		unconditioned stimulus
UO		of undetermined origin
URI		upper respiratory infection
USP		United States Pharmacopoeia
USPHS		United States Public Health Service
ut dict	ut dictum	as directed
UV		ultraviolet
UVR		ultraviolet radiation

Abbreviation	Latin Derivation	Meaning
V		volume
VD		venereal disease
VDRL		Venereal Disease Research Laboratory
VHF		very high frequency
vid	vide	see
viz	videlicet	namely
VLF		very low frequency
V/O		verbal order
VPC		volume packed cells
v/v		percent volume in volume
W		white (race)
w		weight
w/		with
WBC		white blood cell(s)
WDWN		well developed, well nourished
wk		week
W/V		weight per volume
X	unknown crossed	

NAMING OPERATIONS

An operation may be named either for the person(s) who originated or perfected it (called an eponym, e.g., Blalock-Taussig operation) or for the anatomical part(s) involved and the specific action taken on it (them).

Other than eponymal terms, then, most operations have one of these appropriate roots:

term	meaning	example
-centesis	needlepuncture to draw fluid	amniocentesis (puncture of the fetal covering)
-desis	fusion, binding	arthrodesis (fusing joint surfaces)
-ectomy	to cut out	appendectomy (removal of appendix)
-nyxis	puncture	scleronyxis (puncture of the sclera of the eyeball)
-ostomy	making an opening	colostomy (making an artificial opening from the outside to the colon)
-pexy	fixing, fixation	gastropexy (stabilizing the stomach surgically)
-plasty	surgical repair	rhinoplasty (plastic surgery on the nose)
-rhaphy	surgical sewing	blepharorrhaphy (sewing the eyelids together)
-rhexis	fracturing a bone	anarrhexis (deliberate fracturing of a bone for restructuring)
-scopy	examination by use of instruments	laryngoscopy (examining the windpipe, larnyx, with a special tube)
-tomy	cutting, making an incision	laparotomy (cutting through the flank)